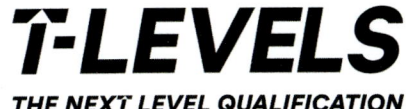

HEALTHCARE SCIENCE

CORE

Stephanie France, Stephen Hoare,
Mary Riley, Gemma Roberts

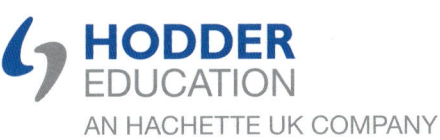

'T-LEVELS' is a registered trade mark of the Department for Education. 'T Level' is a registered trade mark of the Institute for Apprenticeships and Technical Education. The T Level Technical Qualification is a qualification approved and managed by the Institute for Apprenticeships and Technical Education.

Every effort has been made to trace all copyright holders, but if any have been inadvertently overlooked, the Publishers will be pleased to make the necessary arrangements at the first opportunity.

Although every effort has been made to ensure that website addresses are correct at time of going to press, Hodder Education cannot be held responsible for the content of any website mentioned in this book. It is sometimes possible to find a relocated web page by typing in the address of the home page for a website in the URL window of your browser.

Hachette UK's policy is to use papers that are natural, renewable and recyclable products and made from wood grown in well-managed forests and other controlled sources. The logging and manufacturing processes are expected to conform to the environmental regulations of the country of origin.

Orders: please contact Hachette UK Distribution, Hely Hutchinson Centre, Milton Road, Didcot, Oxfordshire, OX11 7HH. Telephone: +44 (0)1235 827827. Email education@hachette.co.uk Lines are open from 9 a.m. to 5 p.m., Monday to Friday. You can also order through our website: www.hoddereducation.co.uk

ISBN: 978 1 3983 6128 7

© Stephen Hoare, Stephanie France, Gemma Roberts and Mary Riley 2022

First published in 2022 by
Hodder Education,
An Hachette UK Company
Carmelite House
50 Victoria Embankment
London EC4Y 0DZ

www.hoddereducation.co.uk

Impression number   10 9 8 7 6 5 4 3 2 1

Year   2026 2025 2024 2023 2022

All rights reserved. Apart from any use permitted under UK copyright law, no part of this publication may be reproduced or transmitted in any form or by any means, electronic or mechanical, including photocopying and recording, or held within any information storage and retrieval system, without permission in writing from the publisher or under licence from the Copyright Licensing Agency Limited. Further details of such licences (for reprographic reproduction) may be obtained from the Copyright Licensing Agency Limited, www.cla.co.uk

Cover photo © Seventyfour - stock.adobe.com

Typeset in India by Integra Software Services Pvt., Ltd.

Produced by DZS Grafik, printed in Bosnia & Herzegovina

A catalogue record for this title is available from the British Library.

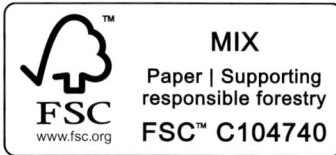
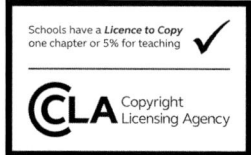

Contents

Acknowledgements iv

Photo credits v

Guide to the book vi

A1 Working within the health and science sector 1
A2 The healthcare science sector 14
A3 Health, safety and environmental regulations in the health and science sector 50
A4 Health and safety regulations in healthcare science 62
A5 Providing person-centred care when working in healthcare science 72
A6 Infection prevention and control in healthcare science settings 119
A7 Managing information and data within the health and science sector 140
A8 Managing information and data 161
A9 Good scientific and clinical practice 182
A10 Good scientific practice 196
B1 Core science concepts: Biology 210
B1 Core science concepts: Chemistry 242
B1 Core science concepts: Physics 259
B2 Further science concepts 282

Core skills 347

Assessment 365

Glossary 372

Index 381

Answers can be found online at: www.hoddereducation.co.uk/subjects/health-social-care/products/t-level/healthcare-science-t-level-core

Acknowledgements

Stephen Hoare

I would like to thank my wife, Janet, for her patience and forbearance during all the hours I was tied to the computer. Also to Rachel and her colleagues at Hodder Education for their support. Finally, to the NCFE reviewers for their helpful and constructive criticisms and suggestions.

Gemma Roberts

I would like to thank Rachel and the rest of the team for their constructive feedback whilst working on this project.

A special thank you to my husband, Karl, for his continuous support, patience and understanding throughout this process.

Photo credits

The Publishers would like to thank the following for permission to reproduce copyright material.

p.1 © kasto/stock.adobe.com; Fig 1.1 © halid994/stock.adobe.com; Fig 1.2 © milkovasa/stock.adobe.com; p.14 © Darren Baker/stock.adobe.com; Fig 2.3 © Jane/stock.adobe.com; Fig 2.5 © Sved Oliver/stock.adobe.com; Fig 2.6 © Dario Lo Presti/stock.adobe.com; Fig 2.7 © Kzenon/stock.adobe.com; Fig 2.8 © blueringmedia/stock.adobe.com; Fig 2.9 © BalanceFormCreative/stock.adobe.com; Fig 2.12 © ThisIs/stock.adobe.com; Fig 2.13 © Institute for Apprenticeships and Technical Education; p.50 © Wirestock/stock.adobe.com; Fig 3.1 © Rainer Lesniewski/Shutterstock.com; Fig 3.2 © Sherry Young/stock.adobe.com; Fig 3.3 © khampiranon/stock.adobe.com; Fig 3.4 © Government Open License; p.62 © pressmaster/stock.adobe.com; Fig 4.2 © Christian Horz/stock.adobe.com; Fig 4.3 © Resuscitation Council UK; Fig 4.4 © Resuscitation Council UK; Fig 4.5 © Андрей Котомин/stock.adobe.com; Fig 5.1 © Rawpixel.com/stock.adobe.com; Fig 5.2 © zinkevych/stock.adobe.com; Fig 5.3 © DC Studio/stock.adobe.com; Fig 5.4 © DC Studio/stock.adobe.com; Fig 5.5 © mjowra. -123RF; Fig 5.6 © Roger Utting/Shutterstock.com; Fig 5.7 © Andrey Popov/stock.adobe.com; Fig 5.8 © manassanant/stock.adobe.com; Fig 5.9 © auremar/stock.adobe.com; Fig 5.10 © Studio Romantic/stock.adobe.com; Fig 5.11 © BillionPhotos.com/stock.adobe.com; Fig 5.12 © wavebreak3/stock.adobe.com; Fig 5.13 © Rawpixel.com/stock.adobe.com; p.120 © maximimages.com/Alamy Stock Photo; Fig 6.1 © Crown copyright; Fig 6.2 © spiderrain08/Shutterstock.com; Fig 6.3 © lightpoet/stock.adobe.com; Fig 6.6 © PHOTOLIFESTYLE/stock.adobe.com; Fig 6.7 © romaset/stock.adobe.com; Fig 6.9 © Crown copyright 2007 283373 1p 1k Sep07; Fig 6.10 © David FR/Shutterstock.com; Fig 6.11 © Gagarin Iurii/Shutterstock.com; Fig 6.12 © Komsan Loonprom/Shutterstock.com; p.141 © milatas/stock.adobe.com; Fig 7.1 © MonkeyBusiness/stock.adobe.com; p.162 © Tryfonov/stock.adobe.com; Fig 8.1 © busayamol/Shutterstock.com; Fig 8.2 © ROM/stock.adobe.com; Fig 8.4 © shoenberg3/stock.adobe.com; Fig 8.8 © Monet/stock.adobe.com; p.183 © Elenathewise/stock.adobe.com; Fig 9.2 © Tyler Olson/stock.adobe.com; Fig 9.3 © James Thew/stock.adobe.com; Fig 9.4 © DavidBautista/stock.adobe.com; Fig 9.5 © angellodeco/stock.adobe.com; Fig 9.6 © StratfordProductions/stock.adobe.com; p.197 © Prajakkit/stock.adobe.com; Fig 10.1 © Rido/stock.adobe.com; Fig 10.2 © PRILL Mediendesign/stock.adobe.com; Fig 10.3 © katrin_timoff/stock.adobe.com; Fig 10.4 © eplisterra/stock.adobe.com; Fig 10.5 © Forance/stock.adobe.com; Fig 10.6 © Stephen/stock.adobe.com; Fig 10.7 © ahoi!/stock.adobe.com; p.211 © Keith R. Porter/SCIENCE PHOTO LIBRARY; Fig 11.1a © Biophoto Associates/SCIENCE PHOTO LIBRARY; Fig 11.2a © Keith R. Porter/SCIENCE PHOTO LIBRARY; Fig 11.3a © Medimage/SCIENCE PHOTO LIBRARY; Fig 11.4a © Biophoto Associates/SCIENCE PHOTO LIBRARY; Fig 11.5a © Dr Jeremy Burgess/SCIENCE PHOTO LIBRARY; Fig 11.19 © Gunilla Elam/SCIENCE PHOTO LIBRARY; Fig 11.22 © gritsalak/stock.adobe.com; Fig 11.23 © sveta/stock.adobe.com; Fig 11.24a © Martin Shields/SCIENCE PHOTO LIBRARY; Fig 11.24b © Peter Bond, EM Centre, University of Plymouth/SCIENCE PHOTO LIBRARY; Fig 11.26 © toeytoey/stock.adobe.com; Fig 11.27 © Alvin Telser/SCIENCE PHOTO LIBRARY; Fig 11.28 © arcyto/stock.adobe.com; p.243 © totojang1977/stock.adobe.com; p.260 © Ruslan Gilmanshin/stock.adobe.com; Fig 13.6 © wittayayut/stock.adobe.com; p.283 © STEVE GSCHMEISSNER/SCIENCE PHOTO LIBRARY; Fig 14.1 © vecton/stock.adobe.com; Fig 14.6 t © STEVE GSCHMEISSNER/SCIENCE PHOTO LIBRARY; Fig 14.8 © vecton/stock.adobe.com; Fig 14.14 © VectorMine/stock.adobe.com; Fig 14.16 © VectorMine/stock.adobe.com; Fig 14.17 © Olga/stock.adobe.com; Fig 14.19 © STEVE GSCHMEISSNER/SCIENCE PHOTO LIBRARY; Fig 14.24 © vonuk/stock.adobe.com; Fig 14.34 © JYFotoStock/stock.adobe.com; Fig 14.35 © macrovector/stock.adobe.com; Fig 14.36 © sabelskaya/stock.adobe.com; Fig 14.42 © Brian Jackson/stock.adobe.com; Fig 14.43 © angellodeco/stock.adobe.com; Fig 14.44 © Monkey Business/stock.adobe.com; Fig 14.45 b © AJ PHOTO/SCIENCE PHOTO LIBRARY; Fig 14.47 © RFBSIP/stock.adobe.com; Fig 14.48 © Proxima Studio/stock.adobe.com; Fig 14.49 © Goffkein/stock.adobe.com; Fig 14.50 © Pee Paew/stock.adobe.com; Fig 14.51 © fresnel6/stock.adobe.com; Fig 14.54 Genome Research Ltd. Francesca Gale

Guide to the book

The following features can be found in this book.

Learning outcomes
Core knowledge outcomes that you must understand and learn. These are presented at the start of every chapter.

Key term
Definitions to help you understand important terms.

Reflect
Tasks and questions providing an opportunity to reflect on the knowledge learned.

Test yourself
A knowledge consolidation feature containing short questions and tasks to aid understanding and guide you to think about a topic in detail.

Research
Research-based activities – either stretch and challenge activities, enabling you to go beyond the course, or industry placement-based activities, encouraging you to discover more about your placement.

Practice point
Helpful tips and guidelines to help develop professional skills during your industry placement.

Case study
Placing knowledge into a fictionalised, real-life context. Useful to introduce problem-solving and dilemmas.

Health and safety
Important points to ensure safety in the workplace.

Project practice
Short scenarios and focused activities that reflect one or more of the tasks that you will need to undertake during completion of the employer-set project. These support the development of the four core skills required.

Assessment practice
Core content containing knowledge-based practice questions at the end of each chapter.

Answers can be found online at: www.hoddereducation.co.uk/subjects/health-social-care/products/t-level/healthcare-science-t-level-core

A1: Working within the health and science sector

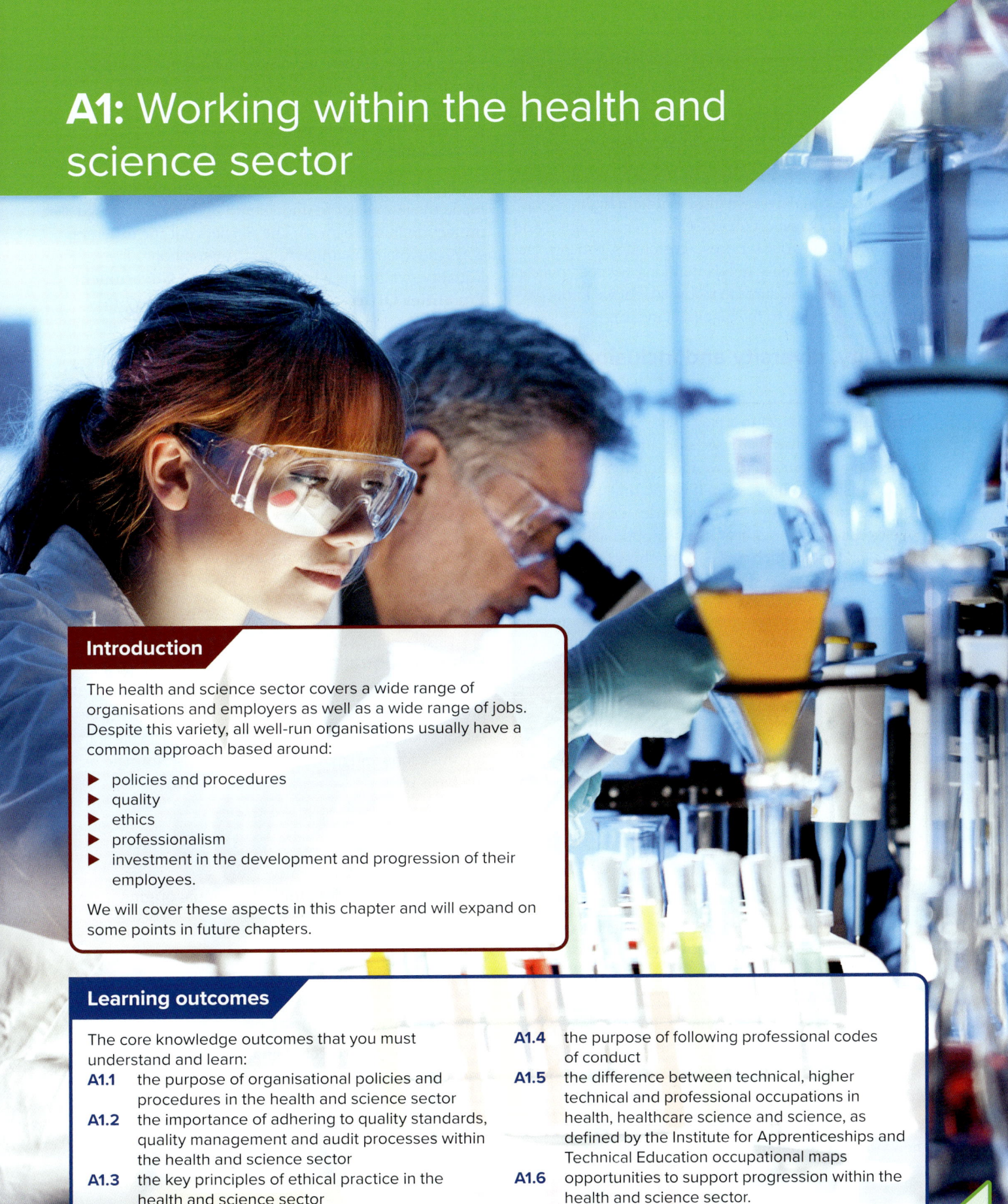

Introduction

The health and science sector covers a wide range of organisations and employers as well as a wide range of jobs. Despite this variety, all well-run organisations usually have a common approach based around:

- policies and procedures
- quality
- ethics
- professionalism
- investment in the development and progression of their employees.

We will cover these aspects in this chapter and will expand on some points in future chapters.

Learning outcomes

The core knowledge outcomes that you must understand and learn:

- **A1.1** the purpose of organisational policies and procedures in the health and science sector
- **A1.2** the importance of adhering to quality standards, quality management and audit processes within the health and science sector
- **A1.3** the key principles of ethical practice in the health and science sector
- **A1.4** the purpose of following professional codes of conduct
- **A1.5** the difference between technical, higher technical and professional occupations in health, healthcare science and science, as defined by the Institute for Apprenticeships and Technical Education occupational maps
- **A1.6** opportunities to support progression within the health and science sector.

A1.1 The purpose of organisational policies and procedures in the health and science sector

In our professional lives we must maintain high standards out of respect for ourselves, our colleagues and those who require our services – customers, patients, etc. It is not enough to have good intentions; we need policies to consult and procedures to follow so that we know we are always working to the highest standards.

Equality, diversity and inclusion policy

Sometimes we can act in a way that is discriminatory without even realising it. If we stop and put ourselves in the other person's place, we might realise the effect our actions would have. Even if we do that, we may still have room to improve. That is why we have policies that cover equality, diversity and inclusion in the workplace which make it clear how to behave (Figure 1.1).

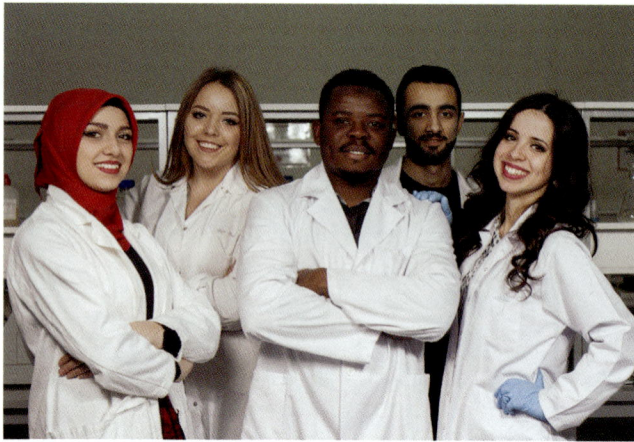

▲ Figure 1.1 Equality, diversity and inclusion should be central to our professional lives

Complying with legislation

One very good reason for having policies that cover equality, diversity and inclusion is to ensure that we comply with the relevant legislation. The main piece of legislation in the UK is the **Equality Act 2010**.

This gives legal protection from discrimination in the workplace and in wider society. Before this **law** came into force, there were several laws that covered discrimination, including:
- Sex Discrimination Act 1975
- Race Relations Act 1976
- Disability Discrimination Act 1995.

Replacing these and other laws with a single Act made the law easier to understand and gave increased protection in some areas. The Act sets out the different ways in which it is unlawful to treat someone. The Equality Act 2010 is administered by the **Government Equalities Office**, which has produced an easy-to-read publication called 'The Equality Act – making equality real'. You can find this by carrying out an internet search using this title.

> **Key term**
>
> *Laws:* legislation passed by parliament that state the rights and entitlements of individuals and provide legal rules that have to be followed. The law is upheld through the courts. If an individual or care setting breaks the law by, for example, inappropriately sharing or inaccurately recording information, they can, in certain circumstances, be fined, dismissed or given a prison sentence.

Ensuring equality

The Equality Act places responsibility on employers, providers of goods and services, caregivers, public sector bodies, private clubs and associations, voluntary organisations and many others not to discriminate on the basis of:
- age
- disability
- gender reassignment
- pregnancy and maternity
- race – this includes ethnic or national origins, colour and nationality
- religion or belief
- sex
- sexual orientation.

Eliminating discrimination

These are called **protected characteristics**. By having policies in place to cover these aspects of equality, and promoting diversity and inclusion, organisations can ensure that they comply with the law and also benefit from treating everyone fairly and equally.

We should also be aware of **indirect discrimination**. This is where there is a practice, policy or rule that applies to everyone in the same way but could have a worse effect on some people than others. Here are two examples of indirect discrimination:
- A woman has been on maternity leave. On return to work, she makes a flexible working request so that she can reduce her hours and look after her child instead of using childcare. Her manager refuses her request and says everyone doing that job must work full-time. This could be indirect sex discrimination.
- A Jewish woman works in a large store. She is told that because of a change in shifts, she now must work one Saturday a month. She explains that, as an observant Jew, she cannot work on Saturdays (the Sabbath). Her manager tells her that it would be unfair to everyone else if she were allowed not to work on Saturdays. This could be indirect religious discrimination.

Safeguarding policies

Safeguarding means ensuring individuals are protected from harm. The NHS England website is a useful source of information about safeguarding in the context of healthcare. Its definition of safeguarding is worth consulting:

> 'Safeguarding means protecting a citizen's health, wellbeing and human rights; enabling them to live free from harm, abuse and neglect. It is an integral part of providing high-quality healthcare. Safeguarding children, young people and adults is a collective responsibility.'
>
> Source: www.england.nhs.uk/safeguarding/about

Note that the policy specifies 'children, young people and adults' – basically, everyone. We probably think of children and young people as being in greater need of protection. However, adults can also be vulnerable and require protection, such as people with learning difficulties or those with a physical or mental disability.

That is why safeguarding policies are required in all organisations, not just in those dealing with children, young people or the elderly. Organisations in the science sector also require proper safeguarding policies covering employees, customers and others they come into contact with, including visitors.

> Section A5.21 covers safeguarding in more detail (see pages 97–99).

DBS checks

There are many situations where you might be working with children or vulnerable adults, such as in healthcare, childcare, education or a voluntary organisation such as Scouts or a youth club. In such situations, the employer or organisation is responsible for checking whether you have a criminal record. This is done through the Disclosure and Barring Service (hence the term DBS check – previously known as CRB). Different levels of DBS check are available, depending on how sensitive the job or role is:
- A basic check just shows any unspent convictions and conditional cautions. Convictions become 'spent' (i.e. they no longer appear on your criminal record) after a period of time, depending on age and length of sentence (if any).
- A standard check shows spent *and* unspent convictions, cautions, reprimands and final warnings.
- An enhanced check shows, in addition to the standard check, any information held by local police that is considered relevant to the role.
- An enhanced check with barred lists shows the same as an enhanced check plus whether the applicant is on the list of people barred from doing the role, e.g. someone on the sex offenders register.

You can only request a basic check yourself. For more information, search gov.uk for 'DBS'. Take care, because if you just do an internet search for 'DBS' the top results will be for commercial organisations that want to sell you a DBS check.

Employment contracts

Every employee has an employment contract with their employer. The contract does not have to be written down – in fact, as soon as someone accepts a job offer, they have a contract with their employer. This means that if either side backs out (for example, the employer withdraws the job offer or the employee decides to take a different job), they could risk legal action for compensation. The employment contract is an agreement that sets out:
- employment conditions
- rights
- responsibilities
- duties.

Both employer and employee must stick to the terms of the contract until it ends. That will happen when either side gives notice, i.e. when the employee announces they will be leaving, or the employer decides to end their employment (for example, through redundancy), or an employee is dismissed (they lose their job). The terms of the contract can be changed, usually by agreement between both sides.

Do not confuse an employment contract with a 'contract to provide services', such as when you agree with someone that they will paint your house or mow your lawn. In those circumstances, the decorator or gardener does not become your employee.

The legal parts of a contract are known as the **terms**; these are legally binding on both parties. Contract terms can take different forms:
- a written contract or statement of employment
- a verbal agreement
- in an offer letter from the employer
- in an employee handbook, on a company noticeboard or intranet.

Some terms are required by law, such as the requirement to pay at least the National Minimum Wage to all employees over 18 years of age (and the rate called the National Living Wage for people aged 23 and over), or the right to a minimum of paid holiday.

> **Practice point**
>
> You can find the minimum wage for your age group on the Gov.uk website:
> www.gov.uk/national-minimum-wage-rates

Some contracts are based on **collective agreements**. This is where the employer or employers negotiate agreements with trade unions or staff associations which represent a group of employees.

Some terms might be **implied** rather than clearly agreed. Examples include:
- Employees should not steal from their employer.
- Your employer must provide a safe and secure working environment.
- If a job provides a company car, the employee needs a valid driving licence.
- Something that has been done regularly over a long period of time, such as paying an annual bonus or certain days off.

When you start a job, your employer is obliged to give you a **written statement of employment particulars**. This is not an employment contract. There are two statements of employment particulars. The **principal statement** must be provided on the first day of work and covers things such as:
- the employer's name, the employee's name, job title (or description of work) and start date
- how much and how often you will be paid
- your hours and days of work and how they might change – as well as if you are expected to work Sundays, nights or overtime
- how long the job is expected to last (or, if permanent, that it is indefinite), and the end date if it is a fixed-term contract
- if there is a probation period, how long it will last and what its conditions are, e.g. to achieve satisfactory performance
- other benefits, such as childcare vouchers or free lunches
- any obligatory training.

As well as this, on day one an employer must give the employee information about:
- sick pay and procedures
- other paid leave, such as maternity and paternity leave
- notice periods, both from the employer and the employee (they may be different).

Within two months of starting work, the employer must give a **wider written statement** that covers:
- pensions and pension schemes
- any collective agreements (see above) that might be in place
- any right to other (non-compulsory) training provided by (or on behalf of) the employer
- disciplinary and grievance procedures (see page 5).

Performance reviews

How do you know that you are doing a good job? You might think you are doing well, but does your employer agree? That is why organisations usually have regular performance reviews for staff. However, this is not just a one-way process.

Performance reviews have several objectives:
- Evaluating work performance against standards and expectations: you might have been given targets to achieve or, if you work in a highly regulated sector, you might have formal standards to maintain or strive for.
- Giving feedback: a performance review gives your line manager (the person who manages you directly, i.e. your boss) the opportunity to help you improve your performance. You should expect feedback to be supportive and encouraging.

- Providing opportunities to raise concerns or issues: performance reviews are not simply about the organisation evaluating your performance, you can also raise any concerns or issues that you have. Try to be non-confrontational – telling your manager exactly what they do wrong and how you could do it so much better might be a career-limiting move!
- Contributing to continuing professional development (CPD): this might mean identifying areas where you need more training or education so that you can develop in your work.

Disciplinary policy

If your employer has concerns about your work, conduct or absence from work (including sickness absence), initially they should raise these concerns in an informal way. However, they can go straight to formal **disciplinary** or even dismissal procedures. A disciplinary procedure is a formal way for an employer to deal with an employee's unacceptable or improper behaviour (this is known as misconduct) or their performance (lack of capability).

Part of this process is that the employer should set and maintain expected standards of work and conduct. You need to know what is expected of you before you can be disciplined for not achieving it!

The disciplinary policy should also ensure consistent and fair treatment of all employees; there should be no favouritism, nor should individual employees feel picked on or bullied.

There should be a process for disciplinary action. This will be part of the disciplinary policy that all employers must have. You should have been given details of this process as part of the wider written statement of employment particulars that you receive within two months of starting work. This should say what performance and behaviour might lead to disciplinary action and what action your employer might take. It should also include the name of someone that you can speak to if you do not agree with your employer's decision.

Your employer's disciplinary procedure should include the following steps:
- A letter setting out the disciplinary issue.
- A meeting to discuss the issue; the employee should have the right to be accompanied by a colleague or trade union representative at this meeting. Some employers may have a policy of allowing a wider range of people to accompany you, such as a friend or relative.
- A decision about the disciplinary issue. This might result in no further action, a first or final written warning, dismissal (i.e. losing your job) or some other sanction.
- A chance to appeal the decision.

Grievance policy

In a well-run organisation, there will be open communication and consultation between managers and their staff. This means that problems and concerns can be raised quickly and settled as part of the normal working relationship.

However, anyone working in an organisation may have problems or concerns about their work or working conditions; they may have problems in their relationships with colleagues. These are all **grievances** that employees want to be addressed and, if possible, resolved. As well as this, the management will want to resolve any problems before they develop into major difficulties.

> **Key term**
>
> *Grievance:* any concern, problem or complaint you may have at work. If you take this up with your employer, it is called 'raising a grievance'.

Issues that may cause grievances include:
- terms and conditions of employment
- health and safety issues and concerns (see Chapter A3)
- relationships with colleagues and management
- bullying and harassment
- working practices, particularly when new practices are introduced
- the working environment
- changes in the organisation
- discrimination – or perceived discrimination.

However, there may be occasions where an employee has a grievance against their line manager and this needs a different approach.

As with disciplinary procedures, all employers should have a written grievance procedure. This should explain what to do if you have a grievance and what happens at each stage in the process. It should provide opportunities for employees to confidentially raise and address grievances. There should be a sequence for raising and resolving grievances. This will usually involve a meeting to discuss the issue. As with disciplinary procedures, you can appeal if you do not agree with your employer's decision.

> **Research**
>
> **Acas**, the Advisory, Conciliation and Arbitration Service, is an independent public body funded by the government. Acas works with employers and employees to improve relationships in the workplace. It has produced several codes of practice that set out the minimum standards of fairness that employers should follow. These include:
> - disciplinary and grievance procedures
> - collective bargaining with trade unions
> - requests for flexible working.
>
> An **employment tribunal** will use the Acas codes of practice when deciding cases. Employers do not need to follow these codes of practice but if they do not and you take your claim to an employment tribunal, your compensation might be increased, so it is in the employer's interest to follow the Acas codes of practice.
>
> There is more information on the Acas website (**www.acas.org.uk/advice**). Do you think the information they give is helpful? Does it help you understand your rights as an employee?

> **Key term**
>
> **Employment tribunals:** responsible for hearing claims from people who think an employer has treated them unlawfully, for example, through unfair dismissal or discrimination.

A1.2 The importance of adhering to quality standards, quality management and audit processes

Adhering to quality standards should be central to any organisation's way of working. Those standards may be national or international standards such as British Standard or ISO (the International Organization for Standardization) or the organisation's own internal quality standards. In the health and science sector, quality standards help improve the quality of care or service provided.

Ensuring consistency

One reason for adhering to quality standards is to ensure **consistency** – always obtaining the same, high-quality outcome.

> **Reflect**
>
> Quality and consistency are terms you will encounter a lot, both in this book and in your working life. Think about how we should always strive for both quality and consistency. If you go to a restaurant, you want the food to be consistently good. If it is consistently bad, you probably will not want to go. But what about a restaurant that is inconsistent? You might occasionally get a good meal, but is it worth a gamble? An organisation should always strive to achieve consistently high quality.

Maintaining health and safety

You will learn, in subsequent chapters, how adhering to proper procedures can help avoid (or at least reduce) accidents and harm to employees, service or care receivers or the general public.

This is covered in most detail in Chapter A3 Health, safety and environmental regulations in the health and science sector.

Monitoring processes and procedures

It is not good enough to intend to do something properly, you must do it. This applies to doing a favour for a friend but is even more important in the workplace. That is why there will often be a check sheet on the wall of a public toilet showing that it has been cleaned according to the required schedule.

This will be covered in more detail in Chapter A9 Good scientific and clinical practice.

> **Case study**
>
> In the summer of 2015, the Smiler roller coaster at the Alton Towers theme park crashed, causing life-altering injuries to four riders (two teenagers had to undergo amputations). The Health and Safety Executive (HSE) report found that there were no mechanical failings in the track, the cars or the system designed to keep the cars separate. The investigation identified a number of human errors that led to the crash. However, the HSE investigators found that Merlin Entertainments (the operator of the theme park) had multiple failings in not performing an adequate risk assessment and not having proper procedures to prevent a series of errors by staff, leading to harm to the public. As a result, Merlin Attractions was fined £5 million.
>
> Do you think 'human error' is ever a valid defence or excuse when harm is caused to employees, patients, care-receivers or members of the public?

Facilitating continuous improvement

Continuous improvement means making many, often small, improvements over time. The success of the GB Olympic cycling team in recent years has been due, in part, to an approach that looks for many tiny performance improvements – in athlete training, equipment or clothing, for example. Each one might shave a hundredth or even a thousandth of a second off a lap time. Cumulatively, they have contributed to many gold medals being won.

We can take the same approach in a science, health or healthcare environment. It starts with adopting quality standards and adhering to them, monitoring performance against those standards and then looking for ways to improve performance.

Facilitating objective, independent review

Audit processes might be a legal requirement – see Chapter A9 for examples. But an audit really means asking the question: 'Did we achieve what we set out to achieve?' We need to have processes that ensure we ask that question in an objective and independent way so that we get useful answers. If we did not achieve our objective, what can we do to achieve it in future? If we did achieve our objective, are there ways we can improve further?

> **Practice point**
>
> **Quality control** (QC) means the testing of a product to ensure that it meets required standards. The QC department in an organisation will be responsible for testing products before they are sold. Any product that fails QC tests will have to be reworked or scrapped.
>
> **Quality assurance** (QA) means having procedures in place that ensure that the product will always meet the required standards.
>
> Which do you think is more important, QC or QA?

A1.3 The key principles of ethical practice in the health and science sector

We are probably all aware of medical ethics – the need for medical professionals to adhere to a set of values or moral principles. This provides a framework for analysing a situation and deciding on the best course of action to take. We will expand upon that in this section. However, aspects of ethical practice are important in all areas of health and science, as we will see.

Beneficence

Put simply, **beneficence** means 'doing good'. All healthcare professionals need to follow the course of action that they believe to be in the best interest of their patient. However, 'doing good' is often too simple in the real world. It is better to think of beneficence as ranking the possible options for a patient, from best to worst, taking account of:

- Will the option resolve the medical problem?
- Is it proportionate to the scale of the problem?
- Is it compatible with the patient's individual circumstances?
- Are the option and its outcomes in line with the patient's expectations?

Several of these points are related to the patient's circumstances or expectations. This forms the basis of patient-centred or person-centred care. This will be expanded on in Chapter A5: Providing person-centred care when working in healthcare science settings.

Nonmaleficence

If you have seen the 2014 Disney movie 'Maleficent' you can probably work out that **maleficence** means 'doing harm', so **nonmaleficence** must mean 'not doing harm'. In that sense, beneficence (doing good) and nonmaleficence (not doing harm) go together. In the science and healthcare sector we all have a duty of both beneficence and nonmaleficence to those we are responsible for.

You can think of nonmaleficence as a threshold for treatment. In other words, if a treatment causes more harm than good then we should not consider it. That is different to beneficence, where we consider all the valid treatment options and then rank them in order of preference or benefit to the patient. A treatment could still be the most beneficial and cause more harm than good.

Another difference is that we usually think of beneficence in response to a specific situation – what is the best treatment for a patient? However, nonmaleficence is something that should always be considered in a healthcare setting. If you see someone collapse, you have a duty to provide (or seek) help for that person. Because we must try to prevent harm, it will be better for that person to receive medical attention than to be left there. Even if you are not qualified or able to help, you can at least make sure that help is given or called for (e.g. by calling 999).

We have described beneficence and nonmaleficence in the context of a doctor providing medical treatment. However, the same principles apply to all health workers who are providing care.

> **Reflect**
>
> Here are some factors to consider in the context of nonmaleficence:
> - What are the risks associated with intervening or not intervening?
> - Do I have the skills necessary to help this person or carry out this action?
> - Are any other factors (staff shortages, lack of resources, etc.) putting the person at risk?
> - Is this person being treated with dignity and respect?

Autonomy and informed consent

Autonomy means that everyone has the right to make the final decision about their care or treatment. That means that, as caregivers, we cannot impose care or treatment on any individual, with some limited exceptions (see below).

This has not always been the case – there have been many instances of 'doctor knows best' in the past and some people might still feel the need to defer to what they see as an authority figure.

Informed consent means that before making that final decision, a person receiving care or treatment has the right to be given all the relevant information about the care or treatment. This might include the benefits, the potential risks and what might happen if the care or treatment is not given.

In some cases, the person may not have the **capacity** to give informed consent. To have capacity, the person must be able to:
- understand the information they are given
- retain that information long enough to make a decision
- weigh up or assess the information to make a decision
- communicate their decision.

If the person does not have capacity to give informed consent, the principles of beneficence and nonmaleficence should be applied. In some cases, for example, with children, the parent or guardian would have to give consent.

According to UK law, adults are over 18 years. However, 16- and 17-year-olds are considered able to give informed consent without the need for a parent. Children under 16 can also give informed consent, provided they have sufficient capacity – intelligence, competence and understanding.

In some cases, the beliefs of a parent (e.g. religious beliefs) may lead them to oppose a course of treatment that healthcare staff believe to be in the interests of the child. In such cases it might be necessary to obtain a court order to overrule the parent's wishes. Of course, this might not be possible in an emergency. In such cases, the principles of beneficence and nonmaleficence should be applied. However, this might result in the parent taking legal action. Ethical issues are not always straightforward!

A1: Working within the health and science sector

Truthfulness and confidentiality

Confidentiality is central to the relationship between patients, care-receivers or the general public on the one hand and science and healthcare staff on the other. Lack of confidentiality may lead to loss of trust; if a patient feels their confidential information may be disclosed without their consent, they may withhold necessary information or even avoid seeking treatment – either way, they are less likely to receive appropriate treatment.

Truthfulness is an obligation on the part of science and healthcare staff. We have an obligation to be truthful, whether that is answering a patient's questions or reporting the results of experiments or analysis. Being truthful with patients is important, even if it might lead to them deciding against a course of action or treatment that we think will be beneficial for them. This is a consequence of informed consent that healthcare staff must accept.

> ### Reflect
> How would you apply the principles we have covered to help you deal with the following situations?
> - A colleague has told you that they have a drink problem, but that it does not affect their work. You, however, are not sure because you have noticed that they are not always fully attentive and even show signs of being drunk on duty.
> - A friend has asked if you can access their partner's medical records as they believe the partner is having an affair and they are worried about STIs (sexually transmitted infections).
> - A patient tells you that they have been using illegal drugs.

Justice

Justice can mean fairness, equality and respect for all. Therefore, when we decide whether something is ethical or not, we must think about:
- Is it legal or compatible with the law?
- Is it fair?
- Does it respect the person's right and equality?
- Does it show respect for all concerned?

A1.4 The purpose of following professional codes of conduct

Whatever area of science, health or healthcare we work in, it is likely that we will be expected to follow specific professional **codes of conduct**. It is not enough to have good intentions; we need to achieve good outcomes – codes of conduct are one way to help ensure that.

Professional codes of conduct may be written by professional societies or organisations. Some examples, covering a diverse range of professions, include:
- The Nursing and Midwifery Council (NMC)
- The Royal College of Nursing (RCN)
- The Health Care Compliance Association (HCCA)
- The Royal Society of Chemistry (RSC)
- The Institute of Food Science & Technology (IFST)
- The Science Council
- The Royal Society of Biology (RSB)
- The Society of Radiographers (SoR)
- The Health and Care Professions Council (HCPC)
- The British Association of Sport and Exercise Sciences (BASES)
- The Institute of Biomedical Science (IBMS).

There are many more. Members of these societies or organisations are expected to follow the code of conduct.

In addition, many organisations in the science, health and healthcare sectors have their own codes of conduct:
- government agencies, such as the Care Quality Commission (CQC)
- private companies, such as HCA Healthcare UK
- employer-led bodies such as the Sector Skills Councils, including Skills for Care and Skills for Health.

Professional codes of conduct will usually follow the same format:
- They clarify the missions (aims) of the organisation and its values and principles.
- They clarify the standards that everyone must adhere to.
- They outline expected professional behaviours and attitudes.
- They outline rules and responsibilities within organisations.
- They promote confidence in the organisation and profession.

Healthcare Science T Level: Core

> **Research**
>
> An internet search or your tutor will help you find examples of professional codes of conduct relevant to your particular field of work. Are these codes of conduct helpful and easy to understand? Will they help prepare you to achieve good outcomes in your work?

> **Key term**
>
> **Levels:** in this context, a way of grading a qualification or set of skills and the corresponding occupations. The levels used today are based on the National Vocational Qualifications (NVQ) levels 1 to 5 developed in the 1980s. Over time, more emphasis has been given to the degree of difficulty or challenge of the qualification rather than the level of occupational competence in the workplace. There are now eight levels, and they cover academic qualifications such as GCSEs, A Levels and undergraduate and graduate degrees, as well as vocational qualifications such as T Levels and apprenticeships – see below for examples.

A1.5 The difference between technical, higher technical and professional occupations in health, healthcare science and science, as defined by the IfATE occupational maps

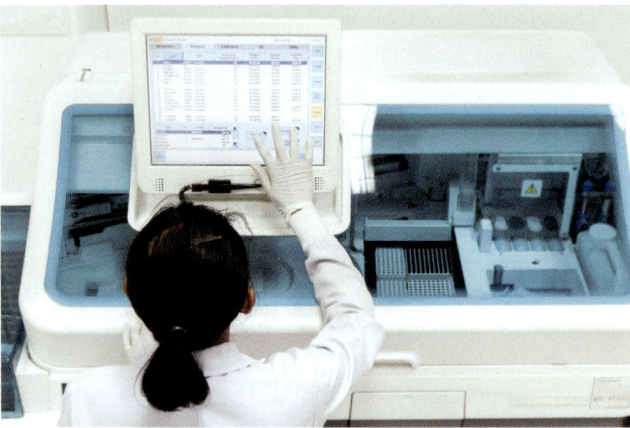

▲ Figure 1.2 Modern laboratory equipment needs qualified and highly trained staff

The Institute for Apprenticeships and Technical Education (IfATE) is an employer-led organisation sponsored by the Department for Education. A key element in the work of the Institute is to support employer groups in developing apprenticeships.

The Institute also maintains the **occupational maps** that underpin technical education. These occupational maps show where technical education can lead. They group occupations that have related knowledge, skills and behaviours into **pathways** so that it is easier to see opportunities for career progression within a particular route. Within each pathway, occupations at the same **level** are grouped into clusters to show how skills you have learned can be applied to other related occupations (Figure 1.2).

This is a small selection of the qualifications available at each level:

- Level 1 qualifications:
  - GCSE grades 3 to 1 or D to G
  - Level 1 NVQ.
- Level 2 qualifications:
  - GCSE grades 9 to 4 or A* to C
  - Intermediate apprenticeship
  - Level 2 award, certificate or diploma.
- Level 3 qualifications:
  - AS/A Level
  - T Level
  - Advanced apprenticeship.
- Level 4 qualifications:
  - Higher apprenticeship
  - Higher national certificate (HNC).
- Level 5 qualifications:
  - Foundation degree
  - Diploma of higher education (DipHE)
  - Higher national diploma (HND).
- Level 6 qualifications:
  - Ordinary or honours degree, e.g. BA, BSc.
- Level 7 qualifications:
  - Master's degree, e.g. MA, MSc, MChem, Meng.
- Level 8 qualifications:
  - Doctorate, e.g. PhD or DPhil.

For a full list, visit **www.gov.uk** and search for 'What qualification levels mean'.

Technical

These are skilled occupations that a college leaver or an apprentice would be entering, typically requiring qualifications at levels 2/3. Examples include:

- adult care worker/lead care worker
- healthcare support worker

- dental nurse
- food technologist
- laboratory technician.

Higher technical

These are occupations that require more knowledge and skills. This could be acquired through experience in the workplace or further technical education. They typically require qualifications at levels 4/5. Examples include:
- lead practitioner in adult care
- healthcare assistant practitioner
- nursing associate
- dental technician
- food testing/laboratory manager
- technician scientist.

Professional

These are all occupations where there is a clear career progression from higher technical occupations, as well as occupations where a degree apprenticeship exists (level 6). Examples include:
- social worker
- healthcare science practitioner
- registered nurse or midwife
- biochemist/biologist/chemist/physicist
- research scientist.

> **Research**
>
> You can view the latest occupational maps on the Institute for Apprenticeships & Technical Education website (**www.instituteforapprenticeships.org/about/occupational-maps**) or search online for 'Institute for Apprenticeships occupational maps'.
>
> Were you able to find relevant information? Will this be a useful resource to help you to plan your career?

A1.6 Opportunities to support progression within the health and science sector

When you were a child, what did you want to be when you grew up? Is that still what you want to do? Some people seem able to plan their careers and then pursue their objectives with single-minded determination. Others may move from job to job without any clear plan. The former group is usually, but not always, more successful than the latter. Whichever category you fall into, the end of your T Level course is just the beginning. It helps if you have a plan as to how you can progress in your career. Even if you are not sure where you want to go, at the very least you should be aware of the opportunities that are available.

> **Research**
>
> Although it is more relevant to the science sector than health or healthcare sectors, the Royal Society of Chemistry offers a 'careers toolkit' of online resources to its members.
>
> Other professional bodies in your field may offer something similar. You should use all the resources and sources of advice and information available to you. Look at the professional bodies listed in section A1.4. Are any of those relevant to your chosen field of work? If so, their website might have useful resources. Make a list of sources of help and information about how to progress your career.

Undertaking further/higher education programmes

As you come to finish your T Level, it is a good idea to have already planned your next move. You will have achieved a level 3 qualification, so you should normally consider moving on to a level 4 or level 5 qualification, unless you decide to change track – in which case there will be a range of other level 3 qualifications that might be suitable.

If you plan to remain in the science, health or healthcare sector, you will probably consider a level 4 or level 5 qualification appropriate to your chosen field of work, such as Higher Technical Qualifications. In some cases this will mean that you have to become registered with a statutory regulator, such as the Nursing and Midwifery Council or the General Dental Council.

Your T Level will be worth UCAS points, so you can continue into higher education (level 5 or 6) at university or with another education provider if you wish.

Undertaking apprenticeship/degree apprenticeship

An **apprenticeship** is a job with training to industry standards and should involve entry into a recognised occupation. Apprenticeships are employer-led, so employers will:
- set the standards the apprentices need to meet
- create the demand for apprentices to meet their skills needs
- fund the apprenticeship, i.e. pay for training

- employ the apprentice, i.e. pay them and give them work
- be responsible for training the apprentice on the job.

The needs of the apprentice are also important. Apprentices are not meant to be simply a source of cheap labour. The apprentice must be able to achieve competence in a skilled occupation. Not only that, but they should also acquire skills that are transferable and offer the possibility of long-term earnings potential, greater security and the ability to progress in the workplace.

A higher apprenticeship (level 4) might lead on naturally from a level 3 T Level, but entry to a level 6 or level 7 degree apprenticeship is also possible. Degree apprenticeships combine working for an employer with studying at a university. Study periods can be on a day-to-day basis or in blocks, depending on the programme and the needs of the employer.

More information about degree apprenticeships is available on the UCAS website (**www.ucas.com**) or the Institute for Apprenticeships and Technical Education website (**www.instituteforapprenticeships.org**).

Undertaking continuing professional development (CPD)

Continuing professional development can take many forms. It is a way in which professionals use different learning activities to maintain, develop and enhance their abilities, skills and knowledge. CPD combines different methods of learning, such as:
- conferences and events
- training workshops
- e-learning programmes
- best practice techniques
- ideas sharing
- shadowing a more experienced professional in the field.

CPD programmes are often run by employers or professional bodies such as those described in section A1.4.

Joining professional bodies

Professional bodies fulfil a number of important functions. As well as being the guardians of professional codes of conduct in their area of expertise, they offer CPD programmes.

In some occupations in the science, health and healthcare sectors you need to be registered with a statutory body, such as one of the professional bodies.

Some professional bodies offer **chartered** status. As well as indicating an in-depth knowledge of the field, chartered status is required in some regulated activities that have to be supervised by a **qualified person**, such as production of pharmaceuticals (see section A9.3 for more information). Examples include:
- Chartered Chemist (CChem) administered by the Royal Society of Chemistry
- Chartered Biologist (CBiol) administered by the Royal Society of Biology
- Chartered Physicist (CPhys) administered by the Institute of Physics
- Chartered Scientist (CSci) administered by the Science Council.

Undertaking an internship

Internships can offer valuable experience in a real work environment – particularly if you have not gained this through an apprenticeship. Internships are usually relatively short and often take place during the summer months, as many are designed for university students. Placements are similar, but generally last longer. Internships and placements are usually offered by large companies, such as GSK (which manufactures pharmaceuticals) or Unilever (consumer products). In some cases, you will be paid at least the UK National Living Wage, but in others it can be much higher than this – though some internships are not paid at all. Bursaries are often available to cover your costs in an unpaid internship. Many of the professional bodies already mentioned will offer help with internships, placements or bursaries. Their websites are the best place to look for advice and information.

Undertaking a scholarship

As well as help with bursaries, many of the professional bodies can offer help with scholarships. These are usually available to help with the costs of obtaining higher qualifications, usually at level 6 or level 7. Educational institutions that offer these qualifications may also offer scholarships or can give guidance on what scholarships and other sources of funding are available.

A1: Working within the health and science sector

Project practice

You are working in a science/health/healthcare organisation (choose one according to your own area of work). You have been asked to produce materials to help new apprentices understand the importance of the working practices of the organisation, as well as to inform them about the ways in which their careers might develop.

1. Prepare a summary of the organisation policies that you are aware of in your organisation, or ones that you know should be in place. Give explanations for the relevance and importance of these.
2. Research the professional codes of practice relevant to your area of work. This might require you to use the websites of any relevant professional bodies to gather information.
3. Prepare a list of the types of CPD that are available or recommended in your organisation.
4. Finally, outline the additional ways in which apprentices can progress in their careers.

You should present the information in the form of a poster or short written document, such as an employee handbook.

Assessment practice

1. What piece of legislation covers the requirement for diversity and inclusion for people with certain characteristics?
2. Who is responsible for obtaining a DBS check for work?
3. What is the name for the legal parts of an employment contract?
4. What are collective agreements?
5. Your employer has a disciplinary policy that includes informal and formal written warnings. You have been found stealing and dismissed. You feel that you have been treated unfairly because you were not given any warnings or a notice period. Are you correct?
6. Give two reasons why an organisation needs an equality, diversity and inclusion policy.
7. Explain, using an example, what is meant by safeguarding.
8. Give two reasons why organisations adhere to quality standards.
9. During the early stages of the COVID-19 pandemic, there were serious concerns that NHS hospitals would be overwhelmed and unable to treat patients. Therefore, hospitals were instructed by the government to discharge any patients who could be transferred back to their care homes. In many cases this led to the introduction of COVID-19 into care homes from hospitals because patients were not tested for COVID-19 or were known to be infected.

   Evaluate this instruction, considering the key principles of ethical practice.

   Your response should demonstrate:
   - reasoned judgements
   - informed conclusions.

A2: The healthcare science sector

Introduction

This unit provides an overview of the purpose of different organisations and care available within the healthcare science sector, and an insight into the diverse range of work environments and job roles available. We will discuss entry requirements needed for different job roles, the scope of the potential career pathways and the progression routes that they can lead on to. Different accreditations and certifications for the range of healthcare science job roles will also be covered, as well as the importance of appraisals and performance reviews when working in the healthcare science sector. The final part of this unit will cover the new technologies now accessible to patients to improve their health and wellbeing, and the benefits that these can bring.

Learning outcomes

The core knowledge outcomes that you must understand and learn:

- **A2.1** the difference between public, private and charitable healthcare organisations
- **A2.2** the purpose of different organisations and services within the healthcare science sector in the UK
- **A2.3** the difference between primary, secondary and tertiary care
- **A2.4** the diversity of working environments within the healthcare science sector
- **A2.5** the purpose of job descriptions, person specifications and the need for entry requirements for jobs within the healthcare science sector
- **A2.6** the range and diversity of job roles within the healthcare science sector
- **A2.7** the links between career pathways and progression routes within the healthcare science sector, as outlined by the Institute for Apprenticeships and Technical Education occupational maps
- **A2.8** the purpose of roles having a clear scope of practice
- **A2.9** the links between registration and scope of practice in relation to activities which can only be undertaken by a registered healthcare professional
- **A2.10** the difference between voluntary and statutory registration
- **A2.11** the role of accreditation and certification in healthcare science sector jobs
- **A2.12** the purpose of appraisals and performance reviews within the healthcare science sector
- **A2.13** the impact of external factors on activities of healthcare science sector organisations
- **A2.14** the benefits of new technology/automation/ artificial intelligence within the healthcare science sector.

A2: The healthcare science sector

A2.1 The difference between public, private and charitable healthcare organisations

Organisations within healthcare science either fall under the public, private or charitable healthcare sectors.

Public sector

The **public sector** refers to anything provided by the state and funded by the government via taxes. An important part of this in the UK is the provision of healthcare services that are free to users at the point of accessing that service (although there are some exceptions, such as dental charges and prescriptions). Public-sector organisations are owned and operated by the government and are funded through **National Insurance**. In terms of healthcare, these can either be national or local NHS (National Health Service) organisations. Public-sector organisations that focus on setting policies and guidelines on a national level include the **UK Health Security Agency (UKHSA), NICE (National Institute for Health and Care Excellence)** and NHS England. Local public-sector organisations include **NHS trusts** and **clinical commissioning groups (CCGs)**. The aim of public-sector organisations is to ensure that the public's needs are being met in relation to healthcare, mainstream schools, police, emergency services and so on, and that these services are accessible to all the public. These services aim to serve the public by providing the care, support and treatment that is needed in local communities.

Public services in the healthcare sector include:
- GP practices
- family planning clinics
- dental practices offering NHS services
- NHS opticians.

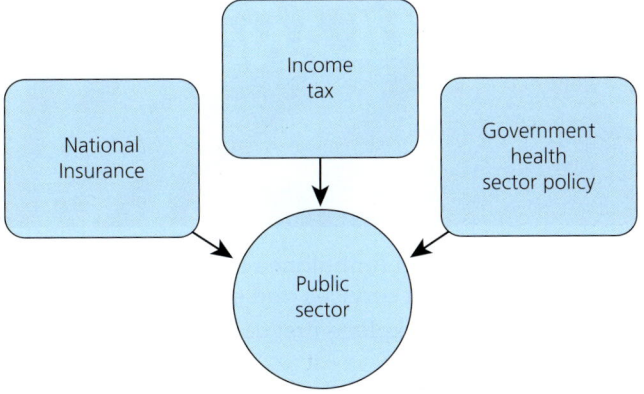

▲ Figure 2.1 How the public sector is funded

Key terms

National Insurance: mandatory payments made by employers and employees in the UK that fund certain state benefits, e.g. healthcare, a state pension and payments for sick and unemployed people.

The UK Health Security Agency (UKHSA): an organisation of the Department of Health and Social Care that is responsible for protecting the nation from the impact of infectious diseases, chemical, biological, radiological and nuclear incidents and other health threats. UKHSA replaced Public Health England (PHE) in April 2021.

NICE (National Institute for Health and Care Excellence): an independent agency of the NHS that offers guidance and recommendations on the appropriate treatment plans for specific diseases.

NHS trust: an organisational unit that provides specialised care in a specific community. Within any community there may be several NHS trusts providing healthcare, such as mental health trusts, community trusts, acute trusts and ambulance trusts.

Clinical commissioning groups (CCGs): NHS services that provide care that is specifically needed in local areas. When specific health needs have been identified, CCGs plan and commission the appropriate care that needs to be invested in and implemented to meet these.

The NHS is the publicly funded organisation that provides healthcare services in the UK. It is made up of several organisations with over 350 roles, and its overall aim is to provide high-quality care and improve people's quality of life using enhancing treatments and support services. It includes:
- **primary care organisations** – independent businesses offering NHS services, including GP practices, dental practices and opticians
- **acute (hospital) trusts** – providers of hospital-based specialised services such as emergency care
- **mental health trusts** – organisations that offer mental health and social care services
- **community trusts** – providers of community-based services, such as district nursing, physiotherapy and speech and language therapy
- **ambulance trusts** – organisations that offer NHS transportation services for emergency and non-emergency care
- **charities and social enterprises** – organisations that provide support services to the NHS, for example Young Minds and Age UK.

Private sector

Private-sector organisations are developed and run by their owners and investors rather than the government or charities. They require those who are using the services to pay for them independently as they charge for these services. In addition to providing a service to individuals, their overall aim is to make a profit for investors, i.e. their shareholders. Private-sector organisations are therefore less restricted by their budgets for the services they offer than public and voluntary sectors are. In terms of healthcare, private (sometimes called commercial or premium) health insurance is sometimes required to use these services, otherwise payment may be required upfront, which can be very expensive. Examples of private-sector services include hospital groups such as Nuffield Health, BMI Healthcare and private residential care homes. Certain services may be offered by private providers that may not be available on the NHS; examples include some cosmetic surgeries and procedures, and treatments such as IVF (*in vitro fertilisation*) where there are limits placed on what the NHS can offer.

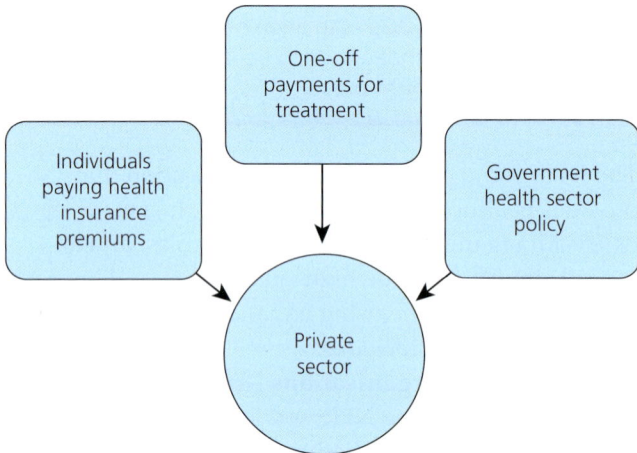

▲ Figure 2.2 How the private sector is funded

Research

Research the private-sector healthcare organisations in your local area. Read about the different services offered.

Are there a range of different services being offered?

Do the services offered meet the physical and mental health needs of your local area?

Voluntary/charity sector

Voluntary or charity-sector organisations are funded through donations, trusts and foundations and government grants that organisations can apply for. Under the Health and Social Care Act 2012, CCGs were granted permission to oversee and support voluntary and charity-sector services. Individual donations and purchases are that sector's main source of income, providing over 40 per cent (around £16.5 billion) of the sector's total income. [Source: www.ncvo.org.uk/about-us/media-centre/briefings/219-the-charity-sector-and-funding] Contracts and grants from statutory bodies generate almost as much of the sector's income.

Voluntary and charity-sector organisations have a distinct purpose: benefiting the healthcare needs of its target audience and the general public. Like private-sector organisations, they are non-government organisations, and their aim is not to make a profit but to provide a benefit to society. Most of their services tend to be staffed by unpaid volunteers; they may have some paid administrative staff, however, especially if they are larger. These organisations generally have a board of trustees that sets the direction of the charity and ensures legislation is being adhered to. Voluntary or charity sector organisations will most commonly undertake fundraising events and activities within communities to raise funds and receive donations.

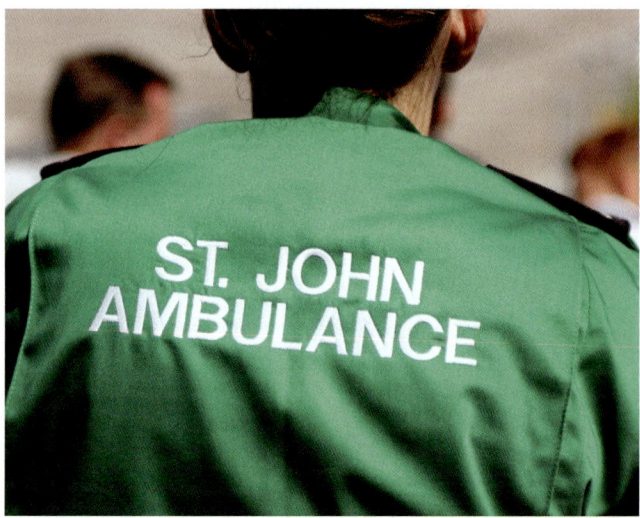

▲ Figure 2.3 St John Ambulance is a charity that provides first aid services and supplies, ambulance services and workplace first aid training

A2: The healthcare science sector

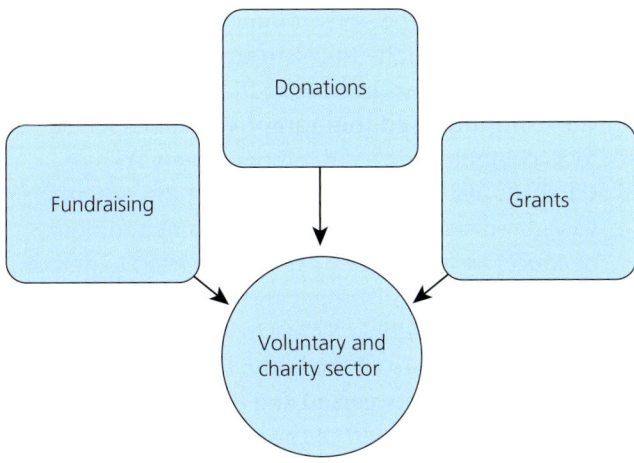

▲ Figure 2.4 How the voluntary/charity sector is funded

> **Research**
>
> Research one voluntary/charitable organisation. This could be one that is personal to yourself – one you have donated to or one that you have an interest in finding more information about.
>
> Read about the organisation's aim, the fundraising it arranges and how it raises awareness. Find out about any fundraising event they may have arranged.

> **Test yourself**
>
> 1 Explain what is meant by a public-sector organisation.
> 2 How are private-sector organisations funded?
> 3 Explain the purpose of voluntary/charitable-sector organisations.
> 4 List three examples of voluntary/charitable-sector organisations.
> 5 Compare the different services offered by the public, private and voluntary sectors.

A2.2 The purpose of different organisations and services within the healthcare science sector in the UK

Different organisations in the healthcare science sector have their own unique purposes depending on the services they provide.

Healthcare science

Healthcare science organisations cover a wide range of different services and teams that are all responsible for providing specialist care in their area. The general purpose of healthcare science organisations includes services such as the collection of specimens for analysis, producing data and images for diagnosis and treatment, and providing health and wellbeing advice for patients with specific health needs.

Collect specimens for analysis

A fundamental part of healthcare science organisations is the collection of specimens from patients for analysis to determine a more accurate diagnosis and treatment plan. **Specimen collection** refers to professionals collecting biological material from patients for **pathology** analysis such as urine, saliva, blood, tissues, organs and other fluids or cells. There are essential steps that go into specimen collection to reduce/eliminate the risk of contamination and/or misplacing them, all varying depending on the specimen material being collected. Hospital personnel are responsible for ensuring these steps are carried out safely and correctly, in accordance with legislations, such as COSHH 2002 (see Chapter A3).

> **Key term**
>
> *Pathology:* the scientific study of the causes, effects and treatment of disease.

> **Research**
>
> Find out the procedure for collecting specimen material for either blood, tissues or organs. Research the good practice principles that hospital personnel must follow.
>
> You may find the *Nursing Times* website useful with your research:
>
> www.nursingtimes.net/clinical-archive/assessment-skills

Produce data and images for diagnosis and treatment

The advancement in healthcare science technologies has enabled the use of data and medical images to reliably detect, diagnose and treat conditions, before a patient's condition can potentially get worse. The information obtained from data and imagery plays a fundamental role in a professional's ability to be able to detect a condition. For many conditions, such as cancer, it is the only **non-invasive** diagnostic method for a patient.

> **Key term**
>
> *Non-invasive:* a medical procedure/treatment that does not break the skin or enter the body.

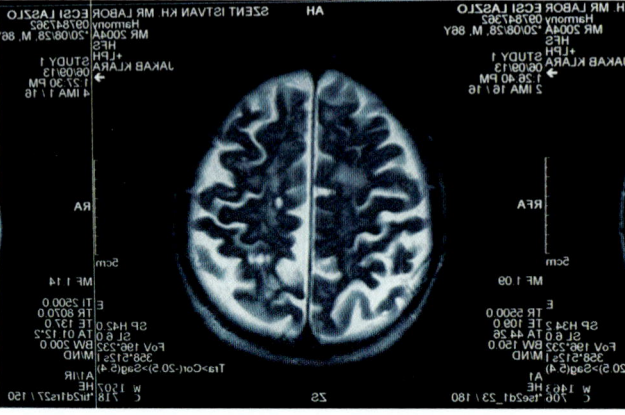

▲ Figure 2.5 CT scan of the brain

Different types of data and imaging techniques may be used by a radiologist to examine a patient and then report back any findings. The most routinely used include the following:

- ▶ **X-rays** – used to diagnose conditions such as bone fractures, breast cancer, arthritis and osteoporosis. It is a type of electromagnetic wave radiation that produces images (radiographs) of the inside of the body to quickly determine a diagnosis. It usually takes around 10–15 minutes depending on the area being focused on.
- ▶ **CT (computerised tomography)** – also referred to as computerised axial tomography (CAT), CT scans are used to diagnose heart disease and vascular disease, as well as to pinpoint a tumour or cancer location. They can also be used to detect muscle and bone disorders and different infections. CT scans use multiple X-rays to create an image of a particular part of the body. They generally take anything between 10 and 30 minutes, again depending on the part of the body being scanned.
- ▶ **MRI (magnetic resonance imaging)** – MRI scans are used to detect conditions such as tumours, spinal cord conditions and strokes. An MRI scan involves the use of radio waves and magnetic fields to produce a detailed cross-sectional image of parts of the body, for example the brain, or certain bones or joints. The procedure can last from 15 to 90 minutes depending on the condition and part of the body being examined.
- ▶ **Ultrasound** – often used for conditions such as breast lumps, prostate issues and monitoring pregnancies. It uses high-frequency sound waves that create images of soft tissues of the body, such as blood vessels, muscles, joints and internal organs, that don't show up well on X-rays. Ultrasound scans take between 30 minutes and an hour.
- ▶ **PET (positron emission tomography)** – PET uses low-dose radiation that checks the activity of cells to create a 3D image of different parts of the body. PET scans are used to detect diseases such as Alzheimer's and Parkinson's, conditions such as seizures and epilepsy, as well as cancer and heart disease. They generally take around 30–60 minutes.

Even with advances in data and medical imagery technologies for detecting, diagnosing and treating diseases, there is research that suggests that the diagnoses drawn from images and data can be imprecise, so sometimes more than one source of examination could be used to help.

Analyse specimens for diagnosis and treatment

Once specimens such as blood, urine and tissues have been collected, they then can be analysed to identify a diagnosis and determine the necessary treatment needed. The diagnoses and treatment have important implications for patient care and for future research, so it is an important role of healthcare science organisations to ensure these are analysed accurately and efficiently. Quality assurance (see section A5.2, page 75) is vital here for a correct diagnosis and treatment plan to be given to a patient. This includes ensuring the highest quality regarding anything from the point of timing of the specimen material, to the preservation and storage of the specimen material, analyses and the patient's data. **Quality management systems (QMS)** and adherence to **standard operating procedures (SOPs)** are essential to a pathologist's role here when analysing specimen material. By taking materials such as blood, urine and tissue cells and analysing them under a microscope, pathologists can compare the material collected to the normal structure and recognisable patterns associated with materials considered to be healthy. Any changes examined at a microscopic level can then be analysed by their structure and identified as a particular disease. This analysis of specimen material, when it is accurate and completed in an efficient timeframe, can provide an effective health outcome for a patient's wellbeing and recovery.

Key terms

Quality management systems (QMS): the implementation of systems, policies and procedures that are designed to ensure high-quality healthcare while minimising the risk of harm to both staff and patients. See section A5.2 page 75 for more.

Standard operating procedure (SOP): written instructions compiled by an organisation that describe how to carry out routine operations efficiently and safely. Healthcare science settings must have SOPs for how to perform jobs that involve potential risks so that they can be carried out safely and in compliance with procedure regulations. See section A9.2 page 184 for more.

Research

Following on from your research on the collection of specimens for analysis on page 17, research the process of analysing your chosen specimen material.

Summarise how the analysis is completed and the steps it includes.

You may wish to use the following NHS website to help you with your research:

www.northdevonhealth.nhs.uk/pathology/departments/microbiology/sample-collection

Provide health and wellbeing advice

Healthcare science professionals represent a broad range of job roles across the sector, all of which have a significant and influential part to play in providing health and wellbeing advice to patients and their health outcomes. Professionals working within the healthcare science sector just within the NHS comprise over 150 service areas and over 56 000 people (NHS England, 2020). [Source: www.england.nhs.uk/wp-content/uploads/2020/03/science-in-healthcare-delivering-the-nhs-long-term-plan.pdf] Through their involvement in services such as diagnoses and treatment, medicine distributions, rehabilitation services, formulating prevention strategies and health improvement plans, and operating and evaluating new healthcare technologies, their specialisms and expertise are vital for the provision of health and wellbeing advice.

The provision of quality health and wellbeing advice is heavily reliant on professionals keeping updated with continuous professional development through education and training programmes. This will ensure they are providing the most up-to-date and relevant advice to patients within their care, for example health and nutrition advice, how to manage emotions, dealing with bereavements and adjusting to illnesses.

By ensuring they are adhering to the standards set by the **Health and Care Professions Council (HCPC)**, healthcare science professionals are involved in making key judgements regarding a patient's diagnostic and treatment plan, many working directly with patients and providing them with advice and resources to help them with their health and wellbeing. An example of this is a cardiologist advising a patient who has been diagnosed with angina on recommended foods to include in their diet. At the same time, professionals will also be developing innovations and research programmes to educate their patients with the hope of improving public health.

Key term

Health and Care Professions Council (HCPC): a UK organisation that aims to protect the public through the regulation of registered healthcare science professionals, ensuring they are meeting clinical standards.

> **Reflect**
>
> The National School of Healthcare Science (NSHCS) is an organisation that supports and implements the delivery of healthcare science training and educational programmes throughout the UK. It facilitates an annual healthcare science week for celebrating and increasing awareness of the broad job roles within the healthcare science sector and the impact they can have on providing and implementing health and wellbeing advice within the UK.
>
> Read about the NSHCS's Healthcare Science Week page using this link:
>
> www.healthcareers.nhs.uk/career-planning/career-advisers-and-teachers/teaching-resources/healthcare-science-week
>
> With a partner, discuss the impact that this annual networking event could have for educating and inspiring a local community about the importance of the healthcare science role.

Pharmacy services

Pharmacies are there to provide products to patients when they need treatment – either because they have a prescription from their GP, or they need a non-prescription item – ensuring any products supplied are legally allowed to be sold and are suitable to support patients' welfare. In the UK, the **Medicines Act 1968** governs the main legal framework for categorising medical products and the supply of these products to the public. Secondary legislation such as the **Human Medicines Act 2012** has provided amendments to this act and more recent guidelines for settings to abide by. **Pharmacists** are responsible for the safe supply of medication and must be committed to ensuring that the quality and supply of **controlled drugs** are in accordance with the law, are suitable for patients' welfare and are in line with the standards set by the **Medicines and Healthcare products Regulatory Agency (MHRA)** and the **General Pharmaceutical Council**.

Pharmacy services include a range of settings from hospital and prison pharmacies to laboratories and the pharmaceutical industry. A pharmacist is expected to work autonomously using their professional judgement. As well as supplying prescription and non-prescription products, they give health and wellbeing advice to patients, and may also sell a range of other retail items, for instance toiletries, food and drink. Pharmacy services are also tasked with providing information and medical advice to patients, confirming whether medicines are safe to use in conjunction with other medications and providing information about potential side effects.

> **Key terms**
>
> **Medicines Act 1968:** the first act of parliament that provided a system for licensing medical products in the UK.
>
> **Human Medicines Act 2012:** an act which was designed to modernise and amend medicines legislation in the UK.
>
> **Pharmacist:** in accordance with the Pharmacy Act 1954, a person who is on the register of pharmaceutical chemists with the General Pharmaceutical Council may be called a pharmacist.
>
> **Controlled drugs:** those licensed with a valid marketing authorisation for use within the UK and come within the Misuse of Drugs Act 1971.
>
> **Medicines and Healthcare products Regulatory Agency (MHRA):** an executive agency of the Department of Health that is responsible for ensuring that medicines are safely manufactured and supplied.
>
> **General Pharmaceutical Council:** the UK's pharmacy services regulator that ensures high-quality services and safe measures are being offered by pharmacy professionals. Pharmacy professionals must meet requirements to remain on the council's register.
>
> **Prescription:** a written order that is presented to a registered professional who has legal authorisation to dispense a medicinal product.
>
> **Prescriber:** a registered healthcare professional with the legal authorisation to prescribe a medical product.

Supply prescription products

Prescription products are the most regular treatment provided to patients in the healthcare science sector. Pharmacies supply these products through **prescriptions** when a patient requires medical treatment. Prescriptions are generally presented to a **prescriber** in a written format and signed by the professional authorised legally to prescribe it (usually a doctor following a GP appointment or other consultation). Any dispensing of prescription medicines must legally only be carried out in response to a valid prescription (unless it is a prescription being made in a hospital, which would then be prescribed following the patient's official diagnoses). The pharmacist must check that the prescription is valid and in date, that the medicine is appropriate for the patient and their individual health needs, and that the labelling on the prescription, and advice to the patient, adheres to the law.

The dispensing of prescription products should be accurate and SOPs must be followed. Pharmacies are responsible for ensuring that they acquire enough stock to supply prescription products efficiently to ensure that patients' needs are being met.

> **Research**
>
> Find out more about the supply of prescription products for pharmacy services with this link from the Pharmaceutical Services Negotiating Committee:
>
> **www.hwlpc.co.uk/wp-content/uploads/2018/06/Pharmacy-Support-Pack-v4-120618.pdf**

Supply non-prescription products

As well as supplying prescription products, pharmacy services also supply over-the-counter non-prescription products; however, this must be done by a registered pharmacist or under the supervision of one. This includes the supply of **General Sale List (GSL)** items, not just **pharmacy medicines**. Non-prescription products can now be purchased online via a pharmacy's website, however certain requirements must be met for a purchase to be completed online, and such purchases can only be made for items on the GSL.

> **Key terms**
>
> ***General Sales List (GSL):*** medicines that can be sold in smaller quantities in most retail shops and are not restricted to pharmacies as they do not require consultations with a pharmacist and/or a medical professional, for example, paracetamol. There are legal restrictions on the quantities of medicines on the GSL allowed to be sold at one time, for example a maximum of two packs of paracetamol per person in England.
>
> ***Pharmacy medicines:*** also known as 'over-the-counter' medicines; medicines that can only be purchased from a registered pharmacy, are kept behind the counter and require discussion with a medical professional such as a pharmacist or a trained member of staff acting under the supervision of a pharmacist.

Pharmacists have a legal obligation to ensure that all purchasing of non-prescription products is done safely and that the patient does not intend to misuse the product in anyway that may cause them harm, for example purchasing of an alarming amount of paracetamol packages could raise concern about the buyer's intentions. Pharmacists are expected to use their expertise and professional judgement when supplying non-prescription products and be confident that the patient is aware of the appropriate use of the medication and any possible side effects that could be experienced.

> **Research**
>
> Further to your previous research on prescription products, conduct independent research into the Human Medicines Regulations 2012 for its regime for the supply of non-prescription products. Summarise the main practices that must be followed in the UK as set out by the Human Medicines Regulations. You could use this link to help you with your research.
>
> **www.legislation.gov.uk/uksi/2012/1916/made**

> **Reflect**
>
> There is much discussion over the legal classification of medicines and determining the level of professional input needed for the supply of medical products.
>
> Consider the potential benefits and barriers of making medicines available for 'over-the-counter' purchasing, rather than requiring a prescription from a GP.

> **Research**
>
> With a partner, conduct research and compile a list of ten medicines that are on the UK's GSL.

Provide health and wellbeing advice

Pharmacies have an obligation to keep updated on medically valid information in order to provide the public with specialised knowledge and professional judgement. Service users require competent advice regarding the appropriate medication or medical product required. Although pharmacists hold the responsibility for the safe provision of supplying prescription and non-prescription products to the public, health and wellbeing advice – such as behavioural support with stopping smoking – can also be provided by a pharmacy staff member, not just a pharmacist. For this reason, it is imperative that all staff members keep up to date with their continuous professional development and training.

Perform retail duties

A large proportion of a professional's roles in pharmacies includes performing a range of retail duties for services to run consistently. Pharmacies that are based in communities have a much broader role than the dispensing of medications correctly, as it also includes educating patients by providing them with health advice, explaining the proper use of medications, answering any questions patients may have and discussing any concerns. Retail duties might include administrative tasks, such as ensuring that stock checks are carried out regularly, and liaising with other agencies, such as GPs. Another important duty of any pharmacy employee is to be able to communicate with patients regarding other services and resources available to them when they are not accessible at that pharmacy.

Optical care services

Optical care services offer specialised advice and urgent eye care treatments such as testing patients' vision and refractive errors, detecting any eye abnormalities, performing retail duties and dispensing prescription eyewear. Optical care services in the UK are regulated by the **General Optical Council**, which has the authority under the Opticians Act 1989 to implement rules and regulations that optical professionals have a duty to abide by in their practices.

Registered **optometrists**, **ophthalmologists** and **dispensing opticians** have a professional obligation to ensure the highest of quality care when performing duties relevant to their specialisms, such as conducting eye and vision tests, diagnosing and monitoring patients' eye conditions, as well as dispensing appropriate treatment to meet the needs of patients. Either through the NHS or privately, professionals working in optical care services must meet the regulations implemented by the General Optical Council when dispensing prescription and non-prescription eyewear, testing patients' vision, and detecting and treating any abnormalities.

> **Key terms**
>
> **General Optical Council:** the UK's regulator for optical care services which ensures the registration of qualified optometrists and dispensing opticians, and that the highest of standards are being practised to protect the eye care needs of the public.
>
> **Optometrist:** a trained professional who undertakes eye examinations to detect vision problems and eye abnormalities and defects. Optometrists provide primary vision care.
>
> **Ophthalmologist:** a professional who specialises in the diagnosis and treatment of eye abnormalities and will prescribe the treatment needed.
>
> **Dispensing optician:** a specialist who fits and supplies patients with the most appropriate spectacles and/or contact lenses from the prescription provided by an ophthalmologist.

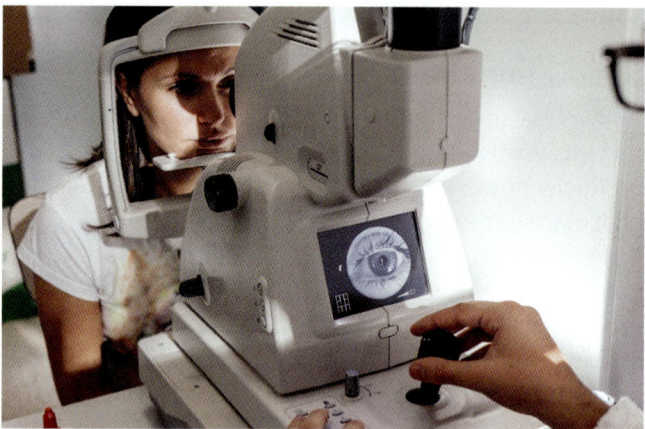

▲ Figure 2.6 An ophthalmology eyesight examination

Dispense prescription eyewear

A dispensing optician is responsible for the designing, dispensing and fitting of spectacles. Once a prescription is received from an optometrist, the dispensing optician will analyse it and discuss the patients' options with them while advising them on the different options for spectacle lenses or contact lenses based on their personal circumstances, e.g. if their occupation requires them to be in front of a screen for several hours a day. Once a decision has been made, the dispensing optician will take the necessary measurements, e.g. facial and head frame, so that the order can be processed. Once an order has been manufactured, the eyewear can then be fitted and accurately adjusted if needed. The patient should be given advice on the use of the eyewear and any aftercare service if applicable.

Test vision and refractive error

A routine eye examination usually involves a vision test, or refraction test, to detect any **refractive errors**. Vision tests can identify whether a patient needs lenses and if they have any conditions, for example **astigmatism**. A patient's eyes are firstly assessed to see if they need corrective lenses with the use of a computerised refractor or even by shining a light through the patient's eye. This enables the optician to measure the patient's refractive score by observing the amount of light coming off their retina. They assess the eyes by observing how light bends through the cornea and the lens of the patient's eyes. From this an optician will then assess what prescription a patient needs by carrying out an individual lens assessment in each eye. To do this, a **phoropter** is used, and the patient is asked, testing one eye at a time, to read out the letters on a chart on the other side of the room. Patients will be asked to start reading out the row with the smallest letters that they can identify first. A score will then be combined from the whole procedure – a score of 20/20 is considered to be perfect vision.

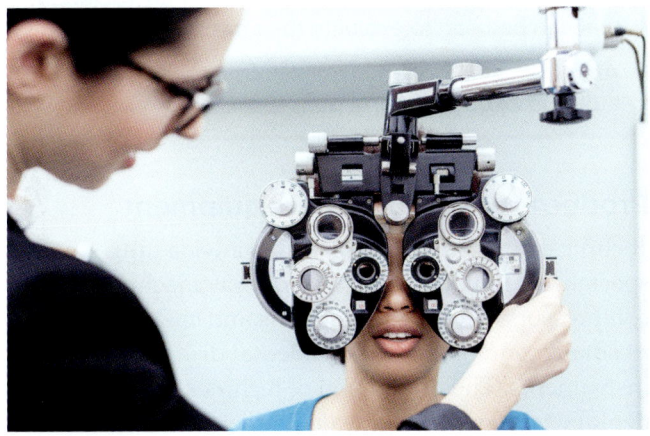

▲ Figure 2.7 An eye examination using a phoropter

Key terms

Refractive errors: also known as refraction errors, are vision problems that make it difficult for an individual's vision to focus.

Astigmatism: a type of refractive error that can bring about blurry vision due to the lens of an eye being more of an oval shape, which means light is more focused on one part of the eye.

Phoropter: a specialised instrument that is used during an eye exam to test patients' individual lenses.

Detect eye abnormalities

Eye abnormalities can be detected in the retina and macula by an optometrist through a routine eye exam. Eye exams such as **optical coherence tomography (OCT)** can also be used to test a patient's eyes. An OCT scans the different layers of the retina and takes images of the eyes, which allows the optometrist to detect any eye conditions. Once eye abnormalities are detected, optometrists are then able to monitor, manage and treat conditions such as glaucoma and dry eye.

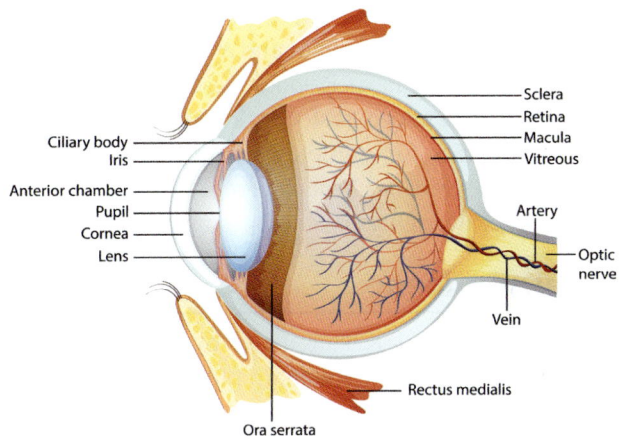

▲ Figure 2.8 The anatomy of the human eye

Research

Conduct independent research and summarise the procedures for one of the alternative eye tests an optometrist could use to test the retina and macula for abnormalities:
- ▶ visual acuity test
- ▶ dilated eye exam
- ▶ fluorescein angiogram.

The following link may help with this research:

www.nei.nih.gov/learn-about-eye-health/eye-conditions-and-diseases/macular-edema

Supply non-prescription eyewear

A dispensing optician or optometrist can supply eyewear over the counter or online where a prescription is not required. This includes non-prescription reading glasses, sunglasses, sports eyewear and contact lenses. Although non-prescription eyewear can magnify vision, e.g. reading glasses, the lenses have no corrective power. Optical professionals also advise customers on the most suitable frames and styles to best suit their features. Any retailer can supply non-prescription eyewear. It is most commonly supplied for reasons such as preventing future eye care, keeping individuals' eyes safe and for fashion purposes.

Perform retail duties

All professionals working in optical services are to ensure that the work environment is clean and visually appealing, and that optical displays are organised and fully stocked with eyeglasses, sunglasses and accessories. Optician services that are based within communities and/or retail shops have a much broader role, which includes providing health advice and answering any questions clients may have. Retail duties also include administrative tasks such as stock taking and liaising with other agencies, for example eye care wards in hospitals when referring clients on for secondary services or GP practices when liaising over prescriptions.

Dental services

Dentistry within the UK is regulated by the **General Dental Council (GDC)**. The main purposes of dental services are to ensure that patients are receiving high-quality preventative care and providing treatment to maintain the health of a patient's mouth. The GDC ensures that dental services provide top-quality and safe general dental treatment, produce technical dental equipment and respond to dental emergencies, as well as prescribing a range of dental products made at dental laboratories.

Provide general dental treatment

Dentists provide a number of dental treatments as a general part of their daily job role. They provide patients with preventative advice and treatments when needed. Such treatments include regular dental exams, cleaning the teeth and checking for gum disease, oral problems and cavities. **Dental X-rays (radiographs)** may also be taken if cavities or any other oral problems are present. Common treatments include the removal of a tooth or tooth filling (**dental restoration**). The removal of a tooth involves the numbing of the tooth and gum tissue, and then loosening and removing the tooth with dental **forceps** (a tool for removing teeth). There are several reasons why a dentist may have to remove a tooth, including gum disease, an **abscess**, tooth decay or breakage of the tooth. A filling might be performed to fill a cavity in a tooth or from breakage or chipping. Filling materials are used to restore the tooth's full shape and function.

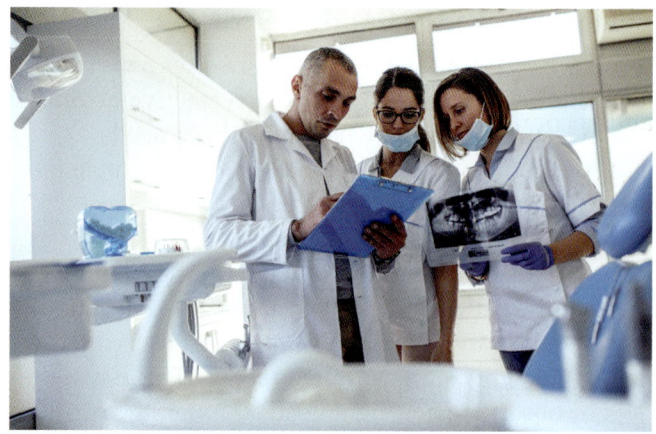

▲ Figure 2.9 Dental X-ray examinations

Key terms

General Dental Council (GDC): the UK-wide independent organisation that regulates and sets standards for qualified dental professionals to ensure that high-quality dental services are being provided.

Dental X-rays (radiographs): digital images of a patient's teeth created by exposure to X-ray radiation that can be used to evaluate their oral health.

Abscess: an infection in a tooth that causes the build-up of bacteria and pus.

Produce technical dental equipment

Technical dental equipment covers a wide range of specialised equipment including X-ray machines, air compressors, dental work stations and chairs, as well as smaller equipment such as dental drills and filling instruments. The production of technical equipment by dental engineers offers invaluable services to patients and enables professionals to conduct specialised treatment. Dental Engineers and Henry Shein Dental are both examples of suppliers that produce technical dental equipment in the UK.

Respond to dental emergencies

Dental emergencies include severe toothache; a patient's tooth being knocked out, broken or chipped; an abscess; loss of a filling or crown and broken orthodontic work. If a patient is experiencing any excessive bleeding or pain involving their teeth and requires immediate treatment, it would be considered to be a dental emergency. Dentists must ensure they are prepared and able to respond to a dental emergency and effectively manage a patient's condition to minimise pain and treat their condition.

A2: The healthcare science sector

While receiving treatment during a routine check-up or for a dental emergency, a patient could be vulnerable to a medical emergency such as collapsing and becoming unresponsive. The GDC states:

> 'A patient could collapse on any premises at any time, whether they have received treatment or not. It is therefore essential that all registrants must be trained in dealing with medical emergencies, including resuscitation, and possess up-to-date evidence of capability.'
>
> Source: www.gdc-uk.org/docs/default-source/scope-of-practice/scope-of-practice.pdf

Research

Complete research into Resuscitation Council UK's quality standards:

www.resus.org.uk/library/quality-standards-cpr/primary-dental-care#1-summary

Read 'Section 3: training of staff' and make notes on the key points of the section for how professionals should respond to medical emergencies.

Prescribe products

Any registered dentist can prescribe products that are on the **British National Formulary (BNF)**. Dental practitioners are able to assess a patient's condition, medical history and prescribe products in their competences and job scope. NHS dental services can only prescribe medical products contained in the 'List of Dental Preparations', which is contained within the BNF. This list does differ in terms of products and measurements, as seen on the following links:

https://bnf.nice.org.uk/dental-practitioners-formulary
https://bnfc.nice.org.uk/dental-practitioners-formulary

Key term

British National Formulary (BNF): a pharmaceutical reference that informs and gives advice on prescribing medicines available on the NHS; it is jointly authored by the Royal Pharmaceutical Society and the British Medical Association (BMA).

Produce a range of dental products made at dental labs

Dental laboratories can customise unique dental products for individual patients. The equipment used by dental lab technicians includes a range of highly efficient digital systems used for fixing or removing dental prosthetics and requires high precision. Dental products that can be made at dental labs include:

- crowns
- bridges
- dentures
- prosthetic products (denture teeth and implants)
- therapeutic products (orthodontic devices).

The manufacturing and production of dental products relies on good communication between dental lab technicians and dentists. The dentist must provide the lab technicians with a prescription detailing the patient's choice of product. Dental lab technicians are responsible for assisting dentists when discussing material choices and designs for specific products. It is important that dentists collaborate with dental labs to ensure high-quality planning and designing of dental products.

Prosthetic and orthotic services

The purpose of prosthetic and orthotic services is to provide specialist care during the rehabilitation process of patients who have absent or deficient limbs by designing, manufacturing and fitting custom-made devices. They are also responsible for repairing and maintaining devices, as well as providing patients with advice on prosthetic and orthotic use.

Design and manufacture custom-made devices

Prosthetic and orthotic technicians are qualified in the designing and manufacturing of custom-made devices for patients based on the prescription provided by a prosthetist or orthotist, and the patients' medical needs and bodily features. Custom-made facial prosthetics include orbital, nasal and auricular (eye, nose and ear) prostheses, while body prosthetics may be made for the limbs and torso area. Custom-made orthotic devices include orthotic splints and bespoke footwear.

Technicians may work for the NHS, an independent company that is contracted to the NHS, or a private company that works directly with patients. The process of designing and manufacturing custom-made devices may happen before a patient has amputation surgery, depending on the condition of the patient.

For orthotic devices such as bespoke footwear, a patient will have an in-depth foot exam and assessment so that an accurate cast of their foot can be formed and sent to an orthotics laboratory. Once in the laboratory, the cast can be used to create orthotic footwear that matches the patient's measurements exactly. Devices should be designed and manufactured to meet the patient's rehabilitation goals in the most effective way possible.

> **Research**
>
> CM Prosthetics is a specialised prosthetic company in the UK that provides services to the NHS and the private sector. Discovery Orthotics produces custom-made orthotics devices.
>
> Using the links that follow to their websites, review the custom-made prosthetics offered by these companies. Find three products offered by each, noting down each device's aims and features.
>
> www.cmprosthetics.co.uk/custom-made-prosthetics
>
> www.pplbiomechanics.com/collections/custom-orthotic-devices

Fit custom-made devices

Once a prosthetic or orthotic device has been designed and manufactured by a technician, it can then be fitted. Staff will work with patients to assess how well the device fits and help them adapt to it. This is important as inaccurate fitting of prosthetic and orthotic devices can lead to further damage and discomfort. With prosthetics, the fitting of custom-made devices usually begins around six weeks after a patient has had amputation surgery and the disturbance to the residual limb has had a chance to heal. At this point, a temporary fitting is used; the final prosthesis will not be fitted until several months after a patient's surgery, so the limb has fully recovered.

The process with orthotic devices is less complex. Once the product has been manufactured and dispatched, the patient's comfort and fitting are assessed.

Patient feedback and follow-up appointments are scheduled routinely for professionals to assess their patients' recovery processes.

Repair and maintain devices

Due to their everyday use, and sometimes the complexity of prosthetic and orthotic devices, they need to be repaired and maintained by technicians regularly so that they continue working efficiently to meet the patients' health and wellbeing needs. Prosthetic and orthotic technicians are responsible for carrying out repairs and any necessary modifications to custom-made devices.

Prosthetic and orthotic use and wellbeing advice

Prosthetic and orthotic professionals have an obligation to ensure that patients are provided with information and advice on their rehabilitation process. Patients also need full understanding of how to use and maintain their devices effectively. Patients will work with professionals throughout their rehabilitation, so clear and effective communication throughout the process is essential to ensure that patients have confidence in the services they are being provided with.

> **Reflect**
>
> Consider the benefits of custom-made devices for a patient's health and wellbeing. How would it help them emotionally? What might these devices do to their confidence in their day-to-day lives? Overall, consider why prosthetic and orthotic services are important for the healthcare science sector.

A2.3 The difference between primary, secondary and tertiary care

Care provision in the healthcare science sector is divided in to either primary, secondary or tertiary care.

Primary care

Primary care is the initial care services accessed in the general community and is often the first point of contact a patient will liaise with for advice and/or treatment. It is the general day-to-day healthcare provided by medical practitioners, who have a broad knowledge base of healthcare conditions. They are trained to co-ordinate the appropriate care needed for patients, and, if necessary, refer them on to a secondary provider for more specialist care.

Primary care is any care that can be accessed directly and is generally the first point of any medical consultation.

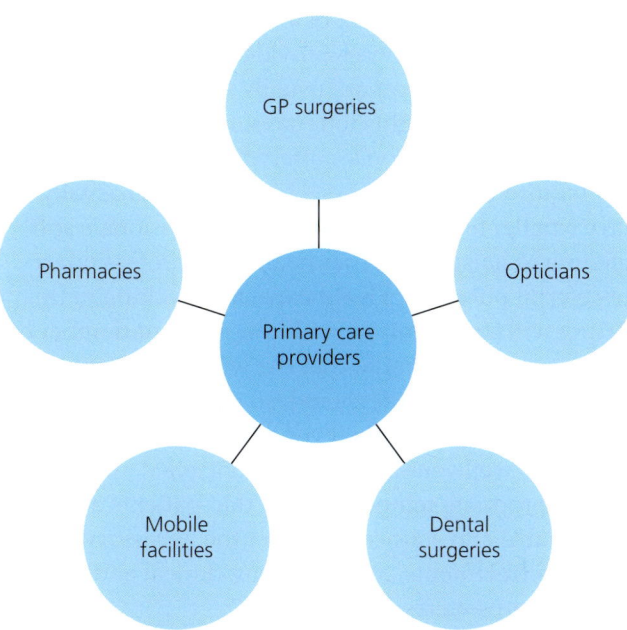

▲ Figure 2.10 Examples of primary care providers

> ### Reflect
>
> Using the link, listen to the NHS podcast 'Primary care networks: Supporting the homeless population to access primary care in Berkshire'.
>
> What are the impacts of the specific services offered here for the homeless population?
>
> Why is it important that initiatives such as this are helping the holistic needs of the homeless population?
>
> www.england.nhs.uk/publication/primary-care-networks-supporting-the-homeless-population-to-access-primary-care-in-berkshire

Secondary care

Secondary care is medical services given by professionals who provide specialised and emergency care that requires a referral from a primary care provider. Secondary care involves services that may be based in a community health setting or in a hospital setting where individuals attend as either **inpatients** or **outpatients**. It involves planned (**elective**) care and emergency or urgent care, as well as maternity services.

Examples of secondary care providers:
- hospitals
- outpatient clinics
- physiotherapists
- occupational therapists
- pathology laboratories.

Secondary care providers can conduct further tests and treatments not available with primary care providers with professionals who specialised in different healthcare science services.

> ### Research
>
> Research and compile a list of the different secondary care services offered in your local area.

> ### Key terms
>
> *Inpatients:* patients who stay in hospital overnight or for a duration while receiving medical treatment.
>
> *Outpatients:* patients who visit a hospital for an appointment but do not stay overnight.

Tertiary care

Tertiary care refers to the provision of highly specialised services that focus on more complex and advanced treatments for specific diseases. These healthcare services require a referral from another specialised health professional, usually a secondary care provider, and requires highly specialised expertise, knowledge and equipment.

Examples of tertiary care providers:
- specialist diagnostic services
- cancer services
- spinal injuries units
- orthopaedics
- burns units
- cardiac sciences
- quaternary care.

Tertiary care services include the use of advanced equipment to conduct treatments such as transplants and neurosurgery. Specialised tertiary care providers include hospitals such as Great Ormond Street.

> **Case study**
>
> Chloe is 41 years of age and has just been diagnosed with stage III ovarian cancer. Chloe had been suffering with constant bloating, feeling fatigued and having severe stomach pains. After visiting her GP, it was discovered that Chloe had abdominal **ascities** so was quickly sent for routine blood tests. The GP consulted back to Chloe that her blood results showed signs of ovarian cancer and that she was being referred to an oncologist. After examining Chloe, an ultrasound confirmed the presence of a tumour and her oncologist very quickly scheduled her to undergo surgery to remove her ovaries and fallopian tubes. Following her surgery, Chloe's oncologist was positive about the progress of her treatment. Next Chloe underwent six cycles of chemotherapy with carboplatin and taxol, then attend outpatients for the next 26 months. On follow-ups, CT scans then revealed no evidence of cancer and Chloe's blood results were good and indicated nothing abnormal.
>
> Generally, patients who have undergone surgery to remove a stage III ovarian tumour have around a 20 per cent chance of achieving the median survival rate of five years. Chloe will have regular health checkups to ensure the cancer remains in remission.
> ▶ Discuss the impact of having specialised tertiary care available in such a timely and efficient manner. How will this impact Chloe psychologically?

> **Key term**
>
> *Ascities:* the abnormal build-up of excessive fluid in the abdomen causing swelling and bloatedness.

A2.4 The diversity of working environments within the healthcare science sector

There are a wide range of working environments in the healthcare sector and this refers both to a professional's physical and psychological working environment. This variety in physical working environments includes factors such as equipment, noise levels, space, colleagues, ventilation and lighting. A professional's psychological working environment is affected by shift durations, organisation of work and whether employees' mental health and wellbeing are supported.

Healthcare science

Hospital clinics

The working environment of a hospital clinic varies depending on the services provided; however, the working hours for staff are usually very structured and are generally eight-hour days, five days a week. Depending on the services offered, some clinics will require weekend hours. Hospital clinics usually have smaller teams, however, with professionals still needing to liaise with other healthcare professionals for referral purposes. Healthcare staff working in this setting will communicate with a significant number of patients, so it is essential that the work environment is welcoming and professional, so patients feel at ease when discussing their conditions. Clinics must be well lit, well ventilated, noise-controlled and at an appropriate temperature so that patients are comfortable and staff can conduct the necessary tests and treatments, as well as any clerical and administrative tasks.

Hospital wards

Professionals working on a hospital ward will engage with a wide range of patients and visitors every day, all of whom are experiencing different health problems, and some who may be very uncomfortable due to the severity of their condition. Staff must be empathetic, patient and professional, with the ability to work in high-pressure situations at a fast pace. They will also liaise with a variety of healthcare professionals regarding the treatment and condition of their patients, whether that be healthcare providers or clerical staff. The working hours on a hospital ward will depend on the particular ward, however, nurses, doctors, healthcare assistants and other occupations present on wards will be working up to 12-hour shifts, with weekends and night shifts being a usual part of their work routine.

Staff often spend most of their shifts moving back and forth between patients, which can have a physical impact. This could be quite challenging when potentially being exposed to difficult situations and circumstances of different patients.

Noise levels on a hospital ward can vary due to machinery, patient pain management, the type of ward and time of day. To ensure patients are comfortable, temperatures between 21 and 24 °C are standard on most wards. Effective lighting is also important for both patients' comfort and suitability for staff to work in; this needs to be dimmed on the wards at night, however, so patients can sleep. All staff working on a hospital ward are required to wear PPE, e.g. gloves and aprons, but the requirements will vary depending on the procedures and treatments being administered.

Laboratories (for example, pathology laboratory)

The work environment of laboratories, such as pathology, may vary with their work hours. Laboratories in healthcare science generally run seven days a week, 24 hours a day. Most employees will work shift work and weekends. Laboratories in healthcare science can be based at public and private hospitals, specialist providers and clinics. Typically, staff working in laboratories are standing analysing microscopy slides and test results, and/or moving around while operating equipment and machinery. However, there may also be extensive periods of time in which they are sat in one position working on a computer, writing up reports. Depending on the setting, laboratories can have a high volume of test results to be analysed and reported on, so the general pace of schedules can be intense and highly structured.

Good lighting in a laboratory is important due to the unsociable hours some employees may be working, and so that test results and reports can be conducted properly. The temperature in a laboratory is usually, depending on the setting, around 20–25 °C, with the correct amount of humidity so that the accuracy of tests isn't compromised. Most employees working in laboratories are required to wear PPE such as safety goggles, visors, face masks and rubber boots.

Patient homes

Healthcare science occupations may require professionals to work in the community and deliver healthcare to patients in their own homes, e.g. district nurses. Work environments can differ from one patient to the next for several reasons, including:

- the patient's condition, e.g. the atmosphere and pressure (stress levels) of the environment due to the pain management needed, patient's responses and communication skills
- socioeconomic factors, e.g. the physical condition of the homes, such as damp, warmth, cleanliness, lighting and ventilation
- demographics, e.g. the geographical area of a patient's home – if a patient is situated in a remote location it could impact on how quickly they can be reached if their condition deteriorates and they need more visits from their district nurse
- time of the visit, e.g. unsociable hours, possibly very early or later on at night, may influence the work environment as the patients could be less welcoming to visitors and be more temperamental towards staff.

Professionals will be faced with different situations daily when working in patient homes, but it also presents an opportunity to develop good patient relationships if you make frequent visits to the same patients. Healthcare science professionals usually make visits to patient's homes with one other colleague who they work closely with rather than with a large team.

> **Reflect**
>
> Can you think of any benefits for patients of having healthcare delivered to them in their own homes? Are there any disadvantages of this?

Medical device manufacturing

Medical device manufacturing refers to the creation of a wide range of medical devices, such as X-ray machines, surgical tools, hearing aids and biomedical implants, for healthcare science sectors throughout the UK. Medical device manufacturers can be NHS-run or privately owned, but products for use in the UK must be approved by the MHRA. Professionals who manufacture medical devices will usually work the standard 40 hours a week; however, some may work overtime on weekends and nights if deadlines are closing in. Most medical device manufacturing is based in laboratories, offices, clinics and hospitals. Staff will be using specialised equipment and machinery so the necessary PPE will be needed to reduce the risk of hazards and injury. Often staff members will be working alongside a team of various professionals, each specialised and trained in their own area of the manufacturing process. In some settings, the work environment will involve the use of noisy machinery, so clear communication between professionals is very important.

Pharmacy services

Hospital pharmacy

Pharmacists and pharmacy technicians who work in a hospital, either the NHS or private, will work directly with patients who have a diverse range of health needs. They will typically work a 37.5–40-hour week, often involving rota work that includes weekends and night shifts, as many hospitals have a 24-hour pharmacy service. Staff will also work closely with other healthcare science professionals to ensure they are liaising over treatments and the administration of medicines; they will also be involved in the dispensing of medicines on the wards so will be communicating with patients daily. Some of the patients that pharmacists are caring for may not be able to be consulted on their medications, so staff will have to make that decision for them.

A large part of the role will be offering advice to other professionals and patients over the dosage of medicines, so staff members must be able to work effectively in a busy, fast-paced environment. For this reason, pharmacists will spend most of their shift moving around and on their feet. Hospital pharmacies should be well conditioned, well lit for dispensing purposes, and sterile and clean to reduce the risk of contamination.

GP practices

Pharmacists working in GP practices will work closely with other healthcare science professionals as part of a **multidisciplinary** team; they will also work directly with patients over medication queries and advice. GP surgeries should be quiet and calm environments as this enables staff members to consult with patients in a professional and empathetic manner, allowing pharmacists to have autonomous clinical responsibility over their case load. Most pharmacists based in GP practices will work no longer than 8.30 a.m. to 6.30 p.m. Monday to Friday, with some GP practices opening on Saturdays for a shorter timeframe.

> **Key term**
>
> *Multidisciplinary:* a combination of a wide range of professionals from different specialisms.

> **Case study**
>
> Elena works as a pharmacist in a GP surgery within a local community. Her case load involves a high proportion of patients with long-term health conditions and complex medication management. Elena has immediate access to patient records, allowing her to advise on any prescription queries that patients may have. Her schedule allows for direct discussions with the patients, bringing them into conversation about their own treatment and agreeing to a course of action that the patients are happy with.
> ▶ Many GPs employ pharmacists such as Elena directly. Explain three benefits that this may have for patients.
> ▶ Highlight the benefits to staff members and GPs of employing pharmacists.

Prison pharmacy

Pharmacies and pharmacy technicians working in a prison pharmacy will work and liaise with a range of different healthcare professionals including GPs, nurses, mental health nurses and physiotherapists. New frameworks within the NHS have initiated a more patient-focused approach in which pharmacies have more face-to-face interaction with prisoners.

Work environments for a prison pharmacy vary depending on the type of prison. Local prisons within the community will rely on prison pharmacies for cases when a prisoner has become ill or has acute health issues and is in need of medication. Depending on the severity and demand for the medication, pharmacies and pharmacy technicians may be under pressure to respond to situations quickly and under intense conditions. The security conditions are very strict, and pharmacists will be contracted to shift work and even night shifts in case an on-call GP requires out-of-hours medication for a prisoner.

Community pharmacy

Pharmacies based in the community are usually accessible on a high street or within a GP practice or health centre (see previously). Staff will usually work in a small team of pharmacy technicians that will be overseen by a managing pharmacist. Staff will be in direct contact with the public and may know those patients with acute healthcare needs quite well. Communication and a professional, welcoming environment are important for both patients and staff.

A community pharmacy should be a clean, well-lit and ventilated, inviting environment in which all health and safety and infection control procedures are being followed. Pharmacists are required to wear the appropriate PPE, such as masks and gloves, when dealing with sterile or potentially hazardous pharmaceutical products. Clearly, the mandatory wearing of PPE due to the recent outbreak of COVID-19 will mean that pharmacists may be required to wear PPE around the public now as well as when dealing with sterile and potentially hazardous pharmaceutical products.

Most high street pharmacies are open Monday to Saturday between roughly 8.00 a.m. and 6.00 p.m.; however, some may have extended hours during evenings and weekends to accommodate the local community. Due to the nature of the job, many pharmacists working in the community spend a high proportion of their time on their feet interacting with patients and overseeing the dispensing of their medications.

Laboratories

Pharmaceutical laboratories usually employ scientists and technicians who are responsible for developing new drug treatments. Depending on the pharmaceutical company, laboratories can include large or small teams of professionals who will generally work on shift rotas. Laboratories contain advanced and sophisticated machinery and equipment that staff must maintain. For this reason, the work environment should be calm so staff can make accurate and precise decisions when working and conducting experiments. The laboratories should also be well lit and ventilated, with a temperature of around 20–25 °C so as not to compromise any scientific experiments. PPE, such as gloves, masks, aprons and goggles, must be worn when in the laboratory to protect everyone.

Pharmaceutical industry

The pharmaceutical industry employs a broad range of different professions including sales representatives, research assistants and pharmaceutical operators. Working hours may differ from department to department, with some working through the day, while others work shifts at weekends and nights due to warehouses operating 24 hours a day. As development and production in the pharmaceutical industry is highly automated, work areas need to be well lit, and workspaces should be kept clear and clean to protect drugs and equipment from being contaminated. Offices and warehouse floors may be noisy due to machinery, telephone calls and the general discussions between members of the team, however, it is important that the work environment remains calm and professional. Some professions will be required to wear the appropriate safety PPE.

Optical care services

High street optometry practice

Optometrists working in a high street practice will have a broad range of clients from the local community, including both NHS and private patients. An optometrist's duty in a high street practice includes conducting detailed eye examinations and dispensing, fitting and supplying spectacles and/or contact lenses. Patients may need to be referred on to a secondary care provider if they need specialist treatment or further complex treatment that is not available at the practice. Optometrists also give patients advice regarding their vision and eye health. The high street optometry practice is one of the most common work environments for an optometrist to work in; they generally work around eight hours a day, Monday to Friday, and usually fewer hours at the weekend.

Hospital clinics (for example, emergency eye care)

Optometrists who work in hospital clinics will treat patients with more urgent eye conditions or injuries. They are more specialised in treating patients with conditions such as glaucoma, and offer artificial eye services, treatment for corneal ulcers, diabetic eye screening and emergency eye care. Hospital clinics providing emergency eye care are staffed by a large team of professionals. They will have clear guidelines to follow in relation to which eye conditions should be dealt with by a nurse and which conditions should be referred to an ophthalmic specialist. It is a fast-paced, busy work environment with lots of liaising with other medical professionals, including ophthalmologists, consultants, nurses and healthcare assistants. Hospital clinics will have equipment for specialised eye care, including a theatre equipped for emergency surgery. They normally operate from 8 a.m. to 5 p.m., Monday to Friday, but will have out-of-hours services to refer patients to in the case of an emergency.

> **Research**
>
> Read the document in the following link:
>
> www.rcophth.ac.uk/wp-content/uploads/2021/12/RCOphth-The-Way-Forward-Executive-Summary-300117.pdf
>
> It was commissioned by the Royal College of Ophthalmologists to identify methods to help meet the increasing demand for ophthalmic services in the UK.
>
> Note down the five common themes highlighted in the report that run through the new models of care. Summarise the importance of each for meeting the increase in demand for ophthalmic services.
>
> The report mentions the development of a **multidisciplinary** eye healthcare team. Discuss how you believe this will help to meet demand in the UK.

Dispensing-only practices

For optical services, dispensing-only practices refer to senior dispensing optical professionals who are qualified and experienced in treating and managing hospital eye service patients. Individuals who use this service include patients with complex dispensing issues, for example a patient who is suffering from dementia or a severe mental health problem. Due to the nature of the patients' needs, dispensing-only practices involve an intense work environment in which professionals have a broad range of patients to treat who all have complex needs. Patients must either have a prescription issued to them or be referred by an optometrist, orthoptist or ophthalmologist to use this service. Dispensing-only practices run Monday to Friday and are usually based in the general eye clinic of a hospital.

Dental services

Laboratories

Dental technicians may work in a dental laboratory with a small team, depending on the size of the organisation, while some dental technicians work alongside dentists, i.e. with patients more directly, and have a smaller scale in-house laboratory. Dental laboratories have a wide range of specialised materials and equipment, including grinding/polishing equipment, hand instruments, electric waxers or, more traditionally, Bunsen burners. Laboratories must be clean for infection control purposes, as well as having efficient ventilation and lighting. Due to the nature of the chemicals and substances that dental technicians are exposed to, as well as the noise levels from machinery, laboratory staff need to wear appropriate PPE while in labs. Laboratory hours would on average include a 40-hour week, but this could be more if self-employed.

Dentists/orthodontists

Professionals working in dentistry and orthodontist practices usually work around 35 to 40 hours per week. The working hours of practices will vary, and some will have evenings and weekend hours to accommodate their patients; unlike other healthcare science occupations, however, there are no added expectations for night work unless the practice has an emergency on-call service. Practices that are based in the community will have a broad range of patients registered of all ages and health needs, including:

- individuals with special needs
- young children
- elderly patients with more complex needs.

Dentists' and orthodontists' practices are patient-focused, fast-paced environments that run on fixed schedules, all differing depending on the treatments offered. Orthodontists either work in dental practices or their own offices. Dentists and orthodontists work in well-lit, well-ventilated and clean office spaces that should be spacious and comfortable for their patients. Treatment areas will be specially equipped with a range of dental and surgical instruments. While working, dentists and orthodontists will wear the appropriate PPE, usually lab coats, masks, safety glasses and gloves. This is to ensure that employees and patients aren't exposed to infections due to their close contact. Communication is a key factor within dentistry and orthodontist practices. Often patients could be experiencing pain or discomfort, so it is important that communication is always direct and professional, whether it is face to face or over the telephone.

Hospitals (for example, emergency dental care)

If a patient requires emergency or specialised dental services, they will access a hospital dental practice such as an emergency dental ward. Hospital practices are more specialised and highly qualified in oral surgery, including **maxillofacial surgery**, orthodontics and restorative services if a patient has a damaged or missing tooth. In hospital practices, dental procedures are carried out in an operating theatre with specialised instruments and equipment. Overnight stays are common in hospitals with emergency dental care due to the nature of some of the treatments, e.g. oral/maxillofacial surgeries. For that reason, professionals working in these facilities will often be contracted to shift work, including night shifts, and will work longer hours than a community dental practice. The physical environment for hospital dental care must be clean, well equipped and well lit for the health and safety of staff and patients.

> **Key term**
>
> *Maxillofacial surgery:* specialised surgery to treat conditions, defects and injuries of the mouth, teeth, jaws and face.

Prosthetics and orthotic services

Manufacturers

Professionals who are specialised in the manufacture of prosthetic and orthotic products often work as part of a large team of individuals who are not likely to come into direct contact with patients but will instead liaise with other healthcare science professionals. Patients' measurements and designs will differ significantly due to the broad and complex range of patients requiring this service. Most prosthetists and orthotists work full time Monday to Friday. Prosthetists and orthotists are at a risk of being exposed to occupational hazards in their day-to-day work environment, such as noise, lighting and chemical/material exposures used in the fabrication process, which could have long-term health impacts. For this reason, staff are required to wear the appropriate PPE, for example masks, ear protectors and safety goggles.

Hospital clinics

Professionals who work in prosthetics and orthotic services are often based within NHS or private hospitals. Staff members who are employed in hospital clinics often work 37.5–40 hours a week, Monday to Friday. Part of the role may include travelling to visit more than one hospital clinic depending on the case load of patients. Depending on the size of the hospital clinic, staff could be situated independently or as part of a large multidisciplinary team, which would require lots of communication between different specialisms. Hospital clinics will be a busy environment involving a high capacity of patient needs and numbers and will require staff to be moving around often when caring for patients. Staff will be required to wear appropriate PPE, e.g. gloves and masks, for preventing contamination.

Laboratories

Prosthetist and orthotist technicians based in laboratories usually work in NHS or private hospitals as well as factories. Staff are usually working alongside several other professionals to consult on findings. Prosthetic and orthotic laboratories are often staffed Monday to Friday with staff working full time around 40 hours per week. They are equipped with specialised machinery and equipment, which staff are trained to use carefully and maintain, often requiring staff to be situated in one position for a long period of time. Laboratories should be well lit, clean and well ventilated to protect any work from being compromised. (Laboratory tests for prosthetics and orthotics include bending and torsional testing which involves the twisting, rotation and bending of products to test their likeliness of failing.) Staff will be working with materials such as metals, plastics, carbon fibres and composites, so are required to always wear PPE, e.g. googles, gloves, masks and protective footwear to reduce exposure and risks linked to potential injury or disease.

> **Reflect**
>
> Think about the work environment at your placement. Consider how it compares to those discussed before. Is the work environment appropriate to meet the needs of the staff and the patients? Give reasons to support your answer, including:
> ▶ details of your work placement environment
> ▶ how the environment is beneficial for the welfare of staff and patients
> ▶ how it compares to any of the above
> ▶ whether there are any aspects of the work environment that could be improved for staff and patients' welfare and why.

A2.5 The purpose of job descriptions, person specifications and the need for entry requirements for jobs within the healthcare science sector

Job description

When any healthcare science job is advertised, it is important that details of the role are included in the advertisement so that any potential applicant has a good understanding of the role and whether it is appropriate for them and their skills. Job descriptions summarise the job role, its purpose and responsibilities, and who an individual would report to. It should give a clear scope of what the role includes, any skills that an individual in that role would require and the overall purpose of the job role.

Person specification

As well as a description of the job role, an applicant also needs to be aware of the person specification and **entry requirements** attached to that role. Entry requirements are formal criteria needed for an applicant to be considered for an interview. Person specifications are descriptions of the traits essential and desirable for any potential candidate in that job role to possess. They generally include qualifications and skills that a candidate is required to (or should ideally have to) apply.

Skills required for a role could be attributes such as an understanding of the specialism involved, good verbal and written communication skills and the ability to work as part of a team. A person specification may also include the necessary experience (e.g. a minimum of two years in a certain position or working at a certain level) required by an individual applying for the job. Some healthcare jobs may require any individual who is successful in securing the job to have a clean, full driving licence, for example, hospital porters.

All person specifications within the healthcare science sector will involve an applicant requiring a sufficient Disclosure and Barring Service (DBS) check to ensure their suitability for the job. The required mandatory training and continuing professional development attached to a particular job role must also be made clear to an applicant when reading the specification, as they will then have a professional responsibility to uphold that.

It is essential that any applicant applying for a job role in the healthcare science sector studies the person specification attached to a job to ensure that the role is suitable for them and their skills and attributes.

> **Research**
>
> Research your own potential job role aspiration and summarise:
> - a description of the role, including a professional's main responsibilities in that role
> - entry requirements including essential qualifications and skills required
> - mandatory training required while in the job role.
>
> You may need to use the NHS website for guidance on this:
>
> www.healthcareers.nhs.uk/explore-roles/explore-roles

> **Case study**
>
> A job advert has been posted online for a healthcare science assistant. Look over the job description and person specification that follows in Figure 2.11, and then answer these questions.
> 1. What do you think the purpose of job descriptions and person specifications are for jobs within the healthcare science sector?
> 2. Do you feel they are important? If so, why?

A2.6 The range and diversity of job roles within the healthcare science sector

Healthcare science

Healthcare science assistant

Healthcare science assistants support a broad range of areas and departments in the sector from pathology to respiratory and even cardiology. The role of a healthcare science assistant is to support healthcare professionals by inputting and analysing data, disposing of hazardous waste, sterilising equipment and ensuring stocktakes are completed regularly. They are responsible for labelling, sorting and storing specimens in line with procedures and in accordance with health and safety requirements. They also support the team by helping with fluid and tissue sample analysis, and loading and operating machinery. More

A2: The healthcare science sector

> **Healthcare Science Assistant**
> **Job description**
>
> **Responsible to: the Manager**
> **Summary of the role**
>
> The Blood Sciences Department has a permanent, full-time vacancy for a Healthcare Science Support Worker (HSSW) Band 2. The role includes working as part of a team within the Blood Sciences specimen reception.
>
> **Main responsibilities**
>
> - Working in a fast-paced environment taking receipt of large volumes of laboratory specimens.
> - Carrying out clerical, administrative and technical duties.
> - Checking and examining electronic and paper requests and transfering requests on to the Laboratory Information System in preparation for sample analysis.
>
> **Person specification**
>
> | | Essential | Desirable |
> | --- | --- | --- |
> | Qualifications | 5 GCSEs or equivalent
IT literate with good keyboard skills | NVQ Level 2 or equivalent in a relevant subject
GCSE (or equivalent) at grade A–C in English, Mathematics and a Science subject |
> | Experience | Experience with laboratory equipment ranging from manual pipettes to automated analysers | Experience in a modern Blood Sciences Laboratory, gained in the last three years |
> | Knowledge | Understanding of health and safety, infection control and good laboratory practice | Laboratory information management system experience |
> | Skills/qualities | Good communication skills
Team player
Scientific or technical skills
Able to follow instructions
Flexible and adaptable
Careful and methodical | Clerical skills, such as cleaning, ordering stock, data processing |

▲ Figure 2.11 Advert for a healthcare science assistant

experienced healthcare science assistants will gain knowledge around putting together chemical solutions under supervision.

Healthcare science associate

Healthcare science associates work with a range of multidisciplinary teams within laboratories, hospitals, general practices and other settings in the healthcare science sector. Their role includes supporting practitioners in performing technical and scientific procedures, ensuring quality control in the technical processing of biological samples and diagnostic tests, performing routine investigations and communicating authorised results by telephone according to protocols. They are trained to be able to support practitioners with the assessment and safe diagnosis of disease and illness, support teams with the development of and adherence to standards and protocols, and perform routine investigations and record results. More experienced healthcare science associates will be responsible for supporting and training junior staff.

Clinical scientist

Clinical scientists are responsible for the research and development of techniques and equipment that will help to prevent, diagnose and treat illnesses. They use their medical expertise to support clinical staff with the interpretation of adult and paediatric biochemistry tests. As laboratory-based professionals, clinical scientists analyse physiological samples, collect data to help develop effective treatments, and research and investigate conditions including organ abnormalities, infertility, genetic disorders, **haematology** and the causes of illness or death. Areas of expertise for clinical scientists include **life sciences**, **clinical bioinformatics**, **physiological science**, and **physical science and bioengineering**. Clinical scientists also work directly with patients to help find ways of improving their health and wellbeing.

> **Key terms**
>
> **Haematology:** the analysis, diagnosis and monitoring of blood-based disorders.
>
> **Life sciences:** the study of living organisms, for example microbes, human beings and fungi.
>
> **Clinical bioinformatics:** the development of methods for acquiring, storing, organising and analysing biological data that affect patients' responses to drug treatments to aid in their prognosis.
>
> **Physiological science:** the use of advanced technologies to evaluate the functioning of different body systems and to diagnose abnormalities.
>
> **Physical science and bioengineering:** measuring what is happening in the body and devising advanced ways to diagnose and treat disease.

Healthcare science practitioner

A healthcare science practitioner's role is to analyse a broad range of diagnostic tests, use their expert knowledge to assess patients' samples, diagnose the presence of disease and identify appropriate treatment plans. They are vital in the monitoring of a patient's healthcare and in the correct choice of treatments, and in using their specialised knowledge to perform patient-sensitive, quality-assured investigations and tests. Healthcare science practitioners are also responsible for the research and development of more effective treatments that will improve the treatment of patients. They will be able to perform a range of complex clinical procedures, and record and interpret clinical data.

Biomedical scientist

Biomedical scientists are highly specialised in conducting a wide and complex range of scientific and medical tests to help healthcare science professionals with diagnosing and treating diseases. Their focus is on the disease process, and biomedical scientists are crucial in the early detection of medical conditions. They play a key part in the screening of diseases and monitoring the effectiveness of medications and treatments. Biomedical scientists are specialised in using a wide range of sophisticated equipment in laboratories to carry out their research into medical conditions such as cancer, meningitis, diabetes and blood disorders. They are generally specialised in areas such as blood, infection and cellular sciences.

Pharmacy services

Pharmacy services assistant

Pharmacy services assistants provide a variety of pharmacy and medicine services to patients under the supervision of a pharmacist or a pharmacist technician. Main duties include helping to supply, prepare and assemble medicines, issuing medicines to patients and assisting the pharmacy team with providing advice to patients regarding their health. Pharmacy services assistants are also responsible for ordering and receiving medicines, as well as their storage, disposal and return. They will be trained in working towards meeting pharmacy SOPs when carrying out routine operations within the organisation and must also be educated in the importance of health promotions and healthier lifestyle choices so they can advise patients effectively.

Pharmacy technician

Pharmacy technicians are under the supervision of a pharmacist and are responsible for ordering, preparing and supplying prescriptions for patients. The role includes ensuring prescriptions are accurate and that a patient's prescription is in line with the guidelines of the General Pharmaceutical Council on the basis of the patient's medical information. Once this has been done, pharmacy technicians will then supply completed prescriptions to patients. Pharmacy technicians check prescription prices to ensure consistency and accuracy, contribute to the daily running of the pharmacy and complete regular inventory stocking. An important aspect of the role is to communicate effectively with the rest of the team and with patients, ensuring they are able to help patients with any questions they might have and also instruct them in the correct way to take their medication. They also have to make sure that they are keeping the safety of the pharmacy team and patients at the forefront of the practice by maintaining health and safety consistently and adhering to policies and procedures, such as infection control protocols.

Pharmacist (dispensing and pharmaceutical industry)

Pharmacists' work in the dispensing and pharmaceutical industry can include conducting research and designing, producing and testing new pharmaceutical goods. They are also involved in the design of packaging, quality assurance and the marketing and sales of new medicines and treatments. The dispensing and pharmaceutical industry often has pharmacists working as representatives for the company to vouch for their medical products, including highlighting any health benefits for patients. These pharmacists often have access to the latest technologies and equipment.

Prescribing pharmacists

Pharmacists work in a range of different settings within communities and liaise with several different professions. A pharmacist's role is to offer expert advice to other healthcare professionals and to advise patients about their prescriptions and the use of medications. Their duties include using their expert knowledge of medicines to provide advice and give instructions on a range of medicines, including correct dosages and medical equipment, and overseeing and supervising the dispensing of prescriptions to patients to ensure that legislation is being adhered to safely. Pharmacists provide healthcare to patients by conducting health checks and completing medical reviews for patients' conditions. They offer screening programmes for patients with conditions such as diabetes and high blood pressure and deliver further healthcare within the community with services such as prescription collection and delivery. They provide information for managing long-term health conditions and potential side effects of medications, and clarify where medications are safe to take with others that a patient may already be taking. Stock ordering and the maintenance of accurate medication records are also regular responsibilities of this role. Pharmacists also recruit and train new staff members, as well as ensuring that they and staff members maintain a clean and safe work environment.

> ### Research
>
> Complete research on the General Pharmaceutical Council using the following link:
>
> **https://inspections.pharmacyregulation.org**
>
> ▶ Gather information on the five principles for the standards set by the General Pharmaceutical Council.
> ▶ Review an inspection report for a pharmacy in your local area.

Optical care services

Optical assistant

An optical assistant's main duty is to help the optometrist to provide vision care and treatment to patients. They are the first point of contact for a customer and their role includes clerical duties such as booking eye examinations and eye health screenings. They also assist customers by measuring eyewear frames, helping them to find the right frames and lenses for their eyewear, and answering any queries that customers might have. Many optical assistants work in private practices; however, some are based in a retail environment.

Ophthalmic nurse

An ophthalmic nurse provides care for patients who are suffering from eye conditions, injuries or infections, for example glaucoma. Ophthalmic nurses must have effective assessment skills to be able to assess patients in a thorough and timely manner. They are responsible for assessing a patient's condition, diagnosing and treating patients, and advising patients regarding their aftercare to avoid the need for further medical intervention. Because a large part of their role involves assessment and educating patients with information about their conditions, excellent communication skills are key. Ophthalmic nurses must be able to instruct patients on how to use their prescribed treatment, such as how frequently drops should be applied, and ensure these instructions are clear and understood.

Dispensing optician

A dispensing optician's role is to advise patients on the most suitable spectacles and/or contact lenses on the basis of their visual needs. Dispensing opticians must be registered with the General Optical Council to be able to practise in the UK, and their specialism enables them to advise patients on prescription sunglasses, UV protection and other requirements such as night-driving eyewear.

Optometrist

Optometrists are primary healthcare specialists trained in examining, diagnosing and treating defects in vision, injury, ocular diseases and abnormalities. They are also able to detect systemic diseases such as diabetes and hypertension. Optometrists also offer medical advice, assess patients' health and prescribe, fit and supply spectacles and contact lenses. They are qualified and trained to use a range of precision instruments and testing tools, and can make referrals to specialists and/or ophthalmologists (eye surgeons).

Dental services

Dental nurse

A dental nurse's role is to work closely with dentists to aid in the treatment of patients by responding efficiently to instructions, ensuring all materials and supplies are readily available before procedures, passing the necessary instruments to dentists and preparing materials needed for procedures such as fillings. They are responsible for the maintenance, decontamination and sterilising of dental equipment, ensuring that patients are comfortable, taking notes throughout procedures and ensuring that patients' information and services are recorded accurately and in concordance with data protection and confidentiality policies. A dental nurse is also responsible for the general upkeep of a surgery by ensuring continuous high standards of cleanliness and control of infection throughout.

Dental technician

Dental technicians are responsible for designing, constructing and repairing a variety of dental devices to help improve patients' teeth. They work from a dentist's prescription to make orthodontic devices such as braces, bridges and crowns. Dental technicians often specialise in areas such as orthodontics, and fixed, removeable or **maxillofacial prostheses**. Responsibilities of a dental technician include constructing models of a patient's mouth and teeth from images transferred over by a dentist, undertaking prosthetic procedures such as producing mouth guards and retainers, treating the loss of teeth by constructing dentures and fabricating veneers, crowns and bridges to restore patients' teeth. Dental technicians also work on the rehabilitation of patients who have suffered an injury, disease or abnormality by fabricating maxillofacial prostheses, as well as ensuring that all relevant records are kept up to date and in accordance with policies and procedures.

> **Key term**
>
> **Maxillofacial prostheses (singular: prosthesis):** products that will reconstruct and restore the function and improve the overall quality of a patient's oral health.

Dental laboratory assistant

Dental laboratory assistants support dental technicians in the manufacturing of dental devices in line with a patients' prescription. Their role is to work under the direct supervision of a dental technician and comply with General Dental Council guidelines. A dental laboratory assistant will contribute to the design and construction of simple dental devices such as mouth guards, gum shields and dental models. They will understand the use of basic materials and have good knowledge of oral anatomy. More experienced dental laboratory assistants may develop the knowledge and skills to aid in the manufacturing of more complex devices such as crowns, dentures and bridges.

Dentist

Dentists provide highly specialised dental care to the public either through the NHS or privately. Their role includes preventing, diagnosing and treating diseases, injuries and malformations. Dentists work as General Dental Practitioners (GDPs) and have excellent knowledge of the human anatomy and of the causes of and treatments for oral diseases. Their role includes assessing patients' oral health, diagnosing and treating oral problems and diseases, and performing general hygiene procedures such as cleaning; they also provide more complex care such as extractions and root canals, and carry out dental and surgical procedures. A huge part of a dentist's role is to communicate informatively and clearly with patients, providing them with expert advice and promoting good oral hygiene to improve their overall healthcare.

> **Research**
>
> All professionals working in dental services need to be practising in accordance with the General Dental Council's guidelines and standards.
>
> Review the standards set by the General Dental Council and complete a table of the nine principles.
>
> Extend your table by adding one standard that you feel is most relevant to your chosen career and why.
>
> www.gdc-uk.org/standards-guidance/standards-and-guidance/standards-for-the-dental-team

Prosthetic and orthotic services

Prosthetic and orthotic technician

Prosthetic and orthotic technicians are responsible for the manufacturing, maintenance and repair of prostheses or **orthoses** (splints). Prosthetics products include artificial limbs, whereas orthotic products include devices such as braces, splints and diabetic footwear, and are designed to replace, support or improve the functioning of a limb or spine. The technician's role is to design devices that aid the movement, reform and improvement of the functioning of a limb or the spine. Patients who require prosthetic and orthotic products are most probably in severe pain and discomfort, have issues with movement and sometimes suffer from medical conditions such as multiple sclerosis, diabetes, stroke or musculoskeletal injury.

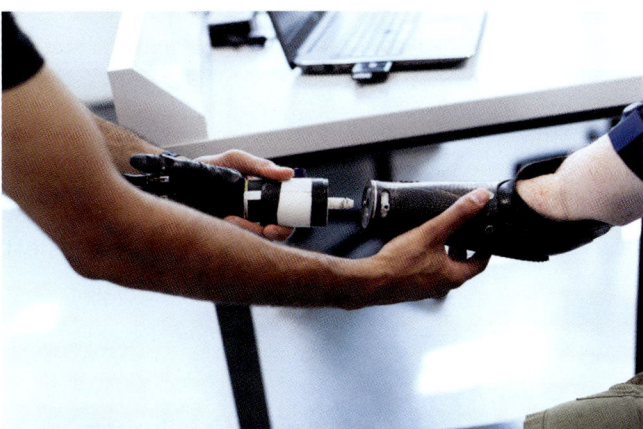

▲ Figure 2.12 Fitting a prosthetic arm

Prosthetists

Prosthetists work with a range of different patients to create and fit artificial replacements for individuals with missing limbs. They prescribe, design, manufacture, fit and modify prosthetics for patients, enabling them with their rehabilitation process. They will assess patients' conditions and create and design products to aid in their recovery. Prosthetists also liaise with other professionals such as surgeons to offer their expert advice. Prosthetists will often work with a diverse age range of patients including children who have been diagnosed with cerebral palsy or born with missing limbs, adults with conditions such as arthritis, individuals who have been involved in serious accidents and military veterans who have been injured in combat.

Orthotists

An orthotist's role is similar to a prosthetist's in the way in which they aid patients' rehabilitation and functioning; however, orthotists specialise in fixing problems or deformities in nerves, muscles and bones.

They make and fit braces and splints (orthoses) for patients who need extra support with movement and function. Orthotists work with patients who have a wide range of medical conditions, from musculoskeletal problems due to arthritis, diabetes or neuromuscular disorders, to spinal injuries caused by a traumatic accident. An orthotist's main purpose is to improve a patient's mobility and function, while relieving pain, correcting impairments and helping them adapt to the products designed for them. They also play an important role in preventing a patient needing serious surgical procedures such as amputation as they can design and fit splints and specialised footwear.

> **Test yourself**
>
> 1 Describe three aspects of a biomedical scientist's role.
> 2 What is the role of a pharmacy technician?
> 3 Identify what an optometrist specialises in.
> 4 Explain the responsibilities of a dental nurse.
> 5 Complete a comparison of a prosthetist's and orthotist's roles.

A2.7 The links between career pathways and progression routes within the healthcare science sector, as outlined by the IfATE occupational maps

As an individual seeking out a career within the healthcare science sector, it is important that you familiarise yourself with the Institute for Apprenticeships and Technical Education occupational maps. This way, you can have well-thought out career pathways and progression routes to aim for.

> **Reflect**
>
> Do you know what is required for your career aspiration and how to get there?

Institute for Apprenticeships and Technical Education (IfATE)

The Institute for Apprenticeships and Technical Education (IfATE) is responsible for technical qualifications, which is the main, classroom-based element of T Levels such as the one you are studying for. It oversees the development, approval and publication of apprenticeship standards as well as the **occupational maps** for T Levels and apprenticeships.

> **Key term**
>
> *Occupational maps:* a visual outline of the pathway an individual will study for technical, higher technical and professional occupations, which also shows potential progression routes.

Career pathways as per the occupational maps

The IfATE website shows where technical qualifications like this one and many other T Levels can lead on to.

www.instituteforapprenticeships.org/occupational-maps

Scroll down to 'Health and Science' and click on the job titles under the heading 'Healthcare Science Pathway' (see Figure 2.13).

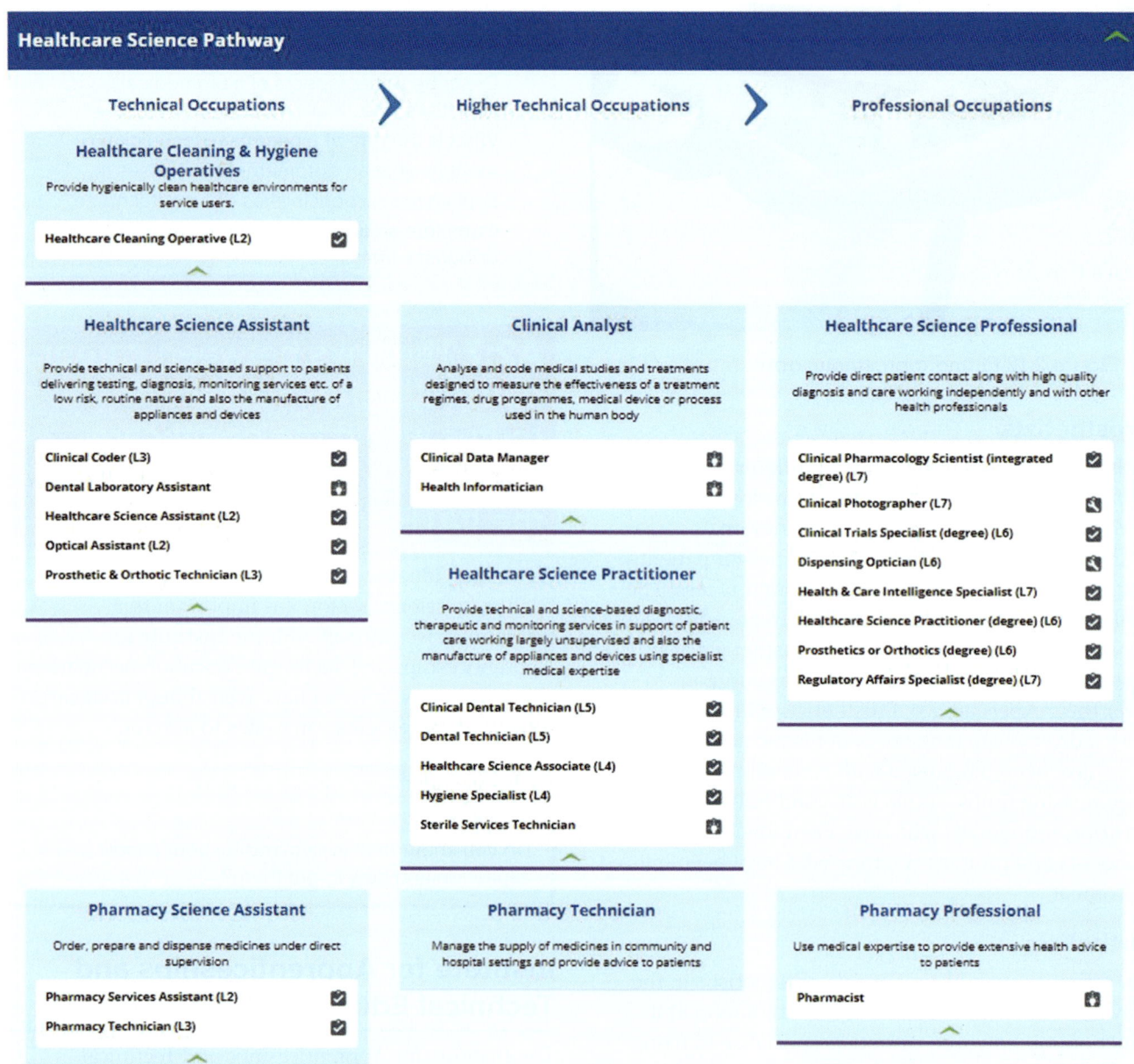

▲ Figure 2.13 Healthcare Science Pathway

A2: The healthcare science sector

> **Case study**
>
> Satvir is an 18-year-old student who achieved very good GCSE results including his L2 Maths, English and Science. However, after a few months studying his A levels, he decided that this route wasn't for him and has redirected himself to progress into the healthcare science sector. His overall aim is to become an Insight and Intelligence Manager and start a Health and Care Intelligence Specialist course.
>
> Using the link, research the following for Satvir's planned career pathway:
> - occupation summary
> - the entry requirements and qualifications
> - the occupation duties
> - knowledge, skills and behaviours of the role.
>
> www.instituteforapprenticeships.org/occupational-maps

> **Research**
>
> Use the link to find out the entry requirements and qualifications needed for one of the three following roles:
>
> **Healthcare Science Practitioner – Clinical Dental Technician (L5)**
>
> www.instituteforapprenticeships.org/apprenticeship-standards/clinical-dental-technician-integrated-v1-0
>
> **Healthcare Science Professional – Prosthetist or Orthotist (degree) (L6)**
>
> www.instituteforapprenticeships.org/apprenticeship-standards/prosthetist-and-orthotist-integrated-degree-v1-0
>
> **Pharmacy Science Assistant – Pharmacy Technician (L3)**
>
> www.instituteforapprenticeships.org/apprenticeship-standards/pharmacy-technician-integrated-v1-0

A2.8 The purpose of roles having a clear scope of practice

Scope of practice describes the minimum knowledge, skills and activities a professional is qualified and competent (and therefore permitted) to perform. Healthcare science practitioners must ensure they are working to a high standard within their scope of practice in order to be deemed professionally competent and to meet the terms of their professional licence. Scopes of practice are likely to change over time as professionals' roles develop and due to advances in the healthcare science sector, e.g. in terms of technology available, to accommodate the most current needs of society.

According to the HCPC, scope of practice refers to:

> 'the limit of your knowledge, skills and experience and is made up of the activities you carry out within your professional role'.
>
> Source: Health and Care Professions Council, www.hcpc-uk.org/standards/meeting-our-standards/scope-of-practice

> **Practice point**
>
> Refer to two different job roles in your placement. For each role, find out:
> - what their scope of practice includes
> - whether it has changed in the last decade and, if so, how
> - why is it important for professionals in those roles to keep up to date with their scope of practice.

A2.9 The links between registration and scope of practice in relation to activities which can only be undertaken by a registered healthcare professional

Dispensing optician

General Optical Council (GOC) registration

As stated previously, the GOC is the UK regulator for the optical professions. It protects patient safety by ensuring that optometrists or dispensing opticians have the competency and appropriate knowledge and skills needed to work in this role. It is illegal for dispensing opticians to practice if they are not registered by the GOC. Activities that registered dispensing opticians can undertake include:
- advising patients with different eye care needs on lenses, frames and spectacle repairs
- completing facial measurements for frames
- ordering a range of optical products, including lenses, from prescriptions and checking them on delivery

- checking that optical products meet the required standards
- supervising and training junior dispensing opticians to the required standards.

Pharmacist

General Pharmaceutical Council (GPhC) registration

In the UK, it is illegal for a pharmacist to refer to themselves as a pharmacist if they are not registered with the GPhC. Anyone who practices and uses the title of 'pharmacist' without registration can be prosecuted. Activities a registered pharmacist can legally undertake include:
- assessing and dispensing medications
- conducting health screenings
- supervising the ordering of medications
- educating patients on the safe intake of medications and side effects
- providing health and wellbeing advice to patients.

Dental technician

General Dental Council (GDC) registration

Dental professionals are regulated and registered to practice within the UK through the GDC. It is illegal for an individual to practice dentistry in the UK without being registered, which includes:
- working with other dental professionals for treatment planning
- following prescriptions to design, plan and make custom-made devices
- modifying devices to follow a prescription, e.g. dentures and crowns
- carrying out infection prevention and control procedures to meet legislations
- keeping up-to-date and accurate laboratory records.

Clinical scientist and biomedical scientist

HCPC registration

Clinical and biomedical scientists are required to be registered with the HCPC to practice professionally. Practice of such activities include:
- investigating and diagnosing illnesses and diseases
- conducting scientific research to improve human health
- carrying out analysis of specimen material
- performing diagnostic testing and developing new and existing treatments.

Prosthetic and orthotic technician

HCPC registration

Prosthetic and orthotic technicians must also be registered with the HCPC for which standards of proficiency are in place that must be met. Standards of proficiency include:
- practicing safely and effectively in line with their scope of practice
- practicing within the legal and ethical boundaries of prosthetic and orthotic practices
- maintaining fitness to practice
- being autonomous in their practice and exercising their own professional judgement
- being conscious regarding culture, equality and diversity in practice
- maintaining confidentiality
- communicating effectively
- working effectively with other professionals
- maintaining records accurately
- reviewing their own practice consistently
- assuring high quality in their practice
- keeping updated with the knowledge base of the prosthetic and orthotic professions
- improving their own practice by drawing on appropriate knowledge and skills
- maintaining a safe practice environment.

> **Reflect**
>
> Why are registrations and scope of practice important for occupations in healthcare science? What impact do they have on professionals and patients? Think about what could happen if they were not required.

A2.10 The difference between voluntary and statutory registration

Healthcare science professionals must be registered to undertake the activities required of their job role. Registration for healthcare professionals includes both voluntary and statutory registration.

A2: The healthcare science sector

Registration	Main points	Examples
Voluntary	• Not a legal requirement for healthcare professionals • Focuses more on professionals committing to their continuous professional development (CPD) • Promotes the highest fitness to practice • **Professional Standards Authority (PSA)** accreditation assists voluntary bodies, and the focus is on maintaining high standards throughout practice	The Society and College of Radiographers The Academy for Healthcare Science
Statutory	• A legal and mandatory requirement for professionals to practise specific activities in their job role • PSA applies the same high standards as voluntary registration, however, they are mandatory for statutory registrations • Provides protected title (for example, biomedical scientist)	Nursing and Midwifery Council (NMC) Health and Care Professions Council (HCPC) General Medical Council (GMC)

▲ Table 2.1 Voluntary and statutory registration

> **Key term**
>
> *Professional Standards Authority (PSA):* a body that sets and promotes standards of regulation for both voluntary and statutory registration for healthcare science professionals. The PSA ensure high standards are being practised to promote the health, safety and wellbeing of the public.

> **Research**
>
> Research one statutory and one voluntary registration within your placement. Summarise both of the registrations you have researched. What actions do the registrations require staff to practice in their job role?

A2.11 The role of accreditation and certification in healthcare science sector jobs

Accreditation is the formal recognition of healthcare science professionals' competencies and their ability to perform activities. This means validating a professional's competency, i.e. ensuring that they have the skills and knowledge to perform adequately in their job role. Professionals are validated on their professional competency once they have been evaluated on their performance of their skills and continue to demonstrate them in their job role. It is effectively the acknowledgement of a professional's status or level of achievement in their role.

Certification is the assurance that a professional has been assessed on these competencies.

Accreditation and certification link to a professional's CPD requirements within their role and the quality expected of their practice. They help to maintain compliance by standardising practice and equality within organisations, increasing the extent to which healthcare professionals are using evidence-based practice. Another advantage is that they also define and outline ethical conduct that employees are required to follow when performing their duties. For example, a healthcare science professional must demonstrate autonomy, beneficence, justice and nonmaleficence in their everyday job roles to protect their patients' wellbeing, so these are assessed as part of the accreditation and certification processes.

National School of Healthcare Science

The NSHCS is part of Health Education England and is responsible nationally for the overseeing of education programmes for all healthcare scientists working in the NHS and for the accreditation process against the standards set by the Academy for Healthcare Science. The Academy for Healthcare Science is responsible for approving education providers within the healthcare science sector and quality assuring the accreditation process undertaken by the NSHCS.

The Academy for Healthcare Science works alongside professional bodies that provide accreditation and certifications to ensure that they are of a good enough standard to deliver and provide accreditations and certificates. They also oversee the registration of healthcare science professionals, for example, the PSA, to ensure the implementation of high standards, education and training, and the safety and wellbeing of patients.

> **Research**
>
> Healthcare science practitioners are accredited by the PSA. Research the answers to these questions:
> ▶ What does the PSA do?
> ▶ Who does it oversee?
> ▶ What is their accredited register programme?

A2.12 The purpose of appraisals and performance reviews within the healthcare science sector

Within the healthcare science sector, professionals regularly participate in appraisals and performance reviews with their line managers, including a review of their performance year on year, to monitor progress, development and contribution to their workplace.

The purpose of a professional's performance review is to reflect on their performance and competency skills needed for their job role over the last 12 months. It is important that performance reviews and appraisals are completed annually so that development can be reviewed, and any areas of underperformance can be identified so that the necessary support can be put in place. Once development and underperformance has been reviewed, professionals can be set individual targets, which should be SMART (specific, measurable, attainable, relevant, time-bound) goals.

An individual's SMART goals should not only be personal to their professional development but also contribute towards the organisation's **key performance indicators (KPIs)** to ensure the organisation is meeting its strategic targets. SMART targets set in appraisals and performance reviews should always identify and facilitate not only their own personal and professional development but also aid progression within that organisation. They should also cover salary and grade reviews, which decide whether employees meet the required criteria for a pay rise, for example if an employee has met the mandatory training requirements to continue their professional development expected of them annually.

> **Reflect**
>
> What is the impact of appraisals and performance reviews on healthcare science professionals?
>
> Why are they important in the healthcare science sector?

A2.13 The impact of external factors on activities of healthcare science sector organisations

As seen with the COVID-19 pandemic, there are several unexpected external factors that can easily and suddenly overwhelm the services of the healthcare science sector in their attempts to provide care for a surge of patients.

External factors

Epidemics and pandemics

Pandemics are the worldwide spread of an infectious disease. Pandemics have profound implications for the population and for healthcare science organisations, facilities and supplies, as well as long-term financial implications. Pandemic examples include the 1918–20 influenza pandemic (Spanish flu) and, more recently, the coronavirus pandemic that began in 2019. **Epidemics**, however – such as the 2014–16 Ebola virus epidemic in West Africa and the 2015–16 Zika virus epidemic in Brazil – are large outbreaks of an infectious disease in one community or region. Epidemics also have a huge impact on healthcare science services and put a sudden strain on a community's access to its services due to a surge in patient care.

Extreme weather

Exceptionally cold or hot weather, or intense storms and intense precipitation (i.e. rain or snow) that causes flooding, are classed as extreme weather. Exceptionally hot weather can have adverse impacts on the functionality of hospitals and other healthcare science organisations, for example with the storage of medicines within acceptable temperature ranges, as well as causing an increase in GP activity with patients, particularly elderly people, needing treatment for cardiovascular diseases that can be intensified in extreme heat. With extreme cold weather, there is an increased risk of hypothermia for patients. Depending on an area's flood risk zone, an area's health facilities and ambulance services could be interrupted causing a lack of access to healthcare for patients. Intense storms could cause power lines to become disrupted, meaning potential disruption to vital equipment and patient care. Evacuations may also not be possible, causing fatalities if patients' conditions worsen. The Australian and Californian bush fires of 2020 are both examples of the devastation and disruption that can be caused to patients and the healthcare science sector.

Infrastructure

The infrastructure of the healthcare science sectors describes the basic systems vital for an organisation to function effectively, such as transportation, buildings and power systems. Any significant damage to infrastructure could affect patient care, causing evacuations to be necessary if certain care is not available. Patients may have to be transferred to another facility, which could cause limitations in the services and treatments accessible and the patients' conditions to deteriorate.

Geographical events

Geographical events may involve fire and floods, resulting in rescue and evacuations of families from their homes and an increase in patient admissions. Fire and floods can affect the accessibility of care services available, causing a huge strain on the services that are functioning. The impact of climate change on the healthcare science sector is becoming more apparent, for example more deaths and illnesses from extreme weather, which can disrupt food systems, cause **vector-borne diseases** and reduce access to health and social care services.

> **Key term**
>
> **Vector-borne diseases:** infections that are transmitted by an infectious agent, e.g. mosquitoes, blackflies and ticks.

> **Research**
>
> Use the link to read the WHO article on climate change and health. Create a presentation on how climate change is affecting health, breaking it down into the short-, medium- and long-term effects. Focus on a particular aspect of climate change, for example storms and flooding, or heatwaves. When you have finished, share with your classmates and tutor for feedback.
>
> www.who.int/news-room/fact-sheets/detail/climate-change-and-health

Impact on activities of healthcare science sector organisations

External factors such as those mentioned previously can have a significant impact on the provision of services in the healthcare science sector.

Impacts of external factors include:

▶ **Service overload**
Any external factor causing a patient surge and a sudden overload of services needed will stretch facilities beyond their means, resulting in an overwhelming attempt to meet these needs and provide the necessary care needed.

▶ **Re-prioritisation of services**
An external factor can have a serious impact on the hierarchy of services that are deemed a priority to the public, meaning other healthcare science services are not prioritised in terms of staffing and supplies. For example, a WHO survey estimated that a reduction in essential maternal and child health interventions could have caused more than one million additional child mortality rates in 2020.
SOURCE: https://www.sciencedirect.com/science/article/pii/S2214109X20302291

▶ **Insufficient staff resources**
Resources and staffing will be stretched due to the surge in patients or through staff illnesses, potentially causing further barriers to the services available for patients if contingencies are not in place to deal with such factors.

▶ **Inaccessible services/supplies**
Services may become unavailable due to the demands of dealing with an external factor. For example, the major disruption to cancer services and decrease in patient referrals or screening for cancer during the Covid-19 pandemic. Supplies such as necessary PPE are at risk of becoming inaccessible due to the surge in demand for them, causing a further health risk to patients and staff. This can have a direct impact on the supply chain for organisations due to the cost of supplies increasing due to supply and demand. If supplies are in short supply, and the demand for them is already high during an external factor, then the delivery capacity of supplies becomes unmanageable, causing further impact on supplies.

▶ **Damage to facilities**
External factors such as floods and fires could cause considerable damage to a building's facilities such as access to clean water and electricity, which is detrimental for the use of services and equipment, and also damage to communications such as telephone lines and internet. This then causes significant impact on the services and treatments accessible and the ability to provide them.

▶ **Additional resource requirements** (equipment, materials, staffing)
Additional staffing may be required to cope with the threat of an external factor due to the surge in patients. Additional materials and equipment

would also be needed due to an increase in patients, or potential damage to materials and equipment. Measures would have to be implemented to ensure these additional necessities are available.

▶ **Contingency plan implementation requirements** (disaster recovery plan, and changes to service delivery arrangements impacting turnaround time and patient services)

Any external factor requires an urgent response and recovery plan to ensure high quality necessary care continues to be offered. Without appropriate emergency planning, the impact could be catastrophic. It is imperative therefore that healthcare science organisations have a suitable **Disaster Recovery Plan** in place and that changes to services are managed effectively so as not to impact on the quality and timings of patients' care being generated.

> **Key term**
>
> *Disaster recovery plan:* a plan created by an organisation that documents detailed instructions for how to respond and recover effectively to an unexpected event.

A disaster recovery plan for a hospital may cover:

▶ **Communications**
How will the hospital be notified of an external disaster and how will this be communicated throughout the hospital? Consider how this might be done if the usual infrastructure is damaged, e.g. if electricity is down.

▶ **Resources and equipment**
Extra supplies should be kept in case of emergency, so that essential activities can continue and patients can be protected.

▶ **Safety and security**
The police may become involved in the event of a disaster, so internal security measures need to be maintained to ensure, for instance, that people entering and leaving the hospital can still be controlled.

▶ **Staff responsibilities**
All staff in the hospital must have received training so that they know what to do in a disaster situation, who will be in charge (chain of command) and any other relevant preparation to keep the system functioning.

▶ **Utilities**
In the event of a disaster, water, fuel and electricity supplies may be disrupted. How will the hospital ensure there is enough oxygen, and that generators will kick in to maintain essential systems?

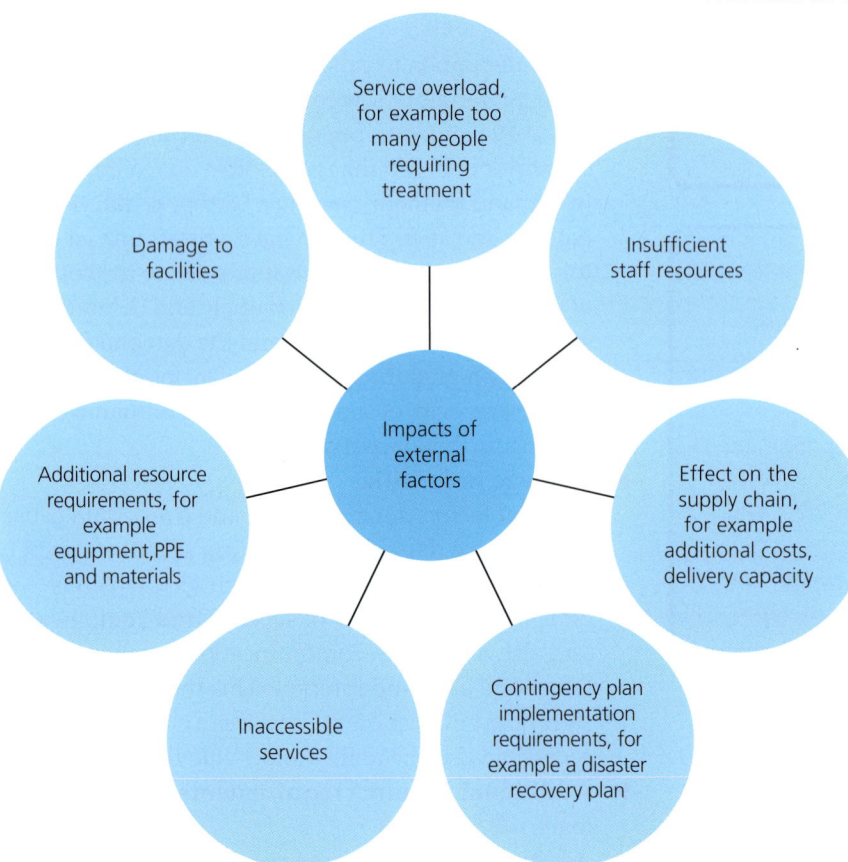

▲ Figure 2.14 Impacts of external factors on healthcare science services

Testing and evaluation of the disaster plan

The hospital should test its disaster plan regularly and note areas for improvement:
- Was it possible to communicate within the hospital and throughout the community effectively?
- Were there enough essential resources and supplies?
- Was it possible to provide for the safety of the patients and staff?
- Were staff aware of their responsibilities during an external disaster situation?
- Was the hospital able to maintain proper patient care throughout?

Test yourself

1. Identify three external factors that can potentially impact on the activities of the healthcare science sector.
2. Describe two examples of the long-term impact of the coronavirus pandemic on the NHS that have already become evident.
3. What is the purpose of a disaster recovery plan?
4. Give three examples of what a disaster recovery plan should cover.

A2.14 The benefits of new technology/automation/artificial intelligence within the healthcare science sector

The digital era of healthcare science is advancing rapidly every year worldwide. The advances in digital technologies benefit the sector and enable healthcare science professionals to offer resiliency, efficiency and better care insights for patients and more complex health issues.

Key terms

Automation: a range of technologies that conduct healthcare services for patients with minimal human intervention.

Artificial intelligence: the simulation of human intelligence in machines. These machines are programmed to think like humans, e.g. learning and problem solving.

New technologies/ automation/artificial intelligence	Definition	The benefits for the healthcare science sector
Personal mobile technology (constant and personal monitoring)	The tracking of an individual's health via a smartphone to enable the consistent monitoring of a person's health and wellbeing	• Improves the diagnostic process due to a more accessible data collection process • Real-time health monitoring in terms of extracting health information, e.g. heart rate, blood pressure
Point of care testing (POCT) diagnostic equipment	Point of care testing (POCT) diagnostic testing is performed with or by the patient for an immediate diagnosis, e.g. pregnancy tests	• Improves the diagnostic process by giving the patient the results immediately • Reduced manual inputs due to automated testing
Digital consultation	A medical consultation between the patient and a medical professional that enables remote communication for monitoring, diagnosing and treating patients	• Improves the diagnostic process by enhancing the care and support for patients, improving both access and sustainability • Remote access so greater access to more services
Computer-aided design (CAD)	CAD is the use of computers to create, modify, or optimise a design. A CAD model can be used before a surgery to accurately model the patient's features	• Increased efficiency of design • Increased precision, e.g. with the use of 3D scans and 3D prints of moulds instead of plaster casts • Reduced manual inputs as designs can be replicated and modified quickly • Increased collaboration opportunities (for example, remote collaboration)

New technologies/ automation/artificial intelligence	Definition	The benefits for the healthcare science sector
Computer-aided manufacturing (CAM)	CAM is the manufacturing of products using computer and robot digital technology	- Increased efficiency of manufacturing, making it easier for manufacturing to be completed on time - Reduced manual inputs and increased repeatability and modification manufacturing times - Increased outputs (for example, units per hour)
Electronic health records	A patient's health information in digital format, e.g. medications, diagnoses	- Makes for a more timely and efficient process - Increased sharing capacity (for example, records shared between different trusts to improve communication)
Miniature scanning equipment	Imaging techniques and sensing technologies that enable the use of portable medical equipment	- Allows individuals to have access to more services - Individuals have the autonomy to track their own health
Automated dispensing cabinet	A computerised medicine cabinet that allows medications to be stored and dispensed near the point of care	- Increased efficiency - Allows for automated stock checking - Reduced manual inputs
Online clinics	A virtual meeting between patients and healthcare professionals	- Providing remote care
Personal health apps	Online programs that enable individuals to collect, manage and monitor their own health information	- Promotes health to individuals - Individuals have the autonomy to track their own health
Augmented reality applications	Digital applications that combine visual and audio content into patients' real-life environments, e.g. Google Glass for new breastfeeding mothers	- Increased usability (for example, choosing spectacles using a photo and changing spectacle frames on screen instead of physically trying them on)
Imaging in healthcare science (MRI, CT scans, X-rays and retinal imaging)	Medical images that allow for healthcare science professionals to have a visual of different parts of the body for diagnostics and treatment	- Using scans of microscopic slides for pathology consultations, which provide a clearer and more accurate diagnosis

Research

Use the links below to access articles on **automation** and **artificial intelligence** in healthcare science. Complete a summary of how this new technology could benefit the sector.

www.automationanywhere.com/company/blog/rpa-thought-leadership/how-automation-impacts-healthcare-and-life-sciences

https://healthcareweekly.com/artificial-intelligence-in-healthcare

www.nuffieldtrust.org.uk/research/the-impact-of-covid-19-on-the-use-of-digital-technology-in-the-nhs

A2: The healthcare science sector

Project practice

From among the staff at your placement and the different healthcare science professionals you work with closely, arrange an interview with a member of staff and compose a list of questions.

Your interview questions should cover the following:
- Ask the member of staff for information regarding their job role and the services they offer.
- There should be some encouragement in your questions for the staff member to discuss their work environment and to establish what is going particularly well in their role.
- Any relevant registrations and discussion around the activities they are qualified to undertake under their registration.
- You could also include questions regarding the use of new technologies/specialised equipment in their job role and how these new technologies/specialised equipment affect their ability to do their role effectively.

Write up your findings to complete a detailed summary of their job role.

Write a critical evaluation of your work.

Assessment practice

1. Describe (a) three similarities and (b) three differences between public, private and charitable healthcare organisations.
2. Explain what is meant by statutory registration. Give at least two relevant examples.
3. Copy and complete the table to give a definition for each of the following types of care and one example for each.

Type of care	Definition	Examples
Primary		
Secondary		
Tertiary		

4. Discuss the role of the Professional Standards Authority in accreditation in the healthcare science sector.
5. List three benefits of job descriptions and person specifications within the healthcare science sector.
6. Explain the role of a clinical scientist, including the link between a clinical scientist's registration and scope of practice.
7. Discuss the benefits of occupational maps for individuals wanting a career in the healthcare science sector. Your answer should demonstrate:
   - reasoned judgements
   - a conclusion about the benefits of occupational maps for individuals.
8. Explain the importance of appraisals and performance reviews for healthcare science professionals.
9. Explain the importance of a disaster recovery plan. Your answer should demonstrate:
   - judgement on the effect on services without such plan
   - a reasoned conclusion.
10. Identify how artificial intelligence is used in a medical setting.

A3: Health, safety and environmental regulations in the health and science sector

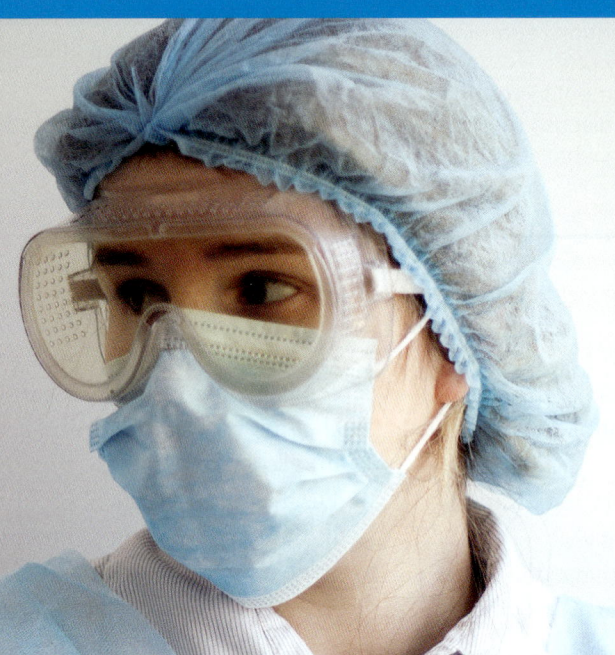

Introduction

When you work in the health and science sector you should feel safe. Your employer must make sure that you have a safe working environment and are not exposed to any unnecessary risks – we say that they owe you a **duty of care**. However, it is also the duty of every employee to play their part. You will need to be aware of the legislation and regulations that help to keep you and your colleagues safe, and to understand your rights, duties and responsibilities.

Laboratory and industrial processes can cause harm to the wider public and to the environment. So, you also need to be aware of your responsibility to help in eliminating (as far as possible) such harm.

This chapter covers the relevant legislation and regulations while Chapter A4 will cover how these are applied in the workplace.

Learning outcomes

The core knowledge outcomes that you must understand and learn:

A3.1 the purpose of legislation and regulations in the health and science sector

A3.2 how to assess and minimise potential hazards and risks, including specific levels of risk, by using the Health and Safety Executive's 5 Steps to Risk Assessment

A3.3 how health and safety at work is promoted

A3.4 how to deal with situations that can occur in a health or science environment that could cause harm to self or others (for example, spillage of hazardous material).

A3: Health, safety and environmental regulations in the health and science sector

A3.1 The purpose of legislation and regulations in the health and science sector

Health and Safety at Work etc. Act 1974

The Health and Safety at Work etc. Act 1974 (sometimes referred to as HSWA 1974 or HASAWA) sets out the duties of employers and employees to ensure the health of anyone at work or who may be affected by work activities. Under HSWA 1974, the employer must ensure, as far as is reasonably possible, the health, safety and welfare of all employees while they are at work.

The employer's specific duties include the following:
- providing and maintaining **plant** and systems of work that are safe and without risks to health
- arrangements for ensuring safety and absence of risks to health in the use, handling, storage and transport of articles and substances
- giving the information, instruction, training and supervision necessary to ensure the health and safety at work of employees
- maintaining any place of work in a condition that is safe and without risks to health
- providing and maintaining all means of entry and exit (i.e. doorways, corridors, walkways, etc.) that are safe and without such risks
- providing and maintaining a working environment for employees that is safe, without risks to health, and adequate as regards facilities and arrangements for their welfare at work.

The legislation recognises that it is impossible to avoid all risk and so all of the above duties are to be carried out 'so far as is reasonably practicable'.

> **Key term**
>
> **Plant:** any equipment used in the workplace, e.g. laboratory equipment.

Health and safety is not the sole responsibility of the employer. Employees must play their part. HSWA 1974 states that it is the duty of every employee:
- to take reasonable care for the health and safety of themselves and of others who may be affected by what they do, or don't do, at work
- to co-operate with the employer to enable the employer to perform their duty under the legislation.

> **Reflect**
>
> HSWA 1974 means that employees have a duty to themselves and to their co-workers. You should not do anything that could cause harm. But not doing something you should have done can also affect health and safety in the workplace. The act says that employees must co-operate with the employer in ensuring safe working practices are carried out. Think about how health and safety in the workplace is a partnership between the employer and the employee – how can you play your part in how you work? Is there anything that you are doing that you should not be doing? Is there anything that you are not doing that you should be doing?

HSWA 1974 is an enabling act – that means that the government can introduce regulations at any time to modify the act or to establish up-to-date standards. Many regulations have been introduced under HSWA 1974. The ones that are most relevant to work within the health and science sectors are covered in the following sections.

> **Research**
>
> The Health and Safety Executive (HSE) is responsible for enforcement of HSWA 1974 and associated regulations. It has a website that is an excellent source of information about all matters related to health and safety in the workplace: www.hse.gov.uk
>
> The COVID-19 pandemic meant there was an increase in the number of people working alone (**lone working**). This includes people working from home as well as those more likely to be alone in the workplace because of COVID-safe practices. Find out what the HSE recommends that lone workers should do to protect their health and safety.

Management of Health and Safety at Work Regulations 1999

These regulations aim to reduce the number and severity of accidents in the workplace, through assessing and managing risks. They make good health and safety management a legal requirement for, and impose duties on, both the employer and the employee. The main duty of the employer is to assess risks to health and safety in the workplace as they affect both employees and any others present (e.g. members of the public, visitors, etc.). The employer must then ensure effective planning, organisation, control, monitoring and review of measures taken to prevent or protect against risk. The employer must also appoint one or more 'competent persons' to assist in carrying out these legal responsibilities – this could be the employer themselves or employees appointed to the role.

The duties of employees under the regulations are to use machinery, equipment, dangerous substances, transport equipment and safety devices in accordance with their training and instructions. Also, employees have a duty to inform their employer and other employees of any dangers or shortcomings in the arrangements.

> **Practice point**
>
> As we have seen, there is a legal requirement for employers to manage health and safety through assessment and management of risk. Good employers will always take this responsibility seriously. However, there will always be some employers who do not do this. When you apply for a job, it is worth considering a prospective employer's approach to health and safety in the workplace.
>
> Similarly, it is your responsibility to abide by the letter and the spirit of these regulations – for both your own health and safety and that of your colleagues. Be prepared to demonstrate to an employer that you understand these responsibilities and can be trusted to follow the regulations.

Control of Substances Hazardous to Health (COSHH) Regulations 1994 and subsequent amendments 2002

COSHH is designed to protect people against risks to health arising from work-related exposure to hazardous substances. It requires assessment and control of risks before any work takes place.

Anyone in charge of, or working in, a laboratory should be familiar with COSHH and actively involved in implementing it. The steps involved are shown in the table.

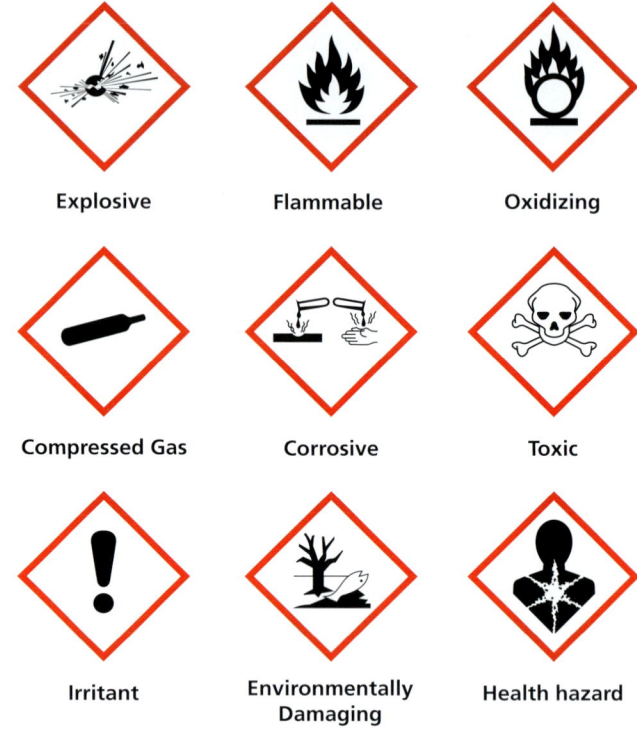

▲ Figure 3.1 The GHS hazard pictograms

Carry out an assessment of the tasks in the laboratory:
• Record the scope of assessment (who the tasks are carried out by, what is being assessed, when the tasks are carried out).
• List significant laboratory tasks.
• List substances involved.

Assess the factors that decide the appropriate control approach:
• What are the hazard categories associated with each task?
• What degree of exposure is likely? (This depends on the quantity handled as well as the nature of the substance.)

Determine the control approach:
• None: open bench working (i.e. not in a fume cupboard or other containment) with general ventilation.
• Intermediate: fume cupboard or other exhaust ventilation.
• High: glove box or similar containment.
• Special: purpose-designed facility.
• Use of personal protective equipment (PPE) for eyes and skin where there is a risk from skin contact or for inhalational protection.

Implement and review:
- Assess other tasks and related risks.
- Planning (how it will be implemented and resources needed).
- Consider safety and environmental risks.
- Consider other aspects of COSHH – monitoring, health surveillance and training.
- Use and maintenance of control measures (including regular checks and reporting defects).
- Set up proper record-keeping and review procedures.

Research

The Royal Society of Chemistry website has a great deal of information about COSHH in chemical laboratories, although this is applicable to many types of workplace in the health and science sectors. Visit www.rsc.org and search for 'COSHH in laboratories'.

Personal Protective Equipment (Enforcement) Regulations (1992; updated 2018)

Managing and reducing risk is always the priority. If a factory roof leaks, it is better to repair it than to issue every member of staff with their own umbrella. Use of PPE should be considered only after everything else has been done to reduce risk. However, in most workplaces in the health and science sectors, some level of PPE will always be necessary. These regulations define employers' responsibilities to provide appropriate PPE to reduce harm to employees, visitors and clients. This can include providing safety helmets, masks, goggles and gloves.

Health and safety

PPE is not always convenient or comfortable. Healthcare staff have spoken about the discomfort of wearing full PPE throughout shifts lasting eight hours or longer during the COVID-19 pandemic. That is one reason why all other steps to remove or reduce risk should be taken before considering the use of PPE. However, the pandemic also illustrated the importance of appropriate PPE when faced with an invisible and potentially life-threatening risk.

Reporting of Injuries, Diseases and Dangerous Occurrences Regulations 2013 (RIDDOR)

The purpose of RIDDOR is to define employers' duties to report serious workplace accidents, occupational diseases and specified dangerous occurrences ('near misses').

RIDDOR puts duties on employers, the self-employed and people in control of work premises (the **Responsible Person**) to report certain serious workplace **accidents**, occupational diseases and specified dangerous occurrences as well as **reportable injuries**.

Reportable accidents are those that result in death, major injury, or being absent from work or unable to do normal work for more than seven days. Accidents that result in absence from work for more than three days but less than seven days must be recorded but do not need to be reported unless they are reportable injuries.

RIDDOR requires employers and self-employed workers to report cases of occupational cancer and any disease or acute illness caused by **work-related** exposure to a biological agent (e.g. bacteria, viruses or toxins). This may take place because of identifiable events or unidentified events.

Key terms

The following terms have a specific meaning in terms of RIDDOR:

Accident: a separate, identifiable, unintended incident, which causes physical injury. This specifically includes acts of violence to people at work.

Reportable injuries: the following injuries are reportable under RIDDOR when they result from a work-related accident:
- the death of any person
- specified injuries to workers (see the HSE website for more information)
- injuries to workers which result in them being unable to work for more than seven days
- injuries to non-workers which result in them being taken directly to hospital for treatment, or specified injuries to non-workers which occur on the premises.

Work-related: an accident in the workplace does not always mean that the accident is work-related – the work activity itself must contribute to the accident. An accident is 'work-related' if any of the following played a significant role: the way the work was carried out; any machinery, plant, substances or equipment used for the work; the condition of the site or premises where the accident happened.

Case study

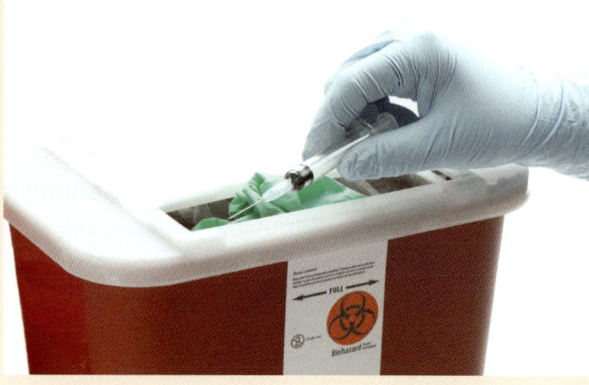

▲ Figure 3.2 Safe disposal of contaminated syringe needles, 'sharps'

Samah made a list of identifiable events in her workplace, including accidental breakage of a laboratory flask, accidental injury with a contaminated syringe needle (Figure 3.2) or an animal bite. She found it harder to think of unidentified events.
▶ Samah read that an unidentified event could be when a worker is exposed to legionella bacteria while conducting routine maintenance on a hot water service system. What other unidentified events could be present in your workplace?
▶ Do you think laboratory workers are more likely to be exposed to identifiable or unidentified events?

Environmental Protection Act (EPA) 1990

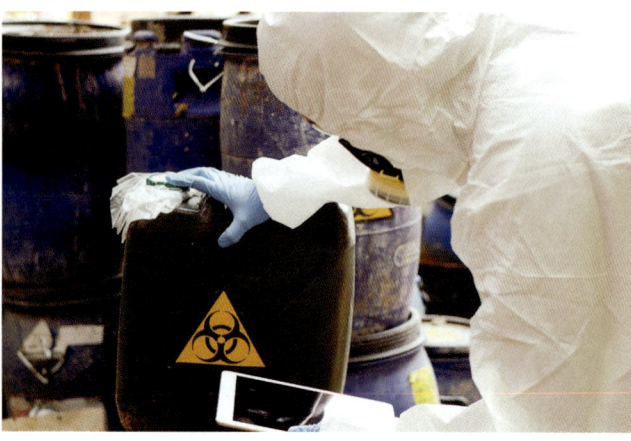

▲ Figure 3.3 Hazardous waste can be harmful to the environment

The EPA aims to improve control of pollution to the air, water and land by regulating the management of waste and the control of emissions.
▶ The EPA enables the Secretary of State to make any process or substance subject to strict controls and to set limits on its emissions into the environment. Carrying out such processes requires approval and there are criminal sanctions against offenders.
▶ The EPA also covers regulation and licensing of the disposal of controlled waste – this has a very broad meaning and includes any household, industrial or commercial waste.
▶ The way in which the EPA is enforced is quite complex. The Environment Agency (EA) or, in Scotland, the Scottish Environment Protection Agency (SEPA), together with local authorities, are responsible for control of processes specified by the EPA.
▶ Local authorities are responsible for the collection of some controlled waste, such as household waste.
▶ Local authorities also regulate and license the disposal of controlled waste from industrial or commercial premises such as shops, offices, laboratories, hospitals, GP surgeries, care homes, etc.

Thus, the EPA 1990 applies equally to the contents of your wheelie bin and to waste or emissions in the workplace.

Other legislation

The table lists some of the other legislation relevant to the health and science sectors and explains the relevance of each.

Special Waste Regulations 1996
Measures relating to: • the regulation and control of the transit, import and export of waste (including recyclable materials) • the prevention, reduction and elimination of pollution caused by waste • the requirement for assessing the impact on the environment of projects likely to have significant effects on the environment.
Hazardous Waste Regulations 2005
Controls the storage, transport and disposal of hazardous waste to ensure it is appropriately managed and any risks are minimised.
Waste Electrical and Electronic Equipment Regulations (WEEE) 2012/19/EU
Aims to reduce the amount of electronic and electrical equipment incinerated or sent to landfill sites. Places onus on all businesses to correctly store and transport electrical waste.

A3: Health, safety and environmental regulations in the health and science sector

Regulatory Reform (Fire Safety) Order (RRO) 2005

Aims to reduce death, damage and injury caused by fire, by placing legal responsibilities on employers to carry out a fire risk assessment. Because of this, all organisations are required to have procedures for evacuation in the event of a fire.

Manual Handling Operations Regulations 1992 (as amended)

Requires employers to assess and minimise the risk to health of employees involved in the manual handling, moving and positioning of an object, person or animal. It also covers workplace ergonomics, i.e. ensuring furniture is suitable and adaptable to different body sizes and types.

Health and Safety (Display Screen Equipment) Regulations 1992

Defines employers' responsibilities in carrying out risk assessments of workstations used by employees, including the use of display screen equipment, to minimise identified risks, such as:
- tiredness caused by poorly designed or adjusted workstations
- repetitive strain injury (RSI) and carpal tunnel syndrome
- eye strain leading to headaches, fatigue and sore eyes.

Test yourself

1. Which act (rather than regulations) listed above controls the disposal of waste in the workplace?
2. Name two sets of regulations that cover accidents in the workplace.
3. Name three sets of regulations that cover hazardous substances.
4. How does RIDDOR define a work-related accident?
5. What is a reportable injury under RIDDOR?
6. Who is responsible for safety in the workplace – the employer or the employee?

A3.2 How to assess and minimise potential hazards and risks

Minimising risk is extremely important in reducing harm in the workplace. Before we can minimise risk, we must first identify the risks. This is generally done by carrying out a risk assessment.

Risk assessment is a part of the risk management process and involves identifying a **hazard** and then deciding on the likelihood of exposure to that hazard (the **risk**). You need to decide:
- how likely a hazard is to actually cause harm
- the severity of that harm – just how serious the consequences could be.

This means that if a highly dangerous substance (i.e. the hazard) is contained so effectively that there is almost no possibility of coming into contact with it, the risk will be low. However, the probability of exposure to a less hazardous substance might be much higher and could pose a greater risk.

The Health and Safety Executive's 5 Steps to Risk Assessment are outlined in the following sections.

Key terms

Hazard: something that has the potential to cause harm.

Risk: how likely a hazard is to cause that harm.

Step 1: Identifying the hazards

Look around your workplace and think about what hazards there are. It is easy to overlook some hazards when you work in a place every day, so it is useful to follow some guidelines:
- Check manufacturers' instructions, particularly data sheets for chemicals and equipment.
- Look at accident or sickness records to see what has caused issues before.
- Think about non-routine activities such as changes in procedures or maintenance and cleaning, for example, when equipment is taken out of service.
- Consider long-term hazards to health, such as high levels of noise or exposure to harmful substances.

Step 2: Deciding who might be harmed and how

Once you have identified the hazards, you can then think about how employees (and others, such as visitors and contractors) might be harmed. That means you identify groups of people that might be at risk, including those with particular requirements (e.g. new employees, young workers, people with disabilities, visitors or temporary workers).

Step 3: Evaluating the risks and deciding on precautions

Risk is a part of our everyday lives and it is impossible to eliminate all risks. What you must do is identify the main risks and what action you need to take to manage those risks. An employer must do everything reasonable to protect people from harm. This means there is a balance between the level of risk and the measures needed to control the real risk.

You need to ask:
- Can the hazard be eliminated?
- If not, what can be done to control the risks so that they are unlikely to cause harm?

Once you have evaluated the risks, you can consider some suitable precautions:
- Try a safer way of doing things.
- Restrict access to the hazards.
- Organise the work so that it reduces exposure to the hazard.
- Finally, once all other precautions have been taken, use PPE.

It is important that all employees are involved in this stage, to make sure that any course of action will work in practice.

Step 4: Recording findings and implementing them, including completing risk assessment documentation

This is important: remember, to be effective, documentation should be simple and focus on the controls needed. The key points that should be recorded are:
- A proper check was carried out.
- Everyone who might be affected has been consulted.
- All the obvious significant hazards were dealt with.
- Reasonable precautions were put in place and any remaining risk was low.
- Employees, or their representatives, were involved in the process.

Step 5: Reviewing your assessment and updating if necessary

Workplaces change and evolve; new equipment is brought in or new substances and procedures are used. This means that a risk assessment has to be reviewed regularly to answer some key questions:
- Have there been any significant changes?
- Are there any improvements that could be made?
- Have any employees noticed any problems?
- Have there been any accidents or near misses that you could learn from?

> **Research**
>
> The HSE website is a great source of advice and information about many aspects of safety in the workplace. You can read more about risk assessment in its guide – download a copy from www.hse.gov.uk/pubns/indg163.pdf or visit www.hse.gov.uk and search for 'risk assessment'. The HSE also produces a risk assessment template in Word or PDF format as well as examples of risk assessments, although these are not so relevant to the health and science sectors.

> **Test yourself**
>
> 1 What is meant by a hazard?
> 2 What are the five steps in a risk assessment?

A3.3 How health and safety at work is promoted

So far, we have seen how health and safety in the workplace depends on everyone playing their part. This is made clear in HSWA 1974 and other legislation, but it should be obvious: an employer must provide a safe working environment, but employees must do all they can to take care of their own safety and that of their colleagues.

Therefore, a good approach to health and safety must become engrained in the workplace. It must become part of the culture, not just something added on or viewed reluctantly or simply as rules to be followed.

For this reason, health and safety must be promoted by providing a framework of good practice and getting everyone to pull together in ensuring a safe working environment. This section will look at ways that can be achieved. Some of this involves following organisational policies and standard operating procedures (SOPs).

Encouraging individuals to take reasonable care of their own and others' safety

Everyone in an organisation must play their part – to increase the safety of themselves and their colleagues. This starts with the need for individuals to be given the knowledge and information about how to keep safe.

Modelling good practice

Management must lead by example, such as washing hands and wearing appropriate PPE. This helps to create a culture of good practice.

This may not be enough in small organisations or where staff often work alone – they may not often be able to see good practice.

Following organisational policies and SOPs, including site-specific emergency procedures

As well as complying with regulations, following policies and SOPs should enhance safety. However, it does mean that these policies and/or SOPs need to be high quality, well designed and with health and safety addressed at every stage. Everyone has a part to play here. If you see any issues or weaknesses, you should raise these with your supervisor or line manager.

Ensuring there is clearly visible information and guidance

The HSE produces a health and safety law poster (Figure 3.4) and it is a legal requirement for any employer to display a copy where it can be easily read. As well as outlining health and safety laws, the poster lists clearly and simply what employers and employees must do to ensure safety in the workplace.

It is human nature that after a while we no longer notice the things we see every day. It can therefore be helpful to use a range of eye-catching and informative posters and other available materials that keep changing to continually promote good practice.

Following processes for recording and reporting issues and concerns

We can all learn from our mistakes – but it is better, where safety is concerned, if we learn not to make those mistakes. Employees must be free to raise issues and report their concerns. But that will be effective only if there are procedures in place to record and, most importantly, act on those concerns.

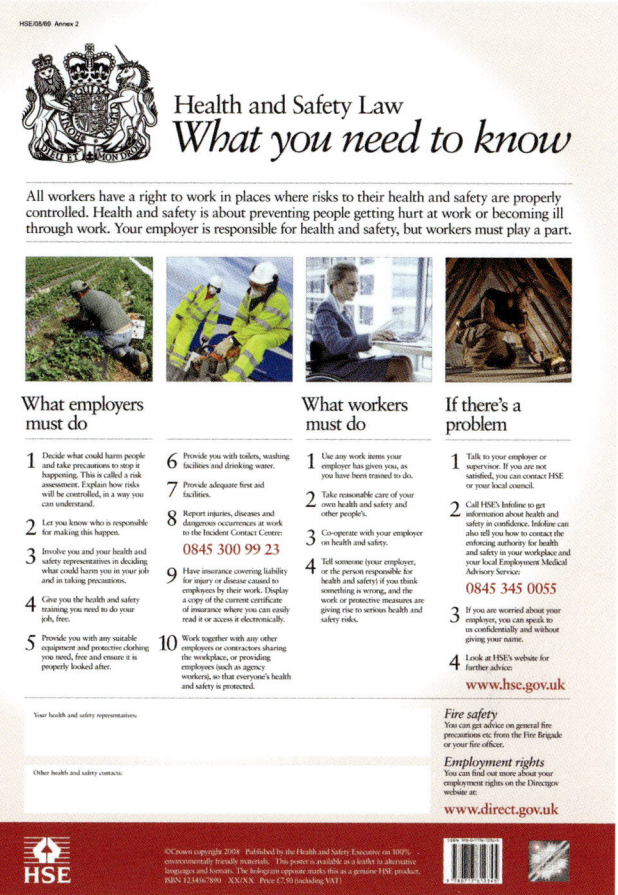

▲ Figure 3.4 The HSE safety law poster

Maintaining equipment and removing faulty equipment

Badly maintained equipment increases the likelihood of failure and can become a serious hazard. Faulty equipment can certainly represent a hazard and should be removed, or at least taken out of use, before it can cause harm.

Following correct manual handling techniques

Manual handling covers a wide variety of activities such as lifting, lowering, pushing, pulling and carrying – these are the cause of over a third of all workplace injuries. When these activities cannot be avoided, the risks of the task should be assessed and sensible measures should be put in place to prevent and avoid injury.

You should take account of:
▶ the strength and capability of the individual
▶ the type of load (box, crate, container for liquids, bulky item, etc.)

- environmental conditions, for example:
  - is the floor or the item being lifted wet?
  - could strong wind cause problems with light but bulky items?
- whether people have received adequate training
- how the work is organised – can it be reorganised to minimise handling or reduce the risk?
  - try to store materials in smaller quantities
  - try to store materials closer to where they are used.

Some points to remember when lifting by hand:
- Avoid, as much as possible, any twisting, stooping and reaching.
- Try not to lift from floor level or above shoulder height – particularly heavy loads.
- Arrange storage areas so as to minimise the need to lift and/or carry.
- Minimise carrying distances.
- Assess whether the load is too heavy – can it be broken down into smaller components, or can a colleague help?

If you have to use lifting equipment:
- use an aid such as a forklift or pallet truck, hoist (electric or hand-powered) or conveyor belt
- consider storage as part of the delivery process, i.e. heavy items could be delivered directly to the storage area.

> **Case study**
>
> Jack works as a technician in a hospital laboratory. Several times a day he collects items from the stores two floors below in a separate building. These include non-hazardous chemicals (such as 2.5, 10 and 25 litre bottles of solvent or 1–25 kg bottles of powder), large cartons of lightweight plasticware and heavy gas cylinders (compressed nitrogen and helium).
> - What risks or hazards would Jack face in handling these items?
> - What precautions should Jack take to minimise the risks?
> - What changes could Jack's employer make to the way the work is organised?

Ensuring working environments are clean, tidy and hazard free

You may have seen signs in various workplaces saying, 'A tidy area is a safer area', and they are displayed for a good reason. Even when obvious hazards are removed, clutter can itself be a hazard:
- Items on the floor can be a trip hazard.
- Unnecessary items can conceal other hazards.
- The need to move items to get at other things can be a hazard.
- Dirty work areas can be a source of chemical or bacterial contamination.

Regular cleaning and tidying are important, and it may not be appropriate to leave the job to regular cleaning staff, for example, if there is specialist equipment or specific hazards. Making cleaning and tidying part of the regular laboratory routine will make for a much safer workplace.

Appropriately storing equipment and materials

The saying 'a place for everything and everything in its place' is an important way of ensuring safety in the workplace. It is the responsibility of the employer to ensure that appropriate storage facilities are provided – but it is everyone's responsibility to make sure that they are used properly.

Storage of hazardous substances is covered by regulations including COSHH Regulations 1994, subsequent amendments 2002, and the Hazardous Waste Regulations 2005.

We also need to think about moving equipment and materials in and out of storage and so the Manual Handling Operations Regulations 1992 (as amended) are also relevant. See pages 52, 54 and 55 for more on these three sets of regulations.

Completing statutory training

Question: who needs training in health and safety? Answer: everyone!

HSWA 1974 requires employers to provide all information, instruction, training and supervision needed to ensure (as far as reasonably practicable) the health and safety of employees.

The Management of Health and Safety at Work Regulations 1999 identify situations where training is particularly important, such as:
- when new people start work
- when there is exposure to new or increased risks
- when existing knowledge or skills have become rusty or out of date.

There are other regulations that include specific health and safety training requirements, for specific industries or for exposure to specific hazards, e.g. asbestos.

If you work with contractors or other self-employed people, they may still be classed as employees for

A3: Health, safety and environmental regulations in the health and science sector

health and safety purposes. This means that they need the same level of protection and appropriate training as regular employees – and they have the same responsibility to ensure their own health and safety and that of co-workers.

> **Research**
>
> The HSE publishes a leaflet, 'Health and safety training: a brief guide'. This is aimed at employers but is also very useful for employees. You can download a copy from **www.hse.gov.uk** – search for 'health and safety training'.
>
> Use the leaflet to identify types of employees who may have particular training needs. Think about whether this would include you.

> **Test yourself**
>
> 1. Identify three ways that management can promote health and safety at work.
> 2. Identify three ways that employees can promote health and safety at work.
> 3. Why is it important that equipment is properly maintained?
> 4. Why is it important that the workplace is kept clean and tidy?
> 5. A delivery of boxes has just arrived. You have been given the task of moving them to the storeroom and putting them onto shelves. Name three things you would have to consider to ensure safe handling.
> 6. Give three situations where the Management of Health and Safety at Work Regulations 1999 says that training is particularly important.

A3.4 How to deal with situations that can occur in a health or science environment that could cause harm to self or others

This is where we can put into practice what we have learned in the previous sections. Health and safety at work is governed by law and regulation (see section A3.1) that requires us to assess and minimise any potential hazards (section A3.2) and do all we can to ensure a safe working environment (section A3.3).

In any workplace, the response to a situation that could cause harm should follow a similar pattern.

Following organisational health and safety procedures

As well as helping to minimise the risk of harm, all organisations should have health and safety procedures that everyone can follow if something does go wrong. You need to be familiar with these and think about how they could prepare you to deal with any situation.

Keeping oneself and others safe, including evacuation as appropriate

In dealing with any situation, the priority is not to make things worse. For example, cleaning up a chemical spillage is important to prevent harm, but it must not be done in a way that exposes you or your colleagues to greater risk. Think about what actions and precautions you would need to take:

- The use of equipment such as a fire extinguisher or chemical spillage kit.
- The use of appropriate PPE.
- Do you have the training and capability to deal with the situation?
- Are you aware of procedures to be followed?

You should also realise that some situations are too hazardous for you to deal with yourself. In such cases, it might be necessary to evacuate the area. That could mean evacuating a room, a building or even a whole site. Are you familiar with the evacuation procedures?

Securing the area

It might be necessary to evacuate a room or building – but you do not want people wandering back in. Even if evacuation is not necessary, it is important to prevent unnecessary access while clean-up is taking place. Assuming that everyone is safe, the next step is to make sure that the situation does not get worse, for example, that a chemical spill is not continuing.

Reporting and/or escalating as appropriate

Even if the situation is relatively minor and fully controlled, you will still need to inform your supervisor, line manager, safety officer or other responsible person. If the situation is more serious than you can control by yourself, you need to know what action should be taken to escalate the response. This might involve bringing in more senior or experienced members of staff, a specialist response team or the emergency services, as appropriate.

Debriefing and reflecting on the root causes, to prevent the situation from recurring

Once the situation has been dealt with, it is important to learn lessons. This means that those involved need to review what happened and why. This will usually mean that management, safety officers or others will debrief those involved in the incident. The purpose is not to assign blame but to learn important safety lessons. It may be that procedures or working practices need to be changed to reduce the risk of future harm.

> **Test yourself**
>
> 1 There is a chemical spillage in a school laboratory. Describe three actions that you would take to deal with it.
> 2 Under what circumstances should you evacuate an area?
> 3 Following a small fire in a chemical store, a debriefing is held for all employees involved. What is the main purpose of this?
>   a To ensure there is no adverse publicity for the company.
>   b To investigate the cause and assign blame.
>   c To investigate the cause and learn safety lessons.
>   d To remind employees that existing procedures must be followed without question.

> **Project practice**
>
> You have been recruited by a newly formed private physiotherapy company. The company has been formed by a group of qualified physiotherapists who have either worked for other private companies or in the NHS. They have formed a management team and recruited a manager with admin and finance experience. Neither the manager nor any of the physiotherapists has any experience of health and safety legislation.
>
> You have been asked to prepare a report for the new company that achieves the following objectives:
> - Makes the management aware of its responsibilities under current health and safety legislation and regulations.
> - Makes recommendations for implementing a health and safety policy in the new company.
>
> You need to complete the following steps:
> 1 Research a strategy.
>   - Carry out a review of the relevant legislation and regulations.
>   - Select the legislation and regulations that are applicable.
>   - Justify why you have selected some legislation/regulations and not others.
> 2 Plan a project based on the legislation and/or regulations you have selected.
>   - Summarise each piece of legislation and/or regulations.
>   - Describe the steps you would need to take to perform risk assessments, including identifying hazards.
>   - Identify the recording and reporting requirements.
> 3 Present your findings in a written report for the management team. You should cover the following areas:
>   - obligations of the company and employees
>   - roles and responsibilities
>   - specific risk areas that need to be considered
>   - how to promote the strategy within the company.
> 4 Discuss the following questions:
>   - Does the company have the necessary information and expertise to prepare an adequate strategy for health and safety?
>   - What further steps should be taken to draw up and implement the strategy within the company?
>   - Who should be responsible for promoting the strategy within the company?
>   - How should the roles and responsibilities be assigned? Think particularly about who should draw up the risk assessments and SOPs.
> 5 Reflection – write a reflective evaluation of your work.

A3: Health, safety and environmental regulations in the health and science sector

Assessment practice

1. Who does the Health and Safety at Work etc. Act, 1974 make responsible for the health of everyone at work?
2. To what extent does the Health and Safety at Work etc. Act 1974 compel employers to remove all risk from the workplace?
3. Which should come first, writing the SOPs or preparing the risk assessment?
4. Which of the regulations, **W** to **Z**, shown in the table, are relevant in each of the situations **A** and **B**? More than one of the regulations might apply to each situation.

Regulations		Situation in the workplace	
W	Management of Health and Safety at Work Regulations 1999	A	A company that does not handle hazardous materials needs to update its health and safety policies.
X	Control of Substances Hazardous to Health (COSHH) Regulations 2002		
Y	Environmental Protection Act (EPA) 1990	B	A technician in a school laboratory needs to dispose of old chemicals.
Z	Special Waste Regulations 1996		

5. A company is reviewing its training policy. All new employees undergo a half-day induction process that includes health and safety training. Half-day refresher courses are offered to all staff every five years. Evaluate this policy and suggest how it could be improved and why.
6. A new company has developed an approach to health and safety that includes the following:
   - The human resources department has the responsibility for carrying out all risk assessments.
   - The production department has the responsibility for preparing all SOPs.
   - Risk assessments and SOPs are made available on the company intranet.

   Assess what might be missing from the company's approach to risk assessment and SOPs. Your answer should include reasoned judgements.
7. Explain why the use of personal protective equipment should be considered only when all other steps have been taken to reduce risk.
8. You have been asked to dispose of large drums of solid and liquid chemical waste. Describe what the following legislation would require the process to include:
   - Environmental Protection Act (EPA) 1990
   - Control of Substances Hazardous to Health (COSHH) Regulations 2002
   - Manual Handling Operations Regulations 1992.
9. A company kept an accident book that was used to record all accidents that led to an employee being off work for more than seven days. Describe what the Reporting of Injuries, Diseases and Dangerous Occurrences Regulations 2013 (RIDDOR) requires in terms of recording and reporting accidents.
10. A technician has been given the task of producing SOPs for maintenance and disposal of scientific equipment. Outline the legislation and regulations that they would need to consider in producing the SOPs.

A4: Health and safety regulations in healthcare science

Introduction

Feeling safe from risks and harm in the workplace is a basic right, regardless of the setting you are based in. Employers have a fundamental duty to protect their employees and mitigate any work-based risks to the best of their ability, providing a safe working environment for all.

As discussed in Chapter A3, an employer has a duty of care, and should ensure their staff are not exposed to any unnecessary risks in the course of their work and that they are abiding by relevant legislations and regulations. It is also the responsibility of employers to educate and train their employees in health and safety, and how it is embedded into their day-to-day activities, whatever their job role may be.

This chapter covers the relevant legislations and regulations related to health and safety, and how they apply to employers, employees and patients specifically within the healthcare science sector.

Learning outcomes

By the end of this chapter, you will understand about:

A4.1 the purpose of specific health and safety regulations, guidance and regulatory bodies in relation to the healthcare science sector

A4.2 the purpose of the Human Medicines (Amendment) Regulations 2019 and the role of the Medicines and Healthcare products Regulatory Agency (MHRA)

A4.3 the purpose of the Misuse of Drugs Act 1971

A4.4 the requirements of national and local/organisational regulations and policies related to first aid

A4.5 the overarching responsibilities of trained first aiders

A4.6 the purpose of the Resuscitation Council (UK) and the guidelines that they produce

A4.7 the functions of the Serious Hazards of Transfusion (SHOT) haemovigilance scheme.

A4: Health and safety regulations in healthcare science

A4.1 The purpose of specific health and safety regulations, guidance and regulatory bodies in relation to the healthcare science sector

Health and Safety (First Aid) Regulations 1981

The regulations set legal guidelines for employers on the provision of adequate and appropriate equipment, facilities and personnel to make sure their employees receive immediate attention if they are injured or taken ill at work. Notice the term 'adequate and appropriate'; this means it depends on the circumstances of the workplace as to what must be provided.

To decide on what is adequate and appropriate, an employer must carry out a **needs assessment**. This will cover aspects such as:
- the nature of the work done
- any workplace hazards and risks
- the characteristics and size of the workforce
- the work patterns of staff
- the history of accidents in the organisation.

On the basis of this needs assessment, the employer will then have to:
- ensure there is an appointed person to take charge of first aid arrangements, or that there are enough trained first aiders
- provide adequate facilities and a suitably stocked first aid kit
- provide all employees with information about the first aid arrangements.

> **Reflect**
>
> Think about your own placement setting. Are you aware of what to do in the event of someone needing first aid in your placement? Are you aware of where the first aid kits are located?

Employees do not have any specific duties under these regulations. However, it is useful if you make your employer aware of any health issues that you have. This will allow them to take account of your needs and make appropriate provision. For example, if you have a serious allergy that might require you to use an adrenaline auto-injector (often known by the brand name EpiPen®), then (with your permission) first aiders can be made aware and, if necessary, receive extra training to help you if you have an allergic reaction at work.

Health and Social Care Act 2012

The Health and Social Care Act 2012 aimed to reconstruct the NHS significantly to tackle national health inequalities. The five main purposes of the act are shown in Figure 4.1.

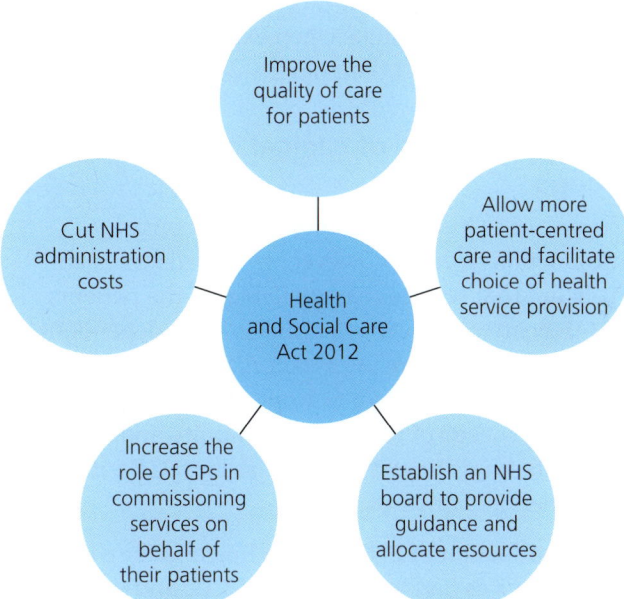

▲ Figure 4.1 Main purposes of the Health and Social Care Act 2012

The act focused on reducing health inequalities by clarifying the specific duties of health bodies such as the Department of Health, clinical commissioning groups (CCGs), Public Health England (since replaced by the Office for Health Improvement and Disparities) and NHS England. The establishment of an NHS board creates accessible resources and guidance for local authorities and practitioners to follow to ensure the most effective care is being provided. The act also aimed to cut NHS administration costs by abolishing health bodies, for example primary care trusts, so that most of the spending went to the NHS for improving healthcare services. For example, out of £190.3 billion of the Department of Health and Social Care in England's budget in 2021/22, £136.1 billion went to the NHS to distribute out to healthcare services. [Source: www.kingsfund.org.uk/projects/nhs-in-a-nutshell/nhs-budget]. In the past, clinicians had to negotiate with primary care trusts over the services required for their patients, but this act enables clinicians to commission services for their patients directly and clinicians are free to innovate to deliver the most appropriate quality services to patients. It also places specific emphasis on local authorities providing services that help prevent individuals developing needs for care and support, or deteriorating to the extent where they need continuing care and support. It ensures that care practitioners and local authorities are trained in line with national standards so that high-quality specialised care is being provided within communities to innovate and empower individuals when experiencing health conditions that affect their day-to-day life.

The introduction of clinical commissioning groups

The role of CCGs has changed since its initial introduction in 2013; however, its overall aim is still to ensure that services are available for the patients that they are responsible for. CCGs are independent organisations that ensure finances are available for the services required; for example, they assess the healthcare needs of the local community and then distribute funds to services such as local GPs, mental health services and hospitals.

The introduction of 211 CCGs in England meant that all GP services had to belong to a CCG, and they were given 60 per cent of the NHS commissioning budget, overseen by NHS England, which enabled them to design specific services required to meet the health needs of their patients. CCGs are therefore responsible for ensuring that the GPs that belong to them are at the heart of commissioning services by giving practitioners the authority to decide what healthcare services their patients need, as well as choosing who will provide other healthcare services to patients on the basis of who will provide the best clinical result. They have a duty to ensure that the services they are arranging meet the necessary requirement available in line with their budgets.

The Health and Social Care Act 2012 remains a very complex piece of legislation with mixed reviews regarding its provisions. Many believe the act was brought about to start the process of privatising the NHS, while others argue its purpose was to increase patient choice by making GPs the driving force of their patients' healthcare needs.

> **Research**
>
> Use the following link to find out more about the Health and Social Care Act 2012 and the structural changes it brought about:
>
> https://assets.publishing.service.gov.uk/government/uploads/system/uploads/attachment_data/file/138258/A3.-Factsheet-Overview-of-health-and-care-structures-240412.pdf

A4.2 The purpose of the Human Medicines (Amendment) Regulations 2019 and the role of the MHRA

The Medicines and Healthcare products Regulatory Agency (MHRA)

The MHRA authorises products for human use by approving the manufacturing, importing, distribution (e.g. to pharmacies), sales or supply, advertising, labelling, safety, efficacy and quality of a medical product.

It regulates medicines, medical devices and blood components that are used for transfusions within the UK. This includes facilitating vaccine production and ensuring they are safe to use through clinical trials. It is responsible for the validation and authentication of medical products for human use. MHRA has a reputation worldwide as one of the main specialised authorities and plays a leading role in protecting and improving public health.

Human Medicines (Amendment) Regulations 2019

The Human Medicines (Amendment) Regulations 2019 were put in place to amend the Human Medicines Regulations 2012. The 2019 regulations required new safety features to appear on the packaging of certain medicinal products and introduced the sale or supply of prescription-only medicines under a 'serious shortage protocol', which means that a pharmacist is able to dispense a different quantity or substitution of that medicine in the event of a shortage.

The amendments also reviewed the exemption for drug treatment services in emergencies involving a heroin overdose. The result is that this is no longer limited to naloxone hydrochloride being distributed through injections via a doctor – organisations that are likely to come across an individual who has overdosed now also have access to naloxone to help prevent deaths.

The amendments introduced two new safety features on the outer packaging of prescription-only medicines for sale in the EU:
▶ a unique identifier 2D bar code
▶ an anti-tampering device to verify the authenticity of the medical product.

These amendments were put forward for the MHRA to be able to operate outside of the EU medicines regulatory network following Brexit.

A4.3 The purpose of the Misuse of Drugs Act 1971

The Misuse of Drugs Act 1971 was brought in with the purpose of controlling the use and distribution of harmful drugs to prevent their misuse. Medical substances, if misused, can have damaging and dangerous consequences for individuals, so the act provided the legislative framework for regulating dangerous drugs. It also brought in a new classification system for drugs according to their relative degree of potential harm if misused. This involved the introduction of Class A (e.g. heroin and cocaine), B (e.g. amphetamines) or C classifications (e.g. as of 2002, cannabis) and introduced maximum penalties for each.

According to this act, each drug is categorised based on:
▶ whether there is evidence it is being misused by patients
▶ whether it is likely to be misused due to its availability
▶ whether its effect could form a societal problem.

The act created the Advisory Council on the Misuse of Drugs and gave the UK Home Secretary the authority to introduce and intervene with stricter standards of security around the misuse of drugs. It also made it unlawful for an individual to be in possession of a controlled drug unless they are a licensed healthcare science professional. The offences covered by the act cover the production, supplying and possession (including possession with intent to supply, which means having something to give to someone else rather than for personal use) of controlled drugs unless you are a licensed professional.

The penalties for offences involving the different categories of drugs at the time of writing (January 2022) are shown in the table below.

	Offences under the Misuse of Drugs Act 1971			
	Producing	Supplying	Possession	Possession with intent
Class A	Life	Life	7 years	Life
Class B	14 years	14 years	5 years	14 years
Class C	14 years	14 years	2 years	14 years

▲ Table 4.1 The maximum penalties for offences classified by the Misuse of Drugs Act 1971

Source: www.gov.uk/penalties-drug-possession-dealing

A4.4 The requirements of national and local/organisational regulations and policies related to first aid

National regulations

In relation to first aid, the Health and Safety (First Aid) Regulations 1981 (see section A4.1) are the UK's national regulations that are responsible for making sure that employers make adequate first aid provision for employees. The standards set by these regulations apply to all workplaces throughout the UK, including self-employed people, to ensure that first aid practices are adhered to nationally. It is also strongly recommended that national standards regarding first aid are used to protect non-employees (such as visitors) also, as with the standards set by the Health and Safety at Work Act 1974, which require that patients, staff and visitors' safety and welfare must be protected (see Chapter A3).

Healthcare Science T Level: Core

> **Research**
>
> Using the link, create a factsheet summarising the requirements of national regulations related to first aid with a specific focus on the Health and Safety (First Aid) Regulations 1981.
>
> www.hse.gov.uk/pubns/priced/l74.pdf
>
> Your factsheet should include:
> - examples of how the size of different organisations affects the first aid provision required
> - the information that should be recorded when a first aid incident occurs
> - a checklist of needs that require assessing when weighing up risks and required number of first aiders
> - the first aid needs of those employees who travel, work in remote areas or are lone workers.

> **Research**
>
> Are you aware of the details of your work placement organisation's first aid policy? Review the first aid policy in your placement and find out the following details:
> - How many first aiders does the organisation have?
> - Who are the first aiders who work in your area?
> - Where are the first aid boxes kept?
>
> Clarify anything you are not sure about with your placement manager.

Local/organisational policies

Local organisations, such as GPs, community centres and hospitals ensure that national regulations are being adhered to within their local communities. These organisations have their own policies for first aid that must meet the requirements of national regulations such as the Health and Safety (First Aid) Regulations 1981, for example having an appropriate number of first aiders for the number of employees within the organisation.

Local healthcare science organisations policies will differ depending on the size of their organisation, number of employees and work environment/hazard rating. Requirements set by national policies such as the Health and Safety (First Aid) Regulations 1981 ensure that employers in local organisations are compelled to take the necessary steps to ensure that patients, employees and visitors have access to first aid treatment in the event of an accident. Some aspects of national policies will have little relevance to a local organisation's policy because of the nature of the organisation, staff ratio and so on; however, each organisation's policy will be unique to their work environment. For example, the first aid policy of a GP practice with 15 employees will differ from a local hospital's policy with over 5000 members of staff, visitors and patients entering the premises every day.

A4.5 The overarching responsibilities of trained first aiders

Healthcare science employers have a duty to provide adequate first aid. This means that there must be a person appointed to take charge of first aid, and that there is an adequate ratio of trained first aiders. For example, the Health and Safety Executive (HSE) suggests that it is good practice to have one first aider to every 50 employees. [Source: 'First aid at work Your questions answered' from the HSE www.hse.gov.uk/pubns/indg214.pdf]

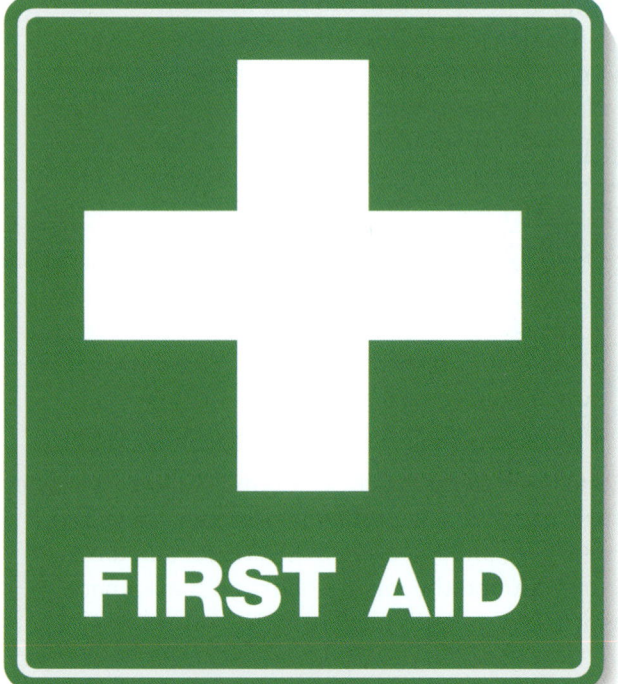

▲ Figure 4.2 First aid symbol

The role of a trained first aider includes several responsibilities:
- providing first aid treatment for minor injuries and illness
- ensuring, where necessary, that the casualty is referred for further treatment if appropriate to the circumstances of the injury/illness; this could be to their GP, an NHS walk-in centre or the A&E department of the nearest hospital
- ensuring that the first aid box/kit for which they have responsibility is kept clean, tidy and appropriately stocked; it is the responsibility of the employer to provide the contents, but the first aider must make them aware when items need to be reordered, or they need to order these themselves (e.g. from a central store)
- any support provided, as far as possible, reflects an individual's needs and does not discriminate against them in any way.

There are different types of first aider that a workplace can provide appropriate training for, and their responsibilities differ as discussed in the table below.

First aider	• Has a higher level of first aid at work training than appointed persons and emergency first aiders, and can handle a range of first aid emergencies and other specific injuries and illnesses • This includes being trained in assessing initial situations for the appropriate intervention needed • Will give appropriate first aid treatment until emergency services arrive (if necessary)
Appointed person	• Has certain first aid responsibilities • Responsible for looking after first aid equipment, e.g. the first aid kit • Maintains first aid records • Contacts emergency services if necessary
Emergency first aider	• Has the practical and theoretical first aid training to handle emergency situations • Can give emergency first aid to an individual until emergency services arrive

Research

Using the link, review the St John Ambulance website for their account of the roles of a first aider. Create a leaflet explaining these roles and discuss them with your tutor.

www.sja.org.uk/get-advice/i-need-to-know/the-role-of-the-first-aider

Practice point

With a manager in your placement setting, discuss the training providers that their first aiders have undertaken training with, for example, voluntary aid societies such as St Andrew's First Aid, St John Ambulance or the British Red Cross, or awarding organisations such as Ofqual.

Apply to complete first aid training with one of these providers.

A4.6 The purpose of the Resuscitation Council UK and the guidelines that they produce

If someone stops breathing or suffers a cardiac arrest, there is a very limited time available before they suffer permanent damage or even death. The Resuscitation Council UK states that, for someone in cardiac arrest, every minute spent without receiving **cardiopulmonary resuscitation** (CPR) and having a **defibrillator** used on them reduces their chances of survival by ten per cent. Therefore, it is essential that they receive CPR as quickly as possible. CPR involves chest compressions to maintain the flow of blood to the brain together with artificial ventilation (mouth-to-mouth resuscitation) to maintain an oxygen supply. A defibrillator (see next) uses a jolt of electrical energy to restart the heart.

Resuscitation Council UK

The Resuscitation Council UK helps to save lives in several ways, including by:
- promoting and publishing high-quality, scientifically informed resuscitation guidelines
- developing educational materials for learning resuscitation methods
- supporting research into resuscitation.

Resuscitation guidelines

The Resuscitation Council UK's guidelines help to ensure that healthcare professionals throughout the country share the same knowledge around teamwork and best practice for resuscitation.

Their updated 2021 guidelines include detailed information about basic and advanced life support for a range of different topics including:

- systems saving lives (factors that can improve the management of cardiac arrest patients, such as community initiatives that promote CPR training for all ages, including in schools)
- adult basic life support (cardiac arrest recognition continues to be a key priority for the emergency response trigger)
- adult advanced life support (it is important that chest compressions and early defibrillation should be carried out; after three defibrillator attempts adrenaline should then be used)
- special circumstances (the identification of circumstances outside the usual cardiac arrest situation, for example mass casualty incidents and cardiac arrest in sport cases)
- post-resuscitation care (greater emphasis is placed on screening cardiac arrest survivors for physical, cognitive and emotional problems, and referring them to appropriate rehabilitation programmes)
- paediatric life support (checking circulation with breathing assessments while performing rescue breaths: chest compressions should follow immediately if there are no signs of life from rescue breaths)
- newborn life support (while managing the umbilical cord, clamping is recommended after 60 seconds for newborns and any babies born premature but after 28 weeks. If newborns are born after 34 weeks, a laryngeal mask can be used if face mask ventilations are unsuccessful)
- ethics (highlighting the discussions about resuscitation for an individual's advance emergency care treatment plan, and discussion with family members and patients about support outcomes for family members who witness resuscitation attempts)
- education (employers are encouraged to provide employees with the opportunity to complete accredited life support courses).

You can learn more about the guidelines and download the most recent version by visiting Resuscitation Council UK's website www.resus.org.uk.

Using an external defibrillator

Section B2.6 describes how contraction of the heart is initiated by regular electrical signals produced by the sinoatrial node (the 'pacemaker' of the heart). In sudden cardiac arrest, these signals become disrupted and disorganised – this is described as fibrillation. Defibrillation uses a jolt of electrical energy to the heart to help restore the heart's rhythm so that it starts beating normally again.

Automated external defibrillators (AEDs) are becoming increasingly common in public spaces (often on the outside of buildings or inside shopping centres, sports centres, entertainment venues), schools and colleges, as well as in many workplaces. They are designed to be used by members of the public without any special training.

The location of an AED will be indicated with a sign (Figure 4.3) and there may also be a poster giving information about its use (Figure 4.4). Many are programmed to give verbal or audible instructions too.

The first course of action, if someone suffers a cardiac arrest, will be to call 999 and ask for an ambulance (large organisations may have their own procedures as an alternative to calling 999). The call handler will be able to guide you through how to perform CPR and will also tell you the location of the nearest defibrillator.

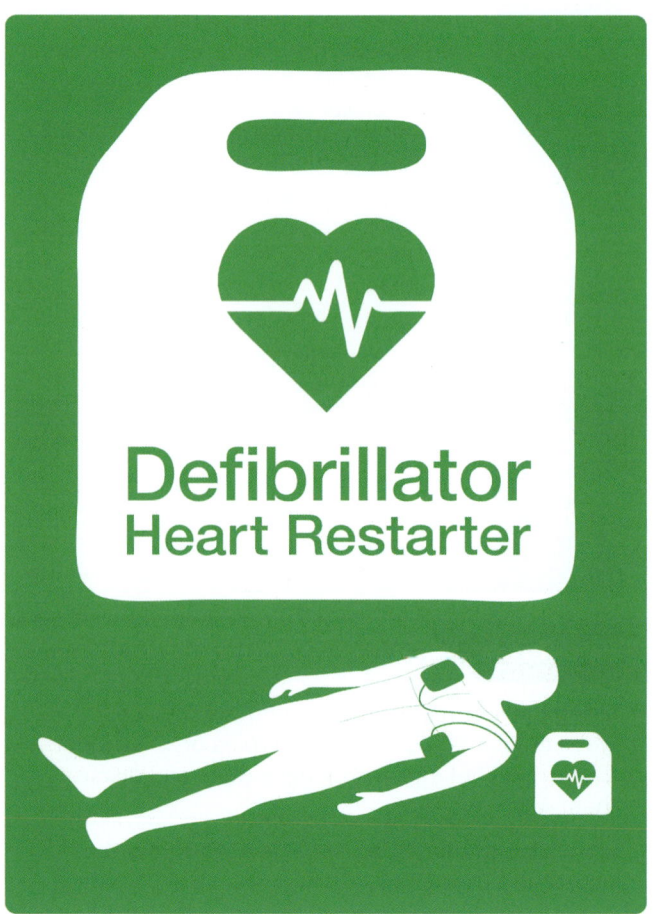

▲ Figure 4.3 Defibrillator sign

A4: Health and safety regulations in healthcare science

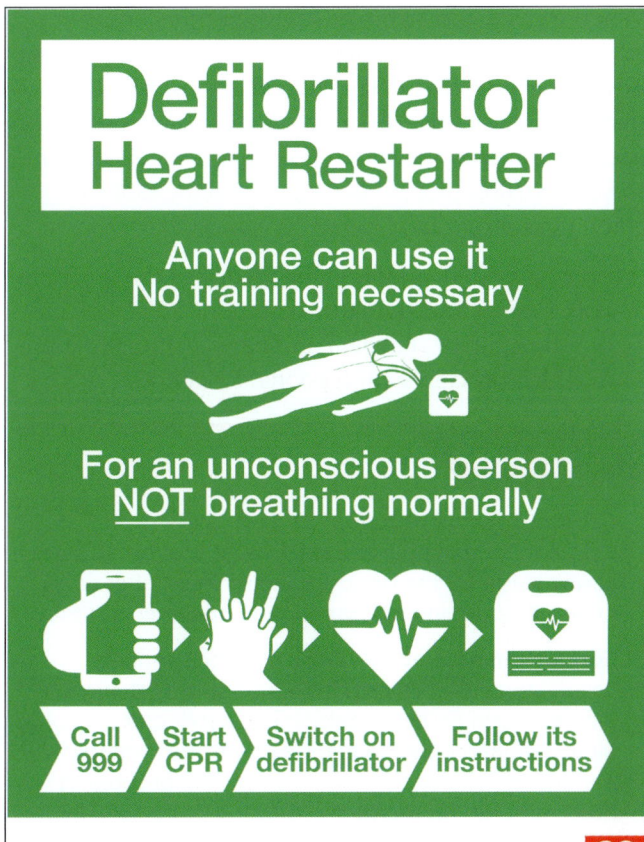

▲ Figure 4.4 Poster giving information about the use of a defibrillator

AEDs or public access defibrillators are designed to be used by the public without any training. When you switch on the defibrillator, it will give you clear instructions and guide you through what you need to do.

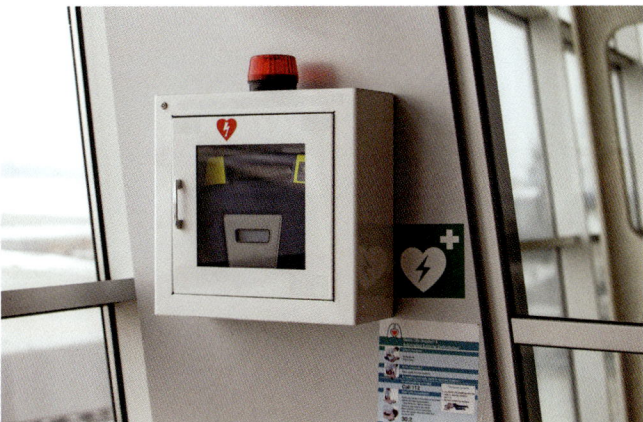

▲ Figure 4.5 Defibrillators are often found in public spaces, schools and colleges, and in some workplaces

Employers are not obliged to provide AEDs to comply with the Health and Safety (First Aid) Regulations 1981 (see section A4.1) unless the needs assessment identifies a need for one. This might happen if:

▶ there is large number of people passing through the site; the larger the number present, the greater the risk
▶ there are more older people present (employees and/or members of the public) as cardiac arrest is more common with increasing age
▶ risky procedures are undertaken – for example, the use of toxic chemicals.

If a need for an AED is identified, it is good practice to ensure that staff are familiar with their use. Grants are available from both the government and charities such as the British Heart Foundation to increase the provision of AEDs in public spaces.

A4.7 The functions of the Serious Hazards of Transfusion (SHOT) haemovigilance scheme

Blood transfusion is a complex process involving several different steps and, if done incorrectly, it could result in severe patient harm and/or death. SHOT is the UK's independent, professionally led **haemovigilance** scheme that focuses on the collection and analysis of blood transfusions and blood components from all healthcare science organisations in the UK.

According to the Department of Health [Source: www.cas.mhra.gov.uk/ViewandAcknowledgment/ViewAttachment.aspx?Attachment_id=102864], the UK national haemovigilance surveillance programme – Serious Hazards of Transfusion (SHOT) – has repeatedly identified that patients are harmed, and some die, as a result of being given the incorrect type of blood.

> **Key term**
>
> *Haemovigilance:* a set of surveillance procedures that cover the blood transfusion process. This includes the donation process, the processing of blood and its components, the provision of transfusions to patients and their follow-up checks.

The SHOT scheme ensures that all organisations involved in the provision of blood transfusions are performing this role safely and effectively. Employees performing the checks must sign to confirm that all steps have been followed. This includes:
- transfusion requests (a patient's clinician requesting a blood transfusion due to loss of blood from an injury or during a surgical procedure, or through illnesses such as anaemia)
- pre-transfusion checks (such as checking the patient's blood pressure, pulse and respiration rate, if the donor is currently on any medication or has travelled abroad recently, and that the donor blood type matches the patient's blood type)
- collection (a patient's identity details are recorded, and the date, time and signatory of a person trained and competency assessed in blood collection is recorded)
- administration (observations are taken at a minimum of every 15 minutes to record a patient's blood pressure, pulse and respiration rate, and body temperature)
- post-transfusion (a patient's blood pressure, pulse and respiration rate, and body temperature are once again taken and recorded).

When transfusion errors or adverse events occur, such as a **serious adverse reaction (SAR)** or **serious adverse event (SAE)**, SHOT produces informative instructions for how these events should be reported and recommendations to improve patient safety with the transfusion process (see the following table for some examples).

A report is issued annually that identifies the most up-to-date figures and statistics, common themes within error reporting for that year and key recommendations for healthcare science professionals to follow.

> **Key terms**
>
> **Serious adverse reaction (SAR):** a response or reaction, for example anaphylaxis, to the transfusion at any stage for the donor or the recipient that could be life-threatening or worsen their health condition.
>
> **Serious adverse event (SAE):** any occurrence associated with the transfusion process that might lead to death or life-threatening, disabling or incapacitating conditions for patients, for example a patient contracting HIV, and so result in or prolong hospitalisation or morbidity.

> **Research**
>
> Here is a link to the safe transfusion practice checklist that healthcare science professionals follow during the transfusion process. Read this checklist.
>
> www.shotuk.org/wp-content/uploads/myimages/Safe-Transfusion-Practice-Transfusion-Checklist-July-2020.pdf
>
> Now read the following document for further information on pre-transfusion sampling and administration essentials.
>
> www.shotuk.org/wp-content/uploads/myimages/Transfusion-aide-memoire-02.06.21.pdf
>
> Once you have read both documents, answer the following questions.
> 1. Identify two steps from the transfusion request checklist.
> 2. State who the unit must be signed by during collection.
> 3. During administration, identify the minimum observations to be carried out.
> 4. State the four essentials for labelling blood samples.

> **Research**
>
> Find and read the 2020 SHOT Annual report, in particular pages 60–5. Make notes to summarise the contribution of human factors in SHOT error incidents.
>
> www.shotuk.org/wp-content/uploads/myimages/Interactive_SHOT-REPORT-2020_V2.1.pdf

A4: Health and safety regulations in healthcare science

Transfusion error	Definition	What to report
IBCT – WCT (Incorrect blood component transfused – wrong component transfused)	Where a patient was transfused with a blood component: a of an incorrect blood ABO/D group b which was incompatible with the recipient c which was intended for another patient but was fortuitously compatible with the recipient d other than that prescribed, e.g. platelets instead of red cells.	Patients receiving a blood component intended for a different patient OR a component of an incorrect group due to clinical and/or laboratory errors in the transfusion process, for example 'wrong blood in tube' (WBIT).
HSE (Handling and storage errors)	Transfusion of the correct blood component to the intended patient, but where handling or storage errors may have rendered the component less safe for transfusion.	Cases of potentially 'unsafe' blood component where there were handling, or storage errors involved, such as transfusion of a time-expired unit.
Near miss	A near miss is an error or deviation from standard procedures or policies that is discovered before the start of the transfusion that could have led to a wrong transfusion or a reaction in a recipient if transfusion had taken place.	Samples or tests rejected following a communication from the clinical area to inform the laboratory of an actual or potential error (e.g. patient misidentified).

Project practice

You are working in a healthcare science organisation (use your own placement setting here) and you have been asked by your manager to produce induction materials to help outline the importance of health and safety regulations in healthcare science industries for new members of staff. Your induction materials should include:

▶ a summary of the organisation's policies and procedures for health and safety, including an explanation of their importance
▶ a list of first aiders at your organisation
▶ the risk assessments that should be undertaken in that organisation
▶ overall evaluative conclusion for how well the organisation follows national regulations and promotes health and safety throughout for staff, patients and visitors.

Assessment practice

1. State two items covered in the needs assessments carried out by employers under the Health and Safety (First Aid) Regulations 1981.
2. Identify three purposes of the Health and Social Care Act 2012.
3. Describe the responsibility of clinical commissioning groups (CCG) under the Health and Social Care Act 2012.
4. Discuss the responsibilities of the Medicines and Healthcare products Regulatory Agency (MHRA).
5. Explain the reasons why a drug may be given a certain classification under the Misuse of Drugs Act 1971. Include an example in your explanation.
6. Discuss the requirements of national regulations and policies related to first aid and how they then influence the requirements of local/organisational first aid regulations and policies.
7. Identify three responsibilities of a trained first aider.
8. Explain why the Resuscitation Council UK's educational materials for learning resuscitation methods are made available for free to the general public.
9. Explain why an external defibrillator would be used and where it might be found.
10. Discuss the importance of employees having a clear transfusion structure/checklist to follow when involved in the provision of blood transfusions.

A5: Providing person-centred care when working in healthcare science

Introduction

In this chapter, you will explore the main components of maintaining a person-centred approach when working with a variety of service users within the health and science sector. In this sector, it is important for professionals to be aware of the values and standards that enable supportive relationships with service users and their families. When providing medical or social care, the individual must be put at the heart of the provision.

Learning outcomes

The core knowledge outcomes that you must understand and learn:

- **A5.1** the National Health Service (NHS) core values and how they underpin the provision of care and support within the healthcare science sector
- **A5.2** the purpose of quality assurance standards within the healthcare science sector
- **A5.3** the importance of placing individuals, their carers and significant others at the centre of their care and support
- **A5.4** the principles of choice and consent
- **A5.5** the consequences of undertaking a procedure without gaining consent
- **A5.6** the purpose of the NHS constitution
- **A5.7** the role of the Care Quality Commission (CQC)
- **A5.8** the purpose of the Care Certificate, and who may best be suited to gain a Care Certificate
- **A5.9** the fundamentals of privacy and dignity of service users
- **A5.10** techniques that can be used to ensure terms/procedures are always clearly explained to service users/carers, taking into account their individual needs
- **A5.11** the responsibilities of employees and employers in relation to equality, diversity and inclusion
- **A5.12** the importance of ethics and research ethics in the healthcare science sector
- **A5.13** the definition of 'duty of care'
- **A5.14** the role of regulating bodies/acts relevant to the 'duty of care' in healthcare science and medical professions
- **A5.15** the consequences of not maintaining 'duty of care'
- **A5.16** the purpose of the relevant legislation in the healthcare science sector, in relation to rights of the individual
- **A5.17** the importance and application of probity and candour in a healthcare science setting
- **A5.18** the consequences of failing to maintain the duty of candour
- **A5.19** the principles of the six Cs
- **A5.20** the relationship between partnership working and the provision of person-centred care
- **A5.21** the principles of safeguarding, found in the Health and Social Care Act 2012
- **A5.22** the signs and symptoms of different types of abuse and harm
- **A5.23** signs and symptoms of radicalisation as outlined in the Prevent strategy (2011)
- **A5.24** how individuals' mental and physical capacity can influence their needs in relation to overall care
- **A5.25** the impact of dementia on an individual's needs
- **A5.26** the impact of learning difficulties on an individual's needs
- **A5.27** how to promote independence and self-care strategies
- **A5.28** the positive effects of promoting independence and self-care
- **A5.29** the overarching principle of the delivery of health promotion through the Making Every Contact Count (MECC) initiative and the risk factors this initiative targets
- **A5.30** strategies for promoting health and wellbeing within all aspects of care
- **A5.31** methods of obtaining feedback from service users relating to their experience of contacts and treatments

A5: Providing person-centred care when working in healthcare science

> A5.32 methods of using feedback obtained from service users to drive improvements in the healthcare science sector
>
> A5.33 the definition of an urgent or immediate referral and factors that would dictate the need for this action
>
> A5.34 the functions of services that work with urgent or immediate referral
>
> A5.35 how to act on urgent or immediate referrals appropriately within limitations of role.

A5.1 The NHS core values and how they underpin the provision of care and support within the healthcare science sector

Patient comes first

Holistic care is important within the healthcare profession to ensure the patients' **physical, intellectual, emotional and social needs** are a fundamental part of the care provided; these are often known as **PIES** within the healthcare profession. Holistic care means ensuring the patient's opinions and choices are considered and discussed during any appointments. All medical discussions should be carried out in a sensitive manner and any complications of medication or surgery should be discussed before an appointment to make sure the patient is able to make their own informed choice. Empowerment is a part of ensuring patients come first within the healthcare sector, meaning they are to be enabled and given the right to choose.

Compassion

Compassion is also part of the six Cs (see section A5.19, page 96). To be compassionate, a professional must be sensitive and show sympathy towards a service user's circumstances and understand how they may feel. Compassion is an important aspect of healthcare to ensure patients' needs are being listened to.

Communication and understanding are key when working within the healthcare sector and, therefore, professionals must be able to use a variety of communication skills, such as active listening. Showing compassion also helps patients who may have no family or friends and may need significant support from the professionals working with them to ensure acceptable care. Compassion is invaluable in healthcare and can be a key element when providing care as it can affect the outcome of the patient's experience. It overlaps with respect and dignity, for example knocking and announcing yourself before entering a patient's room, taking time to explain appointments and procedures, or taking the time to listen to patients' complaints or queries.

> ### Case study
>
> Rafael is a patient of Dr Scholl and he has an exceptionally good relationship with her. Rafael is 54 years old and has had difficulty with his breathing over the last few months. He has asthma and smokes, and feels more breathless than usual. Dr Scholl refers Rafael to the hospital for a chest X-ray and further investigations. There the consultant discovered Rafael has developed emphysema. As the consultant discussed this with Rafael, Rafael did not show emotion even though he was severely upset. The consultant discussed the signs and symptoms of emphysema and told Rafael he should stop smoking immediately as that is a major cause of emphysema. Rafael was then told he would be contacted by his doctor to further discuss results and was sent home. Rafael made an appointment with Dr Scholl immediately; he is furious and upset. Rafael opens up to Dr Scholl and tells her his concerns and the reasons for his emotional state. Dr Scholl spends a long time with Rafael explaining the condition and ways to reduce the progression of emphysema. Dr Scholl also provides advice for groups he can attend to help support Rafael with emphysema and understanding the condition. Rafael leaves feeling more optimistic and thankful for the time Dr Scholl took to discuss his illness with him.
>
> 1. How do you think Rafael felt when the consultant told him that he had emphysema? Why do you think he felt like this?
> 2. How did having a good relationship with Dr Scholl enable Rafael to come to terms with his condition? Explain your answer with relevant examples.
> 3. How did Dr Scholl show compassion towards Rafael? Use examples to explain your answer.

Improving lives

Improving patients' lives is the foundation of effective outcomes in healthcare. Professionals should aspire to provide effective treatment and support to their patients.

This value emphasises the importance of patients reaching their full potential. Part of this, therefore, means ensuring they can make choices about their medical conditions. For example, individuals with additional needs such as physical impairments must be empowered to look after themselves and receive support where necessary. A service user who is paralysed from the waist down may wish to bathe themselves without extra support, for example, and it is important that they are given this opportunity of empowerment from the professional.

It is also important to acknowledge the use of **multidisciplinary teams** where a variety of professionals work together to support patients and their families.

Respect and dignity

Respect and dignity are a part of regulatory standards within the healthcare sector, meaning that it is the professional's duty to act in a respectful way towards patients and uphold their dignity. An example of upholding a patient's dignity would be if a patient was paralysed from the waist down and needed assistance while bathing; the healthcare professional must give the patient the opportunity to bathe themselves after assisting them into a bathtub or shower. This enables the patient to feel empowered and that they still have independence. Healthcare professionals must also ensure they are respectful of patients' wishes and needs. The patient should always have a choice in making their own decisions other than cases where this cannot be applied, for example under the Mental Capacity Act.

The Health and Social Care Act 2008 outlines the importance of upholding dignity and respect within the healthcare profession. The act states regulations that are to be implemented within health and social care settings, such as treating individuals equally and ensuring privacy where needed. Treatment must be autonomous; therefore, professionals must treat patients with a duty of care.

Commitment to quality of care

Quality of care is about ensuring patients receive the best possible care from the professionals and organisations they are working with. A central part of this is that care should be person-centred, ensuring that the patient's needs and preferences are at the heart of the care provision. A professional must always ensure the patient is considered within their care and treatment by providing them with options when making decisions.

Working together for service users

Multidisciplinary teamwork is an essential part of healthcare. This entails working together with other health and social care professionals while supporting a patient.

For example, a patient who may have coronary heart disease will need primary, secondary, tertiary and potentially **palliative care** professionals to work together to meet the patient's needs. The patient may also require support from informal carers such as their family and friends. Good communication between these groups and individuals will benefit patients, as well as save time and prevent misunderstandings.

> ### Key terms
>
> **Multidisciplinary team:** a range of professionals from a variety of disciplines working together to support a patient's care.
>
> **Palliative care:** this type of care can provide support to patients with terminal illnesses to ensure continual monitoring and relief from their symptoms. Palliative care may take place either within the patient's home, a hospital or hospice.

> ### Research
>
> Using the example of a patient with coronary heart disease, research and explain the multidisciplinary team involved in supporting them. Include both formal and informal carers. State which type of care each professional is working in, i.e. primary, secondary and so on. (Refer to section A2.3 if you need a reminder of each of these.)

Everyone counts

Within the NHS nobody should ever be discriminated against on the basis of their personal background or characteristics (especially the nine characteristics protected by the Equality Act 2010 – see section A5.11, page 88). Part of the NHS's principles are to be inclusive of each individual's needs and identities. Inclusivity means each service user is given the opportunity to discuss their needs and preferences. At no point should an individual feel disempowered or disadvantaged because of who they are, for example, their religious views or disability. If a patient or professional experiences **negligence** because they have been discriminated against on the basis of a protected characteristic, it needs to be reported and investigated immediately.

> **Key term**
>
> **Negligence:** when professionals breach their duty of care, which can cause harm to the patient.

A5.2 The purpose of quality assurance standards within the healthcare science sector

Quality assurance increases measures of high standards throughout the healthcare science sector. Quality assurance is carried out by observing processes and identifying strengths or limitations within the way practices are conducted. Professionals are required to uphold standards within each sector to provide consistent and effective care; this can be completed through the use of maintaining policies and procedures within a setting.

Quality assurance framework (Academy for Healthcare Science)

The **Academy for Healthcare Science (AHCS)** is a body that promotes standards and quality within the healthcare science sector. This includes education and training centres. In effect this means that, in these settings, the AHCS measures the use of excellence of standards, i.e. how well they work and whether they may need improvement.

Healthcare science professionals must regularly update their professional knowledge through continuous training, which will also help their career progression. Professionals within this sector must be signed up to an awarding body, such as those working in physiology or the engineering of medicines, to ensure their training and practice is significant within the healthcare science field. The AHCS aims to implement high standards of education and training to ensure accreditation of professionals within the healthcare science industry. The quality assurance framework provides clear information relating to the organisation's aims and mission.

> **Research**
>
> Find out more about the AHCS quality assurance framework at the following website:
>
> www.ahcs.ac.uk/education-training/quality-assurance

Safety for professionals and patients

Providing safe measures within a healthcare or science sector for professionals and patients is essential, otherwise this may result in severe consequences such as malpractice or poor treatment. Examples of safe practice within the healthcare science sector may include adhering to policies and procedures, such as the Health and Safety at Work (HASAWA) 1974 regulations.

Quality assurance provides a specific framework for the high standards of education and training required for professionals, therefore ensuring effective accreditation that should lead to high professional standards and skills. It ensures that the skills of professionals are of a high standard, meaning patient safety comes first and their health is not jeopardised. These professional standards are developed with input from the CQC, Public Health, Health and Care Professions Council (HCPC) and other organisations, such as the IOC, to determine standards of knowledge to be acquired through training.

> **Health and safety**
>
> Re-read section A3.1 on page 51 to remind yourself of the Health and Safety at Work Act 1974 (HASAWA).
>
> Work in pairs and write a summary of how HASAWA is designed to prevent harm to patients and professionals using relevant examples.

Patients must always be at the heart of the service and care provided by professionals. As part of this, professionals must ensure that patients are aware of any potential risks before undertaking any medical trials, treatment or surgery. The benefits of any care or treatment must also outweigh the risk, therefore providing the patient with a beneficial outcome through the use of necessary treatment. Quality assurance safeguards patients with the implementation of professional bodies such as the CQC, IOC and HCPC to standardise methods of treatment and diagnosis, which further ensures that patients' health is a public priority.

Effectiveness of practice

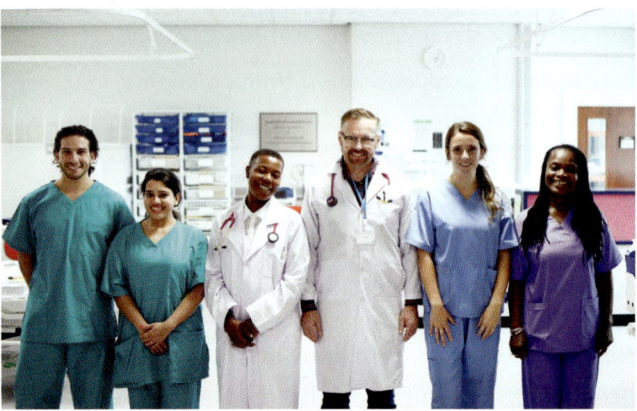

▲ Figure 5.1 Healthcare science professionals

Effective practice is essential within the healthcare and science sector to continually provide high-quality care. This means that any care provided must be the most appropriate method for the patient to achieve the desired outcome. Effective practice within the sector covers a variety of aspects, including communication techniques, following policies and guidelines, and providing person-centred care (see page 80), as well as the use of multidisciplinary teamwork.

Quality assurance helps implementation of effective practice: it ensures high standards of professional behaviour are maintained in healthcare science sectors by ensuring professionals continually develop their professional practice through training courses to identify innovations in working practices. The AHCS ensures patients are at the heart of the provision, providing a holistic approach towards patient care. Organisational bodies such as the CQC, IOC and HCPC provide guidance and informed conclusions from continual research that enables practice within the healthcare and science sector to be updated frequently with new methods.

Provision of best possible experience

To provide the best possible experience within the healthcare and science sector, patients must feel assured that the advice or treatment provided is within their best interest. Any negatives of treatment or medication should always be outweighed with positives. Patients are to be empowered and given the opportunity to discuss their thoughts and feelings, ensuring they receive the experience they desire as much as is within the power of the professionals providing care. Quality assurance ensures professionals are working towards providing effective outcomes through the use of training, observations and mentoring to achieve best practice.

This encourages a platform for effective care and experience within the healthcare science sector for patients, as professionals have a duty of care to uphold the six Cs. The AHCS also promotes quality care within the healthcare science sector by incorporating ethical guidelines within professional practice. Ethical guidelines define practices that are morally right or wrong within the healthcare and science sector; furthermore, these guidelines provide a starting point to identify how professionals should work to support service users. Employees in a healthcare setting should be provided with the organisation's handbook to establish relevant policies and procedures they must adhere to within the setting to provide outstanding care. This relates to quality assurance, as providing new employees with guidance and knowledge of an organisation's working ways ensures they know what is required for effective working practice, for example, how and when to use reporting systems within the setting.

> **Research**
>
> Explain the importance of the implementation of AHCS **ethics** in healthcare practice, using this link: https://ahcs.ac.uk

> **Key term**
>
> *Ethics*: principles that determine morality.

A5: Providing person-centred care when working in healthcare science

As well as consistent guidelines, it is important that all professionals who provide care receive similar training. Therefore, quality of care towards patients requires controllable measures throughout the sector through consistent principles of care outlined by the assessment frameworks, such as within the CQC, AHCS and HCPC.

Quality assurance in healthcare science education

Quality assurance means observing working ways in the healthcare and science sectors to ensure service users are benefited. If services are not meeting the needs of the public, methods must be changed, whether it be technological software, diagnosis methods, medical implementation or treatment. This applies to education providers within the sector as well as practice generally.

Quality assurance

Quality assurance processes aim to ensure high standards are maintained throughout education and training. It also ensures that all healthcare and science professionals undergo a similar education requiring examination boards and educational centres to teach specific topics that relate to current practices. Bodies that ensure significant quality assurance and education of healthcare and science professionals are the CQC, the Institute of Medicine (IOM), Public Health UK and the government. The IOC conducts research into innovative treatment methods and to further understanding of illnesses, diseases and disorders. It works alongside the government to provide guidance and new measures of treatment outcomes. The Office for Health Improvement and Disparities carries out research into healthcare to provide guidance and knowledge of outcomes of diseases and disorders; it helps to implement effective measures within government guidance and healthcare practice. These bodies work together to implement regulatory guidelines and best practice in health and science to ensure effective outcomes for service users such as in the care or treatment received.

> **Research**
>
> Following the links provided, read into the IOC to investigate what each organisation does to help provide effective research and health outcomes for the public.
>
> www.iom-world.org/research

Quality assurance also establishes the importance of consistent training across services and educational organisations to prevent differences of understanding of professional standards and procedures, for example within hospitals, general practitioner (GP) practices and care homes, to mention a few. Educational and training programmes must provide effective descriptions and analysis of procedures, including meeting expectations of patients, maintaining confidentiality where necessary, and monitoring their health and care. Standards of quality assurance are outlined in the following table to establish how to recognise quality or the need for improvements within organisational settings.

Standards of quality assurance	Explanation
Proportionality	Compliance with standards should outweigh any risks. A diverse approach of meeting these standards within the healthcare science sector must also be mitigated within the sectors.
Accountability	Standards within the sector should be continually reviewed to ensure they continue to adhere to expectations of legislative standards, for example, relating to data protection following GDPR 2018 (see page 94). External bodies such as the CQC do this reviewing to ensure standards are high within settings.
Consistency	Consistency is important throughout sectors to ensure there are continual procedures upheld and repeated that are recognisable to all professionals within the sector. Consistency requires the health and science sectors to follow legislative guidelines and organisational policies and procedures that they can integrate into each workplace setting.

Healthcare Science T Level: Core

Standards of quality assurance	Explanation
Transparency	Transparency means openness. When professionals are collaborating with patients as well as their families and other professionals, they must be clear about what they are doing and trying to achieve. Professionals have a duty of care and therefore must be truthful towards those they work with and not withhold information without good reason (note that safeguarding may involve exceptions to this – see page 97).
Targeting	Targeting means using strategic measures such as identifying the correct target audience or segments of research. It can also cover focusing on a particular disease or disorder, for example, to encourage the public to seek medical advice if they experience certain symptoms. An example of this could be encouraging men to seek advice for mental health to reduce suicide and self-harm rates within this group.
Agility	Agility means that professionals are required to respond competently without compromising the health and safety of their patients or themselves. For example, dealing quickly with changes to new legislative guidance.

Quality management

Quality assurance management standards within the healthcare and science sector can be established through the principles of the AHCS. These include proportionality, accountability, consistency, transparency, targeting and agility. **Quality management** means efforts made to ensure the healthcare and science sector continually maintains superior care to the public. Quality managers review factors that may need consideration and investigation in order to provide better products and excellent care. Management of the quality of health and science procedures is essential for conducting effective work within this sector, as a lack of quality management could result in negligence and ineffective methods of care, support and treatment. Methods of quality management include, excellent communication between professionals, supporting and observing one another to ensure procedures are conducted correctly, and identifying problematic areas that require attention.

Quality control

Quality-control processes uphold healthcare and science standards through inspection, setting practice from employees, service user views and the quality of data systems and processes. It is important as it ensures standards are continually observed and maintained by preventing poor practice and stopping trainees who are unable to meet the standards from entering or continuing in the workplace.

Quality assurance supplies a framework for quality control, therefore ensuring high standards are maintained within services. Through this framework, standards are tested and measured against policies and procedures.

Quality-control standards provide requirements and specifications to ensure consistency within healthcare services. This helps to maintain high expectations to meet service users' needs and build trust within the public services. Quality-control measures prevent mistakes and, ultimately, unnecessary deaths from occurring in healthcare industries. It includes the provision of safety guidelines and precise industry-specific education, for example on the disposal of hazardous waste and substances in accordance with COSHH (see section A3.1 for further information).

One example of quality control is the way that medicinal materials are tested and measured through experiments so they can be supplied for use by the public and prescribed by medical professionals. This prevents faulty materials being used and causing problems. If problems are identified through quality control, such as software that may not be up to date within the organisation causing problems in recording information or searching for patient records, these issues can be resolved.

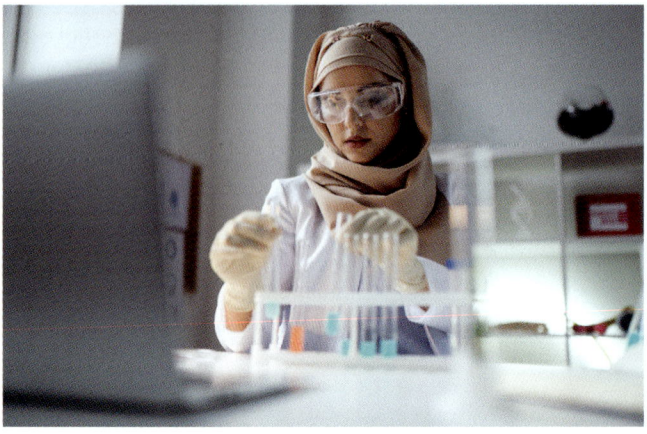

▲ Figure 5.2 A science professional testing in a lab

A5: Providing person-centred care when working in healthcare science

Quality control can be organised through a variety of organisations that observe and investigate standards within the healthcare science sector, for example the CQC. The CQC observes current methods and asks organisations to implement improvements. Professionals within the healthcare science sector must be appropriately trained through standard measures of testing and experience of services provided. The CQC provides regulatory standards that outline how healthcare science providers must ensure they employ competent staff to meet regulations. Furthermore, the CQC states that educational providers must provide essential training and support for ongoing continual professional development (CPD).

The quality of education is also subject to quality control in order to ensure high standards in the workplace, for example through sufficient practical training and **simulated experiences**.

> **Key term**
>
> **Simulated experience:** a useful way to train healthcare professionals, for example through the use of virtual reality or mannequins for first aid purposes. These provide almost lifelike experiences to prepare students for the healthcare industry workplace.

A5.3 The importance of placing individuals, their carers and significant others at the centre of their care and support in order to ensure the following

Any care provided is in the service user's best interest

Patients should always be at the heart of the provision. They must always be consulted within any medical and social care decision to ensure their thoughts are considered (unless they do not have the capacity). They should also have their physical, intellectual, emotional and social (PIES) needs considered. For example, if a patient has just been diagnosed with cancer their thoughts must be considered with regard to their treatment and aftercare plans, such as whether they wish to receive chemotherapy or not. There will be advantages and limitations of any care plan, so patients must be allowed to decide what suits them. There may be extreme circumstances where healthcare professionals need to make an executive decision on a treatment plan, however, such as when the patient is unconscious or in the absence of a 'do not resuscitate' (DNR) order.

> **Case study**
>
> Katie is a 42-year-old woman who has three children aged 12, 18 and 21. She works full time within events management. Katie's working hours vary through the week – she may have to work through the day, night and weekends. She relies a lot on her son, who is 21, for support with childcare as her partner passed away two years ago. Katie has been experiencing memory fog and irritability for a while and, as a result, contacted her GP. Her GP has sent her on to a neurologist to get tested and eventually Katie was diagnosed with early onset dementia.
>
> ▶ Identify the key factors that will affect the care needed for Katie. Consider Katie's priorities, her lifestyle and individual goals.
> ▶ Produce a care plan that will incorporate Katie's PIES (physical, intellectual, emotional and social) needs. Consider the following to help with PIES: employment, social life, hobbies, family life and the impact the illness will have on Katie and her family.
> ▶ Discuss the professionals who will be involved in her care and, for each, explain why they will be involved.

Compliance with the ethical principle of autonomy

Compliance means working within a set of rules, policies or procedures that the organisation has put in place. In this case, this is for healthcare workers to provide quality care to service users.

The principle of autonomy relates to the rights of individuals to make decisions about their own treatment or care through detailed information provided by a healthcare professional. A patient should be provided with the necessary information about their health and any potential care options to enable them to make an informed decision. A professional must explain all the implications to the patient, but also comply with the principle of autonomy by not interfering with the patient's decision about their own treatment.

To comply within healthcare and science sectors, professionals must follow regulations within the setting, and these regulations will include measures that bring practice in line with government legislation. In other words, legislation influences organisational policies and procedures, which promotes effective patient care. If a professional does not comply with these, this may result in forms of maltreatment towards a patient, as well as a greater workload for other colleagues in the organisation in rectifying this.

See section A1.3 to remind yourself of the meaning of the following terms:
- justice
- beneficence
- nonmaleficence
- autonomy.

Engagement with healthcare professionals

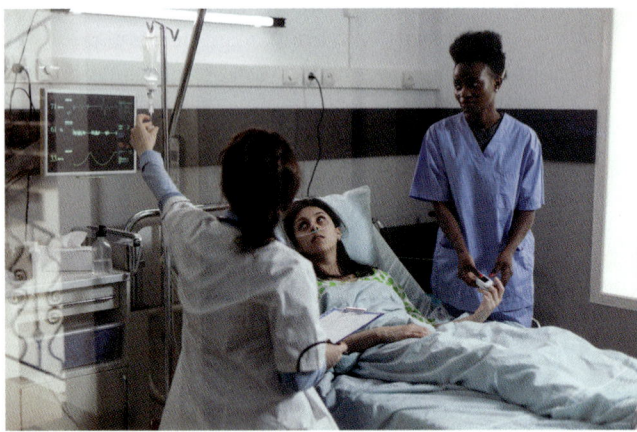

▲ Figure 5.3 Nurses caring for a patient

Patients may encounter a range of healthcare professionals that work alongside them to provide holistic care. A multidisciplinary team will include a range of health and social care professionals that must work together and communicate with one another to support the service user.

Working within a multidisciplinary team will include reporting, recording and communicating need-to-know information (because of the requirement for data protection and confidentiality, see Chapter A8) to other services that the service user may be involved with currently or in the future. Each professional involved in the multidisciplinary team will have a particular area of expertise; professionals may work in primary, secondary, tertiary or palliative care. For example, an individual with dementia will need to visit their primary carer, i.e. a GP, as well as a healthcare assistant, a neurologist, a social care worker and a counsellor, to name a few, all of which are part of secondary care. Tertiary care would only take place during management of the illness, such as surgery, and follow-up appointments. The patient with dementia may eventually need palliative care to support them in their final days if they become physically too weak and more dependent on their support networks. (See section A2.3 for more on the differences between primary, secondary and tertiary care.)

> **Research**
>
> Research the multidisciplinary team involved for one of the following illnesses:
> - Type 1 or 2 diabetes
> - a specific type of cancer
> - multiple sclerosis.
>
> Identify each professional involved with the patient's care and describe their role.

Holistic approaches to individuals' care provision

A holistic approach considers the need to identify the service user's personal needs. If a professional uses a holistic approach, they will consider each of the following areas of the service user: physical, intellectual, emotional and social.

Person-centred planning

Person-centred planning means the patient is able to discuss their personal needs and have them considered during the development of their care plan. A patient being assessed for a particular care plan must be involved with the decisions made to support them and their family. It may be necessary to include the service user's family in discussions as they may also help to support the patient or may need support themselves.

When planning care, a patient must not feel as though they have been disregarded, as it is important for them to have their opinions and needs valued and considered in the most effective and sympathetic manner.

Person-centred care

Person-centred care involves the patient being actively involved in their medical care. It allows the patient to feel empowered, as they are actively involved in looking after themselves with the support of professionals. The CQC states that patient-centred care is one of their fundamental standards.

A5: Providing person-centred care when working in healthcare science

> **Test yourself**
>
> 1. Explain the meaning of person-centred care.
> 2. Review and explain the quality assurance standards. Provide examples of how each standard is linked to effective care.
> 3. Describe the importance of ethical principles.

> **Research**
>
> Research the Care Quality Commission (CQC).
>
> Write a short introduction to the work of the CQC.
>
> Explain their standards of care and how they ensure quality within a variety of healthcare and science sectors.
>
> Then, choose two settings and explain how the CQC works with each to provide regulatory standards and quality. Provide examples and reference your sources.

Advanced care planning

A patient may need **advanced care planning** if they are suffering from a terminal illness and need continued final care, such as either moving to assisted living accommodation or **palliative care**. Palliative care offers the patient comfort and care during their final stages of life. Advanced care planning is about ensuring a continued high standard of life for a patient during this stage of life. It identifies the personal values and needs of the service user involved; therefore, as ever, professionals must actively engage the service user. Families may need to be involved in the care decisions with their relative, not least because they may provide informal care.

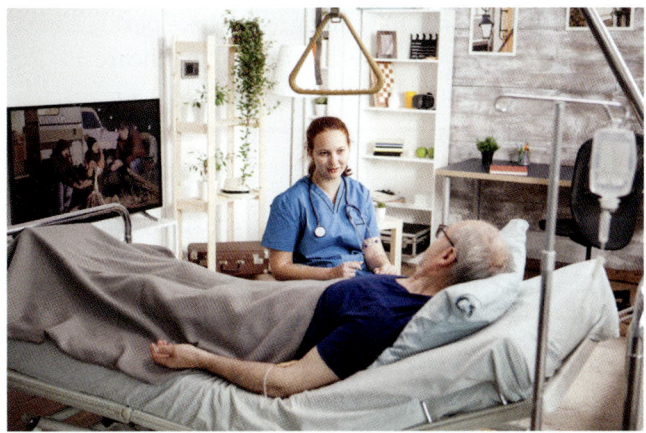

▲ Figure 5.4 A patient being comforted by a healthcare professional

> **Case study**
>
> Winston is 78 years old and was diagnosed with bowel cancer five years ago. Winston has continued working as he owns his own mechanical engineering company. He has become more exhausted over the last few months and experienced loss of appetite and overall weakness within himself. He lives in a three-storey house with his partner, who also works full time.
>
> Winston makes an appointment with his GP as he is experiencing these new symptoms. The GP refers him to hospital where he receives a variety of tests. Winston received the news his cancer is now in the final stages and, unfortunately, he does not have long left. His partner has been helping to care for him when he can as Winston is finding it difficult to move himself and make it to the toilet.
>
> ▶ Create an outline of a care plan that will support Winston's needs. Consider the following: Winston's lifestyle, family, goals and desired outcomes.
> ▶ Provide examples of care and support within your plan and use specific technical terms that are relevant. Consider the following: initial assessment, diagnosis and treatment plans, patient planning, patient goals.
> ▶ Explain how the care plan provides support for the individual.
> ▶ Consider physical, intellectual, emotional and social needs (PIES).

A5.4 The principles of choice and consent

Service users have the right to make choices about their treatment and care (unless incapable of doing so). They must therefore be aware of what their choices are and what they are consenting to at any point. Before a service user can provide **consent**, they must receive adequate information that they understand using their preferred communication methods. Consent must then be obtained from the service user once they are fully aware of any risks or consequences. Alternatively, service users do not have to agree to take part in anything they do not wish to, and healthcare professionals must respect their right to do so.

> **Key term**
>
> **Consent:** permission or agreement, usually for someone to participate in something or to be subject to an activity, such as surgery.

Ethical and legal requirement to gain consent for any medical care, procedure or treatment

Ethics refer to moral principles, such as what is right and wrong in the treatment of an individual or use of data if taking part in clinical trials or research. An individual must also be given the choice as to whether their health records may be shared with third-party companies or other professionals who may be part of a multidisciplinary team. In health and social care, it is crucial to work ethically to ensure patient health is at the heart of the provision.

To **consent** means to give permission; it is therefore important to establish trust within a professional relationship with a patient. A their will always be asked to give consent to discuss their medical history or to pass it on to another medical or social care team, such as a social worker. If consent is not provided, a professional cannot continue with the activity. If they were to do this, it would breach legislation and cause distrust between the professional and patient.

Where procedures or treatment may involve medical examinations, medication or surgery, the patient must be aware of the potential risks, side effects and complications, as well as the intended benefits. Once the patient has been made aware of all of these factors, they are then asked to give consent, and they must be free to agree or disagree to this.

Characteristics of valid consent

To ensure consent is valid, the service user must be informed appropriately. Professionals must give information that the service user can clearly and effectively understand with documentation or diagrams where appropriate. Once the information has been communicated, the professional must check the service user's understanding and ask for verbal or written consent.

Informed

Informed consent means a patient has been provided with full knowledge of the potential risks and benefits of treatment or procedures by the relevant professional.

Freely given

Freely given consent implies individuals are given real choice and the opportunity to say no. Coercing individuals into a choice is inappropriate and unethical.

Given by an individual with capacity to consent

Capacity in this context is the ability to be able to understand information provided and make a decision. The decision made must be communicated effectively. An individual may be unable to make or communicate a decision if they have an impairment such as dementia, severe learning disabilities, intoxication by drugs or alcohol, and/or have suffered from brain damage or mental illness. If an individual is unable to consent themselves due to a lack of capacity, an advocate must be in place.

Provided recently

Consent does not have a specific timescale; however, it must be dated. Professionals must confirm that the patient is still happy to consent closer to the time of treatment or procedure. Consent can also be withdrawn at any time and the patient must be given the opportunity to do this.

Choice considerations

To empower a service user, they must be given options. Choice is a human right that every individual is entitled to. Service users must be given the opportunity to receive information on a range of treatments, support, medications and so on that relate to their illness, disorder or change in lifestyle.

Principles of individuals being able to opt in or out of treatment

The patient must be given the opportunity to continue or withdraw their consent for treatment. A patient can opt in or out of treatment for any reason. The professional must not try to reconvince the patient if they choose to withdraw. It is a legal right and the patient is entitled to change their mind without the influence of others.

Rights of individuals to dictate their care plan

Individuals have a basic human right to make choices and to dictate the paths they choose within their life. A patient must be able to choose the care they wish to receive and the frequency of treatment, medication or professional help and support. The patient is also entitled to change their mind after they have discussed and confirmed a care plan. Finally, the patient is the one who should be given the necessary information and empowered to make their own choices.

A5.5 The consequences of undertaking a procedure without gaining consent

Consent is a legal requirement; service users must be informed of any changes to ongoing treatments for their illness or disorder. If a service user is not given the opportunity to consent or misinformed in any way, legal procedures must be followed to compensate the service user.

Legal ramifications

If the law is broken, ramifications (consequences) are to be expected. **Clinical negligence** means any form of misdiagnosis, mistreatment (for example without legal consent or overuse), failures or mistakes within health and social care, and could result in legal action to ensure the negligence does not continue and that the safety of patients is protected.

Criminal prosecution

Criminal prosecution (i.e. a criminal trial with the power to impose penalties) can take place if there are any health or safety breaches within an organisation, including failure to obtain consent. The Health and Safety Executive (HSE) and the CQC have the authority to prosecute public and independent organisations.

Requests for compensation

If an individual has received maltreatment or their human rights have been infringed, for example through treatment without consent, they are entitled to take legal action and apply for compensation. Should a service user experience clinical negligence, legal action can lead to individuals receiving compensation. If a patient has died due to clinical negligence, their next of kin may be entitled to compensation. Compensation may also be awarded if an individual has faced loss of earning, psychological damage, pain or suffering, or for any adaptations they have had to make to their life due to treatment or care to which they did not consent.

Professional ramifications

If a professional is not following health and social care principles and values, they will be liable for any maltreatment of a service user. They may be suspended or lose their job if there is any implication of harm to service users presently or in the future. However, such actions can also harm the organisation they work for.

Reputational damage

Service providers within the healthcare sector may experience reputational damage due to legal proceedings, for example loss of public trust and faith in their services. This may cause patient numbers to decrease dramatically within a service facing legal action. To overcome reputational damage, the service provider must carry out strategic planning to rectify any problems, develop positive outcomes in future where things have gone wrong and overcome public fear, so that society can identify the improvements made to the services.

Disciplinary action

Disciplinary action is a response to employee misconduct due to inappropriate behaviour. It can take a variety of forms such as informal or formal meetings, or performance reviews that look at the professional's working practices. It is important to ensure professionals are not working in an unsafe way, even if the service user has consented to the treatment.

Dismissal

Dismissal may be appropriate if a service provider has caused harm, whether intentional or not. A worker can be dismissed if they have not obtained appropriate consent from either the service user or an appropriate third-party person acting on their behalf.

Loss of registration to professional body

An organised professional body may be justified in removing an individual's registration if there are issues of inappropriate conduct towards service users. Professional bodies include the Nursing and Midwifery Council (NMC) and the Health and Care Professions

Council (HCPC) to name but a few. Loss of registration will cause difficulty in regaining professional status within a recognised body and may mean that the individual cannot continue to be employed within the health and social care industry.

A5.6 The purpose of the NHS constitution

The NHS constitution lays out the:
- rights of patients, the public and NHS staff
- pledges to patients, the public and NHS staff
- responsibilities of patients and the public
- principles and values of the NHS.

The core values and principles of the NHS are to be upheld by all professionals working within it. All NHS sectors and third-party providers must abide by legislations and the NHS constitution. The constitution sets out key aims, such as the rights of patients and the responsibilities healthcare professionals have in ensuring patients are kept safe in the healthcare system.

Patient rights are emphasised within the constitution. The constitution is set out as a commitment to ensure professionals within the NHS are accountable with regard to decision-making and work carried out.

> **Research**
>
> Visit and find a specific example for each of the bullet points above, i.e. one patient right, one pledge of the NHS and so on. Compare your examples with another student.

A5.7 The role of the Care Quality Commission

The CQC is a government organisation that was set up to protect service users and services. Professionals within the health and social care profession are also protected by the CQC and can seek advice from it.

The CQC is responsible for:
- undertaking inspections/audits
- making grading decisions
- providing recommendations
- making judgements
- distributing fines
- bringing legal action (when required)
- closing down providers that consistently do not meet required standards.

The CQC regulates a variety of care services to ensure standards are upheld throughout the health and social care sector. Professionals must be registered with the CQC to ensure thorough observations and inspections continue to take place within health and social care settings. Data on working practices is gathered along with patient and staff feedback and used as evidence to regulate the effectiveness of the care services. If necessary, the CQC will act if services are required to improve. This ensures professionals are held accountable for any poor care of service users and that this is rectified.

Inspections may differ across health or social care services according to the team and the type of inspection that is carried out. Regular checks are ongoing within services but depend on the level of cause for concern, which will also affect the impact of regular inspections as well as the size. Focused inspections may be carried out if there is a major concern within a particular service or a setting. Another reason for an inspection may be a change of circumstance, such as a takeover of the service.

During an inspection, a report will be produced to include ratings of the service. This provides the public with the ability to make decisions when choosing a service provider and choices of the types of care. There are four different ratings: outstanding, good, requires improvement and inadequate. Ratings will be used when identifying answers for the five key questions, then there will be an overall rating. Evidence is collected to reach judgements about the quality of care. Reports are then published for quality control and to provide action plans where necessary. Action plans will consider areas that are of concern and suggestions for improvements. If an organisation or professional is deemed inadequate, sanctions will be taken, such as fines, suspensions, monitoring and further training.

If services are deemed inadequate, action will be taken immediately against either the person causing harm, abuse or neglect or the organisation as a whole. If a service is graded as 'requires improvement', it will be provided with key areas identified by the inspector that must be improved with the reasoning as to how, why and when. Once the improvements have been made, the inspectors will return to re-evaluate the setting. If a setting is still deemed inadequate, the CQC has the legal power to shut it down.

A5: Providing person-centred care when working in healthcare science

> **Research**
>
> Using the CQC website, identify and explain the five questions used during an inspection.
>
> **Extension**
>
> Evaluate the importance of each question used during an inspection.

A5.8 The purpose of the Care Certificate

The Care Certificate is an assessment against a set of 15 standards that health and social care professionals must ensure they adhere to. Care Certificates are part of the introductory skills that all health and social care professionals must have to demonstrate required standardised knowledge, skills and behaviour. Healthcare professionals must complete and reflect on these standards through a portfolio of knowledge. The 15 standards must be demonstrated through a variety of skills with a thorough observation from a senior leader.

The Care Certificate is widely used in the health and social care sector as an assessment that must be completed on starting in one of the following sectors:
- social workers
- nurses
- community support workers
- other health and social care professionals.

The Care Certificate is reviewed and updated regularly to reflect changes within health and social care and ensure the skills that it assesses are effective. It is important that health and social care services can provide a high quality of care to encourage members of the public to continue to use services and seek care and advice.

> **Research**
>
> Research the 15 principles of the Care Certificate and identify how you will uphold the standards.
>
> If you have not previously been assessed within your placement setting, you should also discuss the Care Certificate with your tutor or placement co-ordinator to discover whether this will be carried out during your course or after.

A5.9 The fundamentals of privacy and dignity of service users

Dignity and privacy are important in healthcare, as we need to ensure the service user is treated with respect and cared for to the best of our ability. It is also important to uphold these to ensure malpractice is avoided. A healthcare worker should use a variety of communication methods to ensure this, alongside understanding and empathy towards service users.

> **Case study**
>
> How could you provide privacy in these three scenarios?
> - A patient, Sally is incontinent and therefore, has to wear an adult diaper (nappy). However, she would rather physically be escorted to the bathroom.
> - A patient, Dean, needs a physical examination during their GP appointment. He has been asked to undress from the waist up.
> - A service user, Luke, is paralysed from the waist down and has to be bathed by a carer. How could you ensure dignity and privacy for him?

Privacy

Respecting the personal space and property of patients and service users

Patients and service users are entitled to privacy. They should be treated with the utmost respect both in terms of their personal space and their property. An example of this could be not entering a person's bedroom without permission in a residential setting, but announcing yourself beforehand and waiting until they allow you to enter. Patient and service user property should also be respected, for example, in a hospital patients should be able to place their belongings by their bed and not have them misplaced by a professional.

Ensuring personal data is processed in a confidential manner

Confidentiality is major component of privacy, especially when working in the health and social care sector. Confidential information will contain personal

85

details such as medication, date of birth, patient address and so on. This information must only be shared on a need-to-know basis; an example could be if patient information from a GP needed to be shared with a specialist, as dictated by data protection legislation (see sections A7.3 and A7.6, pages 149 and 154) and internal policies. The patient must be aware that their information is being shared beforehand. Confidential information can also be shared if a service user or others involved with that service user are in danger of harm (see sections on safeguarding, pages 97–99).

Maintaining service user trust

It is important to maintain service user trust to ensure you are able to work effectively and care for the patient's individual needs. To do this we must ensure confidentiality. Although confidentiality must be broken in a safeguarding incident, this should still be discussed with the service user beforehand so that they are aware and do not feel misled.

Dignity

Focusing on the value of each individual

All individuals should be valued within every setting, whether they are a professional or a service user. To value individual rights, a professional should adhere to the Human Rights Act, which covers the importance of identifying that each person has specific rights that must be upheld. This means we should show care and compassion towards individuals and show genuine sympathy and empathy. Other methods of valuing individuals include empowering them by providing choices and enabling them to make their own decisions. Service users have the right to their own political or religious views, and these should be respected by the professional. Furthermore, a conflict of views should not cause a difference in care, meaning the professional must adhere to care values and treat them fairly, even if they do not agree with the services user's views.

To ensure dignity is upheld, an individual may require a chaperone during certain intimate procedures, for example, if a female service user is having an ultrasound performed by a male radiologist. In this case, a female chaperone must be present to ensure compliance within care values and uphold the dignity of the service user by ensuring they do not feel overly uncomfortable.

Should a service user require an advocate or interpreter due to additional needs or mental health circumstances, the professional must ensure they talk directly to the service user rather than the advocate to ensure dignity and respect is upheld through direct communication.

Respecting an individual's views, choices and decisions

It is an important part of healthcare to value patient choice. We do this by giving patients the opportunity to have their say with regard to their care and treatment. We treat patients holistically and with dignity and respect for their preferences and beliefs. For example, patients who are Jehovah's Witnesses are unlikely to give consent for blood transfusions, while many individuals may request to be seen by a same-gender health professional during a physical examination for religious or other personal reasons.

Working with care and compassion

Providing care and working in a caring manner is a key part of working in a health and social care environment. Service users and patients expect to be cared for appropriately throughout their stages of life. Compassion relates to how care is provided, such as being empathetic when working with a service user and respecting them and their values. It is one of the six Cs discussed on page 96.

Providing a chaperone for intimate procedures

A **chaperone** may need to be provided in circumstances such as during a physical examination or during a child's consultation. A chaperone can provide a service user with comfort and support during an appointment. A chaperone is not always a family member or guardian; they may be another professional.

Communicating directly with the individual whenever possible

The proficient use of verbal and non-verbal communication is essential in the health and social care sector. Professionals must communicate directly with the patient even if they need an advocate. A patient's confidential information may need to be discussed with an advocate, however, the professional must ensure they include the patient in the conversation to ensure they feel valued.

A5.10 Techniques that can be used to ensure terms/procedures are always clearly explained to service users/carers, taking into account their individual needs

Communication needs must be identified when working with service users and other professionals.

Checking understanding/use of appropriate reading material

During a medical appointment, technical jargon can often be used, therefore the professional must ensure the patient has thoroughly understood the conversation through checking understanding. They should do this, for example, by questioning the service user or giving them the opportunity to ask any questions. Other methods may include the use of leaflets or directing the patient to suitable websites that may be useful to gain further information, such as the NHS website.

Use of appropriate jargon/terminology

First, we need to consider formality. Formal communication may be appropriate with other professionals, for example, discussing medication types or surgery for a patient with a team of professionals. You may use technical terminology during this conversation for clarity. More informal communication should be used with the patient or a family member; you will need to avoid using jargon and you may need to expand on the meaning of a term. Informal communication also includes speaking to the patient as an individual and specifically taking care of them and their needs.

Professionals often work in their own specialised language community, which is a community of people that understand the meaning of technical words such as acronyms or jargon.

Health and social care professionals are usually aware of the need to translate technical language into everyday language when they work with people from other professions or the people who use their services. It is important that professionals check that they are not being misunderstood.

Formal communication may help to foster respect and avoid misunderstandings when interacting with unfamiliar professionals in other agencies. Professionals from different backgrounds often work together to assess and meet the needs of people who use their services. It is important not to assume that people from different agencies will understand the same terminology. An example is a home care organiser who might communicate with service users and care workers as well as with community nurses, GP surgeries, hospital services, occupational therapists, voluntary groups, day care groups and many other organisations.

Use of hearing loops or an interpreter/non-verbal communication, including body language

Sensory impairment refers to when a person's senses do not work properly, for example, the eyes or ears. This means adaptations will need to be made when professionals communicate with them.

A deaf person may use BSL but also be unable to communicate with those speaking English; in this case they would need an interpreter who can sign. Professionals should also be aware of cultural variations in verbal and non-verbal communication that can be interpreted differently. Different words and gestures in the English language may vary in other communities and languages.

Some examples of communication techniques that may be required include:
- translators to change recorded/written material
- signers who use BSL/Makaton
- Braille/symbols
- hearing aids – small microphones that increase volume of sounds
- loop system – a type of sound system used by people with hearing aids
- computer systems that verbalise speech for individuals who are unable to do this for themselves.

Being responsive to an audience's emotional state

Professionals must be aware of the emotional state of patients when relaying information. For example a person may become aggressive when feeling threatened in particular situations. On the other hand, depression may be an emotional barrier that may prevent the individual from seeking treatment or feeling positive. A service user facing an emotional and psychological barrier could be a patient with cancer. They may misunderstand information given to them or it may become distorted due to feelings of deep emotion.

Taking into account an individual's capacity to understand information

Professionals must be aware of differences in people's capacity to understand information when they are working with a variety of patients. For example, someone who has a learning difficulty may find it hard to take in a lot of information at one time, therefore the professional must identify this and establish ways to pass on appropriate amounts of information effectively. This may be through the use of an advocate, a family member or guardian sitting in on the appointment with the individual, or the use of materials such as leaflets if applicable. If a service user is in a coma or has recently awoken from a coma, advocates such as family or informal carers should be involved in the discussion of their health and current circumstance; it is unfair to assume that the service user would be able to take in information during that time.

A5.11 The responsibilities of employees and employers in relation to equality, diversity and inclusion

These are professional responsibilities that are promoted through organisational policies and procedures and, ultimately, derive from relevant legislation. We will look at some key pieces of legislation in this area and what they mean for practice.

Equality Act 2010

The Equality Act 2010 builds on and extends the protections of various previous pieces of anti-discrimination legislation.

This act lists nine **protected characteristics**, and it is illegal to discriminate against someone on the basis of these. They are: age, disability, gender reassignment, marriage or civil partnership, pregnancy and maternity, race, religion or belief, gender and sexual orientation.

The act protects both direct and indirect discrimination. Direct discrimination may include openly discriminating against someone because they are, for instance, over a certain age, have a specific religion or are pregnant. Indirect discrimination can include not hiring an employee due to their name if it is perceived to be from a specific ethnic group. All organisations within the UK must incorporate the act into their organisational policies and procedures.

> **Case study**
>
> ### Direct discrimination
> Anya has cerebral palsy and is a wheelchair user studying drama at school. Anya's class is going on a theatre trip to watch a play they have been studying in her English class. Anya's teacher has told her she cannot go as there is no wheelchair accessibility.
>
> Answer the following questions:
> ▶ Why is this direct discrimination?
> ▶ What are Anya's rights in this situation?
> ▶ How should this situation be handled instead?
> ▶ What should the teacher do?
>
> ### Indirect discrimination
> Simon has recently moved into a dementia care home as he can no longer live independently. Simon has overheard his care worker discussing his personal information with another care worker not directly involved with Simon. Simon's son visits him in the care home, and overhears Simon's care worker ridiculing him saying, 'he's too young to have dementia; he should be looking after himself'.
>
> Answer the following questions:
> ▶ Why is this indirect discrimination?
> ▶ What are Simon's rights in this situation?
> ▶ What should Simon's son do?
> ▶ What could happen to the care worker looking after Simon?

Responsibilities

Recognise patients and service users as individuals

Individual needs must be considered at all times, and this includes recognising, as part of person-centred care, the person as a whole including any religious beliefs and other characteristics. Treating individuals fairly does not mean treating them the same: to avoid discrimination you may need to bear in mind individual needs. For instance, individuals who are pregnant or disabled may need adjustments to ensure they are cared for appropriately.

Do not marginalise, label or discriminate

Discriminatory attitudes such as labelling or marginalisation should not be tolerated.

Labelling is a negative form of prejudice that attaches a social stigma to a group of individuals or an individual. Labelling can lead to ineffective care. Discriminatory practice can affect an individual in a variety of ways as it has an effect on the care provided. Service users experiencing discriminatory practice may suffer neglect or abuse. Needs may not be met and, therefore, care values are not promoted causing a lack of self-esteem and a low self-identity. Marginalisation can cause an individual to develop feelings of insignificance; an individual experiencing marginalisation may have restricted opportunities and be a victim of discrimination. Marginalisation can then lead to a lack of opportunity for an individual or group of individuals.

Support client needs whenever reasonable

A professional should support client needs at all times to the best of their ability, by providing adequate care that meets a variety of service user needs. The professional must assess the service user's condition and lifestyle to implement effective changes, treatments and support that will benefit them.

An example of supporting service users' needs could be facilitating the celebration of festivals and holidays within a residential setting, or a hospital that provides food for a range of religious needs, for example to suit Halal, Kosher or vegetarian diets.

A5.12 The importance of ethics and research ethics in the healthcare science sector

Ethics are moral principles for what society deems as acceptable or unacceptable. Ethical principles allow us to balance individual rights with the rights of others.

They are a key factor in research in any context and must be upheld to ensure safe practice and, furthermore, that no harm occurs during the research.

To enable ethical research, the patient/service user should be put at the heart of service provision, e.g. providing active support consistent with the beliefs, culture and preferences of the individual, supporting individuals to express their needs and preferences, and empowering individuals.

Avoiding conflict and using honourable and trustworthy methods is an important factor when research is being conducted to reduce unnecessary harm to participants.

Ethical considerations when conducting research

Informed consent

As explained in section A5.4, informed consent refers to permission being obtained from a service user after they have received adequate knowledge on what they are consenting to. For example, if a patient is to undergo an operation, they need to be aware of the risks, benefits and recovery time. This, therefore, informs the patient of what they can expect during and after the operation. A patient must give written consent to proceed with the procedure – if consent is not obtained it is illegal to go through with the procedure. Informed consent is also required to pass on and discuss relevant information when needed, for instance between other relevant medical teams or for the purposes of research. Before, during and after the research, the participant must have the right to withdraw their part within the research.

Practising beneficence

Put simply, **beneficence** means 'doing good'. All healthcare professionals need to follow the course of action that they believe to be in the best interest of their patient. However, 'doing good' is often too simple in the real world. It is better to think of beneficence as ranking the possible options for a patient from best to worst, taking the following questions into account:
▶ Will the option resolve the medical problem?
▶ Is it proportionate to the scale of the problem?
▶ Is it compatible with the patient's individual circumstances?
▶ Is the option and its outcomes in line with the patient's expectations?

Several of these points are related to the patient's circumstances or expectations. This forms the basis of patient- or person-centred care.

Respect for anonymity and confidentiality

Anonymity and confidentiality are two important ethical principles. Anonymity means ensuring patient records are kept so that they are unidentifiable, i.e. information cannot be linked to them by anyone not working directly with that patient. Records remain anonymous and confidential except for specific circumstances, e.g. for safeguarding reasons if it becomes necessary to share them (see section A5.9 for further information on confidentiality).

Respect for privacy

Maintaining patient privacy is necessary to allow service users and members of the public to trust the care provided and received. A trusting environment is essential for service users to maintain a good perception of care (see section A5.9 for more on privacy).

Importance of research ethics

Promote the aims of the research

Ethics are an essential part of research methods; they are written statements that are referred to as codes. Ethical codes change over time to reflect what society deems as acceptable/unacceptable at that time. Ethical issues arise when a conflict exists between participants' rights and researchers' needs to gain valuable and meaningful information. This conflict has implications for the safety and wellbeing of participants.

Support the values of the research

It is important to continue to develop improvements for individuals within health and social care, so research aims to establish evidence for current and future treatments to continually improve outcomes. Upholding ethics ensures that research is not morally problematic and is valid in discovering the aims and purpose set out by the researcher.

Hold the researcher accountable

Accountability means the researcher takes responsibility for their actions. Researchers should be held accountable during the research and after the release of data to the public. Regulatory bodies such as the Medicines and Healthcare products Regulatory Agency (MHRA), and legislation such as the Medicines for Human Use (Clinical Trials) Amendment Regulations (MHCTR) 2006 ensure this applies to healthcare professionals when research proposals are produced.

Investment is used appropriately

Services and organisations will need to invest money into the development and planning of improvements and changes. Decisions need to be based on accurate, reliable and recent data for investments to be effective.

Planning of services is expensive and research is often carried out over a long period of time (known as **longitudinal** research). For this reason, it is important to ensure the money and time invested in a study are not wasted. Research may need to be **piloted**, meaning a small-scale study (a pilot study) will be planned and completed first to identify strengths, limitations and gaps within the research study.

Offer regulation on a conflict of interest

As noted above, research is regulated by the pMHRA and under the MHCTR 2006. According to these, a thorough plan must be submitted to a regulatory board before research is conducted. This plan must clearly set out the objectives of the research and how it is being conducted.

If the research is funded by external agencies or companies, the funding must be used appropriately and plans of finances should be made evident. The funding company does not need to know detailed or personal information about the participants involved – as this is to remain confidential. The funding company just needs to be aware of the basics, such as what is being trialled and why, to avoid any bias. When regulatory agencies view the application, clear objectives should be stated within a report stating how the research is to be carried out. The researcher should have an open mind when completing the proposal and conducting research to ensure they do not interfere with the outcomes of the research through their own preconceptions or bias.

Ethical principles must be considered and set out appropriately in relation to how the researcher is going to ensure that participants will not be harmed during or after the research. Ethical principles allow the researcher to identify appropriate research methods. Representative samples should be used, meaning that a range of participants must be included within the study to enable a good overview of individual characteristics to be included within the research. This will ensure it has high validity and relevance to the population at large.

Promote trust from the public

Applying ethical principles during research helps the public to trust the health and social care sector.

It reassures the public that the intentions of the study are good and that it will be carried out in a robust and reliable way. They should be able to trust the processes involved and be sure that there are checks in place to ensure the methodology is sound and the results are recorded and documented accurately. Trust is essential in order get the public to agree to try any new or improved treatment methods identified by the research.

Support important social and moral values

Social values are incorporated within the ethics of research. These values are significant in deciding how to develop an outstanding health and social care service that has an effective process for identifying, diagnosing and treating patient needs. Moral values within ethics ensure that researchers are reducing the risk of harm to patients and service users and, instead, discovering effective methods of treatment.

For example, during COVID-19 vaccination trials, participants were given effective information regarding the potential risks and side effects of the study. They were given written information and signed a consent form with the option to withdraw from the study should they want to. Participants were anonymous to protect their identity. They were also screened before they participated in the trial to check for allergies, underlying health conditions, their living and working conditions, and family health history to ensure they were not at risk of serious side effects or death. Participants were also monitored regularly to ensure their health did not deteriorate over time, to identify whether their health did change and if they experienced any side effects. If a participant did experience any major side effects, they were treated immediately and removed from the trial, protecting them from any further harm.

A5.13 The definition of duty of care

Duty of care is a legal obligation under HASAWA 1974, which requires health and social care practitioners to protect service users' health and wellbeing. Prevention of harm is an important aspect of duty of care. Through providing a duty of care, a professional should ensure they adhere to safe practice and balance individual rights with risks, i.e. the treatment and support provided must outweigh any negatives or risks to the patient.

When providing care, staff must also adhere to organisational policies and procedures to protect themselves and the service users. All service users have the right to be treated equally and fairly, and not be discriminated against. Under the Mental Capacity Act 2005, a person who lacks capacity is considered to be unable to make decisions for themselves, for example an individual with dementia. If a service user is unable to do this, they must be provided with an advocate: someone impartial to the setting who can speak on behalf of the service user.

As part of a person-centred approach health and social care professionals must consider the individuals' physical, intellectual, emotional and social needs (PIES). All service users have the right to receive quality of care and be free from harm.

Another important aspect of duty of care is safeguarding. The professionals who work with patients or service users have a duty to raise any safeguarding concerns, not only relating to the service user with whom they are interacting, but with any other service user, colleague or member of the public they interact with during their duty. The professional must report any act of abuse or neglect as soon as possible.

A5.14 The role of regulating bodies/acts relevant to the 'duty of care' in healthcare science and medical professions

Regulating bodies enable standards to be assessed, met and maintained through a variety of health and social care services. There are a range of organisations and regulating bodies that work alongside government legislation to ensure staff and service users are protected. These bodies ensure staff are registered and can seek guidance or advice when needed. The bodies also ensure that the public are aware of what they can expect when they use a health or social care service.

Health and Care Professions Council (HCPC)

The Health Care Professions Council (HCPC) is the main awarding organisation for statutory registration for healthcare professionals. The HCPC ensures professionals are trained appropriately up to their set standards to maintain quality fitness to practice. Any concerns raised about professionals within the organisational body must be investigated with immediate action. During investigation a professional may be required to work only as a desk-based member within a healthcare setting, meaning they are unable to practice on patients. The HCPC sets standards for health and social care professionals. The HCPC regulates education and training standards within health and social care to ensure all professionals train with the right accreditation and professional standards. If a professional does not meet the HCPC standards, then the council or management within the setting will act on this to ensure any irregularities in care are minimised to protect service users.

Academy for Healthcare Science (AHCS)

The Academy for Healthcare Science (AHCS) is a voluntary regulatory body, meaning it is not mandatory for professionals within healthcare science to be registered with this organisation. Although this is not a legal requirement for healthcare science professionals, employers would deem this beneficial for further training and professional development purposes. The AHCS supports the promotion of healthcare science and scientific services. The AHCS ensures that professionals are supported and that they work alongside the professional bodies to enable collaboration across services. The AHCS also ensures that training and development programmes are registered to promote high expectations of professional standards. Finally, the AHCS ensures that those working within healthcare science can gain accredited registration as other professional bodies may not cover their area of expertise.

General Pharmaceutical Council (GPhC)

The General Pharmaceutical Council (GPhC) is a statutory regulatory body for professionals within pharmaceutical companies, whether they are pharmacists or technicians. The GPhC ensures that professionals within this area of healthcare are supported within their roles and sets standards that all professionals within this field must adhere to. If standards are not met, action will be taken. Furthermore, the GPhC sets educational and training standards that must be completed during pharmaceutical training and afterwards, known as continual professional development. The GPhC provides clear conduct for professionals to follow at all times. A complaint of misconduct within a setting must be investigated immediately. Any professional suspected of malpractice will be suspended temporarily while under investigation and if found guilty will be suspended permanently. The GPhC also completes inspections to ensure services are providing safe and effective care.

General Medical Council (GMC)

The General Medical Council (GMC) works to protect patient safety through effective principles and guidance for individuals. The GMC set out regulations using National Institute for Health and Care Excellence (NICE) guidelines. This covers guidance and advice for professionals and the public about the expectations outlined for health and social care settings. The GMC ensures those working within the medical field, such as surgeons and GPs, are qualified to work in the UK. It also oversees training and education standards, provides guidance to professionals and ensures ethics are being maintained within the healthcare field.

Care Quality Commission (CQC)

The Care Quality Commission (CQC) ensures health and social care services provide quality treatment and support, and a safe environment for service users by setting out standards that incorporate individual care. The CQC inspects health and social care services to assess current care quality and arranges for improvements within the services if necessary. The CQC works collaboratively with other organisations to ensure consistency in health and social care.

General Dental Council (GDC)

The General Dental Council (GDC) is a statutory regulatory body that sets standards across dental services for education, training, performance, future developments and professional conduct. The council ensures those within the dentistry professional are regulated and fit to work within their practice. The GDC has standards in place that must be adhered to; if they are not upheld, action from higher management or the GDC quality team must be taken to protect service users from harm. The GDC protects patients and the wider public to enable confidence within dental services. Any form of misconduct within dentistry must be investigated immediately by the regulatory body. Any professional accused will be suspended, desk-based or their dentistry license permanently terminated if found guilty of misconduct.

General Optical Council (GOC)

The General Optical Council (GOC) is a statutory regulatory body that sets standards for education and training within the optical service, such as eye testing centres and eye surgeries within hospitals. The GOC regulates professionals and ensures they are accredited as well as trained to the required standards. The GOC maintains a register of professionals to ensure regulation and monitoring across optical services, including both optometrists and student optometrists. As with other regulatory bodies, the GOC will investigate any form of misconduct. Any professional accused will be suspended, desk-based or their optical license permanently terminated if found guilty of misconduct.

> **Research**
>
> For each of the regulatory bodies discussed in section A5.14, research and answer the following questions.
> 1. Who are they?
> 2. What do they do?
> 3. What professionals are registered to that body? Provide examples and summarise their role in health and social care.
> 4. Is the regulatory or registration body statutory or voluntary? Explain your answer.

A5.15 The consequences of not maintaining a 'duty of care'

In section A5.13, the definition of duty of care was discussed. Now we will focus on the consequences and disruption to patients and service users if it is not upheld.

If professionals breach their duty of care, they are putting service users and their job at risk. It could lead to a potentially life-threatening illness or injury, or psychological and emotional damage to the service user. In that scenario, the service user is within their rights to sue the person or organisation as they have breached their responsibilities within health or social care. The service user may be awarded compensation, and the professional may lose their job.

The organisation may face the loss of service users if the community no longer trusts the care that they provide. This may have implications for other public health services, which may become overcrowded as a result. Furthermore, if the public lacks trust within services they may not wish to attend appointments or seek health or social care and, therefore, their health and wellbeing will decline.

Poor working practice in health and social care has led to a number of major high-profile cases, causing new legislation to be brought in and regulatory bodies to become further involved in maintaining high-quality care.

A5.16 The purpose of the relevant legislation in the healthcare science sector, in relation to rights of the individual

There are a variety of laws that health and social care settings must abide by to ensure high standards are set.

Legislation is legally binding information that must be upheld in all organisations. The reasoning for much of the legislation relevant to this sector is to ensure staff and individuals' rights are protected. All service users have the right to be treated equaly and fairly within health and social care settings to ensure they receive exemplary care that meets their specific needs.

Employment Relations Act 2004

The Employment Relations Act 2004 provides standardised rights within employment for health and social care workers. The act enables workers to work full-time or part-time hours within a setting and still receive the same number of rights: the number of hours should not determine the protection of individual rights. Professionals may register with a union and a regulatory body to gain support and advice when needed. This act outlines the requirements around the recognition of trade unions in a workplace. Furthermore, the act entitles employees to certain expected working conditions, a specific amount of notice related to their **termination** (losing their job) or contract or if they are to hand in their resignation, and holiday allowances within the year.

Employment Rights Act 1996

The Employment Rights Act 1996 protects employees from being dismissed from their jobs in an unfair way or without any reason. It protects employee rights and requires any dismissal to be thoroughly justified by the employer.

Data Protection Act 2018 (GDPR)

The Data Protection Act 2018 incorporates the General Data Protection Regulations (GDPR) from the EU into UK law. This act controls how personal information may be used and maintained. Personal information must be kept secure and should only be shared among those who require it, for example a multidisciplinary team if necessary to provide a variety of care to a service user: here, the service user must be informed that the information is going to be used, shared and stored. Furthermore, individuals have the right to access the information that an organisation holds on them at any time, and to request that it is deleted after the period when it is no longer needed. The information must not be used for any other purpose than what it is collected for, or shared with anyone who does not need to be aware of a service users' circumstances, i.e. it cannot be shared across medical professionals or organisations that are not directly linked with the patients' care.

Public Interest Disclosure Act 1998 (PIDA)

The Public Interest Disclosure Act 1998 (PIDA) enforces protection against any wrongdoing within the public services. If staff or the public experience any form of wrongdoing or victimisation, they are entitled to disclose this information publicly, to raise concerns to appropriate sector management and seek support from lawyers or the justice system, and to receive compensation from the company that did any wrongdoing. PIDA is therefore designed to protect both service users and health and social care workers who experience risk to their health and safety.

> **Reflect**
>
> For each piece of legislation in section A5.16, explain what it is and why it is needed within health and social care. Use specific examples that relate to a chosen health or social care setting. Ask your tutor for help if you need it.

A5.17 The importance and application of probity and candour in a healthcare science setting

All health and social care professionals must be open and honest with their patients and service users. If something was to unfortunately go wrong with patient care, the professional must inform the patient or their advocate. The patient should then be given a full explanation of the short-term and long-term implications of the incident, receive an apology and, finally, be provided the correct support.

Demonstrating integrity and building trust with service users

Integrity means being honest; a professional within health and social care services must always uphold this. Integrity also means to have moral principles; a professional must demonstrate this to maintain effective relationships with patients and colleagues. Without trust, service users may lose faith in their services, which may affect whether they seek advice from health or social care services in the future. A professional will face many challenges but they must remember to be transparent; it is essential that the professional builds a strong, trustworthy relationship with the individuals they work with in order to have effective outcomes.

Trust is a fundamental part of health and social care. Patients need to be able to trust the professionals they work with for assessments, treatment and further support. Trusting relationships improve patient outcomes – if patients believe the information being provided they are more likely to follow guidance given.

Acting without discrimination

Anti-discrimination policies are an integral part of health and social care. All service users have the right to receive appropriate care according to their needs. A service user should not be discriminated on any grounds that are protected by the Equality Act 2010 (see Chapter A1 for further information on this). Discrimination may be open and direct towards the service user, or indirect and less obvious, but both are unacceptable. Different cultures, religions or other beliefs should not affect the care given to a service user.

> **Test yourself**
>
> 1. Identify the nine protected characteristics in the Equality Act 2010.
> 2. How does the Equality Act cover maternity needs for new mothers?
> 3. What action can a patient take if they feel they have been racially discriminated against?

Respecting service users' dignity and choices

Service users should be empowered and able to make their own choices, whether it be about their clothing, if they receive daily support, or in terms of treatment and care. Dignity refers to respect and maintaining privacy, as demonstrated by respectiing a service user's space and handling personal hygiene activities in a sensitive manner. For example, if a service user may require support with personal hygiene, a professional should ask them whether they require support first and, if they do, the professional must explain how they will help beforehand. If a patient is able to wash themselves, they should be allowed to do so: the professional should not take away their independence but instead they should ask and consider the service user's needs.

Respect for service users' choices and preferences is an integral part of non-discriminatory practice and providing excellent care to patients. For example, professionals must respect how patients wish to be addressed or any cultural choices, and this should not affect the quality of care provided. Other examples include respecting individual diet choice, whether for cultural or religious needs such as Kosher or Halal, or personal preference.

Being open and honest with service users

All service users have the right to receive open and honest answers to their questions, and a professional must be transparent with patients. For example, if anything goes wrong during patient care or surgery, the patient must be made aware, even if this is uncomfortable for the professional. If a patient's health deteriorates even though they have received specific treatment to prevent or mitigate this, a professional must be honest about the condition. Honest, supportive relationships help to build trust. Being open is also important between professionals; for example, if a professional requires support or has mistreated or misdiagnosed a patient, they must discuss this with their superior to prevent further damage or health conditions.

A5.18 The consequences of failing to maintain the duty of candour

As discussed in section A5.17, candour incorporates the duty of being honest and transparent with individuals. Failure to maintain the duty of candour can be detrimental to trust and can lead to negative patient outcomes.

The impact of failure of duty of candour:
- failure to build rapport with service users
- decrease in open and honest communication with service users
- poor patient outcomes
- organisational reputational damage or failure
- professional reputational damage
- decrease in public confidence
- economic impact.

If a professional does not maintain candour within their setting, this may cause a barrier between them and service users, or between themselves and other professionals. Barriers can create tension and, therefore, decrease any relationship building due to the lack of trust and feeling valued. The service users are then more likely to discontinue using that service in particular, or further health and social care services in general, which can consequently decrease positive patient outcomes and cause deterioration of a service user's health.

Economic impact applies to the wider effects of failure of duty of candour. Poor quality of care causes issues within wider care, for example patient information may not be shared adequately or the patient's health may deteriorate due to a misdiagnosis, therefore causing more strain on specialist services.

A5.19 The principles of the six Cs

The six Cs are principles that professionals uphold to ensure service user outcomes are at the forefront of care. They incorporate six different areas of importance:

- care
- compassion
- communication
- courage
- commitment
- competence.

The six Cs help to support strategies in health and social care settings by underpinning a supportive culture and positive practice.

Care

By providing a caring atmosphere, professionals can build positive relationships. Service users expect to be treated with the utmost care through supporting methods and techniques. This helps the individual and improves the health of the whole community.

Compassion

Respect and dignity ensure the patient is given privacy when needed and that their choices are respected. Professionals must value service users' rights and show empathy. To uphold respect and dignity, service users must be provided with their own personal space, they should be able to dress how they want, to go to bed at their desired time and eat according to their dietary preferences. Service users should be given the opportunity to spend their day how they wish; professionals should not force service users into tasks or events they do not wish to take part in. Professionals must also ensure they address service users in the way that they wish to be addressed, for example by their first name or by their title and surname.

Communication

We have already discussed many ways in which good communication is central to care: see section A5.10 for instance. Remember that listening carefully is a key part of communication. It also involves written communication, for instance, keeping records and other documents up to date and complete to the right level of detail.

Courage

To show courage is to be brave. Courage enables professionals to identify any poor practice within a healthcare setting and report any incidents or concerns where necessary.

Commitment

Quality care is about providing the necessary measures for each patient and striving to provide patient-focused care. To do this it is important that employees are trained effectively and have the necessary qualifications that support their role.

Competence

Competence means the ability to do one's job or a given task. It includes the ability to identify and understand a range of service users' physical, intellectual, emotional and social needs. A professional must be competent while working with service users in their settings. Competent care results in effective care and treatment, as it ensures professionals are working according to their roles and responsibilities.

> **Reflect**
>
> Consider a time when you have used the six Cs during work experience.
> - Think about how you displayed the six Cs.
> - Consider whether there were any areas of improvement for future practice.

A5.20 The relationship between partnership working and the provision of person-centred care

Person-centred care uses a holistic approach that promotes choice and empowerment for service users. To provide holistic care for a patient, the collaboration of a multidisciplinary team (a range of professionals working together to benefit the needs of a service user) may be necessary.

How and why practitioners work in partnership

Multi-agency work means organisations working together to meet a service user's needs.

Multidisciplinary work means health and social care practitioners with a variety of disciplines work together while upholding their individual roles and responsibilities. This ensures professionals work together effectively to meet a service user's needs. Practitioners working together must share need-to-know information (as permitted by legislation and policy), use effective communication skills, manage risks, refer where necessary, carry out assessments and ensure service users are provided with advocacy if required.

Inter-professional learning refers to observation of practice and education within a healthcare or science setting. For example, trainee GPs or newly qualified GPs will work closely with advanced, qualified GPs to observe their practice and the key skills needed to make sure they are able to use theoretical knowledge alongside practical skills within their work. Observation and collaborative practice encourages patient-centred focus, as it provides an opportunity for professionals to work together and gain further skills and confidence throughout their career.

Advocacy enables patients to be given a voice and, if necessary, a third-party person to speak on their behalf. For a third-party person to ensure adequate communication on behalf of the patient, there must be individual patient goals in place in their care plan so that the advocate can clarify and negotiate the best outcome for the individual.

Roles and responsibilities of practitioners within partnership working

Partnership is about ensuring that healthcare professionals work together effectively. This may be with a variety of teams including both health and social care professionals. Partnership work can also include the patient's family and close friends who may provide care for them.

Professionals must be able to communicate with honesty and openness when working with other teams and departments to support a service user's needs. Professionals working in a partnership will have a range of expertise and therefore should share appropriate knowledge when required. Professionals must also be aware of their limitations and seek support and refer patients where necessary.

All professionals involved in a patient's case must be aware of any safeguarding risks (see section A5.21) in order to protect the patient or others from harm.

Information must be communicated effectively across teams and services when working with a patient. Multidisciplinary teams must work together to provide effective outcomes for service users. Information should be shared according to confidentiality policies and procedures within organisations; patient records must be shared using encryption or confidential mailing, for example. Information must be recorded in a timely manner and accurately, so that other professionals can review and discuss it with the service user.

Referrals may be necessary should a patient require specialised or immediate care, for example, a GP referring a patient to a radiologist for an X-ray, or referring a patient to counselling to help with depression or anxiety.

Finally, partnership working requires the input of service users themselves. They must be able to make their own choices and be informed of any referrals, assessment or treatment. A service user may need an advocate to support them in making decisions. Reasons for an advocate may be due to the patient being under legal adult consenting age, mental capacity or communication needs.

A5.21 The principles of safeguarding, found in the Health and Social Care Act 2012

The Health and Social Care Act 2012 provides an outline of how the range of services within the NHS and private practices must meet standards to protect vulnerable service users, staff and the general public. Members of health and social care organisations must adhere to the provisions within the act to provide good practice and work towards upholding excellent standards of care. It is also useful to help ensure any malpractice is identified, reported and dealt with immediately.

The six principles of adult safeguarding

Safeguarding ensures the protection of all vulnerable individuals and is supported by a range of legislation. Six key principles are upheld by the Health and Social Care Act 2012 specifically, and so are maintained in health and social care services. These are:
- empowerment
- prevention
- protection
- partnership
- proportionality
- accountability.

Empowerment

Providing opportunity and choice in health and social care is important to ensure the service user is cared for appropriately and holistically. Empowerment is a key aspect within this sector to ensure service users are supported to be independent. If choice is restricted, service users may suffer from inefficient care and their needs may not be met. Having service users make their own decisions helps them to take control of their own wellbeing. Service users and patients must be able to discuss their views and beliefs without these being challenged by the professionals working with them. To do otherwise may lead to abuse or neglect.

Prevention

It is more effective to take action before harm occurs, so prevention is a major responsibility in safeguarding. Professionals working within the health and social care sector must be aware of their responsibilities of prevention when working closely with vulnerable patients, no matter what their age may be. For example, during a check up with a child in a GP surgery, if the nurse or doctor examining them is concerned with bruises on the child's torso, they must respond to this concern immediately, in line with the setting's safeguarding policy, including reporting it on the relevant system to ensure it is appropriately followed up.

Protection

A professional has a duty of care to safeguard their service users, and this includes enabling service users to live free from harm or abuse. It is a human right for individuals, no matter what their protected characteristics may be, to be provided with effective care and support on a daily basis. Protection is a key component for professionals who work within health and social care services as there are a variety of vulnerable individuals involved.

Service users also have the right to appropriate representation should they require it. For example, if a child has been removed from their home due to abusive parents, child protection services will be responsible for them and act on behalf of the child to ensure their protection against harm. Support and appropriate service teams, including a legal and social care team, should enable the child's case to be dealt with appropriately.

Partnership

As discussed previously, multi-agency working means organisations work together to meet a service user's needs.

Proportionality

Proportionality considers aspects of safeguarding for individuals of all ages. Professionals working with vulnerable service users need to ensure they are aware of the safeguarding policies and procedures for the organisation they work in. When dealing with a safeguarding issue, it is important to approach it in a sensitive way that ensures the service user is not put in a difficult position and it is not unnecessarily disruptive. Professionals should ensure they ask appropriate questions, not be overly intrusive and, finally, make sure they report and record all evidence accurately. The service user must be aware when, due to safeguarding, information will need to be passed on to other relevant professionals to support the service user, and that it therefore cannot be kept entirely confidential.

> **Practice point**
>
> Consider a scenario where you may need to break confidentiality for a valid reason, for instance safeguarding.
>
> Explain the scenario to your partner and discuss whether this would indeed be necessary in that situation.
>
> Be sure to not use names of any real people or places in your examples.

Accountability

Accountability is about ensuring we are responsible for our actions or those that we have omitted to do. All professionals must play a part in ensuring they safeguard their service users by following safeguarding policies and procedures. Regulatory bodies ensure healthcare professionals are accountable for their actions, so professionals should be able to identify the actions they have taken and know they have done all they can.

Everyone within a service has a role to uphold; the roles within the organisation should be clear to ensure staff are aware of their expected responsibilities. However, everyone working within healthcare science services must make it their responsibility to be aware of any concerns or changes within patients' lives that may impact them or cause harm.

> **Case study**
>
> Emmet is 68 years old. Emmet's wife recently had a stroke and needs to spend time in hospital recovering. Emmet found a lump in one of his testicles, which was recently diagnosed as cancerous. Emmet and his wife have two children who are now 35 and 38 years old. Emmet's dad died of cancer at the age of 70, and he now fears the same happening to him. Emmet has developed severe depression and finds it difficult to socialise with family and friends. He used to enjoy visiting his golf club and saw his children and grandchildren regularly; this has stopped within the last six months, however. Emmet refuses to attend his follow-up appointments with the GP and surgeons at the hospital. Emmet's wife has found search history on Emmet's computer about euthanasia.
> 1. Name at least two professionals that should be involved with Emmet's care.
> 2. Identify any alarming signs of Emmet's health and wellbeing within this scenario. Explain your reasoning.
> 3. Discuss ways you could implement care into Emmet and his family's life that will support his own as well as his family's health and wellbeing.

A5.22 The signs and symptoms of different types of abuse and harm

Abuse and harm can take many different forms. When someone is abusive towards another person, it is a way to show power and control. The abuser may humiliate and belittle their victim to show a hierarchy of power. Within healthcare science it is important to be able to identify abuse and harm to prevent any serious or continuous maltreatment to service users or staff. Employees within the health and social care sector must receive adequate training on a regular basis to equip them to recognise signs of abuse and neglect. The Prevent programme incorporates safeguarding within health, social care and public services with respect to terrorism and vulnerability to radicalisation. We will now explore the various types of abuse and some ways to spot the effects in individuals.

Types of physical abuse and harm

Breast ironing

Breast ironing (also known as breast flattening) is a practice that occurs in some cultures where, to delay the process of breast growth in young girls approaching puberty, hot objects are used to 'iron' the breasts to try to stop breast tissue growth. Another form may be bandaging young girls' chests. The reasoning behind this is to prevent young girls being seen as sexual objects and therefore help prevent rape, abduction or early forced marriages, and to instead enable them to stay in education for longer.

Breast ironing can have serious long-term and short-term effects on a child's health such as infection, tissue damage, uneven development of breasts, cysts and abscesses. There may be an increased risk of cancer as a result of this form of abuse.

There is no specific legislation relating directly to breast ironing; however, it constitutes child abuse and it may be prosecuted under assault or child cruelty offences [Source: www.cps.gov.uk/cps/news/breast-ironing-recognised-child-cruelty-and-assault-cps]. There are signs and symptoms professionals should be aware of to identify potential breast ironing, such as the avoidance of medical examinations, a refusal to get changed in front of anybody, disruptive behaviour, withdrawal, signs of feeling uncomfortable, difficulty lifting arms and walking or sitting hunched over.

Female genital mutilation (FGM)

The Serious Crime Act 2015 was introduced to make practices such as **female genital mutilation (FGM),** domestic violence and coercive control specific criminal offences.

FGM is a form of female circumcision that involves the removal of all or some of the female genitalia. This practice is more common in Africa and Asia, but it can also take place in the UK; women and girls may also be taken to different countries to have this completed. It is a major concern within the Prevent strategy.

Sexual

Sexual abuse involves any sexual act carried out on an individual without consent. Sexual abuse can be a violent act in which the perpetrator coerces the victim into performing sexual acts against their will, but any act that is not agreed to or where the individual does not have the freedom to not agree to it (including children or adults lacking capacity to consent) is considered to be without consent. Rape is just one form of sexual abuse. Taking pictures or video recordings focusing on sexual acts can also be a form of sexual abuse or harassment as it humiliates and degrades the individual involved. Sexual harassment does not have to be in person: it can also take place over social media, voice recordings or text messages.

Hitting

Hitting is a form of violent abuse that deliberately causes harm to the victim. This can take place in the context of domestic violence by a partner, causing physical trauma. However, physical abuse can happen to a variety of individuals; anyone can be a victim of physical abuse no matter what age or gender, and regardless of their relationship with the abuser. Someone suffering from physical abuse may show signs and symptoms such as unexplained bruises, marks, scar or burns. Victims of physical abuse may become withdrawn or flinch when around other individuals.

> **Research**
>
> Research one of the following widely reported incidents of child abuse. Use the links below as a starting point and refer to reputable sources.
> - Baby P, www.bbc.co.uk/news/uk-11626806
> - Arthur Labinjo-Hughes, www.bbc.co.uk/news/uk-59519562
>
> Using your chosen case study, complete the following questions:
> 1. Identify the signs and symptoms related to abuse and neglect within the case study.
> 2. Identify the professionals involved in each case.
> 3. Identify what went wrong in the investigations, if there were any, before the death of the child.
> 4. Outline actions that should have been taken.

Gaslighting

Gaslighting may occur in an abusive relationship. It describes manipulative tactics used by an abuser to distort the victim's sense of reality, for example by denying that abusive behaviour has happened. The victim may question themselves as to what is real, begin to doubt themselves and eventually blame themselves for the abuse they receive. The perpetrator will mislead the victim into a vicious cycle of guilt and blaming themselves. This is a covert method of abuse, meaning it can be difficult to identify signs of it.

Belittling

Belittling can cause an individual to feel undermined and insignificant and therefore feel inferior and humiliated. It is a type of emotional and psychological abuse.

Bullying

Bullying can take a range of different forms, such as emotional, psychological or physical abuse. A perpetrator may cause a victim to feel embarrassed or scared. A bully may pick on an individual's specific characteristics, or an individual's looks, height or weight to cause insecurities. Bullying causes the victim to feel intimidated and vulnerable.

Verbal abuse

Verbal abuse is a type of bullying where words are used that can cause intimidation and manipulation of the victim. The perpetrator may ridicule their victim and concentrate on a particular characteristic of the victim. Verbal abuse may cause the victim to feel powerless and as if they have lost control of their own voice.

Possible signs of emotional/psychological abuse

Depression

Depression results in an individual feeling persistently down (hopeless, lacking motivation and losing interest in things they enjoy) for a long period of time. When an individual is emotionally abused, they may feel fear and guilt, causing an emotional oppression. Emotional abuse causes the individual to feel as though they are at fault rather than the perpetrator.

Low self-esteem

Low self-esteem is when someone has persistent negative feelings about themselves and lacks confidence. Low self-esteem may be the result of emotional or psychological abuse, for instance through constant criticism or being made to feel guilty. However, existing low self-esteem can make it easier for a perpetrator to emotionally abuse an individual. If the individual does not have a positive image of themselves, it makes it easier for an abuser to identify factors that cause further distress to them.

A5: Providing person-centred care when working in healthcare science

Types of organisational abuse

Organisational abuse is where abuse is perpetuated throughout an organisation as part of its culture. This includes the maltreatment and negligence of service users at residential settings.

Some examples of organisational abuse may include habitual mistreatment of service users, no choices at mealtimes and not respecting or upholding cultural and religious rights.

This can also include removing the right to empowerment and choice. Forcing a service user into a decision is a violation of their rights and can have serious implications for their mental and physical wellbeing.

Possible signs of neglect

Neglect means not meeting the sufficient caring standards. There are two main forms of neglect: self-neglect and neglect due to others.

Self-neglect is where an individual neglects their own basic needs. This may include hygiene, clothing, starving or overeating, or neglecting to take medications that they have been prescribed. For example, an individual consistently looking unkempt or not bathing for several days in a row is a form of self-neglect.

Neglect due to others is related to failure to appropriately care for another individual. The signs of this are similar to self-neglect, but it occurs when a person is unable to independently take care of themselves and, therefore, requires help. An example would be not providing the service user with a substantial healthy meal on a regular basis, which may lead to malnutrition.

If any signs of abuse or neglect are identified within health and social care, the organisational policies and procedures must be followed.

Test yourself

An elderly service user was seriously scalded and injured during bathing.
1. What legislation would you need to follow to report this?
2. What actions should you take if you suspected abuse or neglect within your organisation?
3. Describe organisational abuse with a clear example.
4. Explain how emotional/psychological abuse may result in an individual feeling depressed and anxious.

Types of financial abuse

Financial abuse can entail withholding or taking a service user's money or financial assets in order to control them or restrict their freedom of choice. If professionals accept overly expensive gifts from service users it may be seen as financial abuse, as it could become an expectation for the service user to continually provide expensive and elaborate gifts, or a sign of coercion, where the professional manipulates them into doing this. Signs of financial abuse can include a service user getting into debt, missing or losing belongings, or a sudden lack of money. Financial abuse will be described within organisational policies to ensure professionals are aware of gift acceptance limitations to ensure professional boundaries are not crossed.

A5.23 Signs and symptoms of radicalisation as outlined in the Prevent strategy 2011

Prevent is a government programme focusing on ensuring terrorism is challenged and that any concerns about potential **radicalisation** are dealt with promptly. Prevent strategies are designed to help identify when individuals may be drawn to terrorist groups or cults, and protecting those who are vulnerable to this. In health and social care services (as well as among others, such as faith leaders, teachers and medical professionals) it is important to acknowledge signs of radicalisation and to refer the individuals to the local Prevent body.

Signs of radicalisation in an individual

Radicalisation involves extreme views that are related to social, political or religious beliefs. It involves the coercion of an individual or a group of individuals into changing their views. Radical groups create fear among their followers and can therefore lead them to violent action. One result of radicalisation could be terrorism.

An individual with extremist or radicalised views may be unwilling to discuss their views out loud with a group of individuals outside of their organisation. The individual may also display discriminatory behaviour towards others due to their gender identification, sexual preferences, religious beliefs or social beliefs. They may become easily agitated and overtly angry in some situations.

As professionals in a heathcare setting may encounter radicalisation or extremism, it is important to be aware of and able to identify the signs. If an individual has concerns over a service user or another professional, they must report this. This can be done via their line manager, Prevent officer, whistle-blowing or to their organisational body.

Terrorist or extremist groups may target individuals with vulnerabilities such as low self-esteem, confusion about their faith, victims of bullying or individuals suffering from anger due to feeling unfairly treated by society.

It can be difficult to identify when an individual is at risk of being exploited and manipulated into extremist ideologies. Signs may include increased secretive behaviour; 'script talking', meaning speaking as if they are being told what they can and cannot say; hostility towards others; changing of friendship groups and withdrawal from loved ones. Individuals who are exposed to radicalised views may also be unwilling to discuss their individual opinions as they need to remain inconspicuous and hide that they are part of a terrorist group.

Individuals who are part of radical and terrorist groups may show extreme levels of anger and disregard for others' opinions, beliefs and values. They will not want to discuss their beliefs openly with those who are not involved in their group as there is no form of trust with others outside of their group. Therefore, they may begin to be disrespectful to family members, teachers, professionals and friends if they disagree with their ideologies.

Isolation may be a key sign that an individual is being radicalised. They may spend a lot of time alone, in private locations or in their room in order to carry out secretive research on the internet or use chat rooms.

A5.24 How individuals' mental and physical capacity can influence their needs in relation to overall care

Mental and physical capacity relates to an individual's ability to do things. A service user may have been born with or have experienced an injury that causes them to have limited physical or cognitive ability. Therefore, the service user will require support from relevant services, depending on their condition.

Mental health capacity

This relates to the ability of an individual to process and understand information. An individual may not have the metal capacity to make decisions and therefore require an advocate to speak on their behalf, but others may just need different ways to communicate and for this to be facilitated. Lack of capacity is determined through measures outlined in the Mental Capacity Act 2005 and is dependent upon the severity of conditions.

Conditions that involve lower mental capacity include:
- dementia
- brain damage
- cognitive impairment
- certain mental health illnesses
- stroke
- severe learning disabilities or difficulties.

The following link gives further information about the criteria and procedures in cases where there is a lack of capacity: www.nhs.uk/conditions/social-care-and-support-guide/making-decisions-for-someone-else

Neurodiversity conditions

Neurodiversity is a concept that recognises the differences between the brains of different individuals and that these are seen as normal. Individuals who are **neurodivergent** (as opposed to **neurotypical**) experience the world in a unique way. Increasing awareness around this helps to reduce stigma and, therefore, causes others to identify diversity and accept others.

Common neurodiversity conditions are outlined in the following table.

Condition	Description
ADHD (attention deficit hyperactivity disorder)	Attention is affected, such as the feeling of restlessness, impulsive actions and behaviours.
Dyspraxia	Dyspraxia is also known as developmental co-ordination disorder (DCD): a child may appear to be clumsy; physical co-ordination is affected, preventing a child from performing as expected at different developmental ages.
Dyslexia	This learning difficulty can cause a variety of problems for an individual in reading, writing and spelling. It is often characterised by confusion of letters in words, such as their order or putting letters the wrong way round.
ASC (autism spectrum conditions)	Autism spectrum conditions, as the name suggests, are on a continuum with a lot of variety in how individuals with them present. The individual may have difficulty socialising and communicating effectively with others. Repetitive behaviours may also be apparent in those with ASD.

A5: Providing person-centred care when working in healthcare science

> **Research**
>
> A few neurodiverse conditions are mentioned in the table above. Research other conditions that are also considered to be neurodiverse. Choose two and explain how they manifest themselves in an individual.

Learning disability (for example, Down's syndrome, cerebral palsy, global developmental delay syndrome)

Individuals with learning disabilities have a variety of different and complex needs, and they may not be able to live independently. Learning disabilities may be caused by a variety of factors such as complications during pregnancy, lack of oxygen at birth, genetic factors, illnesses or severe accidents. An individual with learning disabilities may have profound needs and require support with many elements of their life such as eating, bathing, communicating and general personal care.

Condition	Description
Down's syndrome	This is caused by extra chromosomes in a individuals' cells. A child with this condition may take longer to reach developmental milestones and need further support throughout their lifetime. Other related characteristics may include heart defects, other learning disabilities and distinctive physical features.
Cerebral palsy	Cerebral palsy covers a group of conditions affecting an individual's balance and posture due to a dysfunction in the brain causing weakness in the muscles. The individual's brain development is abnormal or may be damaged; this normally happens at or shortly after birth or while a child is developing the womb.
Global developmental delay syndrome	This is an umbrella term for when a child takes longer to reach certain developmental milestones than other children of their age. Individuals will be delayed cognitively and physically, which therefore affects their **motor skills** (muscle movements, such as walking), speech, cognitive skills, social and emotional development.

Physical capacity

Condition	Description
Spinal cord injury	Damage to the spinal cord or nerves can cause permanent changes in bodily functions and an individual's strength. Their ability to control limbs may be affected dependent on the type and severity of the injury. Paralysis may also occur from spinal cord injury.
Arthritis	The most common types are osteoarthritis and rheumatoid arthritis. Arthritis causes pain and inflammation in the joints. It can develop at any age and can severely restrict movement and cause muscle wasting.
Musculoskeletal injury	Some examples of musculoskeletal injuries and disorders include tendinitis, carpal tunnel syndrome and lower back injuries. These injuries and disorders can affect any individual at any age, causing difficulty in the individual's movement and severe pain.

> **Research**
>
> Research and complete a revision poster on two types of arthritis.
>
> Research and complete a revision poster on at least two different types of musculoskeletal disorder.

Communication and comprehension considerations

Communication needs must be considered when supporting an individual with learning disabilities. Many individuals will prefer face-to-face communication. Clear use of vocabulary and concise wording is also essential. Professionals should avoid using jargon when communicating: if technical terms are used, the professional should clearly explain their meaning. It may be worth considering the use of imagery or written language to enable a service user to understand, or the use of an advocate.

When working with an individual who is neurodivergent, professionals should avoid sarcasm to avoid confusion. Direct and concise sentences should be used to enable clear understanding, and elaboration on conversations may need to happen to check understanding. Written instructions or diagrams may be useful when communicating with someone who is neurodivergent as they may understand visual communication more than verbal. Non-verbal methods such as gestures and the use of touch will also need to be considered as some individuals may find it unnerving, unpleasant or confusing.

The use of imagery such as icons may enhance understanding in addition to enabling communication building.

An individual may have additional care needs, such as hearing or visual impairments. Professionals must consider techniques that enable these individuals to communicate effectively, for example the use of sign language, imagery, **augmentative and alternative communication** (**AAC**) or Braille.

AAC is often used by individuals who have communication difficulties. This system includes the use of communication boards and books, signing (such as British Sign Language) and Makaton, which uses signs, speech and symbols as well as voice output communications (VOCAs). Comedian Lee Ridley ('The Lost Voice Guy'), who has cerebral palsy, uses an automated voice on his iPad to speak to his audience.

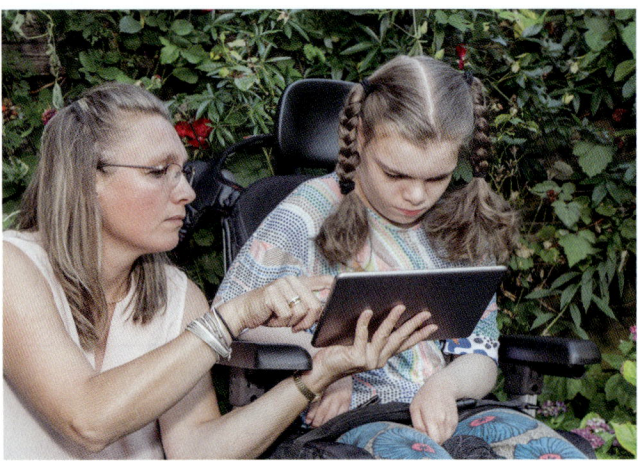

▲ Figure 5.5 Augmentative and alternative communication

Extra monitoring and specific care needs

When identifying that an individual has needs due to neurodivergence or another condition, it is important to make adjustments to accommodate their needs. Professionals should be patient when communicating and understand that it may take longer for them to understand the conversation. Professionals should also be aware of sensory sensitivities among neurodivergent individuals, e.g. smells, bright lights and loud noises, which can distress an individual; the setting should therefore be appropriate for the service user before they take part in communication.

If a service user requires medication, a professional must consider their needs and background history. It is important to investigate any allergies or illnesses that may affect future medication. Administration of medication must also be considered – it may be that a parent, guardian or carer needs to administer the medication, but the service user must be aware of this. For example, a child would need a parent or guardian to administer the correct dose of medication to them for safety reasons.

Consent

Consent of the patients is imperative to ensure the service user is happy with the treatment they are receiving. They must also be aware of any implications of treatment or side effects. Professionals must take any additional needs of the service user into consideration to identify whether they require an advocate or parent/guardian to consent for them.

> ### Case study
>
> Damien is a four-year-old boy who has a delay in social skills. He has demonstrated repetitive behaviours such as hand flapping while frustrated. Damien's preschool teacher has also noticed him biting his classmates and spitting. His teacher brought this up with his parents who are also concerned and have taken him to see his GP.
>
> Answer the following questions:
> ▶ Suggest one neurodiverse condition that Damien may be diagnosed with.
> ▶ Assess the range of professionals that may need to be involved in Damien's care, as well as support groups that could be beneficial.

A5.25 The impact of dementia on an individual's needs

Dementia is the loss of an individual's cognitive functioning, which affects their thinking, memory and skills such as reasoning. Short-term memory is affected; people will often notice that someone with dementia will still be able to recall long-term memories however. An individual with dementia may also find it difficult to control their emotions, meaning they may have sudden outbursts of frustration, anger or distress. It can be difficult for an individual with dementia to remain completely independent as the condition will deteriorate. Therefore, they may require assistance or daily care to help support them with everyday tasks.

May require support with day-to-day living

Daily routines may become difficult for an individual with dementia because they may find it difficult to cope with tasks involving accurate short-term memory. An individual with dementia may require care to help them with daily living tasks such as eating, bathing and mobility. A care professional can provide support by introducing the individual to social events and activities that will help them to engage with others. Short activities can also be useful to help ease distress for a patient with dementia. If the patient's welfare becomes a major concern, they may need to go into 24-hour care living to prevent any hazards from occurring.

Simple instructions and conversations should be considered when communicating with a patient with dementia to ensure understanding. For example, use simple sentences and easy questions such as closed questions if applicable. Closed questions give the individual an opportunity to answer with a simple, yes or no answer.

Treatment requirements and support

There is currently no cure for dementia; however, there are treatments available to ease the effects and progression of the disease. At the time of writing, commonly used drugs include rivastigmine, galantamine, memantine and donepezil. These drugs are known as cholinesterase inhibitors; they all work in a similar way but each have different side effects and work differently for each individual. Individuals with Alzheimer's disease have low levels of acetylcholine, which helps to send messages between nerve cells. These cells become damaged, causing the disease to progressively become worse and an individual's brain to deteriorate. Use of these drugs can help to improve communication between nerve cells, therefore easing some symptoms.

Therapies can also be helpful for individuals suffering from dementia, such as dance therapy, massage or aromatherapy. Therapies can be useful to help with memory training and prevent frustration.

There are a variety of organisations and charities, such as Alzheimer's UK or Age UK to name a few, that help to support individuals with dementia. They provide group support, medical and non-medical solutions, as well as extra care support. It is also important to recognise the importance of supporting family members and friends whose loved ones have been diagnosed with Alzheimer's or dementia, as it can be challenging to manage the changes these diseases cause.

Trials and medical research

Trials and research are ongoing for dementia as there is still no known way to prevent the disease from occurring. Drugs are continuously tested and trialled to support further understanding of current treatments and develop new and improved treatments for dementia. Non-drug interventions also are continually trialled and tested to improve outcomes.

Research into preventative methods includes investigating individual behaviour, social factors and lifestyle choices. For example, preventative methods to reduce the major impacts of early onset dementia include quitting smoking, reducing alcohol intake, keeping active, socialising and maintaining a healthy balanced diet. Recommendations can be developed as a result of a series of large-scale and repeated clinical trials to establish probable causal relationships between lifestyle choices and the risks of developing this condition.

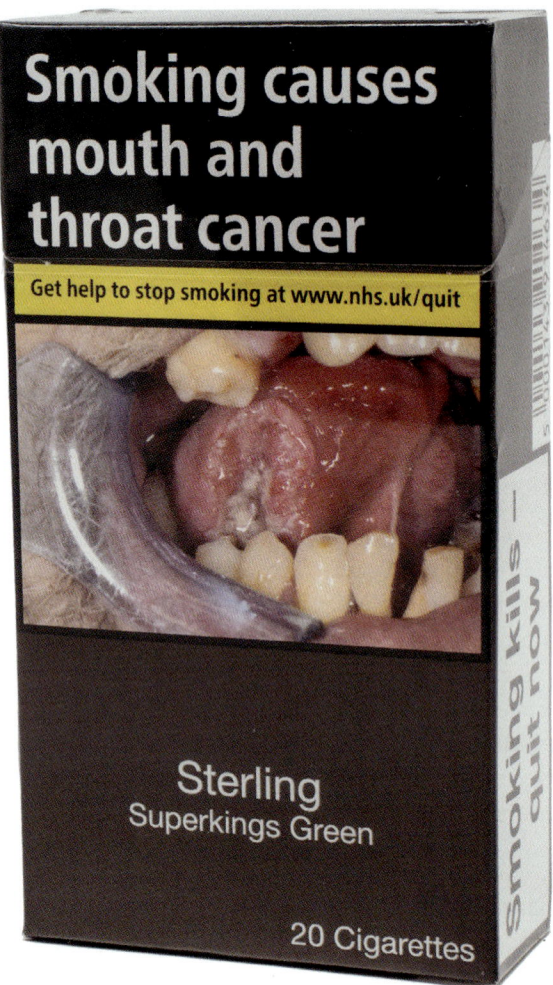

▲ Figure 5.6 Cigarette pack health warning

Clinical trials are continually ongoing to investigate new methods and preventative measures for illnesses and disorders. Relevant charities fund research into illnesses such as trials for cancer medication or cures, arthritis cures or prevention, Parkinson's cures or prevention. The NHS website also features trials and research into medical conditions and preventative methods. Results for research can be reviewed in a variety of ways such as through the government websites, charity websites, the NHS website and organisational bodies such as the HCPC.

When an individual participates within a trial, they must provide informed consent and make family or care members aware they are taking part in a trial in case anything goes wrong and they need further medical help. However, those not involved directly within the trial must not be given extensive details of the trial for confidential reasons. The participant has the right to withdraw from a trial at any point should they wish to (see section A5.4 for further information on this).

> **Practice point**
>
> During your course and any other higher education you may complete, you will be required to research and review a wide range of journals and articles.
>
> Here are some tips and hints to support you with this:
>
> ▶ Your college library or your virtual learning platform may have access to electronic journals and articles.
> ▶ Google Scholar is a great platform for searching a wide range of free electronic journals and articles.
> ▶ Charity websites often refer to a wide range of research to improve and prevent medical conditions. Look at websites such as the British Heart Foundation, Cancer Research and Age UK to review research journals and articles.
> ▶ Use organisational body websites or government websites to review current investigations into medical, clinical or preventative trials, such as https://gov.uk, www.nmc.org.uk, www.hcpc-uk.org or www.cqc.org.uk.
> ▶ Local community centres or hospitals may also conduct research into specific areas related to health conditions that need addressing within the community.
> ▶ Look for medical or psychological databases when investigating appropriate journals.

> **Research**
>
> Using the link that follows and wider research, complete a written report answering the following:
> ▶ Explain and evaluate the current medications for dementia.
> ▶ Investigate and describe current trials relating to dementia.
>
> www.alzheimersresearchuk.org

Appropriate person with power of attorney (financial and medical) and their implications for care

An individual with dementia has the right to make their own decisions as long as they have legal capacity; however, a **power of attorney** will need to be assigned for when the individual reaches mid- to final-term dementia. An individual with power of attorney will be able to make decisions on behalf of the individual with dementia. This should be considered at very early stages of the individual being diagnosed with dementia to enable them to appoint someone they trust.

> **Key term**
>
> **Power of attorney:** a legal document whereby an individual gives another person, usually a family member or friend, the official authority to make decisions in relation to health and welfare on their behalf, such as types of medical and non-medical care. This legal document only comes into effect once an individual with dementia has lost their capacity to make their own decisions.

As an individual's dementia progresses, a lasting power of attorney appoints at least one person as a trusted attorney to be responsible for making decisions on their behalf.

A5.26 The impact of learning difficulties on an individual's needs

Learning difficulties can affect individuals in a variety of ways. As ever, when providing care it is important to consider individual needs, such as physical, intellectual, emotional and social. (See section A5.24 for further information on some types of learning disabilities.) Providing person-centred care is imperative to ensure service users with learning disabilities are provided with effective support and understand communication effectively. The severity of the learning difficulty may affect a number of different aspects of an individual's life. For example, wellbeing may deteriorate more over time due to the individual becoming more aware of their learning difficulty and potential limitations this may cause. However, it is important to note that individuals with learning difficulties or disabilities must be empowered and provided with opportunities, otherwise this constitutes discrimination. The needs of an individual's condition should be reviewed by the appropriate professional to ensure support is in place where necessary, such as at home, work, in education or use of other services.

Requirement to adopt appropriate communication methods

Communication must always be clear and concise; be wary of using jargon and technical language. Consider the use of both verbal and non-verbal methods such as gestures, touch and the use of written language or pictures, such as AAC, for individuals with autism spectrum disorder, physical disabilities, cognitive impairments or cerebral palsy. Due to an individual's learning difficulty their understanding of written or verbal methods may vary (see section A5.24). Use of communication methods may include different use of colours on written forms of information for individuals with dyslexia, or use of space and body language to ensure the service user is comfortable. Pictures or verbal enhancement methods such as hearing aid loop systems could be suitable for those hard of hearing.

Tailor care appropriately to capacity and condition

All individuals have the right to the same opportunities, and valuing people in healthcare is essential to ensure inclusion. As such, it is important to communicate clearly when discussing the approaches and support being provided to service users with learning difficulties. Multidisciplinary working is also essential, so the patient should understand the meaning of this and the variety of professionals that may need to be involved. The service user should be aware of their conditions and the support and treatment that may need to be required.

Empathetic support

Empathy means being able to understand the emotions of others. Empathetic support is crucial when working with service users as they are each effectively experiencing diverse or difficult situations. A professional must remain objective and be able to put their own thoughts and feelings aside to provide empathetic support. A non-judgemental approach is also important when working with individuals with learning disabilities. A professional must work to support and listen to their needs. A professional should also remain patient with a service user if it takes the individual a longer time to communicate or understand the information.

Social and community support

Types of support can vary from charities and carers to religious communities. Social and community groups are good for encouraging service users to socialise with others who may be going through similar circumstances. Depending on the local area, there should be a variety of support groups available that a service user or someone supporting the service user should be able to research. Often healthcare workers will be aware of local support groups and can advise on this. A service user may find it useful to join one of their local community support groups; they provide an integrated approach for those who may need to discuss their thoughts and feelings.

Point of care testing requirements

To test a service user's learning disabilities, intelligence tests known as IQ tests are carried out. Point of care testing means that testing is carried out in the service user's home setting or living space. This helps to break down any barriers a service user may feel.

A5.27 How to promote independence and self-care strategies

Promotion of independence is a key aspect within health and social care as choice and opportunity for the patient should be at the forefront of care. A service user must feel as though they are effectively involved in their care and provided with necessary information that is communicated according to their needs.

Promotion of independence and self-care can help to boost service users' mental health as well as their physical health outcome. It allows confidence to develop and enables the service user to feel less dependent on others.

Education and empowerment of the service user

Empowering patients supports improved health and independence. When patients are educated about their illness or disorder, they can further engage with their own care. Ideally, if patients are aware of how their illness or disorder affects them, they should be able to incorporate useful lifestyle changes for further positive outcomes. Empowerment provides individuals with choices and opportunities to discuss their needs.

Emotional intelligence means the ability to understand one's own emotions. Being able to understand and manage your own emotions in positive ways is an important coping mechanism. A professional must also have emotional intelligence towards service users in order to empathise and communicate effectively.

Understanding health and wellbeing means it is possible to promote useful techniques for healthy lifestyles. It also encourages positive attitudes and provides the opportunity to take part in supportive methods such as exercise.

Self-care is also an important part of empowerment; a service user must be given the opportunity to take care of themselves independently where they can. If a service user requires support, for example when bathing, the professional must make the service user aware of the methods they will use and how they will support them. The service user is entitled to have preferences or to say no to any support offered; likewise, the professional must respect a service user's decisions when providing help with self-care.

Health tracking

If a patient is sufficiently educated, they can track their own illnesses and make any lifestyle changes and improvements that may be necessary. Tracking one's own health can improve upkeep of beneficial habits, such as maintaining a certain step count each day, healthy eating habits, exercise and good sleeping patterns. Encouraging a patient to track their own health and routine can improve the longevity of changes and enable more awareness of their own health conditions. Technology such as smartwatches; pedometers; applications on mobile phones and smart scales that monitor weight loss/gain, muscle mass and body water can be used to track and monitor health conditions and allow an individual to take control of their own health.

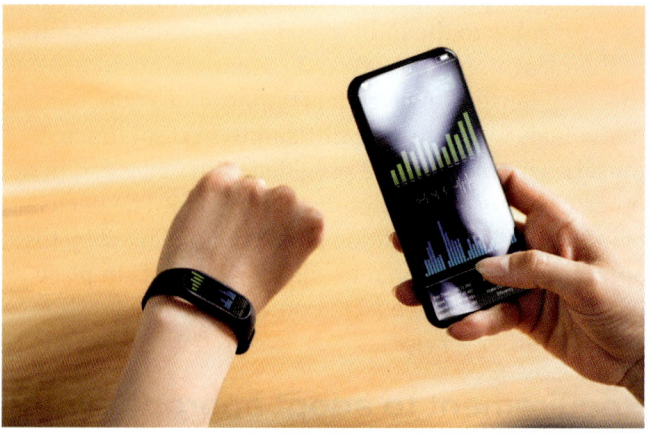

▲ Figure 5.7 Ways to monitor health and track exercise

A5: Providing person-centred care when working in healthcare science

Effective communication to patients/service users

Explaining strategies clearly

Strategies to promote independence must be effectively communicated to service users via a variety of methods. Use of clear techniques and strategies helps to provide understanding and knowledge of how a service user can still live independently with support where required. For example, the use of modifications around the home can enable service users to live independently, for example stair lifts or grab rails inside and outside the home to help with balance.

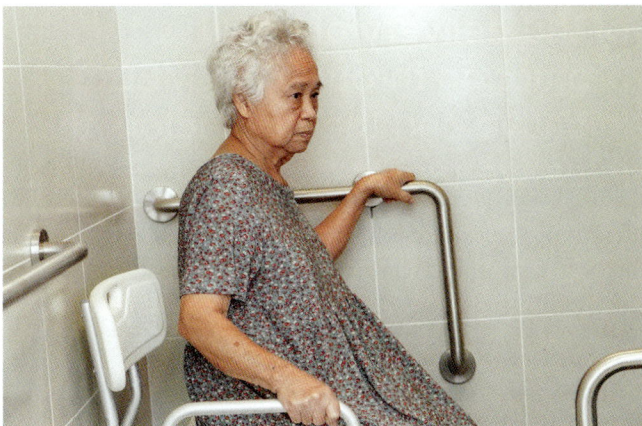

▲ Figure 5.8 Rails that can be placed in the bathroom to help with balance

Signposting to useful groups and resources

Support is essential for service users who may be undergoing major changes within their life. Professionals should provide advice and information on support groups either locally or nationally as service users may find this useful to further understand their own illness or disorder. Professionals can also provide service users with leaflets, telephone numbers and websites that will be useful for their condition. A range of support groups can be accessed, for example Child and Adolescent Mental Health Services (CAMHS) or Macmillan Nurses for cancer support.

Positive role modelling

A role model is a person that someone looks up to; in this context positive role models are useful for changing behaviours to promote positive outcomes. Support groups and charities help service users to identify positive role models who will help them to follow healthy lifestyles, change and overcome any barriers or potential health and wellbeing problems.

A5.28 The positive effects of promoting independence and self-care

Promotion of independence and self-care is important when working with service users as it helps to maintain a sense of control and develop positive relationships between them and professionals.

Service users need to be supported, but that does not mean taking their independence away from them. It is important to ensure that service users have choices and can make their own decisions when they need to. Lack of promotion of choice and empowerment may cause resentment and strained relationships between the service user and professional.

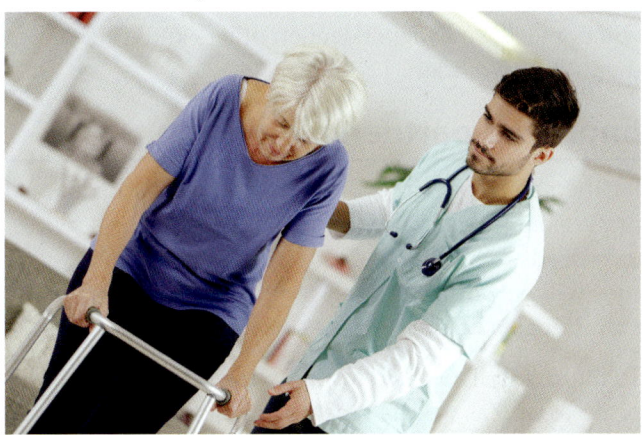

▲ Figure 5.9 A supportive moment between a healthcare professional and service user

Improved active participation

When a service user feels empowered, they will actively participate in their own care and find positive techniques and methods that enhance their daily lives. Independent living encourages the individual to control their actions and discuss their needs.

Enabling service users to recognise their rights and identify their involvement within their own care is an imperative part of providing services. Through active participation, the service user will be involved in their own planning and care, giving them the ability to discuss their own preferences for the care they wish to receive.

Improved self-esteem and independence

Choice and empowerment motivate the service user to become confident in their day-to-day routine. Professionals should encourage service users to be as independent as possible and to continue as much of their previous lifestyle as possible, ensuring they do not feel overly restricted and promoting good self-esteem.

Being viewed as a whole person – with consideration of physical, intellectual, emotional and social needs – provides the service user with positive feelings and outcomes. Independence supports high self-esteem as it encourages the individual to strive and achieve more; for example, if a service user is trying to build up daily strength to move themselves around with limited support, this will help to build their self-confidence. When a service user has high self-esteem they can build positive relationships with their carers, as they will not feel overly dependent on others and consider themselves a burden.

Improved partnership working

Partnership working involves service users and professionals working together effectively. The service user needs to be able to trust the professionals as they will be working closely together to help build a maintainable lifestyle for the service user.

To improve partnership working, the service user and professional, as well as other formal or informal carers, should work together harmoniously to provide the best support and care for the individual's needs. A service user needs to be able to share their ideas in relation to the care and support they receive. When the service user feels empowered and able to choose the care, they will respect the professionals they work with and trust the suggestions they may make in the future.

Improved healthcare staff time efficiency

Being efficient increases productivity and the ability to improve work for the benefit of a range of service users. With efficient working, professionals can also gain more personal satisfaction from the work they do; they will not feel as pressured or under as much stress as they may have previously. Empowering service users can help to relieve the workload for professionals, and managing time effectively enables a realistic schedule, realistic daily workload and reduction in work before it becomes overwhelming and has a knock-on effect on others. Keeping patients aware of timings such as when to take medication, meeting times and appointments also helps the patient to work out their own ways of completing these tasks.

Healthcare time efficiency supports maintainable workloads for professionals. Professionals should support service users to live as independently as possible so they do not become over-reliant on the professional. If a professional does not enable the service user to take care of themselves where possible, it can result in over dependency.

A5.29 The overarching principle of the delivery of health promotion through the MECC initiative and the risk factors this initiative targets

Health promotion of long-term illnesses is an important factor to maintain awareness of within society.

> 'Forty per cent of the UK's disability adjusted life years lost are attributable to tobacco, hypertension, alcohol, being overweight or being physically inactive.'
>
> Source: www.makingeverycontactcount.co.uk

Promoting the reduction of negative lifestyle habits such as smoking or excessive drinking can help to reduce the number of people with long-term illnesses and the detrimental effects this may have on an individual. Helping individuals to improve their health can be through the use of campaigns and support groups.

Using brief and very brief interventions whenever the opportunity arises

Making Every Contact Count (MECC) is an initiative from the UK government.

It is designed to be a simple approach to support individuals with mental health and wellbeing by providing opportunities to make positive changes to their lifestyle. This may be through routine appointments, such as with a GP, for example. MECC is useful to ensure individuals discuss their health and important factors that may be affecting this. The MECC approach is used in organisations like healthcare settings and social care settings such as schools; anyone is able to use the approach, whether it be service users, professionals or a patient's family members. Every individual should have the opportunity to discuss their health and wellbeing as it is an essential part of day-to-day life. Health advice may also be shared in schools and workplaces by providing wellbeing advice as well as healthy options with food and opportunities for exercise.

MECC enables organisations such as those listed previously to identify ways that individuals can seek and receive support throughout the transition of their lifestyle change. The use of support affects individuals in a positive way as it enables them to plan and continually monitor their progress.

Highlighting risk factors

Risk factors that MECC focuses on include:
- smoking
- poor diet
- alcohol consumption
- physical activity levels
- mental health and wellbeing.

When promoting health interventions, risk factors are identified that will impact an individual's health. The list above was chosen for the following reasons:
- Individuals who smoke may be more susceptible to illnesses such as cancer, stomach ulcers, heart disease, high cholesterol and many more debilitating long-term illnesses.
- Poor diet can increase the likelihood of heart disease, high blood pressure and high cholesterol due to lack of nutrients and increased pressure on organs due to increased fat in certain parts of the body.
- High alcohol consumption can lead to excess weight, liver disease, memory loss and other cognitive implications.
- Lack of physical activity can also increase the chance of obesity-related problems and increased fatigue.
- Mental health and wellbeing may be impacted by all these factors; however, external factors such as work, family life and long-term illnesses can also have a detrimental effect and emotional impact.

Social prescribing

Social prescribing means referring individuals to non-clinical settings for mental health and wellbeing services. The use of these services enables a wide range of measures to be implemented to provide positive outcomes for those seeking advice and guidance on their health and wellbeing.

Social prescribing allows individuals to take control of their own health and have the opportunity to seek support when they feel they need to. A professional who may identify the need to refer a patient on to a health and wellbeing service can do so by contacting local services in the community and providing the information to service users to contact them if they wish to. This gives the service user the opportunity to think about the benefits of contacting such services and whether it will be helpful for them.

Other ways to support individuals may be to signpost them to specific services. This may include writing a referral letter (with the service user's permission) to a health and wellbeing clinic. A service user may require support or therapy to help them overcome specific problematic areas. If a professional recognises this, they should provide the service user with information on where they can seek help.

When providing health information, such as advice on healthy eating and lifestyle changes, professionals need to consider factors such as access and the cost of these activities. Not all individuals have the same access to gyms, for instance, as they may be too expensive. Therefore, organisations and councils have started to implement ways to incorporate healthy living into individuals' daily lives, for example cheap gym memberships, access to gym equipment, and access to healthy food choices at work or other organisations such as schools.

A5.30 Strategies for promoting health and wellbeing within all aspects of care

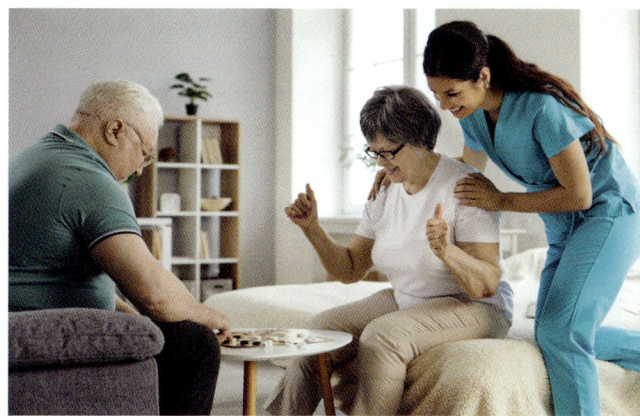

▲ Figure 5.10 A good relationship

Health promotion is an important factor for improving knowledge in a variety of areas. The information can be presented in a variety of ways such as guidance from health professionals, public health promotions and campaigns, charity organisations and through education.

Making Every Contact Count (MECC)

MECC is a useful approach for promoting health and wellbeing within health and social care services, as it provides information on how strategies can be implemented in a variety of services.

As discussed in section A5.29, the identification of potential risk factors to individual health is important when supporting service users to make health improvements. Individuals should have the opportunity to converse realistically with professionals; similarly, professionals should have the opportunity to discuss their thoughts and feelings with the organisations they work for and be signposted to supporting services or therapies if required.

Conversations on healthy eating, regular exercise and reducing health risks are important within the health and social care sector to prevent long-term illnesses and high death rates. Individuals should feel empowered to discuss their thoughts and feelings around these factors to help build their confidence in making positive, long-term changes within their life.

Signposting to appropriate services

As discussed in section A5.29, it is useful to signpost (point) individuals in the direction of appropriate care services and support groups. Preference may vary depending on how an individual wishes to receive support, such as individually, as a family, with a group or with the support of another professional. When someone identifies that an individual needs support with their health and wellbeing, suggestions should be made and advice given; however, it is important to note that it is an individual's choice as to whether they take the suggestions and advice to change their lifestyle.

> ### Research
>
> Using relevant reputable sources, research local community groups in your area that provide health promotion and support for individuals.
>
> Choosing one of the local groups, address the following points:
> ▶ Explain how the group works.
> ▶ Explain the lifestyle changes that can be made.
> ▶ Identify the individuals who may wish to seek these services.

Promoting public health

Health promotion is about improving lives and, therefore, is an important factor in ensuring individuals can maintain quality lifestyles. The Office for Health Improvement and Disparities focuses on specific factors each year that help to prolong life and support good health. It investigates areas that need improvement, such as particular illnesses, geographic areas, age ranges and so on, to identify problems and ways to improve health. Prevention is a key factor when implementing healthy lifestyles such as reducing alcohol consumption, maintaining an effective work–life balance, quitting smoking and eating healthily. Public campaigns to prevent bad habits will encourage people to seek advice about health conditions and identify support networks around them to improve their lifestyle.

Primary prevention is the intervention of health promotion and legal amendments before ill-health factors continue to rise. It is a key factor in the prevention of ill health. An example is legislation to ban or control products, such as cigarettes and banning smoking indoors. The idea was that this ban should deter smokers in the hope they will quit or reduce their nicotine intake, as well as to prevent non-smokers from acquiring illnesses due to passive smoking.

> ### Research
>
> Using the link, research and identify a particular area of research interest by the Office for Health Improvement and Disparities.
>
> https://www.gov.uk/government/organisations/office-for-health-improvement-and-disparities
>
> ▶ Write an overview of the illness or factor you are focusing on.
> ▶ Detect the impact of the illness or factors, giving examples of relevant statistics on its effects.
> ▶ Explain the prevention tactics the government has used to prevent further cases.
> ▶ Identify the legislation that has been put into place to reduce health risks (if any) and explain the impact of this on the public.

A5.31 Methods of obtaining feedback from service users relating to their experience of contacts and treatments

It is important to carry out research within health and social care settings to determine useful factors and statistics to help find methods of improvement within services. There are a variety of ways to successfully conduct research to gain feedback from service users, such as:
- surveys
- verbal feedback
- treatment success/visible results.

Surveys

Surveys are forms of questioning with the use of open or closed questions. Open questions enable service users to elaborate on their answers, whereas closed questions require a simple yes or no answer. Surveys can take the form of questionnaires or use rating scales. For example, patients can answer the question 'How was your experience at this hospital?' by rating it good, adequate or poor. They are often used to ask about customer experience. Surveys provide a simple way to collect data in a timely manner and analyse the results to identify trends and statistics.

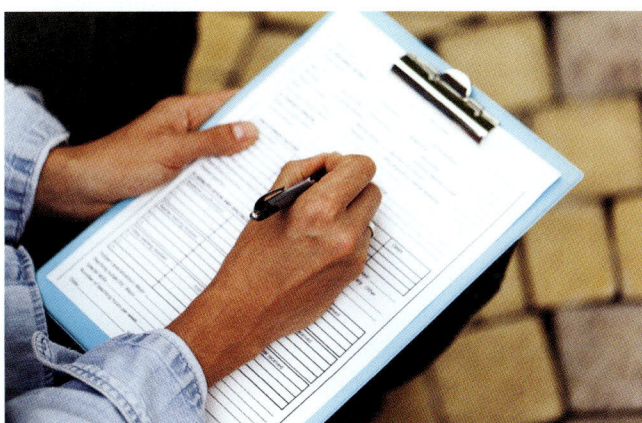

▲ Figure 5.11 A questionnaire

Verbal feedback

Professionals may ask service users for verbal feedback to determine the impact of their treatment or service provided. The use of verbal feedback helps to establish positive or negative factors during a review of the service provided. This helps organisations and professionals to improve their working practice and establish better patient outcomes. Feedback is critical for the development of quality of care and to identify the need for changes to improve services in the future. Without feedback it would be difficult for professionals and services to establish how patients perceive them and the care given.

Organisations may also ask service users to provide written feedback or quotes via a website, or pictures showing effective treatment results or surgery. This enables the public to establish the impact of an organisation and identify whether the organisation is suitable for them. Effective feedback helps to build confidence within the wider public as reviews can be effective for helping others to ask for services needed.

A5.32 Methods of using feedback obtained from service users to drive improvements in the healthcare science sector

Improvements within the health and social care service are important to ensure that the care given and received meets the needs of the public. Feedback is imperative for identifying areas for improvement. It also helps to establish the need for future improvements or more services that may be beneficial to particular demographics and locations.

Introduce service improvement

Feedback from service users provides informative views and insight into the perception of health and social care services. Analysing feedback establishes key trends that either have a positive impact or are particular areas for improvement. Information on the quality of working relationships between service users and professionals, as well as further multidisciplinary work, can also be gathered. People using services must have the ability to review their care or make complaints where necessary; consequently, this must be dealt with in the correct manner to ensure services continue to improve. Once improvements have been made, these should also be reviewed to ensure they are adequate.

Monitor performance

Organisations will follow policies and procedures that have been established to comply with relevant legislation in order to monitor performance throughout the service. Services will be monitored internally as well as externally through organisational bodies such as the CQC. The CQC regulates health and social care services in England. They closely observe and monitor the working relationships throughout an organisation, and may focus on particular areas or departments to gain an overview of the work produced and the effectiveness of care and treatment provided. The CQC will rate a health or social care organisation on a scale of 'outstanding' to 'requiring improvement'; if any improvements are required, they must be completed promptly.

Some organisations may seek the perceptions from families of a patient to ensure that the patient's care is being reviewed properly and the care provided is effective in meeting the patient's significant needs.

Individual monitoring or departmental monitoring may take place regularly throughout the year to ensure departments are working effectively and providing adequate resources for service users. If a professional or department is under scrutiny and requires improvement, this will be closely monitored over a set period of time. If improvements are not made, professionals may be placed on disciplinary or improvement plans.

Budgeting

Budgeting in health and social care consists of a process that enables particular funds to be spent on particular services. Maintaining existing services is normally the starting point, but some services may require updating or improvement and, therefore, will need to be the focus for that budget year.

Funds may need to be applied for, such as when organisations or a particular health or social care sector requires improvement, or to introduce new services, treatments or equipment. Budgeting is a long process that requires significant understanding of costing and equipment measured across a variety of health or social care factors. Poor budgeting may have implications when planning the services provided, which may further impact the policies and procedures the organisation follows, resulting in a lack of effective care and planning.

The budget for health and social care services is provided by public and private funds. Throughout the planning of spending funds, it is important to consider the measures that must be taken to improve services to the public.

Introducing new services

Healthcare science services must change over time to reflect changes in ill-health trends and new, innovative treatments or advances in surgery. Changes usually cost money, therefore services must apply for government funding to enable these changes to happen. New services do not happen quickly – instead they must be planned effectively and over a period of time to identify the strengths and potential implications of introducing them. Before the introduction of new services, surveys may be shared with the local population to gather a consensus of the need for new services.

A5.33 The definition of an urgent or immediate referral and factors that would dictate the need for this action

Urgent care is treatment in life-threatening circumstances; therefore, any service user requiring it will need to seek treatment immediately.

Definition of urgent or immediate referral

Urgent referral will be offered if a professional is concerned with a service user's observations, blood results or current signs and symptoms. If an urgent referral is required, it may happen on the day the patient has been seen, for example by their GP, or within the following days. On the other hand, referrals can sometimes take weeks, dependent on the reason for the referral or the type of service needed because a patient will be put on a waiting list.

The patient's GP will refer the patient to another service, so patient records will need to be sent over to ensure the services referred to are aware of the patient's condition and what they are investigating. In an emergency, for example if a patient is undergoing observations within the accident and emergency service, an immediate referral may need to take place. An example of this may be if a patient seeks help for signs and symptoms that relate to pancreatitis (inflammation of the pancreas), in which case the doctor will immediately refer the patient for an ultrasound. Other conditions that may be severe or life-limiting will also require immediate referral.

Consideration of underlying health conditions

Underlying health conditions may cause an immediate problem. For example, if a service user already has a long-term illness, such as cancer, but it is becoming progressively worse, it may require immediate referral due to the spread of the cancer or the service user's rapid deterioration. Long-term conditions such as asthma are normally monitored by the patient's GP. This may be reviewed every six months to ensure the patient is taking the right treatment and dosage of their inhaler.

A5: Providing person-centred care when working in healthcare science

If the patient's asthma becomes progressively worse or they suffer with further symptoms, such as continual breathlessness or a tight chest, they may need to be referred to a pulmonologist to further investigate any internal or external factors causing the patient problems.

Furthermore, underlying health conditions such as a chesty cough, internal abdominal pain and heart palpitations may be ongoing problems, but these may worsen overtime. Therefore, if the symptoms worsen, the patient should be referred to the appropriate professional to determine why this is happening. This should provide the patient with an understanding as to why their symptoms have become progressively worse, and consequently the patient should receive the treatment or care plans necessary.

Referral to the correct services is an important requirement for professionals. For example, a patient's regular GP works with a variety of illnesses and will have a wide knowledge of the signs and symptoms relating to diseases and disorders. However, they must be aware of their scope of practice and must work within their means; therefore, when a GP no longer has the ability to treat the patient or investigate signs and symptoms with routine observations, they must refer the patient to the right specialist.

> ### Research
>
> Investigate the following professionals and explain their roles and responsibilities.
>
> Provide examples of the service users that each professional may work with.
> - GP
> - angiopathologist
> - cardiologist
> - dermatologist
> - endocrinologist
> - epidemiologist
> - neurologist
> - pulmonologist
> - radiologist
> - urologist
> - pathologist
> - physiologist
>
>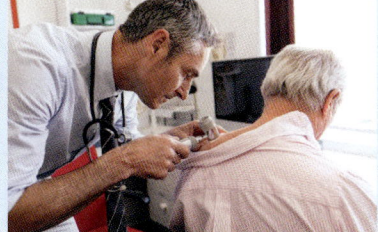
>
> ▲ Figure 5.12 A dermatologist
>
> ### Extension
> Once you have explained each professional's job role and expertise, configure a scenario where a range of these professionals may need to work in partnership to support a service user's needs. Explain and analyse each professional's role in supporting your example service user.

A5.34 The functions of services that work with urgent or immediate referral

There are a range of services that help to provide urgent and immediate care, including:
- NHS Urgent and Emergency Care (UEC) services
- NHS Accident and Emergency (A&E) departments
- NHS Urgent Treatment Centres (UTCs)
- NHS 111.

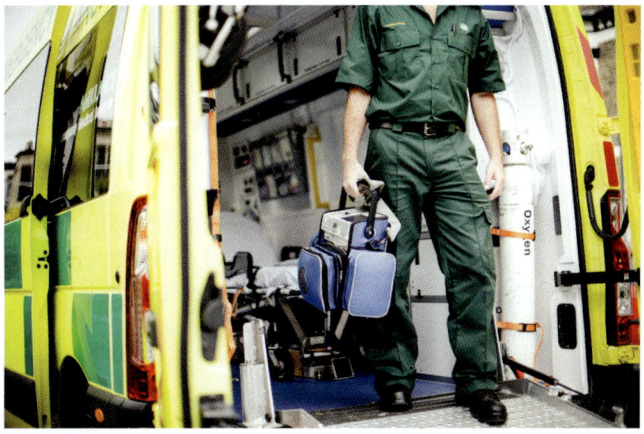

▲ Figure 5.13 A paramedic

NHS Urgent and Emergency Care (UEC) services and Accident and Emergency (A&E)

Urgent and emergency care services respond urgently to patients who require immediate care. Emergency care may be required when the patient is experiencing life-threatening symptoms, intensive treatment, an urgent illness or urgent care after an accident.

Some hospitals have been able to implement plans that help support A&E such as the use of walk-in centres. Walk-in centres enable service users to receive a quick assessment and treatment without the need for an appointment and without the need to go to A&E. GPs will investigate the service user's symptoms during a walk-in appointment. Walk-in centres are an effective way to reduce pressure on A&E departments. They help to support the workload but also ensure patients are seen quickly and treated, diagnosed or referred where necessary.

Before a service user presents themselves in hospital, they may call an NHS service such as NHS 111 (or use the web form) before visiting an A&E department. NHS 111 will help the patient to establish the seriousness of their current situation and whether it requires immediate attention or can be treated via their GP, pharmacy or another relevant service.

If a patient visits the A&E, they will sign in with reception and provide a short overview of their symptoms, unless they have been referred by 111 or an ambulance service, in which case these should be on record on arrival. The service user will need to be seen by the triage nurse to investigate simple observations such as blood pressure, oxygen levels and temperature. Depending on the severity of the symptoms or illness, they may be immediately referred to a specialist within the A&E centre or discharged if appropriate. Diagnosis may be possible if test results can be obtained immediately, therefore explaining the nature of the illness or reason for the symptoms the patient is experiencing. Once the patient is diagnosed, they are able to receive the treatment necessary for their illness or disorder. If the patient is discharged (let out) immediately, the triage nurse may ask the patient to review their symptoms with their regular GP the following day.

> **Test yourself**
>
> 1. Consider signs, symptoms or illnesses that may require urgent care and attention. Explain why and give examples.

NHS Urgent Treatment Centres (UTCs)

Urgent treatment centres are led by GPs and normally offer same-day appointments. These centres may be a 24-hour service where a service user can first call 111 to discuss symptoms and potentially be referred to the urgent treatment centre rather be admitted to hospital. The GP in these centres can assess and potentially diagnose the service user without any further referral, and they can also provide immediate prescriptions for treatment. If the service user requires further care, assessment or immediate treatment due to a life-threatening illness, then the GP will refer the service user on to immediate hospital care. On the other hand, if the patient does not require immediate or urgent care, the GP may ask them to review their condition with their own doctor within the next few days or weeks.

NHS 111

NHS 111 is a service that provides online or telephone support. A service user may ask for advice and support from 111 if they are unsure of the urgency of their medical symptoms. Depending on the situation, a 111 operator may refer the service user to the appropriate type of service for further assessment and treatment, such as urgent care centres or A&E. An NHS 111 operator will ask the service user a series of questions relating to their symptoms, such as the type of symptoms and the severity of each. Once the service user's situation is assessed, the 111 operator will provide guidance on further steps to take such as whether they need immediate medical attention or not.

NHS 111 can also be accessed online where the service will ask a series of questions, similar to those asked via a telephone operator. The questions are set out like a survey and, once the service user has followed and answered all the questions appropriately, the results will advise the service user on their next steps, such as receiving a medical telephone call or visiting urgent care.

A5.35 How to act on urgent or immediate referrals appropriately within limitations of role

Acting in the appropriate way during urgent referrals is important to establish the procedures to be taken to provide effective care and beneficial outcomes for the service user. Identifying the service user's condition is important to establish the timing and measures taken when providing urgent care. Professionals must also know the limitations of their role, meaning that they must be aware of when they are not qualified to advise and be able to identify when a referral to another professional needs to be made.

Understanding of the steps and procedures involved

As discussed in section A5.34, there are particular steps that can be taken to ensure the right methods of care are provided to a service user who is seeking advice and support for their condition. For example, in A&E, a triage nurse will check the patient's details such as name and age. They will then discuss the patient's symptoms and their severity. The triage nurse will then make initial observations that will support them in determining the next steps for that patient, such as what type of treatment and care will be needed and the urgency for it. This therefore helps to determine when the patient should be seen by the next professional within an A&E service, as some patients' conditions may be more severe than others: this determines which service user will be assessed and treated next in terms of waiting times. Professionals need to understand the limitations of their service to enable the patient to receive the appropriate care and referral where necessary. This helps to ensure the best outcomes for service users.

Communication of process to service users

To ensure effective treatment to the service user and efficient use of time, good communication is essential during the assessment and treatment of service users. During emergency care, processes will be quick, therefore communication needs to be simple and accurate. For example, if a service user calls 111 to discuss their symptoms and the operator refers the patient to an ambulance service, the operator must clearly report and record accurate information to the ambulance service to provide them with an understanding of urgency needed to deliver effective care. Another example is a service user seeking support from A&E: they report first of all to reception where they provide their name, date of birth and home address, and they will then discuss their symptoms. The receptionist will record this on their medical records to be efficiently and accurately passed on to the triage nurse, any specialists that may need to be involved and, finally, to the service user's regular GP to ensure information is on record appropriately and any further action that may be needed can be monitored.

Duty of care to service users

Factors of duty of care in urgent care include:
- duty to refer
- care and compassion.

All professionals have a duty of care when providing services to patients. As part of this, it is important to be able to identify the need for referral where necessary. If a patient does need a referral, the professional must be able to determine the urgency of the referral – whether it is immediate or may be referred to a waiting list will depend on the condition. Furthermore, professionals must provide appropriate care and be compassionate when working with all service users.

During urgent care, it is important for professionals to understand that it can be a nervous and anxious time for patients; therefore, professionals must be understanding when discussing the condition with the patient. In an urgent situation, it may be difficult for the patient to understand information being provided, either due to the condition, symptoms or feelings of anxiety and stress; therefore, professionals should be willing to repeat any information and guide the patient accordingly.

Confidentiality

It is important to uphold confidentiality during all situations and in all settings. Information must be recorded accurately and in a timely manner so that patient records are updated efficiently. Data must be sensitively dealt with during urgent care; therefore, patients should have the opportunity for their assessments or treatments to be discussed privately. A&E services can be exceptionally busy, and during busy periods service users may be asked to use beds in a shared area; however, any discussion between patients and professionals must be sensitive and private. A range of professionals will be working with service users, and working shifts may start or finish during a patient's treatment in urgent care; therefore, patient information must be passed on appropriately during a handover from professional to professional. Again, this must be done in a secure area. If professionals are unable to communicate face to face, telephone calls or scanned information should be discussed privately, and any materials sent online must be encrypted.

Follow up

Follow-up appointments, such as a phone call or face-to-face appointment may be required depending on the severity of the condition or illness. Information, therefore, should be recorded accordingly with accurate dates and times to enable a professional working on a patient's case to identify their condition and needs. Follow-up appointments may be days, weeks or months later; therefore, information must be accurate to identify changes in the patient's condition, whether it be positive or negative. This means that the patient can then receive further appropriate treatment or referrals.

Healthcare Science T Level: Core

Project practice

Write a report explaining the use of person-centred care when working in partnerships with a service user. In your report, you should refer to the case study below and address the following issues. Use a range of sources from relevant websites, journals and articles to support your information.

Priya has discovered she is four weeks pregnant and has been to the doctor to discuss this. The doctor has informed Priya she will need to visit the hospital for her 12-week scan. Priya has expressed her fear of hospitals and says that she refuses to enter one. The doctor explains to Priya that she will have to continually visit the hospital and medical centres throughout her pregnancy, to enable professionals to regularly check up on the baby and Priya's progression. Priya is not convinced of the benefit of visiting these centres during this time.

Using your knowledge on the importance of placing individuals at the centre of their care, explain how Priya can be supported during her pregnancy with regards to her phobia of hospitals.

Explain your duty of care with relation to Priya and her baby.

Consider and identify effective ways to promote and implement health and wellbeing for Priya.

Discuss possible complications if Priya does not attend her hospital and medical appointments regularly whilst she is pregnant.

Investigate and explain methods to help support Priya. Consider other professionals that can also support Priya during her pregnancy and help her overcome her fear of hospitals.

Assessment practice

1. Identify and explain the NHS core values.
2. Explain and evaluate person-centred planning.
3. Identify the purpose of the Care Certificate.
4. Explain one appropriate method of alternative communication.
5. Using examples, explain the difference between indirect and direct discrimination.
6. Discuss the importance of two ethical principles in healthcare science research, providing relevant examples.
7. Describe the meaning of duty of candour.
8. Provide a summary of the Equality Act 2010 and describe a relevant example of how to uphold the act in a healthcare setting.
9. Choosing one regulatory body, explain their roles and responsibilities in promoting duty of care.
10. Identify and summarise three of the six Cs.
11. Discuss the advantages and potential implications of partnership working, considering both inter-professional and patient working.
12. Identify and explain three different types of abuse and harm. Provide signs for each type.
13. Define radicalisation.
14. Describe the meaning of mental capacity, identify relevant legislation and provide a summary of this.
15. Describe MECC and explain how it promotes healthy lifestyle changes.
16. Analyse the four services that work with immediate or urgent referrals.

A6: Infection prevention and control in healthcare science settings

Introduction

Infection control can have a significant impact in healthcare science settings and failure to comply can have a detrimental impact on the safety of patients and staff. Many individuals accessing healthcare science services are especially vulnerable to infections, so the prevention and control of transmission of these is very important.

Following the COVID-19 pandemic, the increase in guidance on methods that should be implemented to prevent and control the spread of infections has highlighted the importance of such practices and the impact they can have on the transmission of diseases. This chapter details standard techniques to be used and procedures that must be followed by staff in healthcare science settings to abide by the requirements of legislation in relation to infection prevention and control. It also discusses the responsibilities of practitioners when antimicrobial resistance occurs and the correct actions to take to respond to it.

Learning outcomes

The core knowledge outcomes that you must understand and learn:

A6.1 techniques for the prevention and control of infection in healthcare science settings, including use of appropriate personal protective equipment (PPE), appropriate cleaning and disinfecting

A6.2 the difference between single-use and multiple-use products and the main reasons for using single-use products

A6.3 the scientific principles of cleaning, disinfecting, sterilisation and decontamination

A6.4 the principles of a range of sterilisation techniques and the effect of sterilisation on materials

A6.5 the importance of effective hand-washing techniques

A6.6 the impact of antimicrobial resistance on infection prevention and control

A6.7 the process of waste management and waste streams, taking into account how to reduce waste

A6.8 considerations that must be made when deciding upon appropriate waste streams for various types of special and hazardous waste products

A6.9 the types of spillage that can occur and the associated risks

A6.10 corrective and preventative actions that can be taken in relation to spillages.

A6.1 Techniques for the prevention and control of infection in healthcare science settings, including use of appropriate PPE, cleaning and disinfecting

In March 2012, the National Institute for Health and Care Excellence (NICE) published guidelines on 'Healthcare-associated infections: Prevention and control in primary and community care', laying out **infection** prevention and control measures that should be followed by all healthcare science workers involved in care of patients. It applies to care in the community, such as general practice (GP surgeries) or residential care settings, as well as in patients' homes (domiciliary care). The guidelines state that, as a minimum, any healthcare science workers in these settings should be educated about standard principles of infection prevention and control.

Techniques for infection control

The hands can pick up germs from one place and pass them on to another, passing on infections. For this reason, the best way to prevent the spread of infection is to keep the hands clean by washing frequently with warm water and soap. The importance of this basic step should not be underestimated and should become part of your and everyone's routine.

Use of PPE

Personal protective equipment – known as **PPE** – is used to protect healthcare workers while performing specific tasks that might involve them coming into contact with infectious materials.

Disposable gloves are worn when performing or assisting in a procedure that involves a risk of contact with body fluids, broken skin, dirty instruments or harmful substances such as chemicals and disinfectants. This includes procedures that involve:
- a risk of being splashed by body fluids (blood, saliva, **sputum**, vomit, urine or faeces, for instance)
- contact with the patient's eyes, nose, ears, lips, mouth or genital area, or any instruments that have been in contact with these
- contact with an open wound or cut
- handling potentially harmful substances, such as disinfectants.

Aprons are not needed to carry out many normal aspects of day-to-day care with patients, such as helping them to go for short walks, but they will be needed for:
- performing or assisting in a procedure that might involve splashing of body fluids
- performing or helping the patient with personal hygiene tasks, such as washing
- carrying out cleaning and tidying tasks in the patient's living space, such as bed-making.

Healthcare science workers routinely use face masks as part of their PPE. However, these do not protect the wearer from inhaling small particles that can remain airborne for long periods of time. Face masks are effective barriers for retaining large droplets that can be released from the wearer through talking, coughing or sneezing. They are useful in many patient care areas as they may reduce wound site contamination during surgical or dental procedures. Face masks cannot be used as a protection from all hazardous airborne materials, however, and are often used in conjunction with a face shield.

Since the COVID-19 pandemic the UK Health Security Agency (UKHSA) has updated its advice for the protection of healthcare staff. It states that: 'Any clinician working in a hospital or primary care within 2 metres of a COVID-19 patient should wear an apron, gloves, surgical mask and eye protection.'

> **Practice point**
>
> Practice putting on and removing PPE. The following chart from the NHS Infection Prevention Control website will help you:
>
> www.infectionpreventioncontrol.co.uk/content/uploads/2020/07/Correct-order-for-putting-on-and-removing-PPE-July-2020.pdf

> **Key terms**
>
> *Infection:* the process of bacteria, viruses or other micro-organisms (such as fungi or parasites) invading the body, making someone ill or diseased.
>
> *Sputum:* mucus or coughed-up material (phlegm) from the lower airways (trachea and bronchi).

A6: Infection prevention and control in healthcare science settings

Appropriate order of PPE donning and doffing

The type of PPE required will vary depending on the healthcare science setting and level of precaution required, e.g. risk of droplet or airborne infections occurring. The donning (putting on) and doffing (removal) of PPE should be tailored to the specific type of PPE required. However, Figure 6.1 outlines the general order of donning and doffing in line with best practice in healthcare science settings from general national guidelines. Not all of the steps may be relevant, so practitioners should bypass steps that are not relevant to themselves and their organisation.

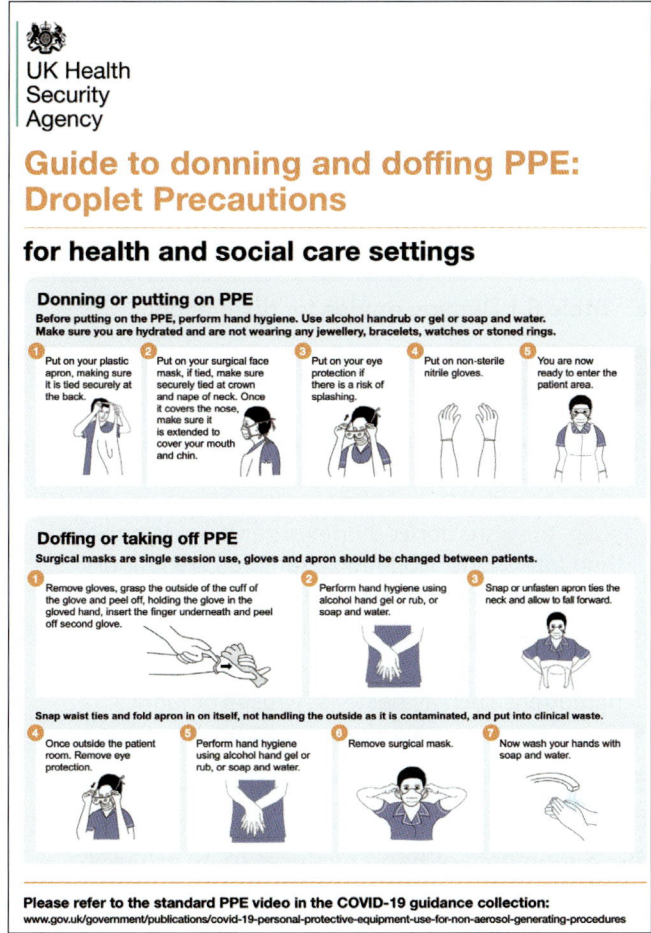

▲ Figure 6.1 The donning and doffing of PPE

Donning

1. Perform hand hygiene, ensuring hands are thoroughly dry after.
2. Put on shoe covers (if required).
3. Put on plastic apron, ensuring it is tied securely at the back.
4. Put on surgical mask/respirator, ensuring that it is securely tied at the crown and the back of the neck, and that it covers the nose, mouth and chin.
5. Put on eye protection (if necessary due to a risk of splashing).
6. Put on the appropriate types of gloves, for example non-sterile nitrile gloves.

Doffing

1. Remove gloves by grasping the outside of the cuff of the first glove and peel it off; while holding that glove in the gloved hand, insert a finger underneath the other cuff to peel off the second.
2. Perform hand hygiene, ensuring hands are thoroughly dry after.
3. Unfasten plastic apron around the neck first and then at the back.
4. Remove eye protection (if applicable).
5. Remove surgical mask.
6. Perform hand hygiene again, ensuring hands are thoroughly dry after.

Appropriate fit and quality control of face masks

As discussed before, face masks are a routine part of a healthcare science worker's PPE and are effective barriers for contamination. There are different types of face mask that can be used depending on the setting and type of procedure being carried out. For example, medical masks (surgical masks) are designed to protect an individual from the risk of splashing from blood and other bodily fluids that could lead to the spread of infections. For this reason, medical masks contain multiple layers of non-woven material and need to be worn so that the material fits over an individual's nose, mouth and chin.

Another type of face mask commonly used is a respirator, which protects individuals against the inhalation of airborne particles through filtration. They are designed to form a seal around an individual's nose and mouth.

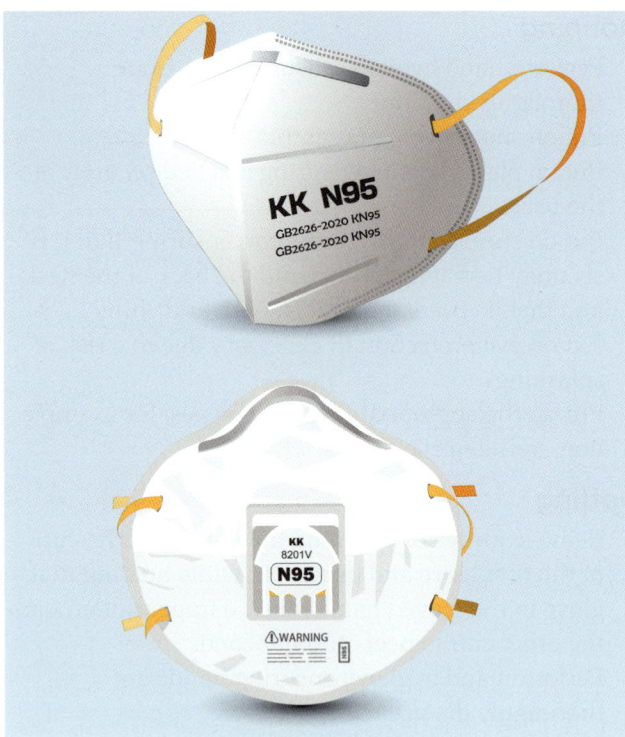

▲ Figure 6.2 A respirator face mask

Any gaps in the seal of a face mask around an individual's nose and mouth can allow airborne particles or droplets to be absorbed. For this reason, it is important that the correct size and appropriate fit of face mask is worn. Inadequate fit of a face mask heightens the risk for individuals and reduces the protection provided. The following factors can affect the appropriateness and quality of the fit of face masks:
- facial hair
- facial piercings
- weight loss or gain
- facial changes such as scars, moles and ageing effects.

Use of cleaning and disinfecting agents

Cleaning must be carried out before disinfecting begins. Cleaning will remove contamination (blood, vomit, faeces, etc.) and many micro-organisms using **detergent**, for example, washing-up liquid and warm water. Disinfection can then take place. Care must be taken as the misuse or overuse of chemical **disinfectants** may result in damage to the user, patients or equipment, and may also result in the development of antimicrobial resistance.

When using any cleaning or disinfecting agent, the healthcare science worker must be sure to:
- follow the manufacturer's instructions for dilution (never just guess how much to dilute a disinfectant)
- wear personal protective equipment
- ensure adequate ventilation
- never use two disinfectants together
- not add anything to a disinfectant (including detergent), as this may result in a dangerous chemical reaction
- discard disinfectant solution after use
- not 'top up' solutions of disinfectant with anything
- dispose of any unused solution.

Best practice for disinfection is to use a diluted chlorine-based product such as household bleach.

Area contaminated with blood or blood stained
Household bleach 10 parts per million (ppm) available chlorine
Dilution of 1 in 10, for example 10 ml of household bleach to 100 ml of water OR
100 ml of household bleach to 1 litre of water

Area contaminated with body fluid (not blood or blood stained)
Household bleach 1000 ppm available chlorine
Dilution of 1 in 100, for example 10 ml of household bleach in 1 litre of water

▲ Table 6.1 Dilution guides for disinfection

> **Key terms**
>
> **Detergent:** purifying or cleansing agent that increases the ability of water to break down grease or dirt. Detergents act like soap but, unlike soap, they are derived from organic acids rather than fatty acids. Common examples are laundry detergent and washing-up liquid.
>
> **Disinfectant:** a substance that destroys, inactivates or significantly reduces the concentration of pathogens such as bacteria, viruses or fungi.

Effective hand-washing techniques

The World Health Organization (WHO) introduced the '5 moments of hand hygiene' in an attempt to reduce the occurrence of healthcare-associated infections. Many NHS trusts in England adopted this model of hand hygiene, which prompts healthcare workers to clean their hands at five distinct stages of caring for a patient. Cleaning hands is the simplest, cheapest and most effective way of preventing germs being passed from one person to another. The five moments for hand hygiene are shown in the following table.

A6: Infection prevention and control in healthcare science settings

Moments	When	Why
1. Before patient contact	Always clean your hands before touching a patient.	To protect patient against germs on the healthcare worker's hands.
2. Before a clean/aseptic procedure	Clean hands immediately before any clean/aseptic procedure as this prevents contamination. An aseptic procedure could be a change of dressing or bandage for the patient.	To prevent harmful germs from both healthcare worker and patient entering the patient's body if dressing is not kept sterile.
3. After body fluid exposure risk	Clean hands immediately after exposure to body fluids (and after glove removal).	To protect healthcare worker and environment from harmful germs.
4. After patient contact	Clean hands immediately after touching a patient and their immediate surroundings.	To protect healthcare worker and environment from harmful germs.
5. After contact with patient surroundings	Clean hands after touching any object or furniture in the patient's immediate surroundings when leaving – even if patient has not been touched.	To protect healthcare worker and environment from harmful germs.

Adapted from: https://cdn.who.int/media/docs/default-source/integrated-health-services-(ihs)/infection-prevention-and-control/your-5-moments-for-hand-hygiene-poster.pdf

> **Key term**
>
> **Aseptic:** free from contamination caused by harmful bacteria, viruses or other micro-organisms; surgically sterile or sterilised.

Good personal hygiene

To prevent infection among patients, it is essential that uniforms are clean. The Royal College of Nursing advises that there must be sufficient uniforms provided to enable freshly laundered clothing to be worn for each shift or work session, with access to spare clothing if staff clothing items become contaminated (for example, splashed with blood and/or body fluids). They also suggest that uniform fabrics must be capable of withstanding water temperatures of at least 60°C (which is high enough to kill bacteria and viruses) and tumble drying.

Tying hair back, if it is long enough, is essential in health and social care as it can contain bacteria that could cause infection. Furthermore, cross-infection (transferring infections from one place to another) could occur if the hair is allowed to trail into body fluids when a healthcare worker is cleaning up a patient or serving food on the ward. Besides this, long hair that is not tied back would get in the way of many tasks, risking getting caught or impairing vision.

'Nothing below the elbow' in clinical situations

Each organisation will have its own policy on uniforms in clinical situations (which includes any situation with patient contact, such as diagnosis, treatment and procedures); however, the 'bare below the elbows' policy was introduced in the UK in 2007 through the NHS. This is an infection prevention method designed to decrease the transmission of pathogens from healthcare workers' contaminated clothing on to patients. The policy outlined how employees' uniforms should comply with good hand hygiene and wrist washing by keeping arms bare below the elbow when delivering direct care to patients. This is because there is a risk of sleeve cuffs becoming contaminated with micro-organisms and infecting patients when coming into contact with them.

> **Reflect**
>
> The NHS issued guidelines for 'bare below the elbow' as part of a larger plan to reduce infections due to methicillin-resistant *S. aureus* and *C. difficile* in healthcare science settings.
> From your experience on placement so far, reflect on the impact that following the bare below the elbow guidelines has had on reducing transmission of infections. Has anyone on your placement explained these guidelines to you and the importance of following them?

Isolation period when sick, where applicable

Healthcare science staff are more susceptible to becoming unwell due to being around infectious pathogens. If an employee becomes unwell, especially with an infectious illness, their setting's sickness policy will usually require them to isolate at home for a specific period until they are free from their symptoms. This will be for a minimum of 48 hours, regardless of the disease, to ensure the individual is no longer infectious and will not spread any pathogens. When returning to work following an isolation period of sickness, an employee's line manager should conduct a return-to-work meeting to ensure that the member of staff is fit to return and to establish the original cause of their ill health.

> **Reflect**
>
> Are you aware of the sickness policy in your placement and the isolation period required for different diseases? Have you read the policy? Are the other members of staff you work with aware of the policy?

Laboratory-specific infection control measures

Laboratory-specific PPE

Healthcare science staff working in laboratories must ensure that infection control measures are being followed and that they minimise the risk of the transmission of infections by wearing laboratory-specific PPE. The minimum requirement for PPE in any laboratory setting where there are potential risks from biological or chemical hazards would include protective eyewear, a lab coat, nitrile or chemical-resistant gloves, long trousers and closed-toe protective shoes (i.e. covering the entire foot, not sandals).

Containment barriers should be put in place for environments in which an employee is at a high risk of being exposed to hazardous substances. The extent and size of the containment depends on the level of risk of potential contamination and exposure. When conducting work that involves containment barriers, staff must ensure they are wearing the essential PPE mentioned above as well as equipment such as a filtering respirator or breathing apparatus to further protect them from exposure to infectious agents or toxins.

> **Key term**
>
> **Containment barrier:** a physical barrier that prevents the spread of infections by enclosing and managing the infectious agents, therefore reducing or eliminating exposure.

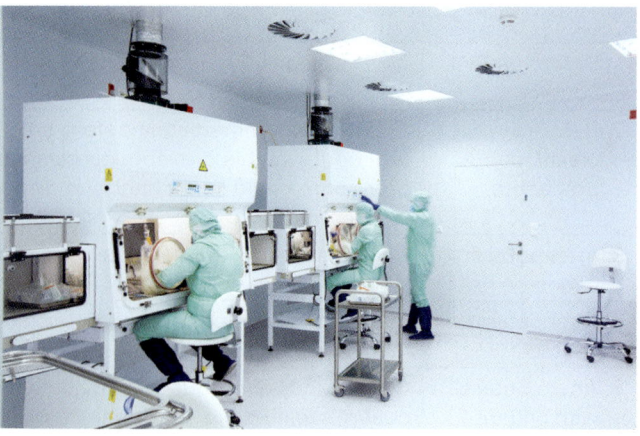

▲ Figure 6.3 Laboratory containment in COVID-19 vaccine production

Other laboratory-specific infection control measures include the use of air pressure and air flow cabinets. Air flow cabinets are designed to protect the environment that the actual micro-organism/sample being tested is in. The cabinet provides insulation for the inner environment and encloses the sample; air is drawn in through a **high efficiency particulate air (HEPA) filter** and flows out of the cabinet in the direction of the individual conducting the test. This keeps the inner environment consistent for the sample.

In contrast to air flow cabinets, which are designed to protect the sample, safety cabinets are designed to provide further protection to the laboratory staff by creating an enclosed and ventilated workspace where they can safely work/conduct tests on contaminated pathogens. The class of safety cabinets used is dependent on the organism being handled and the risk it poses:

▶ category 1 poses a minimal risk to an individual
▶ category 2 poses a moderate potential risk to an individual.

As with containment barriers, employees working with air pressure/air flow cabinets and category 1 and 2 safety cabinets must ensure they are conducting their work wearing nitrile or other appropriate chemical-resistant gloves, safety glasses/goggles, a lab coat and a disposable gown. Such PPE is needed when preparing to use safety cabinets but also when using items specific to these methods (for example, closing lids on analysers) and shouldn't be discarded until all work has been completed and staff are out of that environment.

A6: Infection prevention and control in healthcare science settings

Why control measures are important to prevent the spread of infection within the healthcare science setting

Prevent harm caused to both patients and health workers

As mentioned above, good standards of personal hygiene are essential to ensure the health and welfare of both patients and staff. Poor personal hygiene causes the spread of more diseases than anything else. For example, influenza and colds are spread by people coughing and sneezing without covering their face. Unwashed hands after using the lavatory spread germs such as **norovirus**.

Poor infection control is responsible for **healthcare-associated infections (HCAIs)**, which can develop either as a direct result of healthcare interventions such as medical or surgical treatment, or from being in contact with a healthcare setting. The term HCAI covers a wide range of infections including those caused by methicillin-resistant *Staphylococcus aureus* (MRSA) and *Clostridium difficile*. HCAIs pose a serious risk to patients, staff and visitors as they are easily spread from one person to another. They can result in significant extra costs and workload for the NHS and cause significant **morbidity** (likelihood of disease) to those infected. As a result, infection prevention and control are a key priority for the NHS.

> **Key term**
>
> **High efficiency particulate air (HEPA) filter:** a mechanical air filter that removes/eliminates harmful bacteria and toxins from the air.
>
> **Norovirus:** very infectious virus common in the winter that causes diarrhoea and vomiting.
>
> **Healthcare-associated infections (HCAIs):** infections that occur as a result of having surgical or medical treatment in a hospital.

Local dress code policy

It is important that an employee's appearance is always smart and professional when working in the healthcare science sector, especially when having face-to-face contact with patients. A bad impression can be made instantly, which can affect trust in the organisation, so an employee's appearance needs to be appropriate for the role, professional and smart. Each organisation will have their own dress code policy, for example a uniform or dress expectation such as 'smart attire'. This will be specific to that organisation and must be followed by all staff.

Uniforms should be kept clean and, when worn in clinical settings, should be washed after every shift to reduce the risk of transmission of infections. In addition, they should not be worn in public places to reduce the risk of infections to the general public. Uniform sleeves should be kept above the elbow or be rolled up (see page 124 for more on 'nothing below the elbow' in clinical situations). Each organisation's dress code policy will have its own guidance on name badges/staff ID and how it must be visible on staff. Hair should be kept tidy and clean and, in most clinical settings, should be tied back off the collar. Head coverings (e.g. turbans or hijabs) are acceptable if they are required by an individual's culture or religion. Jewellery, especially hand and wrist jewellery such as watches and rings, should be removed when on shift due to the risk of the jewellery harbouring micro-organisms and impacting with hand hygiene. There are certain exceptions, however, such as a plain wedding ring or the Sikh Kara (a bracelet).

> **Test yourself**
>
> 1. Choose two pieces of personal protective equipment and explain how they can protect the healthcare worker.
> 2. State why healthcare science workers' uniforms must be washed at 60°C.
> 3. Explain the meaning of 'aseptic'.
> 4. Explain three of the 'five moments of hand hygiene' as a method of infection control.
> 5. Discuss why an employee working in a laboratory setting would use a containment barrier.

A6.2 The difference between single-use and multiple-use products and the main reasons for using single-use products

Single-use products

Single-use products are designed to be used on an individual patient during a single procedure and then disposed of immediately after use. They are not designed to be reprocessed (cleaned, disinfected or sterilised) for further use. They have not undergone the appropriate testing to ensure that the products are safe to re-use and are at risk of damage, material alteration and cross-contamination. The materials used in single-use products are also prone to absorb (soak up) or adsorb (hold molecules on its surface) chemicals, which could potentially build up and come in to contact with a patient and cause them harm.

All single-use products will be clearly indicated with the symbol shown in Figure 6.4 to ensure that staff are aware that the product is for single-use only.

SINGLE USE ONLY
DO NOT RE-USE

▲ Figure 6.4 Symbol indicating single-use only products

> **Research**
>
> Research the Medicines and Healthcare products Regulatory Agency report 'Single-use medical devices: Implications and consequences of reuse' using the link below. Summarise the key points, including an explanation of the products that it includes, which legislation the report covers and a conclusion for the consequences of re-use of single-use medical products.
>
> https://assets.publishing.service.gov.uk/government/uploads/system/uploads/attachment_data/file/956268/Single_use_medical_devices.pdf
>
> Add to your summary using additional research from other sources. One source to consider could be this from the *Nursing Times*:
>
> www.nursingtimes.net/roles/nurse-managers/the-implications-of-reusing-single-use-medical-devices-07-12-2006

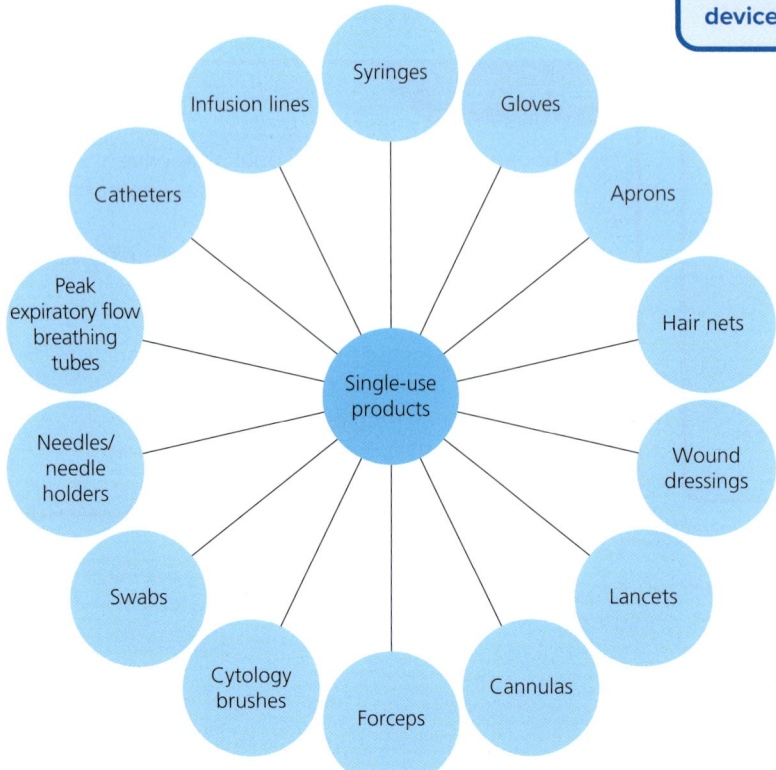

▲ Figure 6.5 Some common examples of single-use only healthcare products

Multiple-use products

Multiple-use products are designed to be used on several different patients, but they must be cleaned, sterilised and/or disinfected (reprocessed) after each use. Multiple-use products do become contaminated with micro-organisms during procedures so they are designed (for instance, in terms of the material used to make them) for safe use several times following a multi-step, rigorous disinfection or sterilisation process that they are able to withstand repeatedly. Failing to follow the cleaning, sterilisation or disinfection process on multiple-use products could result in patients' blood and other biological fluids or debris, such as tissue, being absorbed and transmitted to another patient, resulting in contamination and HCAIs. Clearly this can have serious consequences for patient health.

Examples of multiple-use products include:
- surgical instruments, e.g. clamps, forceps
- blood pressure cuffs
- centrifuges when analysing samples in a laboratory
- endoscopes: long, thin tubes with a camera that are used to visualise areas inside the body, e.g. bronchoscopes, colonoscopes (a doctor will insert a colonoscope through the anus to view the colon and large intestine)
- accessories for medical procedures, such as graspers and scissors.

Main reasons for using single-use products

- It reduces the risk of infection and cross-contamination and so improves patient safety and quality of care.
- It is more efficient and convenient due to being ready to use and the immediate disposing of the products after use.
- Arguably, it is more cost-effective as there is no cost of reprocessing products after use.

> **Reflect**
>
> Consider any disadvantages of using single-use products over multiple-use products. Why are all products not single-use? Discuss with your class.

A6.3 The scientific principles of cleaning, disinfecting, sterilisation and decontamination

Ensuring a clean environment within a healthcare science setting contributes towards the prevention of HCAIs. Requirements from legislations such as the Health and Social Care Act (2008) ensure that healthcare science settings are provide and maintain a clean environment in order to prevent infections spreading. The cleaning process within healthcare science settings is designed to be rigorous and is crucial for the reduction of micro-organisms that can cause harm if transferred.

The scientific principles

Cleaning

Accumulations of dust, dirt and liquid residues will increase infection risks and must be kept to a minimum by regular cleaning. Cleaning reduces the presence of micro-organisms that may be present on surfaces and instruments by removing visible foreign matter, and this minimises the risk of the transfer of micro-organisms. The environment (e.g. door handles, toilet flush handles, taps) plays an important role in cross-infection during outbreaks. Therefore, special attention must be paid to these high-touch fittings and any surface that people have contact with, particularly during outbreaks of infectious diseases such as norovirus. Good design features such as numerous, convenient hand-washing sinks with automatic soap dispensers should also be used in healthcare science buildings.

A written cleaning schedule should be devised for each area, based on the Control of Substances Hazardous to Health (COSHH – see page 52) requirements, including the regular removal of dust by damp dusting both high and low horizontal surfaces. As well as this, all health and social care settings should have a decontamination policy in place and a cleaning schedule stating how and when to clean the different areas, fixtures, fittings and specialist equipment (for example a hoist); what products and equipment to use when cleaning; what to do and what products to use if there is a spillage of blood or body fluids; and what training staff need to implement the policy. It should describe individual responsibilities for cleaning.

Disinfecting

Disinfectant is used to reduce the number of micro-organisms on surfaces to a level that is considered safe, but which may not necessarily destroy some viruses or bacterial spores. Disinfection is usually acceptable for items that pose a medium risk of infection if these devices cannot be sterilised effectively. Chemical disinfection is not as effective as heat disinfection. Heat disinfectants – such as dishwashers, washing machines and washer-disinfectors – clean the item and then expose it to hot water for the required time to achieve thermal disinfection:

- 65 °C for 10 minutes
- 71 °C for 3 minutes
- 80 °C for 1 minute
- 90 °C for 1 second.

While most chemical disinfectants are capable of inactivating bacteria and certain types of viruses (those which have an 'envelope', an outer layer), many are not so effective against other micro-organisms, for example the hepatitis viruses, cysts (dormant bacteria) and bacterial spores.

Sterilisation

Sterilisation is used for food, medicine and surgical instruments, but some items are too fragile for sterilisation as the temperature is too high for them to withstand. To sterilise means to kill all microbes and their spores – whether harmful or not – present on a surface or object, and thus is more effective than disinfection. This can be done by machines called **autoclaves** (see section A6.4), which use high-pressure steam heated to 121–34 °C. Extreme care must be taken when using these machines as steam can scald the skin. Another method is to use direct heat, which can include incineration, boiling in water and dry heat, which inactivates and kills micro-organisms in objects such as glass and metals. Items that can get damaged by heat are subjected to chemical sterilisation, e.g. biological materials, fibre optics, electronics and plastics.

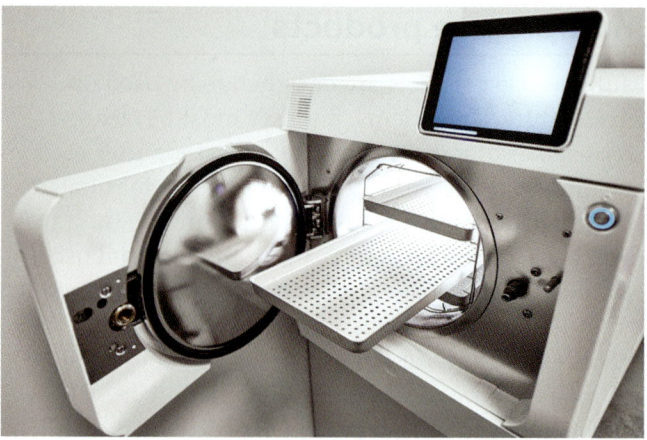

▲ Figure 6.6 Autoclaves are use for sterilising equipment

Irradiation, high pressure and filtration are other techniques used in the sterilising process. Irradiation can be used for aseptic work areas and for sterilising surgical equipment. High-pressure sterilisation is used to sterilise contaminated instruments. Filtration can be used to sterilise fluids, such as drugs solutions, which would be damaged by heat, irradiation or chemical sterilisation.

> **Key term**
>
> *Irradiation:* when objects are exposed to different types of radiation. It may be used to penetrate various materials and can be used to sterilise surgical instruments.

Decontamination

Decontamination is a process or combination of processes such as cleaning, disinfecting and sterilising that removes or destroys contaminants so that infectious agents cannot cause infection. If a piece of equipment is contaminated with blood or other body fluids, it should be removed from service immediately. It must be decontaminated as soon as possible, but best practice is to do it immediately, away from busy areas in the healthcare setting. Decontamination is essential to lower the number of cross-infections between people and to prevent HCAIs.

> **Research**
>
> Research the cleaning schedule at your work placement and bring a copy into your centre. Compare it with another setting, e.g. if you are in a hospital you need to compare your cleaning schedule with another student's cleaning schedule from a different hospital setting. What are the similarities and differences?

Test yourself

1. Explain what disinfecting an item/area means.
2. Explain the most effective method of disinfection.
3. Explain what is meant by decontamination.
4. Describe the purpose of an autoclave.

A6.4 The principles of a range of sterilisation techniques and the effect of sterilisation on materials

Autoclaving wet/dry methods

As mentioned in section A6.3, autoclaving is a method of sterilisation that uses high-pressure steam at 121 °C for 15–20 minutes to decontaminate or sterilise equipment and some consumables, often in a microbiology or clinical laboratory. This method is used to sterilise heat-resistant laboratory and medical equipment and items that are used in close contact or invasive procedures, for example surgical instruments. Autoclaving is one of the most effective methods of sterilisation. The dry/wet methods refer to the relative dryness or wetness of the steam during the process (the amount of liquid water droplets contained within it). Steam of around three per cent wetness is frequently used to create the best outcome for sterilisation.

The process of autoclaving includes the following steps:
1. Put all the items that need to be sterilised inside the autoclave and lock it shut.
2. All the air is then sucked out of the autoclave chamber using a vacuum pump to create a very low-pressure environment.
3. Steam is then pumped at a high pressure into the chamber, with a temperature ranging from 121 to 134 °C. The temperature can depend on the length of the cycle, which usually lasts anything up to 30 minutes.
4. The steam continuously covers the equipment, killing bacteria and microbes.
5. Once the cycle has completed its designated time, the steam is released from the chamber and a short drying period takes place (the length of the drying period depends on the wetness of the steam).
6. Once the drying period is complete, the chamber can then be opened, and the equipment can be removed.

Not all materials can or should be autoclaved. The following table is a general guide:

Example of compatible autoclave materials
• Surgical Instruments • Glassware • Pipette tips • Petri dishes • Polypropylene (PP) and polycarbonate (PC) plastics • Stainless steel • Nomex (rubber) gloves
Examples of incompatible autoclave materials
• Materials containing bleach • Materials containing solvents, volatile or corrosive, or flammable chemicals • Acids, chlorides or chlorine • Polystyrene (PS), polyethylene (PE) and high-density polyethylene (HDPE) plastics • Non-stainless steel • Household glass

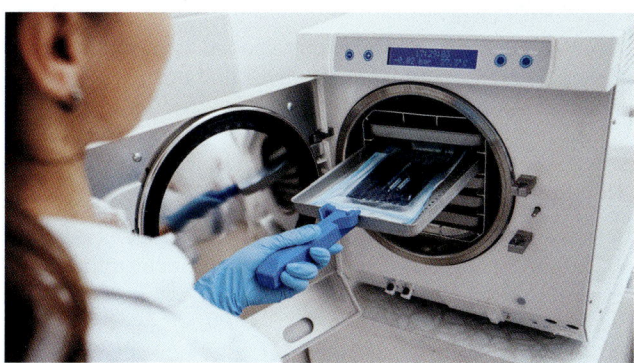

▲ Figure 6.7 An autoclave being used to sterilise medical instruments

Chemical sterilisation

Chemical sterilisation is the process of using gaseous or liquid chemicals to remove residues and sterilise equipment and surfaces. **Gaseous sterilisation** involves exposing the equipment to gases in an enclosed chamber to kill all micro-organisms present, whereas **liquid sterilisation** involves submerging the equipment in a liquid solvent and diluting it with water to kill the micro-organisms. Out of the two, gaseous sterilisation is argued to be the more effective as the gases are able to pass through smaller orifices (holes) so therefore have more of an impact when sterilising than liquid.

Chemicals typically used for sterilisation include:

Gaseous:
▶ formaldehyde
▶ plasma
▶ ozone

- ethylene oxide
- nitrogen dioxide (NO_2).

Liquid:
- hydrogen peroxide
- bleach
- hypochlorite
- phenolics
- heavy metals, e.g. silver.

The effectiveness of chemical sterilisation depends on the temperature, contact time, chemical used and concentration of the chemical. Chemical sterilisation is often used for equipment and materials that are too sensitive for the intense heat of autoclaving and that could become damaged with radiation sterilisation.

> **Research**
>
> Choose one liquid and one gaseous method of chemical sterilisation and summarise each process. How effective are each of these methods? When is each used?

Radiation sterilisation

Radiation sterilisation is the use of ionising and non-ionising radiation to deactivate and kill micro-organisms so that medical equipment is clean and safe to use. It is used on products such as needles, prosthetic implants and syringes. The clean, but not bacteria-free, items are sealed in an airtight bag. The bag is then placed in a radiation chamber; the radiation then penetrates the bag and kills the micro-organisms on the product.

Ionising radiation	Types of ionising radiation
A type of high-energy radiation released by atoms in the form of short electromagnetic waves that destroy micro-organisms.	- high-energy ultraviolet light - X-rays - gamma rays - neutrons - high-energy protons
Non-ionising radiation	**Types of non-ionising radiation**
A type of lower-energy radiation that uses longer wavelengths; it is only used to sterilise surfaces rather than clinical equipment.	- thermal - ultraviolet light - microwaves - very low frequency (VLF) radiation - extremely low frequency (ELF) radiation - visible light - infrared radiation - radio waves

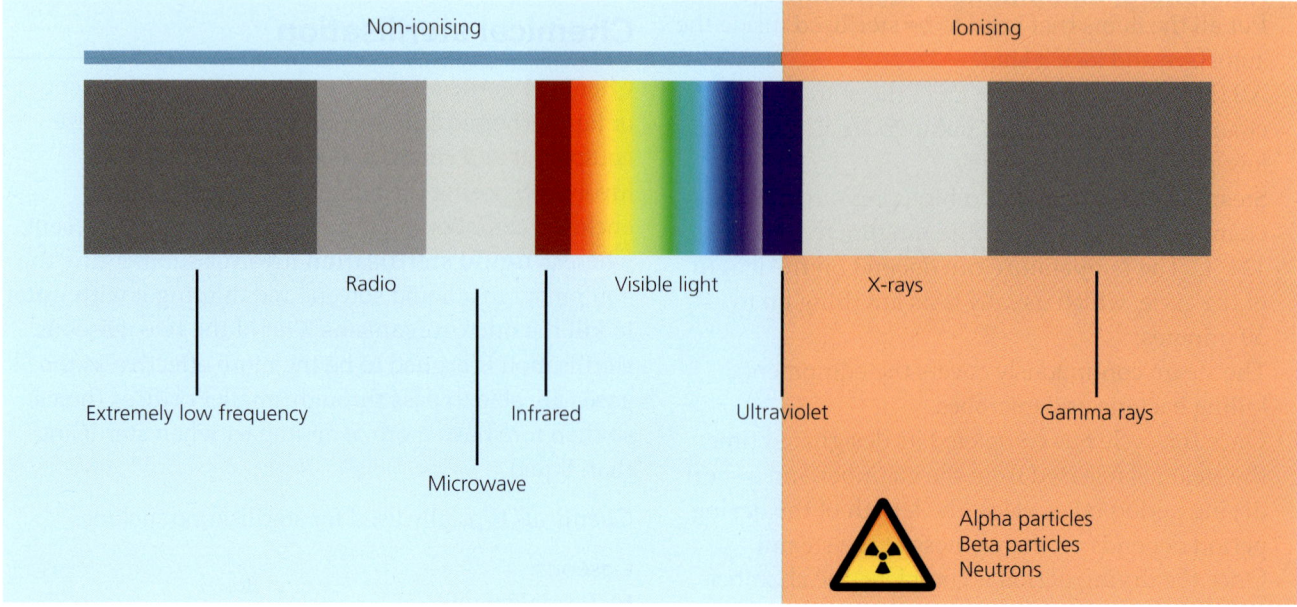

▲ Figure 6.8 The difference between ionising and non-ionising radiation

A6: Infection prevention and control in healthcare science settings

A6.5 The importance of effective hand-washing techniques

One of the most effective ways to help prevent and control the spread of diseases is to wash our hands frequently and thoroughly. Look back at section A6.1 to remind yourself of the WHO's five moments of hand hygiene. Poor hand hygiene is the most common cause of transmission of infections in most healthcare settings. Maintaining good hand hygiene with soap and water is thus very important for staff, patients and visitors in order to reduce the risk of HCAIs, which are more likely to be contracted or spread due to social contact while carrying out clinical care activities.

Current NHS guidance is that effective hand washing should take around 20 seconds (see Figure 6.9 on page 132). Doing this will help stop viruses and bacteria being spread from person to person and causing illnesses such as diarrhoea, influenza and food poisoning. It also helps to maintain sterile healthcare environments and ensures equipment is as clean as possible for patient and staff safety.

A continuous and rigorous routine of hand washing can leave staff susceptible to dry skin conditions such as dermatitis or irritated skin from alcohol-based soaps/hand rubs. Staff should be advised to use **emollient** hand cream both on and off duty to mitigate this. Alcohol-based hand rubs containing emollients in their formulation can also be used to keep hands hydrated.

> **Key term**
>
> **Emollient:** a medical moisturiser used to treat eczema and soften rough, dry and irritated skin.

It is important that staff, patients and visitors follow effective hand-washing techniques, particularly in the following situations:
- before handling medication
- after using the toilet
- when changing and cleaning incontinence nappies/bedpans
- when eating, handling or preparing food
- during physical examinations/tests/manual handling/treating a cut or a wound on a patient
- after blowing their nose, sneezing or coughing
- if they are a patient suffering with diarrhoea and/or vomiting, coughing or any symptoms of influenza (flu)
- if they are a visitor seeing a patient who is experiencing any of these.

A6.6 The impact of antimicrobial resistance on infection prevention and control

Antibiotic stewardship

Antibiotics have made a significant impact on public health worldwide. However, due to **antibiotic resistance** (see next) increasing and the pace of developing new antimicrobial drugs slowing down, not enough new antibiotics are being produced to fight resistant bacterial.

Antibiotic stewardship is the systematic effort to guide and measure improvements in how clinicians prescribe antibiotics for treatments, improving patient outcomes by protecting them from unnecessary prescribing of antibiotics and, in doing so, combating antibiotic resistance. Antibiotic stewardship programmes are, therefore. of the utmost importance globally.

The World Health Organization (2021) published details of the ten stewardship interventions most commonly used by front line clinicians to tackle antibiotic resistance. They are outlined in the following table, which continues on page 133.

Stewardship interventions prior to or at the time of prescription
1. Clinician education – appropriate to all clinical settings via prioritising continuous professional development (CPD), e.g. educational events, mini review seminars with recent updates for evidence-based practice, regional workshops and learning resources such as MEDtube.
2. Patient and public education – education and guidance for the proper use, administration, storage and disposal of antimicrobials, e.g. through mass educational campaigns advertised and available online, or via direct face-to-face clinician/patient contact regarding a specific medical condition.
3. Institution-specific guidelines for the management of common infections – local guidelines can be adapted from national or international evidence-based guidelines that target programmatic interventions, for example respiratory tract infections and urinary tract infections (UTIs). Guidelines outline a standard approach for staff to follow and provide a benchmark for appropriate antimicrobial use that can be used in audit and feedback.
4. Cumulative antibiograms – these reports summarise how susceptible strains of pathogens are to a variety of antibiotics. This enables monitoring of trends in antibiotic resistance.

Healthcare Science T Level: Core

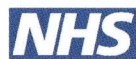

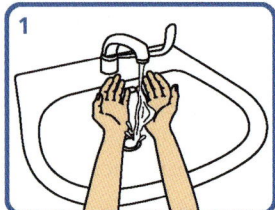	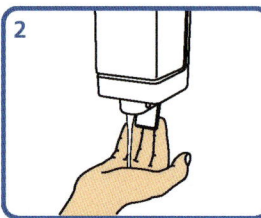	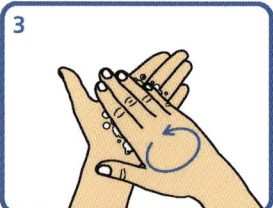	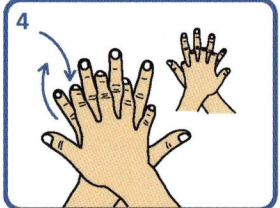
1. Wet hands with water	2. Apply enough soap to cover all hand surfaces	3. Rub hands palm to palm	4. Rub back of each hand with palm of other hand with fingers interlaced
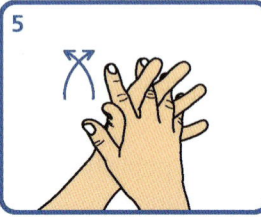	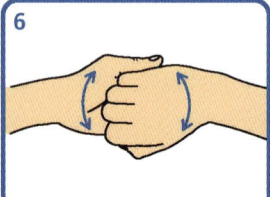	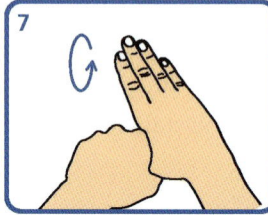	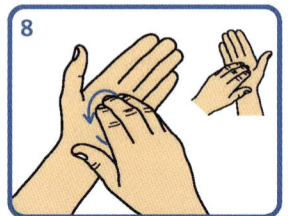
5. Rub palm to palm with fingers interlaced	6. Rub with back of fingers to opposing palms with fingers interlocked	7. Rub each thumb clasped in opposite hand using a rotational movement	8. Rub tips of fingers in opposite palm in a circular motion
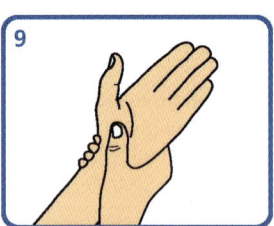	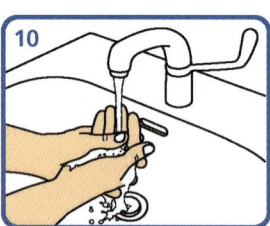	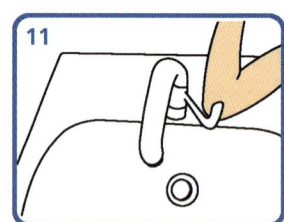	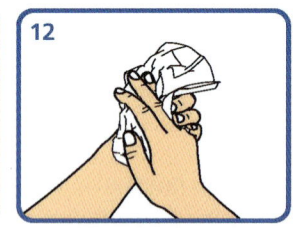
9. Rub each wrist with opposite hand	10. Rinse hands with water	11. Use elbow to turn off tap	12. Dry thoroughly with a single-use towel

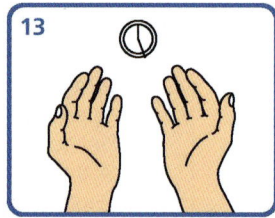

13. Handwashing should take 15–30 seconds

cleanyourhands campaign

NHS National Patient Safety Agency

© Crown copyright 2007 283373 1p 1k Sep07

Adapted from World Health Organization *Guidelines on Hand Hygiene in Health Care*

▲ Figure 6.9 NHS hand-washing technique with soap and water

A6: Infection prevention and control in healthcare science settings

Stewardship interventions prior to or at the time of prescription
5. Prior authorization of restricted antimicrobials – approval must be granted for specific antimicrobials by antimicrobial stewardship members, pharmacists and infectious diseases physicians before they can be released for administration to patients. If a specific antimicrobial is deemed inappropriate, alternative treatment will be recommended.
6. De-labelling of spurious antibiotic allergies – the separation of patients who are at significant risk of adverse allergic reactions or those of little risk is very important. The direct removal of an antibiotic allergy is then recommended for those patients who are considered low or no allergy risk.
Stewardship interventions after prescription
7. Prospective audit and feedback – this involves the review of individual patient cases by clinicians and pharmacists with infectious diseases physicians following antimicrobial use.
8. Self-directed antibiotic reassessments (antibiotics timeouts) – clinicians can assess a patient's ongoing course of treatment, generally after 48–72 hours, to evaluate if the antimicrobials are working correctly. For example, they can test whether a specific pathogen is identified as the infecting agent and modify antibiotic prescriptions if necessary.
9. Dose optimization – assessing patient's characteristics, e.g. age, weight, overall health risk, severity of infection, to determine the appropriate dose, interval and route of administration of an antibiotic.
10. Duration optimization – through reviewing of data, audits and feedback, the appropriate treatment duration can be assessed, meaning the most appropriate drug and the correct dosage can be administered for the right length of time.

Antibiotic resistance

Antibiotic resistance is when bacteria, viruses, parasites and fungi build resistance and develop the ability to evade the drugs that are designed to kill them. If micro-organisms survive exposure, over time they may mutate their structure to protect it against the antibiotics. These mutated micro-organisms then multiply and spread to other organisms to form an overall resistance. **Methicillin-resistant *Staphylococcus aureus* (MRSA)** is an example of a **superbug** that has become resistant to a number of antibiotics. MRSA is carried on the skin and in the throat and nostrils. Breaks in the skin can cause patients to become seriously ill, and it can even become a life-threatening condition. This puts increasing pressure on healthcare facilities as patients are unwell for longer and their illnesses are harder to treat.

Antibiotic resistance is becoming an increasing public health concern and adds a significant cost to national economies. It restricts the choice of treatments available and means that 'simple' infections such as bacterial pneumonia are becoming increasingly difficult to treat. It also puts patients at an increased risk of further health problems; for example, a patient needing a common surgery such as a Caesarean birth is at a higher risk if antibiotics for the prevention of infections are less effective. It therefore leads to prolonged illnesses and hospital stays and, in some cases, it can also increase mortality.

> **Key term**
>
> **Superbugs:** strains of bacteria, viruses, parasites and fungi that are resistant to several types of antibiotics and other medicines commonly used to treat them.

Antibiotic overuse

Antibiotic overuse refers to the use of antibiotics for a patient's health problems when they are not needed. The overprescribing and overuse of antibiotics has led to resistant bacteria which, as covered previously, can have a huge impact on healthcare science settings for infection prevention and control purposes. The overuse of antibiotics causes them to become less effective and can lead to outbreaks of resistant bacteria, often referred to as superbugs. They are very difficult to treat and have a significant effect on healthcare science providers financially because of the cost of the added medical treatment. They also increase mortality rates.

Healthcare science providers are working together to reduce the overuse of antibiotics, including through antibiotic stewardship. For example, antibiotics are not an effective treatment for viral infections so should not be used to treat chest infections, sore throats and ear infections unless they are caused by a bacterial infection. Professionals are instead advising patients on alternative ways to treat infections and are only prescribing antibiotics to patients when they are needed. When they do prescribe antibiotics, they are educating their patients on their proper use and the importance of completing a course of antibiotics properly, for example using them all over the prescribed period, not using leftover courses of antibiotics and never sharing them with another individual.

> **Reflect**
>
> Using the link read over, 'Contained and controlled: The UK's 20-year vision for antimicrobial resistance.
>
> https://assets.publishing.service.gov.uk/government/uploads/system/uploads/attachment_data/file/773065/uk-20-year-vision-for-antimicrobial-resistance.pdf
>
> Do you think it is achievable? Are there any aspects of the vision that you feel are particularly important? What aspects do you feel will be the biggest challenge and why?

A6.7 The process of waste management and waste streams, taking into account how to reduce waste

The management and reduction of waste in the healthcare science setting is very important. Clinical and infectious waste may be hazardous to any individual who comes into contact with it and, as such, organisations are obliged to dispose of waste in the appropriate manner to reduce these risks. Waste should be separated accordingly, and adequate supplies should be provided to ensure staff can dispose of waste safely.

Types of waste	Disposal method
General waste: waste that is not clinical or hazardous, such as paper hand towels, small quantities of food and paper. This includes recyclable waste such as cardboard, some plastics and packaging.	General waste should be collected on a regular basis and placed in a black plastic sack. They should be kept in wheeled bins or skips awaiting collection. Any confidential waste should be shredded beforehand and recycled. Any recyclable waste should be flat-packed if appropriate, e.g. cardboard boxes, and placed in a separate bin for collection.
Glassware waste: including that which is placed in sharps bins for disposing (see Figure 6.10).	Glassware is split into brown and clear glass and then recycled. Broken glass should be placed in a cardboard box and labelled 'broken glass'.
Electrical waste: broken or obsolete electronic equipment, such as monitors, medical machinery and computers.	Electronic waste must be separated into salvageable waste that can be recovered and used elsewhere, and waste that must be disposed of appropriately, e.g. used batteries. Electrical waste must be decontaminated and any data wiped beforehand (this should be done in accordance with an organisation's data protection policy). Removal should then be arranged via porters for the waste to be transported offsite.

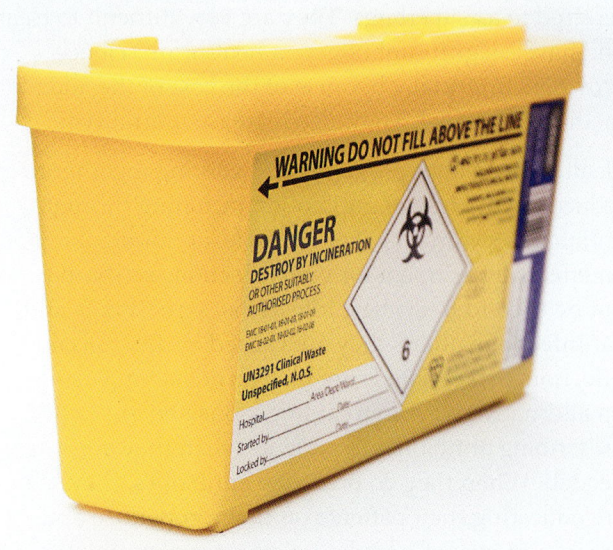

▲ Figure 6.10 Sharps bin

A6.8 Considerations that must be made when deciding on appropriate waste streams for various types of special and hazardous waste products

Waste streams dependent on the type of waste

Infectious waste sent for incineration

According to the World Health Organization (2018), infectious waste is:

> 'waste contaminated with blood and other bodily fluids (e.g. from discarded diagnostic samples), cultures and stocks of infectious agents from laboratory work (e.g. waste from autopsies and

[from] infected animals from laboratories), or waste from patients in isolation wards and equipment (e.g. swabs, bandages and disposable medical devices).'

Source: www.who.int/news-room/fact-sheets/detail/health-care-waste

It therefore poses a risk of infection and contamination to anyone who encounters it. Organisations are required to have policies in place to dispose of infectious waste safely via high-temperature incineration so that pathogens are fully destroyed. Infectious waste is collected and stored in yellow waste streams (i.e. yellow labelled bins) to clearly indicate to staff that it contains infectious materials that must be sent for incineration at a suitably authorised facility.

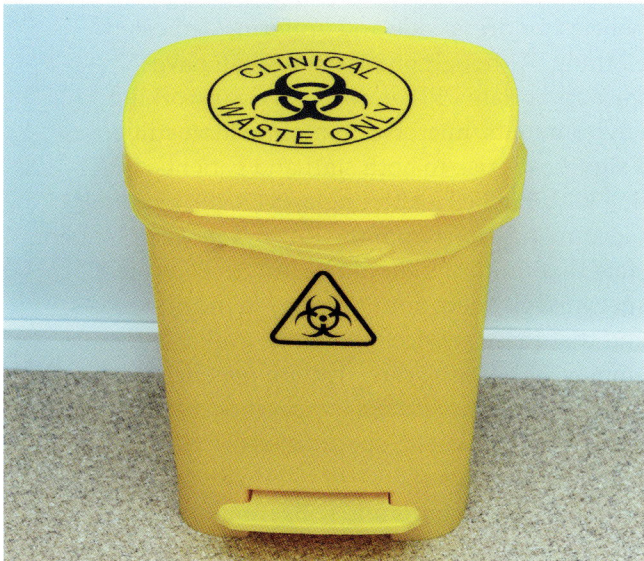

▲ Figure 6.11 Yellow waste stream for infectious waste

Infectious waste sent for treatment to render it safe for disposal

When waste is considered hazardous and poses a risk of infection and contamination, for example PPE such as gloves, masks and aprons, it needs to be sent to an authorised facility to be disinfected so it can then be deemed safe to be disposed of. This waste is identified by the orange waste stream and is generally waste that has been used to treat infectious patients. Infectious waste being sent for treatment to render it safe for disposal is kept in orange bags designed to be leakproof (to decrease the risk of contamination) and then stored in orange-lidded containers.

Cytotoxic or cytostatic waste

Cytotoxic or **cytostatic waste** is very common in healthcare science settings and, if not disposed of properly and individuals come into contact with it, it poses a great risk and can cause individuals to suffer with vomiting, liver damage, abdominal pains and even foetal loss. All healthcare science organisations that produce cytotoxic waste, as per the Health and Safety Executive, are required to have procedures in place for staff to follow to ensure its safe disposal to protect employees, patients and the environment. Cytotoxic waste includes medicine containers containing cytotoxic waste residues, and sharps or swabs used during the treatment of cytotoxic medicines. It should be placed in purple bags or containers. This indicates it is to be disposed of via high-temperature incineration by an authorised and licensed facility. An example of this type of waste is used sharps.

Offensive/hygiene waste

Although **offensive/hygiene waste** does not pose a particularly significant hazard to health, it still must be disposed of appropriately. The tiger waste stream is used for offensive waste, which is the collection of offensive waste into yellow and black striped bags. These bags are clearly labelled so as to not be confused with other waste. They are designed to have maximum impact and to prevent leaks. The bags are stored in offensive waste bins, which are generally operated by a pedal to remove the need to touch the lid and risk contamination with bacteria. It is then collected by an authorised courier who will transport the waste to be recycled at an **energy from waste** facility to be incinerated.

> ### Key terms
>
> ***Cytotoxic and cytostatic waste:*** hazardous or toxic medicines, often used in the treatment of cancers, that pose a serious risk to health.
>
> ***Offensive/hygiene waste:*** non-infectious, unpleasant waste that poses a low risk to health, such as dressings and PPE that are not contaminated with bodily fluids, as well as hygiene and sanitary waste, e.g. incontinence pads. It is waste that is not hazardous but would be unpleasant to come into contact with.
>
> ***Energy from waste:*** the burning of non-hazardous waste as a source of renewable energy.

Anatomical waste

It is important that **anatomical waste** is disposed of in the correct waste stream due to the risk to anyone who may be exposed to it. Anatomical waste should be contained in red stream waste bags, unless it contains sharp needles. Red stream waste bags are highly durable and leakproof so are not easily damaged. They are stored in red-lidded containers and then collected and transported via a licensed carrier to a suitable disposal facility where it will be incinerated.

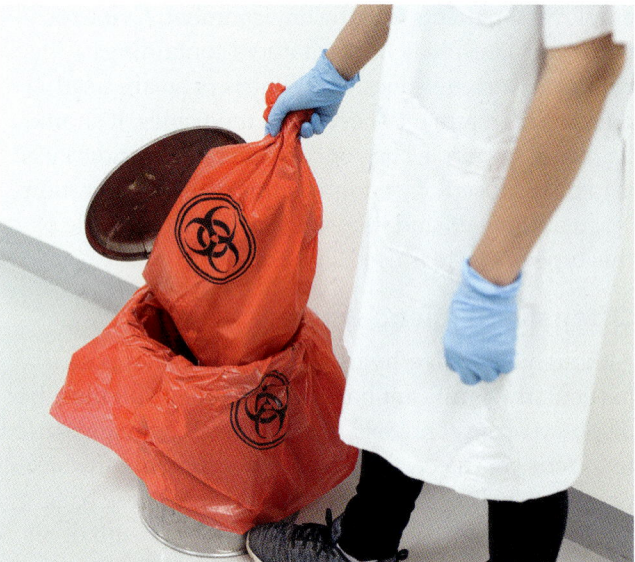

▲ Figure 6.12 Red stream waste bags

Non-hazardous medicinal waste

Non-hazardous medicinal waste makes up a large percentage of healthcare science organisations' waste streams annually. Due to this imposing no risk of contamination or infection, non-hazardous medicinal waste does not need to be sent for alternative treatment to be rendered safe to be disposed of. It is identified using blue waste stream bags and containers and will be taken to a suitable authorised facility for its safe disposal via incineration.

> **Key terms**
>
> **Anatomical waste:** waste that involves human or animal tissue, for instance placenta. It also includes materials soaked in anatomical waste, such as swabs, blood bags, PPE, catheters, IV tubes and dressings.
>
> **Non-hazardous medicinal waste:** waste that poses no physical, biological, chemical or radioactive risk, for example plastic packaging, clean glass and plastic, paper and cardboard.

Dedicated clothing

Professionals working in healthcare science organisations are compelled to follow organisational policies for dress code and uniforms/dedicated clothing. Although professionals will have the appropriate PPE on while in their working environments, microbial contamination still poses a significant risk to both staff and patients. In line with Public Health England (2020), national recommendations from the Royal College of Nursing state that uniforms should be sent to dedicated specialist cleaners or third-party laundry services, and that these services should be available for all employees working directly with patients or hazardous materials to comply with infection prevention standards. Dedicated, specialist services or third-party services can reduce or eliminate microbial contamination, stains and soils from clothing so that it deemed safe for use again. Microbial contamination is reduced or eliminated through the use of high temperatures above 60 °C and bleaching agents such as such as chlorine or activated oxygen bleach.

A6.9 The types of spillage that can occur and the associated risks

Under COSHH guidelines, employers have a legal obligation to protect staff, patients and visitors from hazardous and infectious substances. Organisations have a responsibility to inform staff on the types of spillages possible and associated risks. These can be grouped according to the categories in the following table.

A6: Infection prevention and control in healthcare science settings

Types of spillages	Associated risks
Bodily fluids (for example urine, faeces, vomit)	Contact with pathogens such as norovirus, which causes diarrhoea and vomiting illnesses.
	Any liquid spillage can lead to slips and cause sprains, concussions, breakages and bruises.
Blood	Contact with blood-borne pathogens, e.g. infectious micro-organisms that cause diseases in humans for example, human immunodeficiency virus (HIV) and hepatitis B and/or C.
	Slips and trips which could result in sprains, concussions, breakages and bruises.
Chemical (for example liquid, gas, solid, aerosol)	Injury to the body via damage to the kidneys, liver and other internal organs which then progresses on to other potential health problems.
	Potential burns to the mouth, skin, eyes (potentially causing vision problems) and even respiratory tract.
	Breathing issues such as wheezing and coughing through inhalation of the chemicals – these could also lead to more damaging illnesses such as lung cancer through **asbestos** inhalation.
	Slips and trips that could result in sprains, concussions, breakages and bruises.

Reflect

Are you aware of the relevant waste management processes in your work placement? Has it been explained to you? If so, are you clear on which waste stream is more relevant to your role?

Key term

Asbestos: naturally occurring fibres that provide heat and chemical resistance to environments. Often used in older buildings, but we now know that it poses risks of serious illnesses if inhaled over a long period of time, e.g. years.

A6.10 Corrective and preventative actions that can be taken in relation to spillages

Corrective

Under COSHH (see section A3.1), employers and employees have a duty of care to protect workers from hazards including those caused from spillages. All staff have a responsibility to ensure that correct and safe actions are taken when a spillage occurs, as any occupational exposure to these spillages poses a serious risk of infection. Spillages must be dealt with immediately and the area made safe, for example not letting individuals walk through or near any spillages and displaying any warning signs to ensure individuals are aware that a spillage has occurred and that it is currently unsafe to be in that area.

Staff in a healthcare science setting should ensure that they follow organisational policies and procedures in the event of a spillage to immediately minimise risk of contamination and prevent injury to staff, patients and visitors. Staff should be familiar with the organisation's standard operating procedures (SOPs, see page 183) in relation to spillages so that they have clear step-by-step instructions for carrying out routine operations, including the appropriate PPE that must be worn. Providing staff with appropriate protective equipment is a vital component in establishing a safe working environment with regard to spillages. In line with COSHH regulations, PPE such as protective gloves, eye protection, aprons and boot covers should be available at all times to ensure the highest of protection for staff.

In the event of a spillage occurring that involves potential exposure to staff, patients or visitors, it is essential that the spillage is recorded in line with organisational procedures, clearly explaining the contents of the spillage and the disinfectant products used in the clearing of the spillage. An example of a procedure for reporting spillages would be the completion of a **Datix form** at an employee's earliest convenience (usually within the first 24 hours). Datix forms are incident-reporting forms usually accessed through an organisation's intranet. The incident must then be reported to the organisation's health and safety manager.

Corrective actions for the cleaning of a spillage should be clearly documented in organisational policies in line with COSHH regulations, and should include clear instructions of what measures should be taken to remove each contaminant effectively. Instructions should include a list of approved cleaning products and the appropriate concentration level of detergents when mixed with warm water. For example, according to the Centers for Disease Control [source: www.cdc.gov/hai/pdfs/resource-limited/environmental-cleaning-RLS-H.pdf] chlorine-based disinfectants should be diluted in 5 per cent chlorine-bleach and 95 per cent warm water to ensure maximum reduction of potential risks from spillages.

In line with legislation such as COSHH (1994/2002) and the Health and Safety at Work Act (HASAWA 1974), organisations in the healthcare science sector are obligated to have spill kits accessible in departments so that spillages can be controlled and disposed of safely. The contents of a spill kit usually consist of:

- gloves
- safety goggles
- disposable bags
- signage
- absorbent pads/pillows
- absorbent socks.

> ### Research
> Research a healthcare science organisation's policy and procedure in relation to the corrective actions to take in relation to spillages. Create a short presentation on the organisation's spillage procedure, summarising its main aims and procedures to follow in the event of a spillage.
>
> Complete your presentation by including a step-by-step guide to an infection control SOP at your placement in relation to corrective actions for spillages.

Preventative

It is also important that organisations put in place preventative actions that can reduce the chances of spillages occurring in the first place. For example, with SOPs in place, miscommunication is reduced and compliance with preventative measures should increase. Individuals working in healthcare science settings conducting routine procedures during an emergency situation, for instance, will follow SOPs that minimise the possibility of malpractice and putting themselves and other individuals at risk of harm. If organisations have policies in place to minimise the likelihood of spillages, it should reduce the risk of harm.

SOPs are important to prevent a contamination incident occurring from spillages. Guidelines should be available for staff regarding preventative measures that can be put in place in relation to appropriate storage techniques. For instance, hazardous samples should be stored in safe and secured racks at all times, not kept at a great height to reduce the risk of falling, and only be accessible to the appropriate staff members. Storage should be authorised access only and kept secure to prevent unnecessary exposure and potential spillages.

When staff are responsible for the transportation of hazardous substances that, if spilled, could cause harm, preventative measures should be put in place; for example, to reduce the risk of chemical spillages, chemical jars/bottles should be transported in chemical bottle carriers from site to site and from room to room. Employees should also know how to locate SOPs and guidance for the actions that should be taken to prevent risk and harm from spillages, as well as the location of safety equipment such as chemical bottle carriers and spill kits.

> ### Reflect
> If a hazardous spillage occurs while you are on work placement, observe how the professionals you work with adhere to corrective and preventative actions to clear and reduce the risks of further spillage. What did you learn? How could you use this knowledge to further your understanding of infection prevention and control?

A6: Infection prevention and control in healthcare science settings

Project practice

You work in a hospital as a critical care nurse and, in light of the COVID-19 pandemic, your ward manager has asked you to help mentor the student nurses during their training in relation to infection control. This will include guiding them on how their efforts can reduce the incidence of HCAIs and the importance of good hand hygiene. You are to collate a training pack for the student nurses to read in preparation for your first mentor meeting. Your training pack must include:

- an explanation of common HCAIs and the impact that antibiotic resistance is having on healthcare science settings such as hospitals
- a summary of the correct hand-washing procedure
- a description of methods of cleaning, disinfecting, sterilisation and decontamination for medical equipment.

Include an evaluation of the importance of cleaning, disinfecting, sterilisation and decontamination of medical equipment, as well as highlighting the appropriateness of single- and multiple-use products and their benefits for infection prevention and control.

Assessment practice

1. Identify three different types of healthcare-associated infections (HCAIs).
2. Name three single-use products and three multiple-use products used in healthcare science settings.
3. Explain two differences between the scientific principles of cleaning, disinfecting, sterilisation and decontamination for infection prevention and control.
4. Outline the concept of chemical sterilisation and when it would be used in clinical practice.
5. Assess the importance of staff, patients and visitors maintaining good hand hygiene in healthcare science settings.
6. Explain two methods for reducing antibiotic resistance. Evaluate each method, giving one strength and one weakness for each.
7. Explain the importance of different waste management processes.
8. List four different hazardous waste products and identify the appropriate waste streams for each.
9. Discuss the potential risks associated with a chemical liquid spillage.
10. Identify three corrective and three preventative actions that professionals can take when dealing with a hazardous spillage.

A7: Managing information and data within the health and science sector

Introduction

Before we can think about managing information and data, we have to make sure we know what is meant by the terms **information** and **data**. We often use them interchangeably, as if they have the same meaning – but do they?

Data is a collection of values. These values can be characters or words, numbers or other data types. You may sometimes see the phrase 'units of information' as a description of data.

Information is data that has been processed in a way that we can read it, understand it and use it.

So, managing information and data allows us to use the data to generate useful information that can increase our understanding.

Learning outcomes

The core knowledge outcomes that you must understand and learn:

- **A7.1** a range of methods used to collect data
- **A7.2** the considerations to make when selecting a range of ways to collect and record information and data
- **A7.3** the importance of accuracy, attention to detail and legibility of any written information or data
- **A7.4** the strengths and limitations of a range of data sources when applied in a range of health and science environments
- **A7.5** how new technology is applied in the recording and reporting of information and data
- **A7.6** how personal information is protected by data protection legislation, regulations and local ways of working/organisational policies
- **A7.7** how to ensure confidentiality when using screens to input or retrieve information or data
- **A7.8** the positive use of, and restrictions on the use of, social media in health and science sectors
- **A7.9** the advantages and risks of using IT systems to record, retrieve and store information and data
- **A7.10** how security measures protect data stored by organisations
- **A7.11** what to do if information is not stored securely.

A7: Managing information and data within the health and science sector

A7.1 A range of methods used to collect data

The methods that we use to collect data depend on the type of data. Data types will be discussed in a little more detail in section A7.2.

Focus groups

Focus groups are used widely in health research, as well as in parts of the science sector, as a way of discovering what individuals feel or believe. They can be very useful in understanding and explaining the factors that influence the feelings and attitudes of individuals as well as how they behave.

A focus group interview is usually highly structured. Participants are usually selected on the basis that they will have something to say on the topic – hence the term 'focus' – rather than being randomly selected. The focus group interview will have a facilitator or moderator whose job is to guide the discussion and manage the interactions between the participants. It is important that participants feel comfortable with expressing their views and opinions.

Focus groups can produce huge quantities of data that need to be processed and analysed to give useful information.

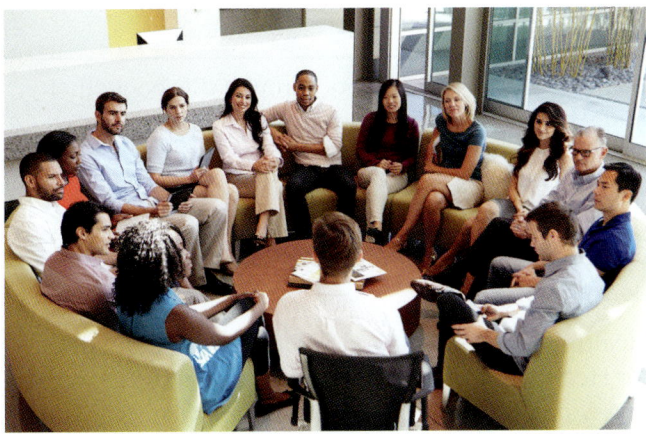

▲ Figure 7.1 Focus groups need a facilitator or moderator to lead the discussion

Surveys

A survey is a way of gathering factual information as well as views and opinions. They can be of two types: **closed-question** or **open-question**.

Closed-question surveys

Closed questions are questions that require a simple answer (see the table for examples). The advantage of closed-question surveys is that they can be quick and easy to carry out and produce a large amount of data that can be analysed quite easily. This can be made even more efficient when the survey is online or in some other electronic format so that the data is already available in electronic format for further analysis.

However, the questions must be carefully worded to obtain reliable data. This might involve giving people information and asking for their opinion, but there can still be ways in which the results might be influenced by the wording of the questions. Consider the following two questions:

1. People under the age of 40 are less likely to die of COVID-19. Do you think the risks of the COVID-19 vaccine outweigh the benefits in this age group?
2. People under the age of 40 are more likely to suffer with 'long Covid'. Do you think the benefits of the COVID-19 vaccine outweigh the risks in this age group?

Do you think you would have given different answers about the risks and benefits if you were asked these two questions?

Open-question surveys

Open questions are questions that require a longer answer or explanation (see the table). The advantage of open-question surveys is that they allow people to provide more information. This can be important when you are gathering information about complex issues or questions that do not have a simple yes/no answer. However, analysis of the data will take longer and be more complex.

Closed question	Open question
Have you been vaccinated against COVID-19?	What is your opinion of the COVID-19 vaccine?
Have you been admitted to hospital for an overnight stay?	What is your experience of staying in hospital overnight?
Who is your GP?	What is your opinion of the service provided by your GP?
When was the last time you were unwell?	How do you feel about your general state of health?

Interviews

An open-question survey can also be carried out face to face, in which case it can become an interview where the person asking the questions has the opportunity to follow up on answers to questions or adapt the interview to the individual. This can improve the quality of the data collected because it may not necessarily impose ideas or opinions on the individual responding to the survey. However, interviews can be even more complex to analyse and draw conclusions from.

Closed-question surveys are probably better at obtaining large amounts of data from a large number of people. Open-question surveys or interviews are probably better when the number of people being surveyed is relatively small.

Observation

This can be a good way of gathering data about behaviour, which explains its widespread use in healthcare and social science or animal behaviour studies (see case studies). It is an important part of the method known as **qualitative research** (see section A7.2).

In clinical and pharmaceutical research, randomised controlled trials are considered to be the most effective and reliable. In these, an experimental treatment or drug is compared either to a **placebo** (dummy treatment or drug) or to an existing treatment or drug. However, it is not always possible or desirable to carry out this type of trial. One example is where it is unethical to give a dummy treatment or drug.

In experimental studies, a researcher will usually have two groups: a test group and a control group. In observational studies, the researcher simply looks at (observes) groups of patients and compares the effectiveness of different types or treatment. An example is the **cohort** study, where a group of people (the cohort) is followed over a period of time. This can allow comparison of different treatment or care pathways to see which is the most effective. Cohort studies can be **prospective** or **retrospective**.

> **Key terms**
>
> **Prospective:** these studies take a group of people and observe them over a period of time. This could involve looking for correlations between factors such as diet or exercise and development of cardiovascular disease. The advantage is that the data collection methods can be tailored to the question being asked. The disadvantage is that these can take many years to complete.
>
> **Retrospective:** these studies look backwards at data from a group of people over many years. This often involves examining published data classifying people according to risk factors or medical outcomes. Although these can give results more quickly than prospective studies, the disadvantage of retrospective studies is that there is little control over data collection. This type of study typically looks at published data from many different sources that might involve different methods of data collection or analysis.

In clinical medicine, observation is very important in making diagnoses. However, the observational method used in qualitative research involves watching people to establish behaviours in a natural setting.

Public databases, journals and articles

You will notice, as you work through this book, that many of the Project practice items at the end of each chapter will start with asking you to research a topic. This is often to search published literature, often for background information, but also to make sure that you are not just repeating work that has already been done.

Health Education England and the National Institute for Health and Care Excellence (NICE) provide access to a wide range of journals and other evidence-based resources for health and social care staff in England. Access to these requires an NHS OpenAthens account; you may be eligible for this if your course involves an NHS placement.

A7: Managing information and data within the health and science sector

> **Case study**
>
> **The Millennium Cohort Study (MCS)**
> The MCS is following the lives of about 19,000 young people born in the UK in 2000–2002. The study collects data on:
> - Physical, social, emotional, cognitive and behavioural development (cognitive development is the ability to carry out conscious mental activities such as thinking, understanding, learning and remembering).
> - Daily life, behaviour and experiences.
> - Economic circumstances, parenting, relationships and family life.
> - GCSE exam results.
>
> The MCS has provided important evidence of how circumstances in the very early years of life can influence later health and development.
>
> Research based on the MCS has shown that children born at or just before the weekend are less likely to be breastfed, because breastfeeding support services are less available in hospitals at weekends. Breastfeeding has been shown to have a strong influence on cognitive development.
>
> The MCS has also contributed crucial evidence on two major health issues facing this generation – obesity and the high rates of poor mental health. There is more information about the MCS on the website: https://cls.ucl.ac.uk/cls-studies/millennium-cohort-study
>
> 1. How do prospective studies like the MCS differ from retrospective studies?
> 2. Do you think a prospective study can produce better quality data?
>
> **Observation of clinical practice**
> Observational research has been used to collect data on errors and potentially harmful events. A UK study on 10 wards in two hospitals showed that almost half of intravenous drug preparations and administrations had at least one error.
>
> This research was an example of an ethnographic study – one where the researcher is immersed in the community being observed. In this case, the nursing staff were told that the observer was investigating common problems of preparing and administering intravenous drugs. The word 'error' was avoided so that the study did not appear to threaten the staff.
>
> Source: K. Taxis & N. Barber (2003) BMJ 326, **684** (https://doi.org/10.1136/bmj.326.7391.684)
>
> 1. Do you think that observational research into patient care is important?
> 2. Is it always possible to build a complete and accurate picture of patient care by comparing outcomes in different hospitals or clinics?

The US National Library of Medicine has an online database, PubMed.gov, that has over 32 million biomedical research articles. Many of these have links to full text content, including free-to-access as well as paid-for content. PubMed is a free resource.

As well as literature databases (books, journals, articles, etc.) there are clinical databases that contain data rather than published research. These include:

- observational data on patients who meet certain criteria, such as disease type or population
- clinical trial data, such as **www.clinicaltrials.gov** (US based).

The World Health Organization (WHO) publishes databases in many health-related fields, including:
- life expectancy
- immunisation and vaccination data
- mortality.

> **Reflect**
>
> From September 2021 NHS Digital (the part of the NHS that designs, develops and operates IT and data services in the NHS) began to collect patient data from GP medical records in England. This data includes information about symptoms, test results, diagnoses and medication as well as about physical, mental and sexual health. The intention is to use this data to improve health and care services through better planning, preventing spread of infectious diseases, help with research and monitoring the long-term safety and effectiveness of care. The data will not include people's names or where they live, but there are concerns that it will not be completely anonymous.
>
> Another concern is that this data will be sold to private companies, such as pharmaceutical companies, as well as being made available to research organisations such as universities and charities.
>
> Do you think that making this type of data available could help in the development of new treatments? NHS Digital plans to charge for access to this data. It says that this covers its costs in processing the data and delivering the service, but some people think that this amounts to selling patient data. Do you think this is ethical? Do you think the benefit of using the data to improve treatment outweighs the risk to patient privacy and confidentiality?

These databases are invaluable sources for health and healthcare researchers.

Carrying out practical investigations

When we think of data, we probably think first about the results of experiments in the lab rather than some of the methods just discussed. Practical investigations in the field of health and healthcare can include laboratory experiments, for example, in basic medical science, using knowledge and techniques that build on the subjects covered in Chapter B2: Further science concepts.

Practical investigations can form the basis of evidence-based practice. These include:
- clinical trials of pharmaceuticals, usually run by pharmaceutical companies
- investigation of different types of care or treatment, such as comparison of drug treatment with talking therapies (talking to a therapist or counsellor) for treating mental illnesses
- investigation of different types of therapy, such as the RECOVERY trial into treatments for COVID-19.

Case study

The RECOVERY trial is the world's largest clinical trial into treatments for COVID-19. It was funded by the Medical Research Council and the National Institute for Health Research and led by the University of Oxford. The trial found one of the world's first effective drug treatments, dexamethasone. This cheap and widely available steroid medicine was shown to reduce deaths of patients in hospital with COVID-19 by one third.

Later the trial showed that tocilizumab, an anti-inflammatory drug used to treat rheumatoid arthritis, also reduces the risk of death in patients in hospital with severe COVID-19.

Do you think that low-cost treatments like dexamethasone would have been found if the investigations had been left to pharmaceutical companies that need to make profit for their shareholders?

Official statistics

Organisations such as the UK Health Security Agency (UKHSA) and the WHO collect and publish statistics on disease, public health, health protection and health improvement. Official statistics are also available from Public Health England (PHE), which was replaced by UKHSA in April 2021, and include those about:
- general public health
- alcohol, tobacco and drug use
- cancer
- cardiovascular disease
- child and maternal health
- chronic disease
- COVID-19
- diet and physical activity
- obesity
- end of life care
- immunisation and infectious diseases
- mental health
- sexual and reproductive health.

The WHO publishes statistics on an even wider range of health-related topics worldwide and by country.

Reflect

Collecting and publishing all these statistics is time consuming and can be expensive. So why do organisations publish official statistics? Think about how such statistics could be used.

Sometimes governments may be embarrassed if official statistics show that policies are not always working. For this reason, it is important that the collection and publication of official statistics is done in a transparent way so that we can have confidence in them.

Test yourself

1. State whether each of these questions is closed or open:
   a. How often do you visit your dentist?
   b. Have you found it difficult to find an NHS dentist in your area?
   c. What type of extra services does your dentist offer?
2. What type of data collection would you use for the following?
   a. To discover trends in the incidence of cardiovascular disease in the second half of the twentieth century.
   b. To compare the amount of exercise taken by 18–24 year olds and 40–50 year olds in a local authority area.
   c. To discover if vigorous exercise increases heart rate more in young people compared to middle-aged people.
   d. To discover if young people are better than older people at using unfamiliar equipment.

A7.2 The considerations to make when selecting a range of ways to collect and record information and data

There are many ways we can collect data and turn it into useful information. If we choose the wrong way, we might discover that it is harder to analyse or present and so we cannot get and communicate the best information and understanding from our data.

Data type

Quantitative data includes measurements such as length, height, age, time or mass. Quantitative data can be either:

- **discrete** (or discontinuous), meaning something that you can count, such as number of patients, number of visits to the GP, number of cases of flu in a year. Discrete data is usually in whole numbers – you cannot have half a patient or visit your GP on 2.75 occasions in a year
- **continuous**, meaning something that can be measured, such as height, weight or blood glucose concentration. Continuous data can have any value within a range and so is usually not in whole numbers – you could have a weight of 94.7 kg or a blood glucose concentration of 5.2 mmol/litre.

Once you process data, for example, by taking an average, it is quite possible for discrete data to no longer be in whole numbers. For example, the average UK household size has been 2.4 for a number of years, but each household will have a whole number of members.

Source: www.ons.gov.uk/peoplepopulationandcommunity/birthsdeathsandmarriages/families/bulletins/familiesandhouseholds/2020

Qualitative data is usually text-based, describing something in a way that may involve numbers (for instance, a rating of how good something is), but will also contain descriptive text. For example, a patient's medical history may contain their age, date of birth and blood pressure (all types of quantitative data) as well as qualitative data such as any diseases or other health conditions they have, operations or medical procedures they have undergone, and other information about their health and wellbeing.

> **Key terms**
>
> **Quantitative data:** is numerical, for example, a patient's age, height or weight.
>
> **Discrete data:** is numerical and can be **counted**. For example, number of patients (you cannot have half a patient). This is sometimes referred to as **integer** (only whole numbers).
>
> **Continuous data:** is numerical and can be measured. It is possible to have any intermediate value, for example, height, mass, length.
>
> **Qualitative data:** is descriptive, for example, a patient's medical history.

The most appropriate method of data collection

A laboratory notebook is the traditional method of collecting experimental data in the sciences and medicine, although paper notebooks are being replaced by electronic versions. These offer advantages in terms of security (e.g. backup of data) and data sharing (e.g. collaboration).

Quantitative data can be collected automatically. For example, a data logger can be connected to a piece of electronic equipment to capture the output (data) and transfer it to a computer. This offers several advantages:

- Data can be collected without the need for a human operator to be present.
- Data can be captured continuously, for long periods if necessary.
- Once captured by the computer, the data can be analysed and processed.

Qualitative data is usually based on observation and so cannot normally be collected automatically. However, qualitative data may be collected via questionnaires or surveys, and these can be set up in electronic format, either on computer, tablet or online. This means that much of the data collection can be automated. As with collection of quantitative data, this allows some (if not all) of the data processing and analysis to be automated.

Application of new technology to collection and analysis of data will be covered in more detail in section A7.5.

Healthcare Science T Level: Core

The most appropriate way to present the information or data

Before considering how to present information or data, we need to think about **dependent** and **independent variables**.

> **Key terms**
>
> **Dependent variable:** (often denoted by *y*) a variable whose value depends on that of another variable. In an experiment, we usually count or measure the dependent variable.
>
> **Independent variable:** (often denoted by *x*) a variable whose value does not depend on that of another variable. In an experiment, the independent variable is usually what we change.

Tables

When we collect data, we usually record it in a table, and this can often be a useful way to present the data.

There are rules to follow when presenting data in a table. This ensures uniformity so that anyone reading the table will be familiar with the layout of the data.
- Put the **independent** variable in the first column; the **dependent** variable should be in columns to the right.
- Put any processed data, such as means, rates or statistical calculations, in columns to the far right.
- Do not include calculations in the table, only **calculated values** (the results of your calculations).
- Head each column with the physical quantity and correct units and separate the units with brackets or a slash ('/'), for example, 'mass (g)' or 'body temperature/°C'.
- Do not include units in the body of the table, only in the column headings.
- Use consistent numbers of decimal places or significant figures throughout (see section B1.64 for more information about significant figures, even if it means writing 20.0 rather than 20.
- Calculated values, e.g. mean or other processed data, should be given to the same number of decimal places as the raw data, or one greater.

The table shows an example of how data should be presented. In this case, four 30-year-old men were asked to walk or run at a steady rate on a treadmill. The subject's heart rate (dependent variable) was measured in beats per minute (bpm) after 10 minutes. Following a period of recovery, the speed of the treadmill (independent variable) was increased and the experiment repeated. This was carried out at eight different speeds. The experiment was repeated for each of the four subjects and a mean value at each angle was calculated.

Speed of treadmill (km/hr)	Heart rate after 10 minutes (bpm)				
	Subject 1	Subject 2	Subject 3	Subject 4	Mean
2	75	78	80	76	77
4	80	82	85	88	84
6	88	89	92	90	90
8	95	98	101	105	100
10	110	105	115	112	111
12	125	100	128	130	128
14	155	158	160	165	160
16	170	175	178	185	177

> **Reflect**
>
> One reason for presenting data like this is that it can help identify anomalous results – ones that stand out as being 'different'. If you look at the highlighted cell in the table (subject 2 at 12 km/hr) you will see that the heart rate is lower than the same subject at 10 km/hr and is much lower than the other subjects at the same speed. Something is obviously wrong – maybe the heart rate monitor was not working properly – and so we discount this result as anomalous, and we have not included it in the calculation of the mean value (you can check that for yourself).
>
> As well as dependent and independent variables, there are **control** variables. These are things that we must keep constant (control) during the experiment. In this case, it means that anything that might affect heart rate, other than the speed of the treadmill, must be kept constant. One control variable would be the angle (steepness) of the treadmill as this makes walking or running more difficult.
>
> What other control variables can you think of?

Graphs and charts

The type of graph we use will depend on the nature of our data as well as what we hope to get from the graph.

Scatter graph

Scatter graphs are used when investigating the relationship between two variables that can be measured in pairs, for example, the age and height of children in a school. The graph can then be used to establish whether there is a relationship between the variables. This could be a **positive correlation** (as variable x increases, variable y increases, as in Figure 7.2), a **negative correlation** (as variable x increases, variable y decreases) or **no correlation** at all. To tell whether the correlation is significant or not you need to carry out a statistical test.

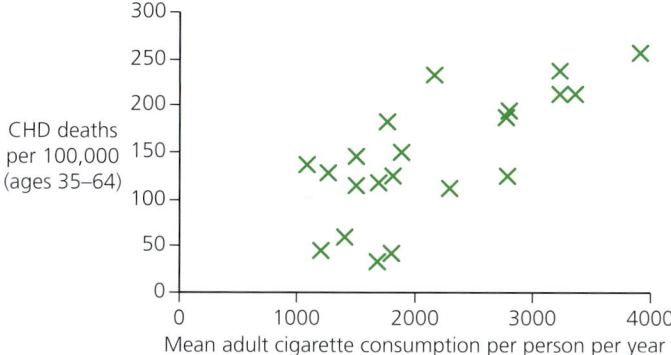

▲ Figure 7.2 Scatter graph showing the correlation between smoking and deaths from coronary heart disease (CHD)

Reflect

Does correlation imply causation?

This question means: just because there is a positive correlation between two variables, does that mean that one causes the other? For example, there is a strong positive correlation between ice-cream sales and deaths from drowning. Does that mean ice cream is a major cause of drowning? Should we ban ice-cream sales anywhere near open water? Or is there some other factor that is correlated with both? Hot weather, for example.

Line graph

Line graphs are used to show **continuous** data (see Figure 7.3). The independent variable, the one that we change, should be on the x-axis (the horizontal axis – think of it like changing a baby's nappy: the thing that is changed goes on the bottom). The dependent variable, the one that changes in response to changes in the independent variable, goes on the y-axis (the vertical axis). You would usually join the points with straight lines. You can draw a smooth curve or line of best fit if you think that intermediate values will fall on the curve/line.

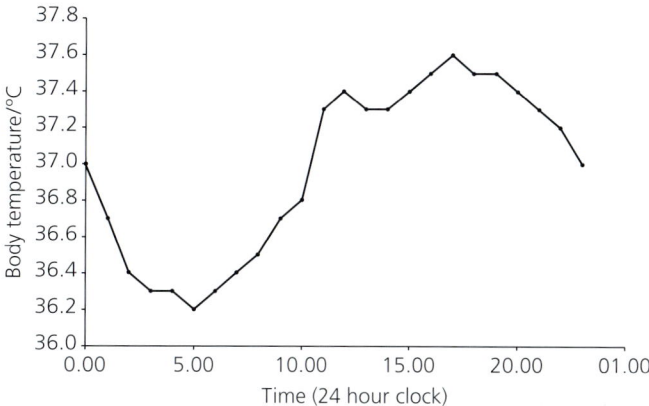

▲ Figure 7.3 Line graph showing how body temperature varies slightly during a 24-hour period

Bar charts and histograms

Bar charts are used to display **categorical data**. If you have an independent variable that is non-numerical (e.g. blood group, ethnic group of patient), then you should use a bar chart. These can be made up of lines, or blocks of equal width, that do not touch (Figure 7.4). The lines or blocks can be arranged in any order, although it can help make comparisons if they are arranged in order of increasing or decreasing size.

Bar charts can be turned through 90 degrees if it is easier to show or read horizontal rather than vertical bars.

Key term

Categorical data: is divided into groups or categories, such as male and female, ethnic group, city or country of residence.

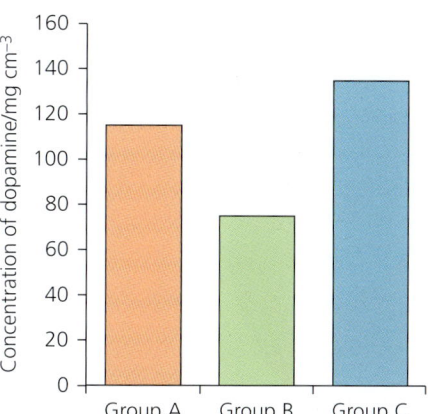

▲ Figure 7.4 Bar chart showing concentration of the neurotransmitter dopamine in three groups of patients

Histograms are sometimes called frequency diagrams. These can be used for either discrete data or continuous data grouped into classes, such as a range of heights or weights. The independent variable is usually on the *x*-axis and is grouped into classes. For example, the height of students in a class could be measured and grouped into 5 cm classes. Height is a continuous variable – students could be any height within a range – and so blocks are drawn touching. The axis is labelled with the class boundaries, e.g. 1600 mm, 1650 mm, 1700 mm, 1750 mm, 1800 mm, etc. and the *y*-axis would show the number or frequency within each class represented by the height of the bar (Figure 7.5).

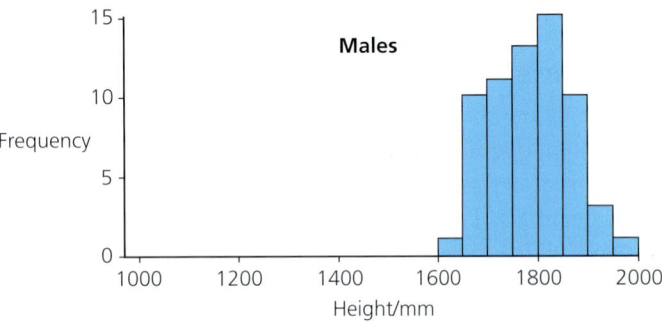

▲ Figure 7.5 Frequency distribution showing height of 18-year-old male students

Pie chart

Pie charts can be used when you need to show proportions or percentages (Figure 7.6). If you are drawing a pie chart by hand, you need to calculate the angle of each sector – divide the percentage by 100 and multiply by 360°, or just multiply the proportion by 360°. However, it is usually much easier to put your data into a spreadsheet and use the chart function to draw the pie chart!

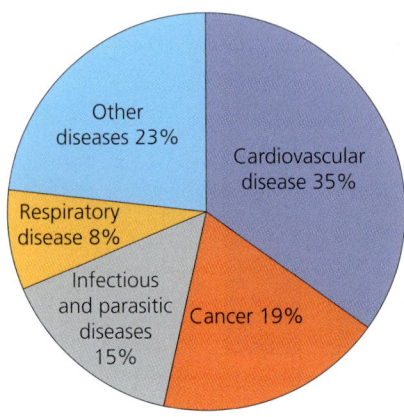

▲ Figure 7.6 Pie chart showing worldwide causes of death from disease, 2000–2019

Source: www.who.int/data/gho/data/themes/mortality-and-global-health-estimates/ghe-leading-causes-of-death

> **Case study**
>
> You have been asked to present data about the incidence (number of cases) of cardiovascular disease in the UK. You have been given the following data:
> 1. Total incidence of cardiovascular disease by age group (21–30, 31–40, 41–50, 51–60, 61–70, 71 and above).
> 2. Incidence of cardiovascular disease by the same age groups but separated into males and females.
> 3. Total incidence of cardiovascular disease (all ages) broken down by ethnic group.
>
> You decide to use a histogram for the first data set. For the second data set, you have two options. You could draw two separate histograms, one for males and one for females. Alternatively, you could use a single histogram and draw two columns for each age group, one for males and one for females.
> ▶ Which do you think would be better?
> ▶ Are there advantages and disadvantages of each?
>
> For the third data set you know that you cannot use a histogram. You could use a bar chart or you could use a pie chart.
> ▶ Think about the two ways of presenting the data. What advantages and disadvantages of each can you see?

Depth of analysis required

Collecting data is the start of the process. To convert raw data into useful information we usually need to carry out some form of analysis. Using graphs and charts can help in analysing the data or they can be the end point, i.e. how we present the data.

The depth of analysis required can determine how we record and present the data. Spreadsheet programs, such as Microsoft Excel or Apple Numbers, are convenient ways of recording data. We could enter the data manually, or even download data collected by a data logger directly into a spreadsheet. Once in a spreadsheet we can use a range of tools to analyse the data:

▶ simple analysis such as calculating the mean (average)
▶ more complex analysis such as statistical tests.

Another advantage of using a spreadsheet to record data is that we can use the graphing tools to present our data in different ways, such as the types of graphs and charts described on pages 147–149.

Qualitative or text-based data, e.g. from observations, surveys or focus groups, would normally be recorded and stored in a database, such as Microsoft Access or Apple FileMaker. Databases can contain huge quantities of data. They can also be used to analyse qualitative data as well as to organise it in ways that helps gain insight into connections, trends or groupings within the data.

Databases also allow others, such as collaborators or the general public, to access the data (if permitted), so this can be a way of presenting and sharing information as well as collecting, storing and analysing data.

The intended audience

This is a consideration largely when deciding how to present our data. Simple graphs and charts can make data and information more accessible to a non-specialist audience. This might be the case with an information leaflet or poster aimed at patients or the general public. Meanwhile, a more specialist audience might require more complex graphs that may give greater insight into the finer detail of the data. This would be the case if we wrote a research paper aimed at fellow health professionals for publication in a scientific or healthcare journal.

Collecting and storing data in electronic format (spreadsheet or database) also allows collaborators to get easy access to the data so that they can use it in their own work.

Storage method

How we store data depends in part on how it is collected and how it is used. Paper-based surveys, questionnaires or records of interviews or observations can, of course, simply be kept on paper. The same is true of results of experiments in a lab notebook. However, if they can be converted to digital format, then we can analyse them in the ways described. Data that has been collected in digital form would usually be stored in that form.

> **Test yourself**
>
> 1. Describe the difference between **qualitative** and **quantitative** data.
> 2. Give two advantages of automated data capture.
> 3. How would you present and process or analyse the following data?
>   a. Raw data from an investigation into blood glucose concentration in diabetics. Each patient had their blood glucose concentration measured every day for a week.
>   b. Measurement of mean blood glucose concentration and body mass index in a group of Type 2 diabetic patients.
> 4. Which would be the most appropriate method to present information about the incidence of the top 20 causes of death in young people to:
>   a. the general public
>   b. a group of health professionals?

A7.3 The importance of accuracy, attention to detail and legibility of any written information or data

There are a few rules we must always follow in keeping written records of our work:
▶ We must be able to understand the record.
▶ It should be legible and contain enough detail for someone else to understand it and be able to repeat the work.
▶ It should be a faithful, honest and accurate record of what we did.

Always write up your work as you go along; do not make notes on scraps of paper and write it all up later – even if you do not lose the scraps of paper, you may not remember all the details. It is always good practice to date all your notes. In some organisations there may even be a legal requirement to do so.

There are numerous reasons why we must pay attention to detail and accuracy in written information or data.
▶ It may be necessary to comply with legal requirements, for example, the General Data Protection Regulation (GDPR) – see section A7.6.
▶ We may need to limit liability, either our own or that of the organisation – for example, by ensuring anonymity and to record informed consent.

- We should be able to provide an accurate account of events. That might be obvious when recording the details of an experiment, but it is also important in a healthcare situation. Knowing exactly what happened in the lead-up to a patient's condition improving or deteriorating can be essential in learning from experience. It might also be needed if there is an investigation into the patient's care.
- It will help collaboration in integrated working and data sharing. You may be able to remember the details of an experiment, treatment or patient's observations. However, unless you record those details clearly and accurately, colleagues may not have sufficient information without asking you for more detail. Sharing of data is essential in multidisciplinary teams, where healthcare professionals with different specialisms must work together.
- It helps to ensure accurate analysis of findings. Accurate analysis begins with good quality data. If the data is poor, then the processed or analysed data will also be poor, and the conclusions may be invalid. Recording a patient's **clinical observations** (see section B2.10 and B2.11 for more detail about this topic) is an important aspect of monitoring a patient. If these observations are not correctly and accurately recorded, it may not be possible to identify whether they are within the normal range.
- It can provide evidence needed in support of audit trails. This could include things as diverse as:
  - keeping a record of a patient's clinical observations
  - providing evidence that a medication or treatment has been given and when.
- To help ensure reproducibility of results. Our work can be reproduced only if it is clear what we did, how we did it and what our results were.

Results are **repeatable** when we carry out an investigation several times in the same place, using the same method under the same conditions, and get the same result.

Results are **reproducible** when investigations are carried out by different people, in different places using different methods or equipment, and get the same result. This means that our findings can be replicated by others.

> **Case study**
>
> A study at a large hospital in England found that nurses sometimes completed documentation retrospectively (after the event) without full knowledge that the recorded care had been completed. One nurse described how a patient had collapsed, but their notes did not contain any information about why they had been admitted. In another case, nurses completed the documentation before they carried out procedures because they were worried about forgetting to complete the paperwork. Accurate record keeping was particularly important for older patients because of the complexity of care that they require and also the problems they may have with communication. However, nurses working with older patients found completing the documentation was very time consuming and took them away from patient care.
>
> The authors of the study recommended that electronic methods of documenting patient care could be used to reduce the amount of unnecessary paperwork as well as to make sharing of information more effective.
> - Can you see lessons for your own practice?
> - Do you feel that there is sometimes a conflict between accurate record keeping and providing care?
> - Should that be the case?

A7.4 The strengths and limitations of a range of data sources when applied in a range of health and science environments

If we are going to be able to draw valid and useful conclusions from data – get good quality information – we need to have an appreciation of the strengths and limitations of the type of data source. Otherwise we risk producing poor quality information based on invalid conclusions.

Results of investigations

Scientific or medical experiments ('investigations') should, if properly designed, give consistent and reliable results. This is because they should be well designed. This includes:
- formulating a clear hypothesis to be tested
- designing an experiment to test that hypothesis
- controlling all variables

- repeating measurements, excluding anomalous results (these are outliers, or results that lie outside of the range of the others) and calculating mean values
- performing a statistical analysis to test the significance of the results.

However, there can be limitations. For example, we might be tempted to apply the results of an investigation done under highly controlled conditions to the more complex situation of the 'real world'. A potential new drug might show promise when tested in test-tube experiments, for instance. However, complex interactions in living systems might mean that the drug does not work as hoped when tested in humans, or it might have unexpected and even harmful side-effects.

Patient history

At its simplest level, this approach involves taking medical histories of patients. This is a skill that many healthcare professionals need to develop. Done well, a medical history will provide detailed information about a patient over a long period. However, the data may be incomplete, particularly if it relies on the patient's memory.

If you consult some of the databases described in section A7.1 you might come across many studies looking at patient histories over time. Some of these will look backwards at patient data – these are known as **retrospective** studies. Others will follow a group of normal subjects (a selection of the general population, perhaps of a particular age) or patients over a long period to look for development or progress of disease over a period of time – these are known as **prospective** studies.

In either case, the studies are likely to involve a **cohort**, which is a group of individuals that have something in common. It could be age, sex, state of health or disease, occupation, etc. Examples of this are the two Whitehall studies. Each of these followed a large group of British civil servants over many years and looked at factors that affected the health of the cohort, in particular cardiovascular disease and mortality rates. One finding was that there was a correlation between employment grade and reduced risk of cardiovascular disease – more senior civil servants enjoyed better health.

The strength of this type of study is that it can provide detailed information over time. However, there are cases where the data may not be accurate or complete, particularly with retrospective studies.

Patient test results

Patient test results usually mean the results of biochemical and other laboratory analysis. These should offer a high level of accuracy. Also, testing laboratories and the tests themselves must usually go through an accreditation process to ensure that they operate to approved standards and give reliable results. This means that test results this week should be comparable with results of tests taken weeks or months ago. It should also be possible to compare test results performed in different laboratories.

However, as humans are complex, a patient's test results will often need careful interpretation. This can introduce an element of subjectivity. Two healthcare professionals might look at the same set of patient test results and make different interpretations or draw different conclusions.

Published literature

The medical and scientific literature is a huge and invaluable resource in the health and science sector. This is the reason why most research projects will start with a literature review, to see what work has already been done and how that can inform and influence the research you plan to undertake. It is also an important tool for learning and diagnosis.

As well as the sheer volume available, another strength of published literature is that it goes through a process of **peer review**. This is where, before it can be published, a research paper is examined by other experts in the field. They might find flaws in the experiments or the logic or interpretation of the results and request that any deficiencies are put right before publication. This process improves the validity of the published research.

This process is not perfect. Professional rivalry means that reviewers are not always impartial. Also, the process can be slow and cumbersome, taking weeks, months or even years. This has led to a trend for **preprints**. These are papers that are published rapidly before peer review. This has the advantage of putting information into the scientific community very quickly. This is important during an event such as the COVID-19 pandemic, because information about new treatments can be made available rapidly in order to save lives.

However, not all published literature is of equal high quality. Some research might be based on studies with very small sample sizes, for example, clinical trials with only a few patients. The methods used in the experiment or study might be biased in a way that produces the results the investigators hoped for. The work might even be based on fraudulent data.

> **Case study**
>
> **Andrew Wakefield and the MMR autism fraud**
>
> Andrew Wakefield was an academic physician who published a paper in the medical journal *The Lancet* in 1998. In this paper, Wakefield claimed that there was a link between the measles-mumps-rubella (MMR) vaccine and autism, based on a study involving 12 children. The publication, and particularly news conferences given by Wakefield, led to a loss of confidence in the MMR vaccine.
>
> After the original publication, other researchers were unable to reproduce Wakefield's findings and it was found that Wakefield had a number of undeclared financial conflicts of interest. As a result, he was charged with gross professional misconduct and in 2010 the General Medical Council's Fitness to Practise Panel judged that Wakefield should be struck off the UK medical register, meaning he would no longer be allowed to practise as a doctor. Following this judgement, The Lancet retracted the paper, stating:
>
> > 'It has become clear that several elements of the 1998 paper by Wakefield et al are incorrect, contrary to the findings of an earlier investigation. In particular, the claims in the original paper that children were "consecutively referred" and that investigations were "approved" by the local ethics committee have been proven to be false.'
> >
> > Source: www.thelancet.com/journals/lancet/article/PIIS0140-6736(10)60175-4/fulltext
>
> As a result of the original publication and the publicity it received, many parents chose not to have their children vaccinated and by 2012/13, cases of measles, mumps and rubella had reached the highest level for 18 years.
>
> Source: www.gov.uk/government/publications/measles-confirmed-cases/confirmed-cases-of-measles-mumps-and-rubella-in-england-and-wales-2012-to-2013

deal of information observing patients or test subjects for a relatively short time. The advantage of this is that we get the data immediately.

Of course, the disadvantage is that our observations might become subjective. **Objective** observations are things that can be measured, such as pulse, temperature or respiration rate. **Subjective** observations are signs that cannot be measured, such as how a person or patient feels. These can be very important, particularly when we observe someone over time and can tell when there is a change in their condition or behaviour. However, we have to take care that we do not misinterpret or over-interpret such observations.

> **Test yourself**
>
> 1. Give two advantages and one disadvantage of using results of experiments or investigations in healthcare.
> 2. Give one advantage of using data or information from published research.
> 3. What is the difference between **objective** and **subjective** observations?

A7.5 How new technology is applied in the recording and reporting of information and data

In section A7.2 we saw the advantages of automated data collection. New technologies are being used to improve both the quality and quantity of data that can be collected, even allowing us to collect new kinds of data. New technology has also transformed the way we can analyse the data collected.

This is particularly true when applied to **longitudinal** research, where measurements or observations are made over a long period. By allowing passive measurement of health-related factors, we can avoid the bias that can occur when we rely on people self-reporting. The widespread use and acceptance of fitness trackers and smartwatches means that these can also be used for monitoring physiological data in subjects that are part of a cohort study or clinical trial.

Real-time observation

Some prospective observational studies can last for many years. However, observation does not need to be carried out over such a long period. We can get a great

AI/machine learning

Big data is a term that you hear more often these days, usually to describe the massive amounts of data collected by companies such as Amazon, Facebook and

A7: Managing information and data within the health and science sector

Google. However, there are many areas of science and healthcare that now generate very large data sets, for example:
- DNA sequences, such as from the Human Genome Project
- proteomics – the study of the proteins produced by the body and how the presence or absence of some proteins is correlated with various diseases
- high content imaging – the automated collection and analysis of microscope images to provide information about processes within cells and tissues
- results from clinical trials
- epidemiology data looking at the spread of diseases (see sections B2.18 and B2.19).

Machine learning is a branch of **AI** (artificial intelligence) that uses computers to imitate the ways in which humans learn. The **algorithm** (a list of rules that a computer follows to solve a problem) can be trained to interpret a sample set of data and then automatically improve the algorithm. This can go through many rounds so that, eventually, the computer is able to interpret very large data sets.

This approach has been used to develop algorithms that can help to interpret medical images, such as those from CT scans or radiography for use in diagnostics, particularly of cancer.

> **Case study**
>
> Research carried out by Moorfields Eye Hospital, DeepMind (part of Google) and UCL uses AI to help identify diseases that can lead to blindness. AI and machine learning technology was trained on thousands of historic eye scans, previously used by specialists to diagnose the disease, to identify features of eye disease and recommend how patients should be referred for care. The AI system can recommend the correct referral decision for more than 50 eye diseases with 94 per cent accuracy. This is the level of accuracy achieved by world-leading eye experts.

Some of these applications come under the general heading of **bioinformatics**. This describes the use of tools and software methods to analyse and process large data sets, such as DNA and protein sequences, genetics, cellular organisation and the mutations that lead to cancer. A related area is **systems biology**, which looks at the chemical and enzyme interactions and pathways within the cell.

Mobile technology and applications

Smartphones and high-speed mobile data networks such as 4G and 5G mean that devices can be connected to the internet almost anywhere in countries with more developed economies – and in many other parts of the world as well. Smartphones and tablets can also be used within a hospital, care home or other healthcare facility to connect to Wi-Fi. This opens up many opportunities for using mobile devices to collect and transfer data.

Health informatics is the use of computer science and AI/machine learning to assist in the management of healthcare information.

> **Case study**
>
> Nottingham University Hospitals NHS trust (NUH) has issued 6500 mobile devices to its clinical staff to allow implementation of electronic observations. Alongside this, NUH developed an app called 'Safer Staffing'. This allows the trust to see the nurse staffing position in real time across more than 85 wards and departments. The nurse in charge of each ward is asked to declare whether they judge that the ward is safe to deliver the required level of care to its current group of patients with the staff on duty. This allows the trust to see where support might be required.

Smartphones also have GPS (global positioning system) receivers built in, which means that they can be used for physical tracking of individuals. This, together with Bluetooth® wireless technology, was used in the NHS COVID-19 app that was the basis of 'track and trace' during the pandemic. If you had been in close contact with someone who tested positive for COVID-19, the app would 'ping' you and you would be told to self-isolate for 10 days. Unfortunately, in the summer of 2021, as lockdown restrictions were eased, the number of people who had to self-isolate grew to such high levels that there were severe staff shortages in areas such as hospitality, transport, retail and healthcare. As a result, there were reports of people deleting the app to avoid being contacted. This was a good example of how technology does not always offer an ideal solution, particularly if it is not properly implemented.

Cloud-based systems

Cloud computing means the availability of computers and computer resources, especially data storage, without active management by the user. Cloud-based systems usually have functions distributed over multiple locations or data centres connected via the internet. This distribution can make cloud-based systems more robust, because they will usually recover quickly if a single server fails. However, it can also make them more susceptible to malicious attacks, as described in section A7.9.

An important application of cloud-based systems in healthcare is the use of **electronic health records (EHRs)**. Because cloud-based systems are accessible to anyone with the appropriate permission, patient data can be available to anyone who needs it across the whole healthcare system. NHS Digital is implementing systems like this – see section A7.1 for an example.

As well as making patient data available to all appropriate healthcare professionals, cloud-based systems mean easier data sharing for further analysis, for example, by AI/machine learning systems that can be used in diagnosis or to gain insight into treatment and prevention of disease.

Digital information management systems

In 2018, the Department of Health and Social Care published a policy paper entitled 'The future of healthcare: our vision for digital, data and technology in health and care'. This addressed many of the areas that we have covered here, such as the use of cloud-based systems, AI/machine learning and mobile technology.

Digital information management systems also offer the advantage of a digital audit trail. This can show, for example, who accessed a patient's records and when, which can help ensure patient confidentiality and protect their personal information (see section A7.6).

Data-visualisation tools

One problem associated with the vast amount of healthcare data that is now available is the difficulty in understanding the complexity of numerical and text-based data. The simplest data visualisation tool is the graph (see section A7.2). Modern technology makes it possible to take multiple data sources, often from cloud-based systems such as patient databases, and present them in a way that makes it easier to understand and interpret them.

Every modern hospital will use data-visualisation tools to manage its in-house processes, such as:
- maintaining electronic medical records to track and monitor patient health
- avoiding diagnosing errors by eliminating human error
- accessing information about patients' demographics (factors such as age or ethnic background) and lifestyles (diet, exercise, smoking, alcohol consumption, etc.) in order to improve care and treatment of the patient.

> **Test yourself**
>
> 1 Explain what is meant by the following terms:
>   a Artificial intelligence (machine learning).
>   b Cloud-based systems.
> 2 Give one advantage of the use of mobile technology in healthcare data capture.
> 3 Give one advantage of using digital information management systems.
> 4 Give one advantage of using data visualisation tools in healthcare.

A7.6 How personal information is protected by data protection legislation, regulations and local ways of working/organisational policies

We have covered the various applications of modern technology in the health sector. We all know that electronic systems are not always secure from all the hacking incidents that have happened over the years. To maintain faith in these different uses of modern technology, patients and staff must feel confident that their personal information will be protected.

This applies equally to personal information stored on paper or in electronic format. In this section we will look at the ways in which personal information is protected. These issues are covered by legislation as well as local policies that most organisations have in place.

Data Protection Act (DPA) 2018

The DPA 2018 revised earlier data protection law passed in 1998, but its main purpose was to implement the GDPR of the European Union (EU). Although the UK has now left the EU, the legislation remains in force at the time of writing.

The DPA 2018 controls the use of personal information by organisations, businesses or the government. The Act is enforced by the Information Commissioner's Office (ICO), which is funded by a charge on **data controllers**, who must register with the ICO. A data controller is a person or organisation that stores or processes personal information, either on paper or electronically. Personal information is defined quite widely, so it includes aspects such as:
- your name and telephone number
- your National Insurance or passport number
- your location data, such as home address or smartphone GPS data – i.e. your smartphone tracking you
- online identifiers such as email or IP address.

However, there are other types of personal data that are also covered by the Act and GDPR, including:
- biometric data such as facial images or fingerprints that can be used to identify you
- health data that can reveal information about your physical or mental health status
- genetic data that can also give information about your health or physiology
- ethnic origin
- political opinions and religious or philosophical beliefs
- sexual orientation.

GDPR 2018

The GDPR came into force within the EU in 2018. It provides a set of principles with which any individual or organisation processing sensitive personal data must comply. There are six legitimate reasons why an organisation may process your personal data:
- You have given your consent for them to process your data for a specific purpose. This must be explicit (for example, you tick a box on an online form saying 'I wish to receive emails from you') rather than default – where you must untick a box to opt out of receiving emails.
- The processing is necessary to fulfil a contract you have entered into. For example, if you place an online order with a company, it has the right to process your personal data so that it can deliver the goods or inform you if there are any delays.
- There is a legal obligation for them to process your data. For example, an employer is obliged to pass employee salary details to HMRC for tax purposes.
- The data processing is necessary to protect you or someone else. For example, if you are admitted to A&E with life-threatening injuries following a road traffic accident, disclosure to the hospital of your medical history is necessary to help save your life.
- Processing is necessary to perform a task in the public interest or for an official function. This applies to any organisation that exercises an official authority that has a clear basis in law. Examples include local authorities, courts and the criminal justice system, and other agencies carrying out duties that are laid down in law. For example, a government agency has statutory powers to research the online shopping habits of consumers. The agency can ask retailers to share the personal data of a random sample of their customers so that it can carry out this function.
- Processing is necessary so that the organisation can pursue its legitimate interests. For example, companies and other organisations need to maintain personnel records.

GDPR includes a number of rights of individuals, for example:
- the right to be informed about the collection and use of their personal data
- the right to have access to their personal data
- the right to have incorrect personal data corrected or completed if it is incomplete
- the right to have personal data erased – but only in certain circumstances
- the right to restrict the processing of their personal data – again, only in certain circumstances
- the right to data portability, so that they can copy or transfer their personal data between different systems, for example, if you have accounts with different banks you may be able to view the details of all of them in a single app
- the right to object to processing of personal data, for example, you can refuse to have your personal data used for direct marketing (sometimes called 'spam' or 'junk mail').

GDPR also regulates the processing by organisations outside the EU of personal data of people within the EU. It prevents transfer of data from within the EU to countries outside the EU (such as the UK) unless those countries have appropriate safeguards in place. If you think about the widespread use of cloud computing described in section A7.5, you can see how easily personal data might be transferred across national borders. Partly as a result of this, the GDPR has become the model for many national data protection laws around the world.

Local ways of working/organisational policies

The DPA 2018 and GDPR are not the only things that regulate and protect personal information. Many organisations have their own ways of working, rules and policies that ensure compliance with legislation and regulations, as well as to protect the organisation (for example, from reputational damage if personal information is misused). The ICO expects organisations to have their own policies in place to ensure that they and their staff will comply with GDPR.

Examples of this include:

▶ ensuring that data is stored securely (electronically or paper-based) so that there will not be any loss of data or loss of confidentiality
▶ restricting the use of mobile devices as ways in which personal information may be misused or divulged. This helps to ensure confidentiality
▶ preventing potential conflicts of interest. For example, organisations must appoint a Data Protection Officer (DPO) who should be relatively senior in the organisation. However, there are some senior jobs (such as Chief Executive, Chief Medical Officer or Head of Human Resources) that would be in conflict with the job of DPO, so the roles should not be combined.

> **Reflect**
>
> Clearly it is essential to protect personal information and ensure patient confidentiality is maintained, but can that be taken too far? A patient's medical history must be kept secure when sharing it with another provider involved in their care, but is there a risk that vital information could be missed if the medical history is kept confidential? Could keeping data confidential from those who need to know put effective care at risk?

> **Test yourself**
>
> 1 Name the legislation and regulation that protect personal information.
> 2 Which of the following are examples of the acceptable processing of personal information?
>   a Collecting contact details from social media so that you can advertise a new patient support group.
>   b Providing a patient's medical history to a life assurance company without the patient's permission.
>   c Providing a patient's medical history to an intensive care doctor when the patient is in a coma.
>   d Transferring a database of patient data to a computer located in an unknown country for analysis.

A7.7 How to ensure confidentiality when using screens to input or retrieve information or data

Having considered the legal framework around the protection of personal data, we should also consider ways in which confidentiality could be lost or compromised through carelessness or poor practice.

Computer systems should always have password-protected access. This helps to protect sensitive personal information from being accessed by anyone without authorisation. It also means that it is possible to see who accessed what information – it provides an audit trail if there is a data breach.

That means that we should always protect login details and passwords. Unfortunately, many organisations insist on the use of passwords that are difficult to remember (although not always difficult for computer hackers to guess). It should be obvious that 'Password1234' is not a secure choice. Nor is it good practice to write your login details on a sticky note on your computer screen. Sadly, both of these – and other – poor practices are widespread.

A7: Managing information and data within the health and science sector

We should always log out of a system when leaving the screen (PC, laptop, tablet, etc.) so that someone else cannot come along and access sensitive personal information. Alternatively, if you have a password-protected lock screen (which is a basic computer security feature), you should lock the screen when you leave it, even if it is just for a minute.

You should also be aware of your surroundings when dealing with personal information. When you get money out of a cash machine, you should be cautious of 'shoulder surfers' trying to see your PIN as you enter it. The same can be true in the workplace where it might be possible for unauthorised people (colleagues, patients, visitors) to overlook you and your screen. For this reason, privacy screen filters can be useful as they make it difficult to read information on screen unless you are directly in front of it.

Another area that is important is the use of secure internet connections. We should all be aware that regular email is not secure – it passes through so many different systems, any one of which could be compromised. Another potential insecurity is the use of public Wi-Fi, such as in coffee shops. Any information shared over a public Wi-Fi network can be intercepted easily. Your home Wi-Fi may not be completely secure either. For this reason, many organisations now use VPN (virtual private network) to access the internet or exchange information safely and privately.

A7.8 The positive use of, and restrictions on the use of, social media in health and science sectors

It is becoming more common for employers to look at the social media of prospective employees. So think carefully before you post pictures of wild nights out on your social media! Of course, social media can offer many advantages as well.

Positive uses

Social media can play an important part, particularly in:
- awareness campaigns and disseminating information – this could be as simple as reminding social media followers to follow common-sense health practices, but it is also possible to target relevant population groups with specific health messages
- correcting misinformation – there is a lot of health misinformation on social media. This might be simply untrue statements. There can also be misinformation in the form of facts presented without context, or in the wrong context. Unfortunately, people are often more inclined to believe information that supports their existing prejudices
- crisis communication and monitoring, for example, during an epidemic or pandemic (such as COVID-19). More people now get their news from social media than from newspapers.

PHE uses a wide range of social media to share news and information about its work as well as public health incidents – the COVID-19 pandemic, for example.

Other uses of social media in the health and science sectors include:
- monitoring public health. People post about everything online, including their health. Hashtags such as #flu can show when diseases are spreading in new locations. Health data from social media has improved prediction of infectious diseases such as flu
- data gathering
- establishing patient support networks. This can be particularly effective among younger people
- recruitment – both of new employees or of subjects for clinical trials and other health research
- marketing by commercial and healthcare organisations.

Restrictions

We have already seen how social media can be a useful tool but can also have disadvantages. To try to minimise the disadvantages, we need to follow some basic rules when using social media in the health and science sectors.
- Do not post sensitive or personal information about yourself or others on social media. This should be common sense, but it is also likely to be covered by an organisation's code of conduct.
- Maintain professional boundaries when interacting with individuals outside the organisation. Again, it should be common sense, but it can sometimes be easy, in the context of social media, to be less professional than you would be face to face.
- Do not share inaccurate or non-evidence-based information. In fact, it is a criminal offence under the Care Act 2014 for care providers who 'supply, publish or otherwise make available certain types of information that is false or misleading'.

More employers in the health and science sectors are implementing social media policies to avoid risks associated with misuse of social media by their employees. These risks can include:
- reputational damage
- infringement of the intellectual property rights of others, e.g. by posting copyright material such as images, videos or music
- liability for any discriminatory or **defamatory** (reputation-damaging) comments posted by employees
- possible unauthorised sharing of confidential information.

A7.9 The advantages and risks of using IT systems to record, retrieve and store information and data

Compared with paper-based systems, IT systems have huge advantages – some of which were discussed in section A7.5. However, while being aware of the advantages, we must also guard against the risk associated with IT systems.

Advantages

The advantages of IT systems in the health and science sectors include:
- ease of access, sharing and transferring data – particularly with greater use of cloud-based systems
- the speed of data analysis as well as the ability to use AI/machine learning (see section A7.5)
- greater data security, for example, when it is password-protected
- standardisation of data. This can be a barrier to be overcome when transferring information and data from old, particularly paper-based, systems to modern IT systems because the older data is likely to be in a variety of non-standard formats. However, moving forward, standardisation can be a great advantage
- the ability to have continuous and/or real-time monitoring of data. This can be particularly important during disease outbreaks such as epidemics and pandemics
- cost and space saving. This is another reason why cloud-based solutions are becoming more widespread
- integrated working, making for greater collaboration between colleagues. It also supports safeguarding practices.

Risks

We have covered some of the risk factors, particularly security breaches – accidental or malicious – that can compromise patient confidentiality. However, there are other risk factors to consider.

There is the potential for corruption of data, making databases unusable. This is one reason why all IT systems need robust procedures for backup of data – although making a backup of corrupted data can just mean that you have a corrupted (and so useless) backup. Organisations need to be aware of the risks of data corruption as a result of ransomware attacks. This is where malicious software is installed on a system (usually by someone in the organisation clicking on a link in an email or on a website) which then corrupts or encrypts all the data held on the system. Some organisations have paid millions of dollars in Bitcoin to ransomware criminals so that they can retrieve their data.

Have you ever called a company, only to be told 'I'm sorry, but our system is down'? That might be annoying when you are trying to find out when you will get the item of clothing you ordered. But when you are trying to access critical patient information, it can be much more serious. This is why many healthcare systems have built-in redundancy – there may be multiple computers handling access to data so that a single failure does not bring the whole system down.

> **Reflect**
>
> It is hard to think about how we managed without modern IT systems. But, do we always appreciate the risks as well as the benefits? We have seen the importance of following policies and procedures, but do we always think about whether that is enough? Are the systems that we use sufficiently secure? Are there procedures to monitor and enforce the policies that are in place? These are questions for management, rather than individual health professionals. However, it is good to ask ourselves these questions, if only to reinforce the need to comply fully with required procedures and policies.

> **Test yourself**
>
> 1. Give one benefit and one risk of using IT systems in healthcare.
> 2. Describe how use of IT systems in healthcare can increase collaboration.

A7.10 How security measures protect data stored by organisations

We have already looked at how security measures can help to preserve patient confidentiality and keep personal information secure. However, that is not the only reason that data must be protected by appropriate security measures. Loss of data can be catastrophic in a modern healthcare setting.

Malicious operators (hackers) may try to access sensitive patient information, or they might have some other criminal intent, such as installation of ransomware. State-sponsored groups have been implicated in various attacks on computer systems in recent years – this has been given the name 'cyber warfare' – and healthcare systems have been targeted. In May 2020, the International Committee of the Red Cross called for governments to take immediate and decisive action to prevent and stop cyber attacks on hospitals, healthcare facilities and organisations, research organisations and international authorities that provide critical care and support for healthcare. This followed cyber attacks against medical facilities in the Czech Republic, France, Spain, Thailand and the United States as well as international organisations such as the WHO.

There are various ways in which an organisation's data can be protected:

- Controlling access to information, for example, through levels of authorised logins and passwords. This can also mean that some staff can access information but not change it ('read only' access). This helps protect against inadvertent change to or deletion of data by inexperienced staff.
- Allowing only authorised staff into specific work areas so that they cannot physically access sensitive computer equipment. In some organisations, the USB ports on computers are disabled so that data cannot be transferred onto USB memory devices.
- Requiring regular and up-to-date staff training in complying with data security. Technology and the methods used by cyber criminals change rapidly, so staff need to keep up to date.
- Making regular backups of files. Often there will be multiple backups so that there is no risk of replacing 'good' backup data with corrupted or encrypted data.
- Using up-to-date cyber security strategies to protect against unintended or unauthorised access. Organisations need to employ good cyber security staff or consultants and make sure that their recommendations are taken seriously.
- Ensuring that backup data is stored externally, for example, cloud-based or on (ideally multiple) servers elsewhere. If there is a fire in the IT suite, you need to be able to get up and running again quickly and this will not be possible if all the backups are stored in a cupboard in the IT suite.

A7.11 What to do if information is not stored securely

Sometimes things go wrong, often due to human error or carelessness. If you discover sensitive information that is not stored securely, you need to take action. This could apply equally to paper-based and electronic patient data.

The first step must be to secure the information where possible. This is mostly likely to be the case with paper records left lying around. However, a colleague might have gone home and left their screen running or still be logged into a sensitive system. In such cases you should log them out and shut the screen down.

Having taken immediate action to secure the information, you must then record and report the incident to the designated person. This will depend on your organisation's policies and procedures, but it might be your line manager or a specialist computer security person or department.

Research

In 2016 the Care Quality Commission (CQC) published a report into whether personal health and care information is being used safely and is appropriately protected in the NHS. The review is available from the CQC website at https://www.cqc.org.uk/publications/themed-work/safe-data-safe-care (or search online for 'safe data safe care').

Think about what the CQC found. Can you see any lessons for your own workplace or professional practice?

There were six recommendations made. Can you see evidence of them being applied in your own organisation?

Healthcare Science T Level: Core

Project practice

You have been asked to prepare a report on data collection, recording and handling in your organisation.

You should research:
- The methods used to collect data.
- The types of data that are collected.
- The way(s) in which data is stored, analysed and presented.

You should also consider how your organisation addresses:
- the use of technology to assist in recording and reporting of data
- the ways in which data is shared amongst those who need to have access to it
- how personal data is protected
- procedures and policies that apply to ensuring confidentiality and security of personal data.

Prepare an evaluation of the methods used, covering:
- ways in which procedures ensure accurate collection and recording of data
- how information sharing is helped or hindered by the procedures in place
- areas that might be improved, such as:
  - reducing the time needed to document activities
  - improving sharing of information
  - increasing security of data and personal information (concentrate on how the systems are used, rather than on the detail of the systems themselves).

Present your report as a written document or slide presentation, infographic or scientific poster.

Discuss your findings with the group.

Write a reflective evaluation of your work.

Assessment practice

1. For each of the following, state whether it is qualitative or quantitative data:
   a. Blood pressure readings.
   b. Responses to a questionnaire about patient perception of the quality of their care.
   c. Height.
   d. Hair colour.

2. For each of the following, state whether it is continuous or discrete data:
   a. Number of weeks that a pregnancy lasts.
   b. Number of children in a family.
   c. Average number of children in families.
   d. Size of the UK population.
   e. Blood glucose concentration.

3. Suggest two security measures that can be used to protect personal data stored on a computer network.

4. Give two advantages of using automated data collection.

5. Discuss the advantages and disadvantages of using surveys to collect healthcare data.

6. Discuss the impact of machine learning on the role of healthcare practitioners.

7. Discuss the importance of having policies to prevent unauthorised access to patient data.

8. Discuss the ways in which security measures can protect stored data.

A8: Managing information and data

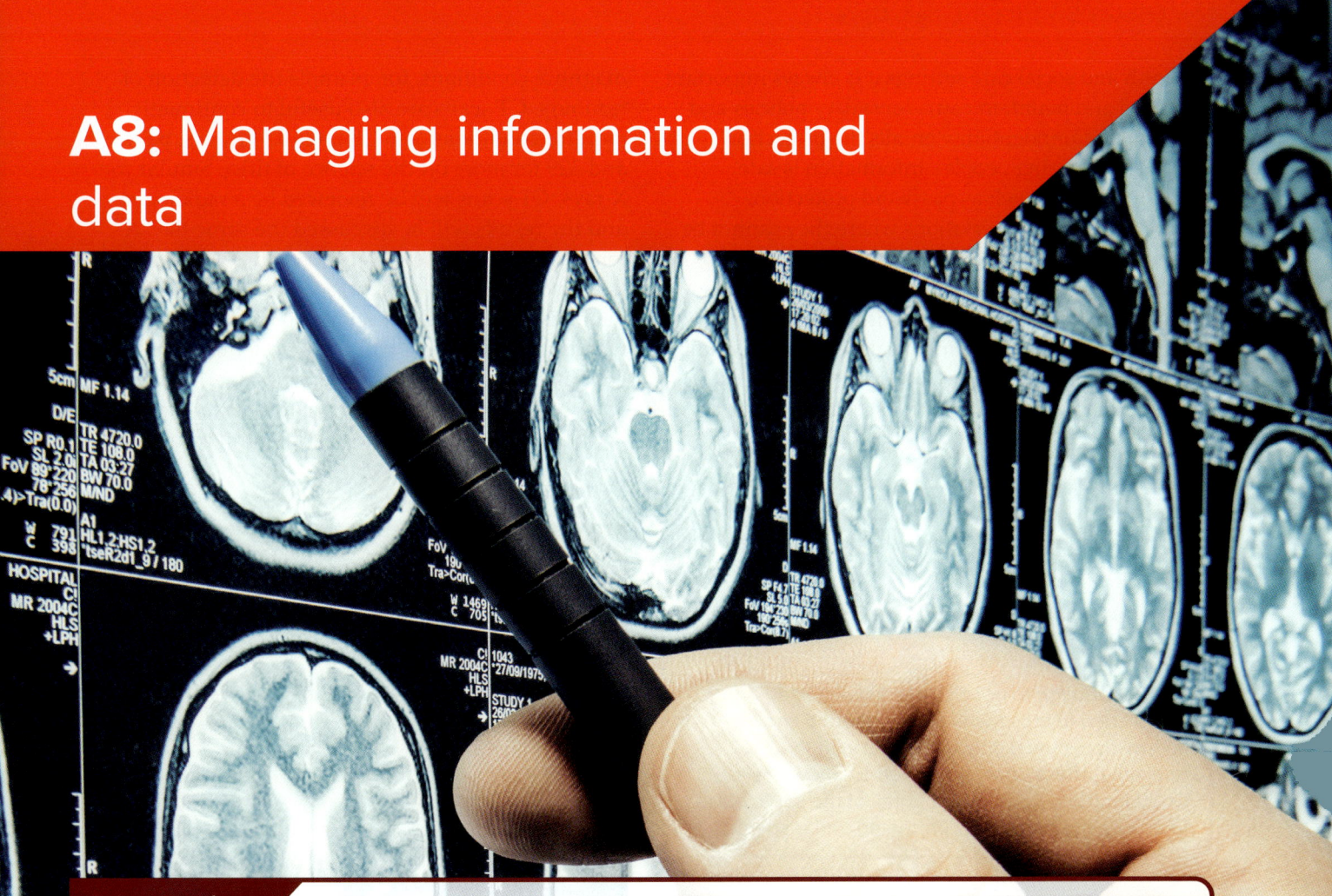

Introduction

Managing data and information within the healthcare science and social care sector is a particularly important role. Important documentation must be correct, while compliance with data protection legislation and regulations is also essential to prevent any breach of confidentiality. If these do not happen, the consequences can be severe: patients' personal information may be leaked, or they may receive the wrong treatment. Information can be presented and stored in a variety of formats, for example verbally, written or in images. It may also include statistical data that professionals may gather and interpret in new ways, leading to new methods and systems being developed to improve services within the healthcare sector.

Learning outcomes

The core knowledge outcomes that you must understand and learn:

- **A8.1** the range of methods of recording and reporting service user information and data
- **A8.2** the responsibilities of employees and employers relating to the safe storage of data and notification of insecure data practices
- **A8.3** the limits of confidentiality where self-harm or harm to others may be involved
- **A8.4** the purpose of different types of statistical databases and software tools used to integrate, analyse and interpret data
- **A8.5** the role of bioinformaticians and data scientists
- **A8.6** the advantages of reporting systems for managing information with regards to incidents, events and conditions
- **A8.7** factors which would dictate the need to escalate issues relating to service user information
- **A8.8** the principles of methods of statistical analysis and interpretation that can be applied to data
- **A8.9** different formats for communicating and presenting data and how to adapt communication style where appropriate.

In health and social care settings it is always important to uphold and maintain **confidentiality** policies and procedures. Confidentiality entails the protection of privacy: ensuring people's information is safe through methods such as password protection, holding sensitive conversations where they cannot be overheard and using locked filing cabinets. Precise policies and procedures may vary depending on the setting, but legislation in the UK is in place to ensure health and social care settings maintain confidentiality and comply with relevant policies and procedures. Breaking these can lead to serious legal consequences.

It is important to understand the difference between data and information: data is significant figures (usually statistics) whereas information is this data given meaningful context, which can be used to make decisions.

> **Key term**
>
> **Confidentiality:** to not disclose service user information to those who do not need to know. Information should only be shared with the relevant professionals on a need-to-know basis. Confidentiality upholds the rights of the service user to ensure their privacy is protected and respected.

A8.1 The range of methods of recording and reporting service user information and data

Physical records

X-rays

X-rays are scans produced by a type of radiation that passes through the body to produce images of the body and identify abnormalities (see Chapter B1 Physics, page 271 for more on the science of this). They can be used to identify abnormalities in the bones, joints and some soft tissue, such as the internal organs. X-rays need to be examined and interpreted by a radiologist. Normally this will be discussed with the patient on the same day. Alternatively, the radiologist may send the X-rays back to the patient's GP who will then discuss the results at an appointment.

Computed tomography

Computed tomography (CT) scans produce more detailed, 3D images that are used to identify and diagnose conditions, for example the detection of tumours. CT scans are also useful to continually monitor conditions (see Chapter B1 Physics, pages 327 and 329 for more on the science of this). Similar to X-rays, CT scans will be reviewed by a radiologist and the results will be discussed the same day. A report will also be sent electronically to the patient's GP. If you are an in-patient, a CT scan normally happens immediately or within the first couple of days, whereas an outpatient will receive a letter to make an appointment through the booking system. Before a CT scan, a patient may be asked not to eat that morning and only drink clear fluids, i.e. water (nil by mouth).

Retinal images

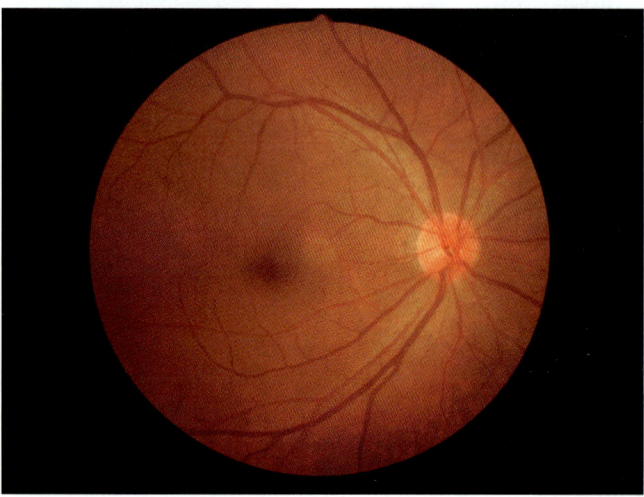

▲ Figure 8.1 A retinal image

Retinal images produce a digital image of the back of the eye. This enables optometrists to investigate and discover diseases or information about the health of an individual's eyes. Individuals who experience blurry vision or have diabetes may need a retinal test. If an individual's diabetes is not controlled appropriately, they may develop retinopathy (disease of the retina), which is caused by damage to the blood vessels at the back of the eye due to high blood sugar and blood pressure levels.

Photographs

Dental moulds

Dental moulds are used to produce an impression of the teeth, gums and other parts in the oral cavity. They are made through the use of a thick liquid material (alginate or polyvinylsiloxane) which is dispensed into a U-shaped guard to fit the mouth and make a significant impression of the person's teeth and

A8: Managing information and data

surrounding areas. A dental mould may be taken when a service user either wears or needs to wear dentures, needs a guard or retainer creating, or perhaps for whitening purposes, or braces.

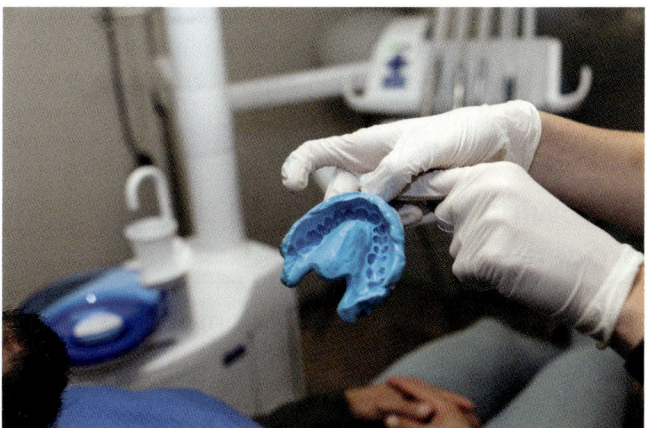

▲ Figure 8.2 A dental mould

Digital and written records

Written records

Professionals will often complete patient notes in a written format that may then be transferred to a digital format.

Written notes must be completed to a high standard and be easy for other professionals to read. Professionals must be able to communicate their notes effectively to ensure others in the multidisciplinary team can understand them, not just those with certain roles. Clear communication is important in all formats – verbal and non-verbal – this includes accuracy in written formats, explaining acronyms or jargon for those who may not understand, and clear gestures and body language. Notes must be recorded appropriately and accurately to ensure that the information passed on is effective.

Modern health and social care settings use electronic systems to keep service users' records, but this may be used alongside written notes. Staff should be aware of the policies and procedures of the settings they work in and have training on using the systems when starting a new job or a new role. Digital records will be password protected to ensure confidentiality is upheld – these must be updated regularly and not shared

Digital notes may need to be sent to other health or social teams that work closely with a service user or if they have been referred to another service. Medical notes should be sent through an encrypted system, which prevents unauthorised access and further upholds confidentiality. An example of this would be the forwarding of X-rays on to a patient's GP from the hospital to ensure medical notes are updated and that the patient's regular doctor has access to the information gained from the X-rays.

> **Research**
>
> Using your previous knowledge and further research of the use of data protection and confidentiality, design a poster for your work placement suggesting how to keep digital records safe.
>
> **Extension**
>
> Create a leaflet on bad examples of security.

A8.2 The responsibilities of employees and employers relating to the safe storage of data and notification of insecure data practices

The Data Protection Act 2018 (see page 94) relates to the processing and storage of personal data and enforces penalties for when this is not done correctly. If data protection is breached at any point, this is considered to be negligence, meaning the individual is liable for sharing information against data protection rules and can be subject to prosecution.

The Care Quality Commission (CQC) is the regulatory body within the health and social care sector that monitors and inspects health and social care services to ensure policies and procedures are in place and upheld. The role of CQC officers is to observe working practices within settings and advise on areas of strength and improvements. The CQC will investigate how the setting upholds data protection regulations and ensures staff are aware of how to do this. The CQC's website sets out their expectations of how settings should handle personal data effectively and according to the laws surrounding this (see **www.cqc.org.uk** for further information).

The Freedom of Information Act 2000 is also an important piece of legislation that outlines the right of service users to access their own personal information.

163

Ensure the safe storage of data

Following recording and reporting requirements

The Data Protection Act 2018 requires that information is stored in a confidential manner. Each setting will have policies and procedures that support staff in identifying specific measures that must be followed. Information that is not stored appropriately or discussed in a private manner may result in a breach of data. A data breach is when information is passed on to unnecessary organisations or individuals and could potentially be misused. A data breach may be unintentional if data is accidentally disclosed.

Each health and social care setting will have different policies and procedures designed to keep service user records safe and secure. Medical records may be recorded in a variety of formats that suit the environment or setting. Records should be accurate and must be kept up to date; if it is not properly recorded, it essentially did not happen. Data protection may be continually amended, so employers must ensure that their employees are thoroughly up to date.

When recording significant information, professionals may use abbreviations or jargon; however, it can be useful to avoid this where possible. If they are used throughout a report, the meaning of each must be made clear at the beginning otherwise other professionals and/or the service user may be unclear and misinterpret information with the report.

Securing information

It is essential information is secured following the correct policies and procedures of the organisation. To comply with UK legislation, organisations must have standardised routines of how to keep information secure. For example, if a professional needs to email sensitive information it must be encrypted and there should be a warning on the email so that the recipient is aware the information is sensitive. Security is an essential factor within data protection and ensuring that service users are protected from a breach of data.

Recording and reporting incidents to the designated person

Within an organisation there should be designated employees who are responsible for duties such as safeguarding and security. The Data Protection Officer (DPO) ensures organisations continue to uphold regulations and process data within legislative rules. If compliance is not upheld, the DPO must take action to address this. Incidents must be reported in a timely manner to ensure that all events can be recalled accurately and so that a timeline can be put together and patient wellbeing restored. If a professional witnesses any malpractice within an organisation they have a 'duty of care' to report it and protect the service user.

Following organisational policies and procedures

Information security management systems (ISMS) procedures

An ISMS is a management system that can be used by organisations to prevent sensitive information from being wrongly accessed. The system enables a healthcare setting to manage and monitor their data with the use of software to uphold security policies. They can monitor how the information is stored and accessed, enabling good practice to be upheld, managed or improved. The software gives professionals limited or unlimited access to information depending on their roles. An ISMS provides healthcare and science settings with the ability to have their information managed and risk assessed accordingly.

> **Test yourself**
>
> 1 What is meant by a data breach?
> 2 Explain the role of the CQC in ensuring secure data practices in organisations.

A8.3 The limits of confidentiality where self-harm or harm to others may be involved

As discussed in section A5.9, confidentiality is a key aspect within the health and social care sector. It forms a key part of the organisational policies and procedures that must be adhered to. Confidentiality must not be breached unless in exceptional circumstances, such as a safeguarding concern, so it is important to understand what those exceptional circumstances might be so that you can act appropriately if these occur. If a service user is at risk of harm to themselves or others, this information will need to be shared with the appropriate professionals and services. Concerns must only be shared on a need-to-know basis. Check your setting's safeguarding policy for the exact details of what must be followed.

Safeguarding

Within health and social care settings there are legal policies and procedures that professionals must adhere to. Safeguarding ensures that vulnerable individuals are kept safe and, therefore, professionals can identify maltreatment, abuse, neglect or self-harm. Safeguarding requires preventative methods: it is important to take action before the harm occurs. Furthermore, safeguarding requires professionals to take accountability of detrimental circumstances when they may arise or when they may be concerned, which is part of the prevention strategy. See section A1.1, page 3, for more on safeguarding.

> **Research**
>
> Prevent is another strand of safeguarding, which relates to the risk of radicalisation. Use the link to create an information sheet on Prevent guidance and how to comply within a healthcare setting.
>
> www.gov.uk/government/publications/prevent-duty-guidance

Liberty Protection Safeguards

The Liberty Protection Safeguards (LPS), which came into force in April 2022, are legal provisions that aim to protect individuals aged 16 and over who may lack the mental capacity to provide consent for care or treatment, such as a patient with severe dementia or certain patients with autistic spectrum conditions.

The Mental Capacity (Amendment) Act 2019 introduced the plans for LPS. It is intended to improve the outcomes for individuals who may need support with decisions or those who may have liberty deprivation, to ensure individuals' rights are at the centre of their care and that any treatments or healthcare plans are in their best interest.

Deprivation of Liberty Safeguards (DoLS) provide support with individuals who may have limited cognitive capacity. DoLS is an assessment that ensures that the care given to the individual is within their best interest. A service user who has dementia, for example, will gradually find it difficult to make decisions unsupported; therefore, DoLS allows the individual to have a representative to authorise decisions on their behalf that incorporate the needs of the service user.

In practice, LPS removes a service users' freedom of liberty, meaning that their safeguarding representative (designated the 'appropriate person') will make choices on their behalf. Before an LPS is approved and authorised, an assessment must be completed on the service user in question. Their mental capacity needs to be established and an overall medical assessment carried out to determine whether an LPS is necessary to prevent harm to the service user and work within their best interests. The LPS representative appointed will depend on where the care is taking place; for example, if the care for a patient with dementia is taking place within a hospital, the hospital manager is likely to represent the safeguarding needs of that patient. In some cases, the appropriate person may be an individual from a local health board – this ensures the representative is a third-party person who can consider the patient's care objectively.

Duty of care

Duty of care is a legal obligation that must be upheld in the health and social care sector. Duty of care entails adherence to legal obligations when taking care of vulnerable service users. As a professional within the healthcare sector, this means that you are responsible for looking after and meeting the needs of the people in your care. You are also responsible for the care of others within that setting, even if you are not working with them directly, should you notice any issues. Compliance with policies and procedures is a key aspect of good practice to ensure effective care for service users and safe practice for professionals. An example of providing a duty of care is to ensure the privacy and dignity of service users when they require help, for example with changing their clothes or feeding.

Consent

Consent means giving permission for procedures to take place or for information to be shared. A patient must be informed thoroughly before they agree to take part in a trial, take medication or undergo surgery, or to their information being shared. When allocating treatment, surgery or therapy to a service user, they must give consent before the service can be administered. The treatment must also be in the best interest of the service user. If an individual is unable to consent, they must have an advocate in place to make these decisions.

Covert administration of medication

Covert means concealed. Covert administration of medication can include the concealment of medication in, for example, food or drink, without the service user's knowledge. When administering medication, the law dictates that service users must have consented to this. However, if a vulnerable service user is lacking capacity, they must have a management plan in place that meets their individual needs and best interests. This may include the covert administration of medication, but this must only be used in specific circumstances. The Mental Capacity Act 2005 allows medicine to be administered through a disguise, such as food or drink, if an individual with lack of capacity refuses to take it. Furthermore, their capacity must be determined under the act. All individuals have rights, and a person's capacity must be appropriately assessed and determined before steps like this are taken.

> **Research**
>
> Research and summarise the main points of the Mental Capacity Act 2005.
>
> Using your knowledge from this:
> - research and identify the key points of covert administration of medication
> - describe one example of where covert administration of medication may need to be used and why.

Compliance with legal requests

This means ensuring that professionals in the healthcare science sector adhere to appropriate legislation, policies and procedures, including those of the organisation, not just national laws. If professionals do not comply with legal policies and procedures, employers have the right to terminate their contracts. Depending on the circumstances, service users or their families can seek legal action to gain compensation from the employee and/or employer.

Legislation ensures professionals are aware of and follow safeguarding and confidentiality policies and procedures. This is to ensure protection of service users and members of the public, as well as the professionals themselves. Compliance in terms of legal requests may include helping those seeking information via freedom of information requests (see below). Note that if a patient is under the age of 18, they are still legally under the care and supervisions of their parents or guardians, unless deemed otherwise by the courts.

Any disclosure of a service user's personal information between professionals in a multidisciplinary team must follow GDPR guidance (see page 94). An example of this could be a GP referring a patient to a hospital. The GP would need to record and report information regarding the current illness or disorder to the surgeon: for example, the patient may need an ultrasound due to high enzymes showing in their blood results. The surgeon needs to acquire the medical history of the patient beforehand; a radiologist will also be involved and need to be aware of the patient's medical notes in order to identify what they are investigating. Once the investigation takes place, the radiologist and surgeon should shares notes to determine any issues, and this information is then shared with the patient and notes will be sent back to their GP. Storing and processing information accurately enables medical professionals to continue to monitor a patient's illness and identify any new or recurring symptoms in the future, but it must be kept securely.

> **Research**
>
> Research and create a short presentation for your team on GDPR regulations and how they may affect your responsibilities as an employee in a healthcare setting.

Freedom of Information Act 2000

This act relates to the disclosure of information from organisations in the public sector, which includes most healthcare science settings, the NHS, schools and government organisations. Service users are entitled to access the information that is held about them by any public organisation. Service users have the right to access information such as medical records, past prescriptions, current prescriptions and other personal information that may be required. Personal information may also contain addresses, date of birth, next of kin and family history. As this is the individual's information, they must be able to view it, and this act lays out their rights in regard to this. Making a request to view this information is often called a freedom of information (FOI) request; this information should be provided to the individual within 20 working days, or a response given to explain when to expect it if longer is needed.

A8.4 The purpose of different types of statistical databases and software tools used to integrate, analyse and interpret data

Statistical databases enable researchers to identify patterns and trends in health and science data. The use of statistics enables the government to allocate funds to certain institutions or geographical areas and to recognise specific needs within the health and social care sector because there is evidence that it should be effective and have a positive effect on the care delivered.

However, statistical analysis has limitations as well as strengths. This may include results being misleading. Although software is able to analyse data effectively, it can only use the information that has been input into the system. If the information is faulty then the analysis of data will not be representative.

Statistical Package for Social Sciences (SPSS)

Statistical Package for Social Sciences (SPSS) is a software suite that helps to collate and analyse complex data through use of visual methods such as graphs and bar charts. SPSS is a useful tool for opening data files, editing data and creating tables and charts showing an overall summary of findings. The use of SPSS has had a positive impact on the monitoring of medical operations and understanding of treatment and diagnosis as it enables a researcher to identify whether their findings are statistically significant. Consequently, SPSS can assist the researcher to draw conclusions from samples of participants that hopefully can be generalised to the wider population.

SPSS uses **inferential statistics** to assist with identifying significant differences between groups used in research. Conclusions can be drawn through a variety of ways, such as analysis of variance (ANOVA), regression analysis and factor analysis.

ANOVA is a test that compares the **means** of two or more groups to determine whether there is a statistical difference; this is important for identifying differences within experimental groups to ensure evidence collected for the groups shows a significant difference, enabling the researcher to compare results and conclude findings. **Regression analysis** enables the experimenter to identify which **variables** have a significant impact on the research topic, meaning the researcher can ignore any other factors considered insignificant to the experiment and focus on the most important areas.

Factor analysis helps the experimenter to identity any underlying factors that may impact the research. These are often difficult to identify and measure. An example of an underlying factor that is difficult to measure is depression; it is difficult to determine one specific factor as to why an individual is depressed as there may be a variety of reasons. Factor analysis aims to summarise and reduce any factors that may not be as significant as others, therefore providing the experimenter with clear conclusions that provide an answer to the topic area or question being researched.

> ### Key terms
>
> **Inferential statistics:** statistics used to predict whether the results of medical trials can be generalised to the wider population.
>
> **ANOVA (analysis of variance):** a checking system for statistical differences and the means of differences in groups.
>
> **Mean:** the average number; all the numbers should be added together, then the value divided by the number of numbers.
>
> **Regression analysis:** determines the relationship between the dependent variable and other variables to distinguish a strength within the data.
>
> **Variable:** a characteristic that can be measured; example include age, gender and ethnicity.
>
> **Factor analysis:** simplifies data by reducing the number of variables, therefore focusing on the most significant variables.

The data input is shown in a spreadsheet view similar to Microsoft Excel; data is in rows and columns. There are a variety of types of **quantitative data** that can be input into SPSS such as **nominal**, **ordinal** and **interval** data. Nominal data is categorical data (see Figure 8.3), such as age, height or weight; an individual can only put one specific answer for this type of data (i.e. you can only have one height).

Healthcare Science T Level: Core

	A	B	C	D	E	F	G
1	Participant	24	Gender	Placebo/Medication	Side effects (Y/N)		
2	1	32	F	P	N/A		
3	2	56	M	M	N		
4	3	Age	F	P	N/A		
5	4	19	M	M	Y		
6	5	65	F	P	N/A		
7	6	43	M	M	N		
8							
9	Key						
10	P = Placebo						
11	M = Medication						
12							
13							
14							
15							

▲ Figure 8.3 An example of quantitative data from an experiment shown in SPSS

Ordinal data is collected with the use of frequency scales showing on a scale of 1–10, for instance how many units of alcohol a person drinks during a week. Interval data is based on units of measurements, for example taking a patient's temperature or measuring their heartbeat. Items are then presented in tables or charts. Nominal data uses the measure of **mode**, ordinal uses **median** and, finally, interval uses the mean.

Figure 8.3 shows the layout of results from participants during an analysis of an experiment. Each heading for each column should be simple and clear, stating what the variables relate to. The use of a key makes it easy for the researcher to simply input a letter or number rather than having to write the whole word, saving time and enabling easy interpretation of the test results.

> **Key terms**
>
> **Mode:** the number that occurs most often.
>
> **Median:** the middle number within an ascending or descending list.

Statistical Analysis System (SAS)

Statistical Analysis Systems (SAS) is a database similar to SPSS as it retrieves and analyses data and enables researchers to report quantitative findings of experiments using graphs and charts. It is used to perform large analyses of medical data to identify areas of concern within healthcare. This software can be used to store large data sets, such as patient records and reports formulated from medical equipment, such as patient observations like blood pressure, oxygen levels and heart rate. SAS can be used in pharmaceutical trials to measure the effectiveness of different drugs.

Software for Statistics and Data Science (STATA)

Statistics and Data (STATA) is another form of software that enables the management and production of data. The software enables professionals to visualise data in graphics. It is a useful program for those studying data patterns in healthcare science. STATA also enables data interpretation for science data; the researcher can manipulate and visualise statistics to report findings effectively. STATA is useful for smaller analyses than SPSS or SAS, which tend to be more useful to analyse and determine data findings for medical science.

Spreadsheets

The benefit of using statistical systems is that it enables those within the health and social care sector to identify important areas that need improvement. Data collection using software enables large-scale studies to be completed, making analysis quicker. Software such as Microsoft Excel or Google Sheets enables the research to be set out effectively and clearly, and for charts and graphs to be produced. This creates a clear summary of statistics and helps to identify specific trends and conclusions.

A8.5 The role of bioinformaticians and data scientists

In healthcare, it is important to continually improve methods of treatment, diagnosis and prevention. Healthcare science enables professionals within this sector to investigate diseases to further understand the effects, monitoring them and potentially finding new ways to treat them. Research in healthcare can highlight areas for further improvement, such as gaps in health provision, informing policies and identifying needs.

Interpretation of scientific data is essential in understanding the development of diseases as well as how to overcome them. Bioinformaticians and data scientists are therefore an essential part of medical science. Their fundamental role is to gather data and design **algorithms** to interpret it. Data scientists help to introduce healthcare industry improvements such as new diagnostic techniques and medications.

Bioinformaticians investigate **genomics** (see section B1.19), which is concerned with the biological structure and function of genomes. Genomes are the genetic components that make up an individual; bioinformaticians use scientific methods to investigate the evolution and mapping of genetic components.

> **Key terms**
>
> *Algorithm:* instructions for solving a problem, especially by a computer.
>
> *Hypothesis:* a prediction of the outcome that will be tested as part of the experiment.

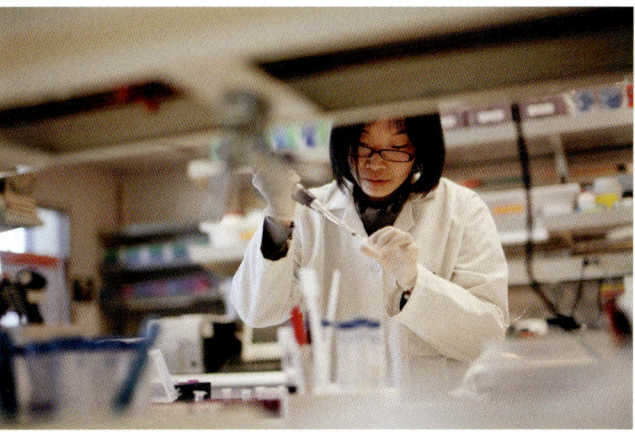

▲ Figure 8.4 A healthcare science researcher in a laboratory

Responsible for bringing together information technology and healthcare science

A bioinformatician predominantly researches areas related to biology, medicine and health. They use computer technology that gathers and analyses data within fields such as genetic and pharmaceutical development, including DNA sequencing (see sections B2.20 and B2.22).

IT and health information are combined by data scientists, who utilise their skills to investigate and manage data gathered by healthcare science organisations.

Clinical trial methodology

Clinical trials are important to gain further understanding of treatments and preventative measures. They are used by scientific professionals to discover and determine findings of health and ill health, and to investigate the effectiveness of potential new treatments.

Each trial has many phases that must be conducted effectively and ethically to ensure there is no intentional harm caused to participants. Participants must be aware of the risks before taking part in the trial, and they must have the option to withdraw from the trial at any time. Clinical trial methods include experimental and observational studies, which must be regulated to ensure safe measures are being used.

When developing clinical methodology, the research must have an aim and objective, known as a **hypothesis**; this is a testable statement where the researcher makes a prediction about the outcome of the research. A hypothesis enables some form of predictability of conclusions before the research takes place to ensure it is worth conducting it. The research will consist of variables, including the **independent variable**, which is manipulated during the experiment to see if changing it has an effect. The **dependent variable** is what is being measured by the experiment.

To understand the difference between an independent and dependent variable in research, read the article in the link below for the following study: 'Hospital healthcare service quality, patient satisfaction and loyalty: an investigation in context of private healthcare systems'.

www.emerald.com/insight/content/doi/10.1108/IJQRM-02-2017-0031/full/html

In this example, the independent variable (IV) is patient view, as the organisation is trying to identify patient thoughts about the private healthcare organisation – the dependent variable (DV).

Once the researcher has defined the aim of the investigation, they must then consider the participants they want to take part in the research. As it is unfeasible to include a whole population, the researcher must choose a sample of the **target population** (the specific group of people the research aims to help). This target population should be **representative**, meaning it should represent the **predictable outcomes** for the wider population.

Predictable outcomes are those predicted by the researcher, meaning particular results are expected before the research takes place.

Clinical trials can allocate random participants that volunteer to take part in the trial, for instance to take a given drug, to avoid any bias in who is selected, which would make the results less reliable. Participants involved in the study may be volunteers or people who have been approached to take part in it due to particular factors, such as age, gender, culture, ethnicity and so on.

Research may first need to be **piloted**, meaning it will be carried out on a small, measurable scale. Once completed, the research will need to identify the strengths and limitations of the pilot. The reasoning behind these **pilot studies** is that research is time consuming and costly; organisations need to invest a lot of money into it, so the research needs to be valid.

Laboratory experiments involve the manipulation of the independent variable under controlled conditions, i.e. where no other environmental factors interfere, which is why they are useful in discovering reliable findings. However, this is not practical or possible for certain experiments. Another method of collecting clinical data is through observational design: observations are about determining behaviours in a simulated real-life situation. A further technique that produces quick and efficient data is the **self-report** method, for instance questionnaires that can be completed in the absence or presence of the researcher. Methods of collection include interviews (structured or semi-structured), observations, questionnaires, focus groups and surveys.

Data may be collected over a long-term period, known as **longitudinal research**, or it can be short term. This depends on the amount and type of evidence needed.

Finally, to conduct research ethical principles must be adhered to (see sections A1.3 and A5.12). They are an essential part of any research in order to ensure participants will not suffer any severe harm. Note that ethics can change slightly over time, however, to fit in with what society deems as acceptable or unacceptable.

Construction of survey methodology for gathering of feedback

Surveys may be developed when healthcare settings or scientists are looking to improve services or diagnostic methodology, or when trialling new medication, software or devices. They are a method of gathering feedback from participants: this can be from people accessing services or those working within the services. Surveys enable service users to express their opinions confidentially to help settings continually improve. Surveys are usually formatted either as questionnaires or scaling methods, for example using a scale of 1–10 or wording scales such as the CQC use, e.g. from 'no improvements' to 'improvements required'. They are used to gather large amounts of information from a wide population and can be used in most circumstances.

In contrast, interviews are mostly used in smaller studies to gain in-depth understanding, for example during a clinical trial. Interviews may be used in clinical trials, for example during the development of a vaccination, to gain a clear understanding of how the individual participating in the trial feels and whether there are any side effects.

Types of survey	Description
Questionnaires	A list of either open or closed questions to be answered either with multiple choice or free answers. For example, questionnaires may be used to gain information for a patient's record in terms of their alcohol intake (the Fast Alcohol Screening Test, or FAST).
Online survey	Questionnaires online via a scale, open or closed questions. An online survey can be used when gathering patient feedback after an appointment.
Open questions	Questions that enable the participant to input their own thoughts when answering.
Closed questions	Specific questions that gather yes or no answers.
Multiple choice	A range of options are given for each question, and the participant will choose one or more. This might be used to list types of activities or eating habits, for example, to gain an understanding of a patient's lifestyle.
Scale questionnaires	Ranking answers such as through numbers or worded scales, for example how satisfied a patient was with the treatment they received.

Collection of healthcare science data

Data collection is the process of gathering information. This allows the information to be measured, a hypothesis developed, questions written and the outcomes evaluated to show whether it supports the hypothesis or not.

Before collecting data, the investigator needs to consider the type of data they want to gather and what they are hoping to find out.

A timeline should then be set to know when the data is to be gathered, collected, interpreted and finalised.

Data collection can be carried out in a variety of ways, and it can be **quantitative** or **qualitative data**.

The method should then be determined, for example how is this data investigation going to be carried out?
- laboratory – experiment takes place in a highly controlled environment, therefore ensuring conditions can be controlled
- questionnaire/survey/interviews
- observations – looking at participants in a natural or unnatural environment and viewing their actions.

Data collection and collaboration should ensure that the public are encouraged to participate in research, which will help to gain a better understanding of wider societal opinions. This also enables improvements in specific areas or particular services. Participants should be informed of the findings from data collected in research they have taken part in. This enables participants to identify how the research has been used and to withdraw if they should wish to.

Interpretation of healthcare science data

Research facilities need to understand how to provide beneficial care and treatment, so it is important to interpret findings correctly and appropriately. Identifying factors of illnesses and diseases earlier can help to prevent fatalities. Furthermore, it helps services to run effectively and to prevent negligence within health and social care services.

Interpreting data can also identify gaps in service provision: as the needs of the public can change over time – such as the increasing age that people now live to or changing environmental factors – healthcare provision must also change to reflect this so that service users can continue to benefit.

Data scientists and bioinformaticians will use a variety of steps to analyse and interpret their data. First, all the information collected should be assembled together and findings should be organised into a variety of relevant categories. The scientists can then begin to analyse it and, from this, develop and summarise conclusions based on any trends identified. Finally, the data will be set out either in written form or with the use of graphs, statistics and tables depending on the type of data (qualitative or quantitative). Once conclusions have been drawn, future developments can then be discussed. Furthermore, any amendments to further research can also be identified and summarised during the final parts of data interpretation.

Data interpretation can take a long time, but this will vary depending on the type of data collected and the number of participants involved. The researcher should have created a timeline before the research began, however, to ensure they work towards particular timescales.

Genomic data can be interpreted through the use of laboratory methods. Scientists can investigate the patients' genetic mapping using gene sequencing to identify any factors such as hereditary disorders or genetic malfunctions. The use of databases and analysis systems enables the professional to reveal genetic complications, if any, and discuss these with the patient.

> **Research**
>
> Using the following link choose a topic related to healthcare.
> www.gov.uk/search/research-and-statistics
>
> Explain:
> ▶ the aim of the research
> ▶ the participants involved: include factors such as age, gender, race, culture, socio-economic status
> ▶ the methodology
> ▶ findings and conclusion of the research.
>
> **Extension**
>
> Once you have completed this task, analyse the findings and consider the impact the research has had on healthcare services.

Development of databases for research purposes

Databases allow for the organisation of important information. Each database should be organised in a way that is effective to locate data sets such as health records. Organisations will have policies and procedures in place that employees must adhere to when working with databases to ensure that these records are accurate and secure. Healthcare organisations use these databases for research to inform future decision making.

> **Test yourself**
>
> 1 Explain the difference between open and closed questions. Give an example of each.
> 2 Explain why questionnaires are often used in healthcare.

A8.6 The advantages of reporting systems for managing information with regards to incidents, events and conditions

Within health and social care settings there is a huge mass of data. Information may include service users' medical history, personal information, family members' information, criminal convictions and healthcare plans. This information must be stored and handled with care and in line with data protection legislation, as it is important that service users are able to trust the professionals that they work with. Legislation (see Chapter A3) must be followed in settings to ensure staff uphold their professional duties.

The advantage of using incident reporting systems such as Datix (see page 138) is that it enables fast and secure communication between services. For example, when a service user requires their GP to refer them on to a hospital, this will be completed through the use of certain IT systems (for example, SystmOne, which is mainly used in primary care settings). All information can be processed via an encrypted referral system and only those who are involved on a need-to-know basis have access to this information. Other incident reporting systems enable practitioners to report accidents, such as if a patient falls during their visit to a hospital, or extreme cases such as giving a patient the wrong medication.

Reduce errors

Technology can help to reduce medical errors. Electronic records are normally backed up through IT systems, therefore reducing the likelihood of missing information or deleted files. Computer-based systems can also enable reminders to be set, informing practitioners of upcoming appointments, reviews or meetings with patients or other service users.

System reports can also highlight any missing fields that may be required (e.g. if a patient's date of birth has not been input), which helps to ensure professionals review information before it is saved. These systems also enable message reports, such as when action may need to be taken. IT systems usually have autosave systems that help to avoid loss of information.

Technology allows information to be reported effectively and in a time efficient manner. This helps to produce rapid information on patients that can be passed on if needed, for instance if a patient's condition deteriorates, their medication is changed or they are referred to another service. Saved information can also help to improve patient safety such as through the reduction of prescription errors. For example, if a GP enters an incorrect dosage of patient medication – say 200 mg per day rather than 20 mg – the IT system will alert the GP before they proceed. IT systems can also reduce errors by identifying any known allergies.

Timely reporting of information

Information must be recorded in a timely manner. If an incident occurs, such as the misuse of medical equipment on a patient or an overdosage of medication, the professional must report the incident immediately and follow the organisation's policies and procedures. The precise timescale may be specified by organisational policy or legislation. For overdoses or other injuries to patients, time is clearly of the essence in rectifying the error and stabilising the patient.

When reporting and recording information it is a requirement that the healthcare professional takes note of the exact date and time to ensure information is accurate. This enables other professionals reviewing patient notes to be aware of significant previous appointments, prescribed medications or referrals, or for information to be reviewed in the future.

Easy access to patient information for tracking and monitoring

It is important for professionals and service users to have easy access to their information. Each organisation will have a system in place that enables professionals to access service user information effectively and monitor their care. Online services are also available for service users to access their information, such as through https://nhs.uk, the NHS app or www.patientaccess.com.

Tracking systems help by ensuring patient information is measured, tracked and monitored accurately. Other information to be tracked and monitored can include hospital room availability or medical equipment availability for surgery. Timings and room allocation will be given out by monitoring systems.

Security can also be enhanced through the use of tracking systems in hospital, for example to identify and allocate patients to beds or specific departments. IT systems can also update schedules and enhance the timing of activities and meetings. Organised services improve patient satisfaction by ensuring appointments happen on time, saving time and money.

Patient information needs to be easily accessible to authorised professionals to ensure efficient time management, effective communication between services and to further reduce any potential errors. Furthermore, professionals who do not generally work with the patient need to be able to access their medical history (when appropriate), so ensuring medical history is updated through IT systems allows the documentation to be reviewed easily.

Practitioners need to routinely monitor patients' health, for instance in the management of a chronic illness, so maintaining accurate records is essential. Monitoring is not necessarily always a weekly occurrence: an example could be an asthmatic patient who needs a review of the dosage for their inhalers and how well their illness is being controlled every six months.

Patient treatment histories and other key information, such as patient referrals and past appointments, need to be recorded effectively to ensure patients and professionals are aware of any updated information in relation to their healthcare.

Insurance

Organisations are required to have insurance policies in place that support them when dealing with claims such as **medical negligence**. When complaints or claims are made against an organisation or a professional, it is important that they have insurance in place to ensure the claiming process adheres to legislation. Reporting systems are useful to have for insurance purposes in order to obtain patient information for medical insurance claims (for example, if patients seek to redeem the cost of surgery).

> **Key term**
>
> *Medical negligence:* when a patient has been directly or indirectly injured or harmed during treatment or care, for example through misdiagnosis or mistakes in surgery.

Patient or professional complaints must be dealt with immediately and in accordance with legislative rules. Insurance helps the parties to deal co-operatively to investigate claims and ensure complaints are dealt with effectively. Insurance companies are outside participants and, therefore, should ensure there is no bias in cases.

A8.7 Factors which would dictate the need to escalate issues relating to service user information

Professionals in healthcare science have a duty of care towards patients that they must continually uphold. If a professional suspects maltreatment or safeguarding concerns, they must act on it immediately. Following legislation and organisational policies and procedures, they are obliged to report any potential issues; in the case of safeguarding, this would be to the person responsible for safeguarding in that setting.

Some service users are deemed as vulnerable and, therefore, the professional must take responsibility for ensuring that the service user is not treated unjustly.

It is therefore extremely important that all professionals recognise what factors indicate the need to escalate issues.

Suspected overuse/abuse of medication

Suspected abuse of medication means that a professional suspects a patient to be using too much medication, i.e. knowingly not in line with medical advice, or that another professional is abusing their power to overprescribe medication to a patient to cause purposeful harm. There are signs that may identify the overuse or abuse of medication, either by a professional or a patient. Behavioural changes may occur if a patient is experiencing side effects to excessive medication. An individual may have irrational behaviour changes or a change of sleeping habits. Other signs may include changes in appetite, speech or breathing difficulties and confusion.

Overuse of medication can cause serious health issues or result in death. If a professional is suspected of abuse of power by overmedicating a patient or secretly medicating them, they must be investigated immediately and their care of the patient must be suspended. If a professional is suspected of malpractice, they must be reported immediately to higher management or organisation bodies such as the CQC.

Breach of confidentiality

A breach of confidentiality means information has been disclosed to a person not authorised to see it, i.e. someone that does not work directly with the service user in question. A breach may also be due to safeguarding concerns when a professional is concerned over a service user's safety or those around them. If a professional is suspected of a breach of confidentiality or misuse of information, they must be reported immediately, for example to a line manager or the organisation director, and investigated. A member of the organisation could also complain to an external regulator such as the CQC or the Information Commissioner's Office (ICO), which deals directly in data privacy and information rights.

The appointment of a DPO is essential within a healthcare organisation. The appointed person is in charge of compliance with data protection regulations and oversees the protection sensitive information. See page 94 for more on GDPR and data protection legislation.

> **Case study**
>
> Sam, a service user, discloses to his key worker that his father and older brother have been abusing him. Sam pleads with the key worker not to tell anyone due to fear of what his family may do. The key worker is confused as he thinks Sam's right to confidentiality may conflict with his right to be protected from harm.
> ▶ What should you do in this situation?
> ▶ What is your duty of care?
>
> Discuss in pairs and each write a paragraph explaining your answers.

Suspected self-harm

Any form of suspected self-harm must be investigated immediately to reduce any further damage to the service user. The way the professional responds to this risk is important so as to not overwhelm the service user; for instance, they should not overreact or act in an angry or shocked manner. If the professional does suspect self-harm, they must ensure the service user is protected from any objects that may be used to self-harm (e.g. blades or medication). Before assuming the worst, the professional must report the matter to a safeguarding officer/person responsible for safeguarding in the organisation before addressing this concern with the service user.

Safeguarding concerns

There are a variety of factors that may raise safeguarding concerns, including abuse, neglect and self-harm. Other types of maltreatment, such as a breach of confidentiality or misusing or mishandling data, are also safeguarding concerns. If a professional notices a colleague misusing or mishandling data, they must report this as it is part of their duty of care.

Types of abuse and harm that would be considered safeguarding concerns:
- Neglect. This can include failure to provide for medical or physical care needs, and failure to give dignity or privacy.
- Physical abuse. This can include hitting, pushing, burning and misuse of medication.
- Psychological abuse. This may include emotional or verbal abuse, humiliation and threats of punishment.
- Sexual abuse. This can include sexual activity where the individual cannot or does not give consent, and sexual harassment.
- Financial abuse. This can include misuse or theft of money, fraud and exploitation of property or inheritance.
- Discrimination. Factors including sex, race, culture, religion, age, ability or sexual orientation.

Healthcare professionals have a duty of care to not cause injury to their patients. A breach of the legal duty of care is referred to as negligence. Negligence may result in damage towards a service user. Clinical negligence details concerns arising from complaints against doctors or healthcare professionals.

How to implement safeguarding in practice:
- identifying people at risk of abuse and neglect
- understanding the importance of observation
- raising awareness of safeguarding implications to employees and service users, providing information, advice and advocacy
- knowledge and understanding of policies and procedures, legislation and regulations
- inter-agency collaboration and multi-agency working to ensure services work collaboratively to protect service users and acknowledge any changes in patient behaviour or circumstances
- staff training and continuing professional development (CPD) relating to safeguarding measures, new legislation and Prevent tactics that are implemented by government bodies and organisations
- promoting empowerment and choice for service users: for example, providing information and guidance on who to communicate with regarding safeguarding issues or concerns, for example if a patient suspects a professional of abusive behaviour or harm towards them.

Information technology (IT)/data breaches

A data breach could occur by accident or be intentional. This may include the release of medical records to unauthorised personnel. Data must be stored confidentiality in line with the organisation's policies and procedures. Not using protective measures, such as passwords and locked cabinets, or disallowing the removal of files from a setting, may result in a data breach. If a data breach does occur, the professional must report this immediately and take action.

Incidents that may constitute data breaches include:
- unauthorised sharing of information online
- inaccurate use of patient information, such as from the wrong patient
- lack of security, such as not locking a computer when leaving the room
- patient files left in sight of others who are not on a need-to-know basis
- sharing information with other organisations or services who are not on a need-to-know basis
- lack of file encryption
- accessing unauthorised data
- loss of data
- misplaced data, such as misplaced information or being unaware of where files are stored.

Safe haven failure

A **safe haven** refers to a safe and secure environment where health data is stored securely by trained members of staff. It involves processing either health-related or non-health-related data that can be used to facilitate medical information and research.

A safe haven failure is any breach in the processing of data that is considered malpractice. If malpractice takes place it must be reported immediately and investigated by organisational bodies and higher management in the service. Insurance companies may also need to be involved in legal proceedings. Furthermore, the patient involved must be informed of the data breach due to their right to have their information protected.

Suspicions of bribery and corruption

The Bribery Act 2010 is a legislation in place to investigate potential bribery. Bribery refers to financial promises, acceptance of money or gifts from service users or unusual activity, for example unlikely purchases on credit cards, in exchange for preferential treatment or favours.

Families or other professionals may suspect a healthcare professional of being involved in bribery or corruption. If this is the case it must be reported and investigated. It can be reported to the police, who will complete questioning and investigative measures. This information will be covered within the specific healthcare science organisation's employee handbook, which should explain the policies and procedures related to legislation that must be adhered to. Any suspicions of bribery or corruption that are identified by other professionals must be reported to a senior member of staff or outside services such as the CQC.

Possible indicators of bribery or corruption include the following on service user documents:

- unnecessary or unlikely purchases from the service user, for example from a range of retailers that are unusual for them
- lack or loss of money from around the house or from a bank account or inheritance
- questionable bills that are out of character or unrelated to the service user, for example random mobile phone bills
- debt from loan companies or credit card companies
- purchases made by others with the use of an individual's bank details, irregular bills and payments on bank statements
- unauthorised purchases
- unauthorised sharing of information online: an example of this may be a professional sharing names or other information that establishes a service user's identity, or any sharing of a service user's photos on social media that identifies the individual receiving care.

Service users may receive letters or phone calls from loan or banking companies indicating abnormal use of finances. Furthermore, documents may ask the service users for approval of loans or purchases.

> **Test yourself**
>
> 1 Identify one type of abuse and explain why it would create a safeguarding concern.
> 2 Describe what is meant by abuse of medication.
> 3 Describe the role of the DPO.
> 4 Explain the term 'financial abuse' and provide an example of this.
> 5 Explain what a data breach is and provide an example of this.

A8.8 The principles of methods of statistical analysis and interpretation that can be applied to data

The use of statistics is important within healthcare science to determine the relative importance of factors such as gender, lifestyle and age, and to identify trends. Gathering data about healthcare outcomes enables us to develop methods to overcome influencing factors that may cause high death rates and illnesses in particular groups. We therefore need to make sure we understand relevant terms and ideas for dealing with statistics.

Descriptive statistics

Descriptive statistics facilitate a clear understanding of research by summarising the data sets that have been investigated. Professionals can collect either qualitative or quantitative data through the use of methods such as observations, questionnaires and case studies. Quantitative data is normally used in descriptive statistics as it is a data set that can be presented in a simple way using numbers to show information. Data can be collected through qualitative methods, but it is usually presented quantitatively also.

The data gathered is analysed and undergos statistical analysis, enabling the investigator to identify trends and make conclusions. Descriptive statistics represent the sample covered in the research, which should be representative of the wider population. The descriptive statistics will help to identify the mean, median or mode. They allow the research to be summarised and presented appropriately to help understanding.

Main types of descriptive statistics:
- measures of dispersion: a variance or range within the data such as a range of intervals or a clear spread of data in a graph
- measures of position: statistics are shown in a rank and statistical scores are compared against one that is considered normal
- measures of central tendency: mean, median and mode (see next) are used to show the most common response
- measures of frequency: percentages or the frequency of numerical data showing how often something occurs.

Mean

The mean in statistical analysis is one form of average. To identify the mean, each piece of data should be added together and divided by the number of units. The mean is thus the centre of a particular variable. An example of this within healthcare could be as follows: if you were calculating the number of patients who had been admitted to hospital due to COVID, you would investigate a representative population of people who had COVID to discover whether they were hospitalised or not, then take the number of patients hospitalised and divide it by the number of participants you had investigated. This will then give you the mean amount.

For example, let us imagine that:
- 500 participants had taken part in a COVID investigation
- 380 of the participants were hospitalised, meaning 120 did not receive hospital care
- dividing 380 by 500 equals 0.76; therefore, for every 100 individuals who had COVID, 76 of them were hospitalised.

Standard deviation

The standard deviation is the mean distance of all the values from the mean (average). The deviation takes all data into account and identifies the most powerful measure of **dispersion**, meaning how the data is spread across the collected findings. This identifies the value of the research from the participants.

The investigator needs to be able to identify how the data is spread and how far it is away from the mean. The mean may identify two sets of statistical analysis, whereas central dispersion (standard deviation) uses the overall numerical data and ignores insignificant data.

With standard deviation, investigators use the **degree of freedom**, known as $n - 1$, where n represents the sample and the -1 represents the division. Therefore, the researcher divides the sample (n) by -1 to gain a larger summary providing an appropriate answer to the equation. This answer will then be representative of the wider population and enable general conclusions.

By using $n - 1$, we obtain a closer estimate of the variability around the mean within the population from which the sample is taken. Therefore, as n (the sample) gets larger, the difference between n and $n - 1$ is reduced.

To calculate standard deviation, we use the following equation:

$$SD = \sqrt{\frac{\sum (x - x_i)^2}{n - 1}}$$

where SD is standard deviation, x means the individual values in your sample, x_i is the mean value, n is the number of values and $\sum$ means the total or 'sum of'.

Figure 8.5 shows the standard deviation against the mean. A and C represent two standard deviations from the mean and B represents the mean. Standard deviation graphs show the variation on either side of the mean.

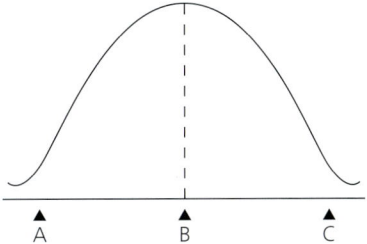

▲ Figure 8.5 Standard deviation

Inferential statistics

Inferential statistics enable generalisation from a variety of data samples. Inferential statistics are used to generalise about a large population, enabling a small target population to be used as a guideline for the larger population (see Figure 8.6). This is less time consuming to conduct compared to larger-scale studies, and findings can be concluded promptly. This is useful in healthcare to discover quick, effective solutions to improve healthcare services, medications and diagnostic techniques. However, as the data has not been fully measured, the reliability of these statistics may be limited.

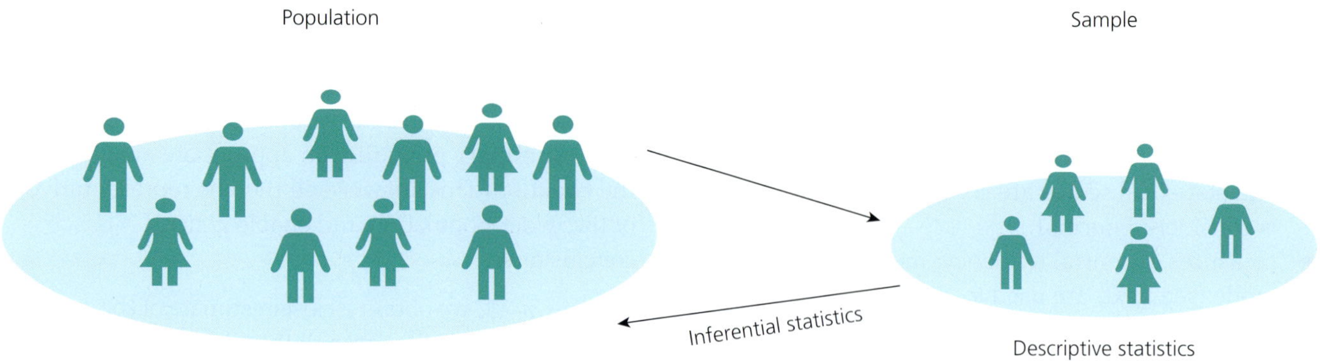

Healthcare Science T Level: Core

Population   Sample

Inferential statistics   Descriptive statistics

▲ Figure 8.6 Inferential statistics

Sampling variation

This involves a small population to record and analyse data. A sample enables a small proportion of data to be collected and measured to provide a quicker analysis. However, sampling may not hold much **ecological validity**, meaning that the overall analysis may be unreliable for a larger population. On the other hand, sampling is less time consuming to gather knowledge within a particular area of research.

> **Key term**
>
> *Ecological validity:* whether the results can be generalised to real-life settings.

Observing errors

Errors cause inconsistency, meaning that measurements may be unreliable. Errors within data can be minimised with repeated measures, meaning the same procedures and methods of data collection can be repeated and used in the future to ensure consistent data conclusions. To minimise errors, research settings must be controlled to prevent unreliable and invalid data. However, the problem with too much control within experiments means it can lack ecological validity, so it does not effectively apply to day-to-day life.

Research is paramount in healthcare science; for example, treatment and prevention methods for cancer are being researched continually to improve knowledge and develop new treatments.

> **Research**
>
> Visit www.hdruk.ac.uk/research/case-studies
>
> Choose the research case study you find most interesting and make notes so you can explain the following points to your classmates:
> ▶ overview
> ▶ challenge
> ▶ solution
> ▶ input
> ▶ output.
>
> Once you have an explanation of each point, evaluate the impact that your chosen case study may have on healthcare provision.

> **Test yourself**
>
> 1. What is the mean?
> 2. What is the mode?
> 3. Explain the difference between quantitative data and qualitative data.
> 4. Sandra is a healthcare assistant and has two service users who require lunchtime care. She has a choice of routes from one person's house to another. She timed her journeys along each route on several occasions and the times in minutes are given in the table.
>
> | Route 1 | 18 | 19 | 23 | 28 | 21 |
> | Route 2 | 16 | 22 | 20 | 22 | 18 |
>
> a Calculate the mean and standard deviation for each route.
> b Which route would you recommend? Explain why.

A8.9 Different formats for communication and presenting data and how to adapt communication style where appropriate

Good communication is essential when working with research and presenting data – we need to understand how to present information in an effective way that allows other individuals to understand it.

The potential audience for the data to be presented will determine how the data is displayed, starting with the simple question of whether it is done verbally and/or using visual methods such as graphs and bar charts. Communication styles may need to be adapted due to additional needs or accessibility issues such as hearing impairments. When communicating information and managing the process of communication, it is important to consider the type of data being shared.

Formats for sharing information

Oral reports

Oral reports include verbal and non-verbal communication. An example of reports being discussed orally may be during a handover where nurses need to communicate information about patients from their shift that they are handing on to the nurse taking over. Oral information must be clear and precise. Other ways in which oral information may be passed on is over the phone, or to a patient receiving information for the outcome of their appointment. If the information is being discussed with a patient, a professional should avoid the use of jargon and any acronyms that they may use with colleagues. The patient needs to clearly understand the language being used. If there are any language barriers, interpreters or other methods must be in place to overcome this.

Written reports

Written reports may include clinical or medical information and could include patient preferences, allergies, conditions and diagnoses to name but a few. Written reports must be accurate and use appropriate and clear language. Dates and times are also necessary on written reports to ensure information is up to date. The report must contain valid information to ensure that any professionals who need to seek the patient's information can identify an accurate timeline of events throughout the patient's life.

Forms and documents

Forms and documents must be precise within health and social care to ensure any information being passed on is accurate. A range of health or social care workers may work with a patient and, therefore, must be aware of their medical history including any diagnosis, symptoms and family history. Forms and documents may need to be passed on through a need-to-know basis, such as for a patient referral. Therefore, the information processed must reflect the patient's needs, personal information and medical history in a similar way to written reports.

Presentations

Presentations may be used in research projects or team meetings. They might include information about innovative areas of healthcare science, as health and social care professionals must keep up to date with any new information. This may include changes in legislation that affects policies and procedures, changes in software systems, changes in medical instruments, and observations and visits from the CQC. Both verbal and non-verbal communication are important during presentations to ensure understanding is clear. Allowing question-and-answer time after a presentation, or during the presentation itself, is useful, as is the use of open body language, verbal techniques such as questioning, and different vocal pitches and volume to help understanding.

Graphs and tables

Graphs and tables ensure research findings are summarised in a clear format. Graphs and tables are used to analyse findings in research and to present a clear picture of data. Visual representations enable others to distinguish clear findings.

An example of a bar chart from an investigation into the waiting times for treatment of patients with cancer is shown in Figure 8.7.

On the left-hand side, which is the y-axis, the number of patients waiting for treatment is shown. On the x-axis, running along the bottom, is each year the research was investigated and analysed. This bar chart clearly shows the number of patients included within the research and the increase or decrease of the patients' waiting times for treatment.

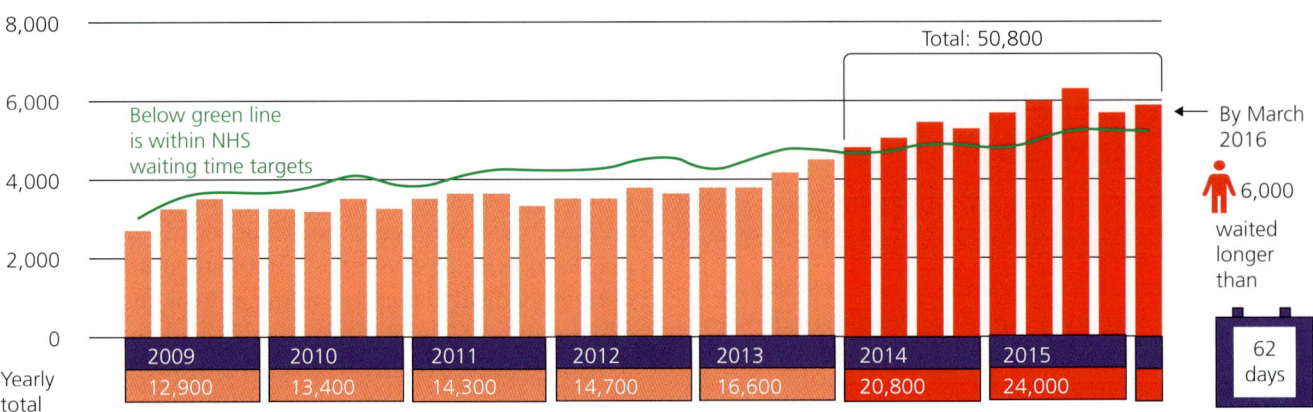

▲ Figure 8.7 An investigation of research on the waiting time for treatment for patients with cancer

Source: NHS England, Provider-based quarterly cancer waiting times data, Oct 2009 - Mar 2016. https://news.cancerresearchuk.org

Leaflets or posters

Leaflets and posters provide precise, summarised information that may relate to health promotion, research or treatment options. Leaflets or posters allow significant information to be presented in a simple format. They may also contain contact information for patients to investigate further queries and seek further information. Too many details may cause confusion or lack of interest for service users; therefore, leaflets and posters should be eye-catching with the use of relevant imagery. Technical language should also not be used; if it is needed, it should be explained in simple terms that enable the service user to understand the information given.

Web pages and social media

Web pages enable patients to access information all day every day. Patients can seek information from a wide variety of web pages and research information when needed. Limitations of web pages may be that patients may misdiagnose themselves or discover information that may be false on web pages that are not monitored. NHS web pages are useful to help service users to research information, for instance about treatment or symptoms. These trusted, updated sites are accessible to all individuals. However, service users should always consult health professionals to confirm any health conditions and not rely on the internet for diagnosis.

Social media can be extremely useful for those wanting to research useful contacts. The limitations of social media are similar to web pages, however, such as inaccurate information, misdiagnosis or potential scamming from fraudulent health insurance companies.

How to adapt communication style to suit the target audience

Choose the appropriate tools to represent the information, including digital and non-digital methods

Understanding patient needs is an essential component in effective practice. A healthcare science professional must be mindful of when other methods of communication need to be used. For example, if a patient is unable to use IT effectively, the professional must make use of non-digital methods such as letters, leaflets and telephone calls to communicate with them.

On the other hand, digital methods are useful for sharing information for many other individuals, such as sending appointment reminders by text or email. They are also helpful for deaf individuals or those who have other access needs that make letters or phone calls impractical. Online prescription services are useful for service users to order repeat prescriptions without having to call their GP or go into the surgery.

Organise information in a logical, coherent way to support the length and purpose of information being shared

Information must be organised appropriately to meet codes of conduct and organisational principles related to data protection and sharing. Sharing information must only be on a need-to-know basis for specific reasons, such as working with a multidisciplinary team when consulting or referring a patient's specific needs to another team.

Information should be structured in a logical manner to avoid misunderstandings or confusion. Information that includes dates (e.g. medical history) should be arranged in a timeline, i.e. chronological order, to help the reader's understanding. There will often be a template used, for instance a form for inputting all of the relevant information that will be needed.

The person presenting the information should not scatter information randomly throughout as this makes it difficult for the audience to understand it. Coherent information is well planned in a sequential manner. There should be a continuous flow of consistent information that covers the main topic in question. Having information organised coherently also enables feedback to be instantaneous.

The presenter should provide clear explanations to ensure general understanding from the audience, such as definitions for jargon or acronyms. They should plan carefully to ensure the audience can clearly identify the meaning of the concepts discussed without confusion.

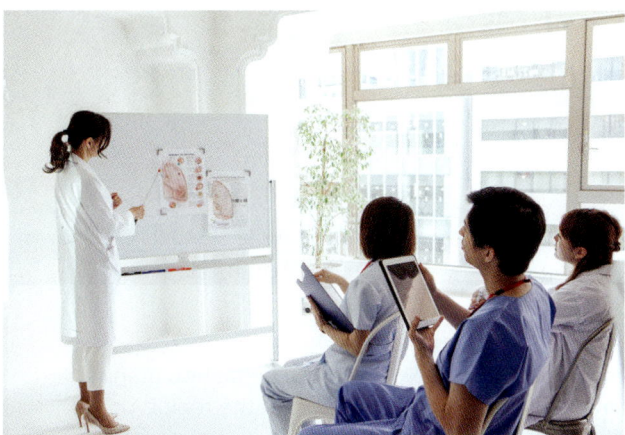

▲ Figure 8.8 Healthcare colleagues communicating through a presentation

An example of clear and coherent written information could be passing on patient information to another service. If the information is sent via a letter or email, the subject or title should include the patient or service concerned, such as:

Subject: Referral of patient Erin Cooper, NHS number 123456789

The main body of the message should then include the reason for the message, such as a referral, the patient's history of the current illness or complications. The letter or email should also contain any relevant dates and times in order of occurrence. Finally, it should contain the name of the sender and correspondence details, such as contact numbers, email, the organisation and the address. Before the email or letter is sent, it should be noted as confidential and for the attention of whom it is intended. If sent via email, this should be encrypted.

> ### Project practice
>
> Research the FOI and write down how you would process a request from a patient to disclose their information. Use the following link to help you research and reference where necessary:
>
> www.gov.uk/make-a-freedom-of-information-request
>
> In your report, include:
> ▶ what an FOI request is
> ▶ what information can be disclosed to the patient
> ▶ how long the process of a request will take to complete
> ▶ what procedures you would have to follow as a healthcare professional
> ▶ advantages and limitations of the FOI referring to the scenario.

> ### Assessment practice
>
> 1 Identify three methods of recording and reporting service user information and provide an example for each.
> 2 Explain Liberty Protection Safeguards and provide an example of when this may be required.
> 3 Evaluate the use of the following three statistical databases: SPSS, SAS and STATA.
> 4 Identify factors that may require safeguarding intervention.
> 5 Describe descriptive statistics.
> 6 Explain the mean and standard deviation.
> 7 Explain the role of a bioinformatician in researching and analysing biological data. Consider the use of biological research in healthcare.

A9: Good scientific and clinical practice

Introduction

If you bake a cake, you follow a recipe. If you strip down and rebuild an engine, you follow a workshop manual. If you have done either of these many times before, then you may not have to keep looking at the recipe or the manual. But if you are new to baking, then failure to follow the recipe carefully is likely to give disappointing results – something that looks and tastes more like a pancake than a light, fluffy sponge. Not paying attention to the workshop manual might result in a few parts left over and a reassembled engine that may never work again.

The same principles apply to our work in science and healthcare. Therefore, we have to follow proper procedures and do our best at all times – particularly when the consequences of getting things wrong can be disastrous. This is why we must always adhere to the standards and procedures that we call good scientific and clinical practice.

Learning outcomes

The core knowledge outcomes that you must understand and learn:

- **A9.1** the principles of good practice in scientific and clinical settings
- **A9.2** what an SOP is
- **A9.3** why it is important for everyone to follow SOPs
- **A9.4** how to access SOPs for a given activity
- **A9.5** the potential impacts of not regularly cleaning and preparing work areas for use
- **A9.6** the potential impacts of not maintaining, cleaning and servicing equipment
- **A9.7** why it is important to calibrate and test equipment to ensure it is fit for use
- **A9.8** how to escalate concerns if equipment is not correctly calibrated/unsuitable for intended use
- **A9.9** why it is important to order and manage stock
- **A9.10** the potential consequences of incorrectly storing products, materials and equipment.

A9.1 The principles of good practice in scientific and clinical settings

Whatever our work environment, whatever branch of science or healthcare, we must aim to achieve:
- consistency
- predictability
- reproducibility
- reliability.

On top of all this, we must ensure the health, safety and wellbeing of ourselves and others.

We can achieve these objectives in several ways, as described in this chapter, but they all share these common principles:
- using standard operating procedures (SOPs)
- effectively managing calibration and maintenance of equipment and work areas
- effectively managing stock
- appropriately storing products, materials and equipment.

The following sections will look at how all of these contribute to good scientific and clinical practice.

A9.2 What an SOP is

A **standard operating procedure** or **SOP** is simply a set of steps or instructions in a sequence that are designed to standardise the approach to a process or action, so that everyone learns to do it the same way. SOPs can be used for everything we do in the workplace, including:
- receiving goods, booking them into stock and informing the accounts department that the invoice can be paid
- cleaning a room in a healthcare facility or a microbiology lab
- producing a batch of a pharmaceutical ingredient
- analysing that batch to make sure it meets standards of purity, activity and safety.

Some SOPs may be just a few lines of instruction, others will be long and complex. They will always aim to ensure that the process or activity is done correctly and consistently.

> **Research**
>
> Find one or more examples of an SOP. Ideally these should be from your workplace, but if none is available, an internet search for 'SOP in healthcare' should provide numerous examples.
>
> Review the SOPs. Are there any common features? Would they allow you to carry out the task without further information? Do some of them require prior knowledge or training, or refer to other SOPs?

A9.3 Why it is important for everyone to follow SOPs

SOPs are created for a reason – to ensure that processes can be followed consistently, which can be crucial in health and science facilities. Ultimately, if you do not follow an SOP, you might get fired from your job, or at least disciplined. Of course, this is not the main reason we must all follow SOPs – failure to follow SOPs might have legal consequences in some organisations, or someone may be injured as a result – but it does illustrate why doing so is so important.

Maintaining health and safety

In Chapter A3 we looked at various health, safety and environmental regulations. You will have learned the importance of following proper procedures, especially in areas that are tightly regulated. Part of this is to perform a proper risk assessment. Every SOP should include a risk assessment of the process being carried out and the steps taken to minimise harm. Following the SOP is essential to reduce harm to employees, the public or the environment.

Enabling consistency of approach

The key word is 'standard'. An SOP should ensure that a process or procedure is always carried out in the same way. The outcome should be predictable. An SOP helps ensure that everything is done in the same way each time, producing consistent outcomes.

Of course, it is important that quality is also built into SOPs. Consistency is no good if all it means is that the product is always consistently poor. Consistency without quality is not enough.

Meeting any legal or organisational requirements

The science and healthcare sectors are highly regulated – for good reason. Companies and other organisations can see the importance of good-quality SOPs that are strictly followed, but some SOPs will ensure that any applicable laws are followed.

Here is a range of examples of how SOPs might be required for organisational or legal reasons:
- cleaning staff writing their initials on a chart to show that regular scheduled cleaning has been carried out
- following government (specifically, Home Office) requirements for storing and issuing controlled drugs in hospitals or care homes
- storing and disposing of hazardous waste (see COSHH Regulations in Chapter A3, page 52)
- carrying out clinical trials of new medicines or therapies
- obtaining regulatory approval for new medicines, medical devices or treatments.

Upholding professional standards

Membership of all sorts of professional bodies from the Royal Society of Chemistry to the various medical colleges (Royal Colleges of Nursing, Midwives, Physicians, Surgeons, etc.) requires adherence to certain professional standards. By following appropriate SOPs, you can show that you are upholding those standards.

Some regulated activities, such as production of pharmaceuticals, have to be supervised by a **qualified person** (**QP**). European Union regulations state that a medicinal product cannot be supplied for sale without a QP certifying that it meets the relevant requirements or standards. A QP is typically a pharmacist (MRPharmS), chartered chemist (CChem) or chartered biologist (CBiol). These roles are administered by the Royal Pharmaceutical Society, Royal Society of Chemistry and the Royal Society of Biology.

Demonstrating compliance for audit purposes

It is not enough to do something properly – you need to be able to show that you did it properly. Having an experienced person watch over you might be useful, but it will not be enough to show that the job was done correctly when your organisation is audited or inspected months or even years later. Having robust SOPs, following them carefully and recording how they were followed provides documentary evidence that will satisfy inspection bodies such as the Medicines Agency, Home Office or Care Quality Commission when they review this at a later date.

> **Test yourself**
>
> 1. What is a standard operating procedure (SOP)?
> 2. Explain two reasons why it is important for everyone to follow SOPs.
> 3. Give two consequences of not following an SOP.
> 4. Explain why SOPs often require you to complete a log or record your actions.

A9.4 How to access SOPs for a given activity

Most organisations should have SOPs for all the procedures and processes that are carried out in the workplace. These should be kept in either hard copy or electronic format and be readily available for use. However, if SOPs are not available, you might need to look elsewhere.

Carrying out detailed index searches (for example, via intranet/manual)

If the SOP is available in your organisation, you might need to search for it. This might involve searching an electronic or paper-based index. SOPs may be held centrally or located in the departments to which they relate. SOPs that are used infrequently might require some tracking down.

Finding SOPs in electronic format via your organisation's intranet or computer network should be quite straightforward – particularly if it has good search facilities, ideally based on one of the online search engines such as Google or Bing.

Completing detailed staff induction and ongoing training

If you wrote an SOP for how to run an efficient organisation, staff induction (processes for getting new employees set up and informed about their new role) and regular training would certainly be very prominent. New staff must be aware of SOPs that affect their area of work – it is not good enough to expect them to learn, sometimes the hard way, 'the way we do things round here'. As well as being part of the induction process for new employees, staff need to be kept up to date with the new SOPs or modifications to SOPs. This should be part of a regular training programme for all staff.

Ensuring the SOP is the most up-to-date version

Using a version of an SOP that was written 20 years ago and has been updated once since then can be worse than useless. Much could have happened in the meantime:
- Methods may have changed.
- Equipment or processes may have been updated.
- Regulations may have changed.
- Roles and responsibilities may have evolved.

It should be obvious that some form of **version control** is needed (for instance, giving each new updated version a new number – e.g. v2, v3, etc.). But it is not enough to know which version you are using – you need to know that you have the latest version. This can be achieved in a number of different ways:
- Controlling the production and distribution of SOPs so that old versions are returned or destroyed when new versions are introduced.
- Maintaining a central deposit (electronic or paper-based) that can be accessed but not removed or downloaded.
- Maintaining a central index or database so that version numbers of SOPs in use can be checked to ensure they are the most up to date.

> **Research**
>
> It is unlikely that you will have responsibility for production of SOPs, at least in the early years of your career. However, you will almost certainly have to use them. You should always know where and how to access the SOPs that cover your work. Find out how your organisation stores, makes available and maintains its SOPs. Think about the tasks you undertake (or are likely to undertake) in your role and obtain copies of the relevant SOPs. Do they provide sufficient information and guidance for you to carry out the task adequately? If not, do you know where to go to get additional help or support?

Ensuring all relevant documentation has been completed and signed

Although people sometimes complain about 'box-ticking exercises', 'mountains of red tape' or 'bureaucracy', good documentation is essential to keep track of:
- what is done
- when it is done
- it being done correctly
- who does it.

These are all essential to make sure not just that things are done correctly but that we can show they have been done correctly. 'Signing off' the records helps to emphasise the importance of following procedures and taking responsibility. It encourages taking ownership of a process.

If something goes wrong and a product does not meet specification, or someone is injured, there is likely to be an investigation. It is important to have good records and an **audit trail** to ensure that lessons can be learned for the future. Learning lessons, in the spirit of continual improvement, is more important than assigning blame. There are examples of this in sections A3.3 and A3.4.

> **Test yourself**
>
> 1. Describe the ways in which an organisation may:
>   a. keep or store its SOPs
>   b. make them available to staff.
> 2. Give two reasons why it is important to use up-to-date SOPs.
> 3. Describe one way in which organisations ensure that the most up-to-date version of an SOP is the one that is used.
> 4. Explain why it is necessary to ensure all relevant documentation is completed.

A9.5 The potential impacts of not regularly cleaning and preparing work areas for use

Risks to health and safety

Some of the more general risks in this area are covered in section A3.3 ('Ensuring working environments are clean, tidy and hazard free', page 58). Other risks can be specific to certain environments or workplaces.

Spread of infection

The COVID-19 pandemic has made us all aware of the importance of hygiene in reducing the spread of

infection. Different micro-organisms can spread in different ways, but regular cleaning and preparation can reduce routes of transmission:
- Contaminated surfaces, known as **fomites**, can transmit bacteria and viruses when touched. These can include:
  - hard surfaces (door handles, handrails, light switches, mobile phones)
  - fabrics such as clothing, towels and furnishings.
- Aerosols, produced by breathing, coughing or sneezing, can transmit infected droplets directly between people. This is why good ventilation is so important. Aerosols can also transfer infectious agents to fomites.
- Accumulations of waste, rubbish, dirt, etc. can provide a breeding ground for infectious micro-organisms or for vermin that can be **vectors** for disease (see section B1.26, page 235).

Production of toxic/dangerous by-products

Aseptic technique is used in microbiology to prevent contamination of bacterial cultures as this can have serious consequences. For example, if a pathogen contaminates the culture, this could lead to disease or even death of anyone who comes into contact with the culture.

In some chemical processes, failure to clean equipment properly can lead to contamination of the product and could also lead to production of hazardous by-products that are toxic, explosive or harmful to the environment.

> ### Health and safety
> Think about the risks we have covered. Do any of these apply in your workplace? Do you need to get more information about precautions to take and procedures to follow? Are there any ways that you could modify your work practices that will help to reduce risks to health and safety?

Invalid results

Contamination can introduce other micro-organisms (bacteria and fungi) that can compete with the one being cultured. This can obviously ruin an experiment. However, there are many other situations in laboratory or clinical settings where contamination, or cross-contamination, can invalidate results.

Here are some examples:
- Environmental samples for water analysis can be contaminated during the sampling process or during transport or storage.
- Analytical reagents can be contaminated. This is likely to invalidate any analysis performed using them.
- DNA samples are at particular risk from contamination – especially cross-contamination. See the case study for more information.

> ### Case study
> The polymerase chain reaction (PCR) is an enormously powerful technique for 'amplifying' DNA or RNA. It uses the enzymes involved in DNA replication to take a few hundred copies of DNA or RNA and create billions of copies. PCR is used in many applications in research (genetic engineering), forensics (DNA samples from crime scenes) and diagnosis (the PCR test for SARS-CoV-2 virus). However, it is also highly susceptible to contamination and so precautions must be taken to prevent this. Use of DNA in evidence in a criminal trial could be invalidated if there were any possibility of 'foreign' DNA being introduced.
> - What precautions should be taken to minimise risk of contamination when working with PCR? Think about use of SOPs and staff training.

> ### Reflect
> Have you ever taken a COVID-19 PCR test? Did you notice any signs of an SOP being followed, or precautions being taken to avoid contamination during collecting the samples?
>
> If you have taken a COVID-19 lateral flow test, think about the instructions provided. Do they have the characteristics of an SOP? Is the information provided sufficient for you to carry out the test correctly?

Inefficient working practices

'Time is money' is a saying you are likely to encounter many times in your working life, largely because it is true. Lack of efficiency means that the job takes longer – and that means it is not just your time that is being wasted but other people may be waiting on your work, so they are wasting time as well. This means higher staff costs as they have to be paid for more hours. And inefficiency is not just about waste of time – it could mean a waste of valuable materials or resources, some of which could be incredibly difficult to obtain.

Damage to equipment

Not following an SOP can have many consequences, including breaking essential and/or expensive equipment. Once again, it is likely to cause your organisation extra costs – such as repair or replacement – as well as increasing the time it takes to get the job done.

> **Reflect**
>
> Think about a workplace you are familiar with. Make a list of all the things that have gone wrong or could go wrong. Now think about the costs and delays that might be incurred as a result.

> **Test yourself**
>
> 1. Describe the ways that regular cleaning can prevent spread of infection.
> 2. Describe how inadequate cleaning can lead to invalid results.

A9.6 The potential impacts of not maintaining, cleaning and servicing equipment

All of the factors that we considered in section A9.5 about not cleaning and preparing work areas apply just as much to not maintaining, cleaning and servicing equipment properly:

- Risks to health and safety:
  - increased risk of injury
  - spread of infection.
- Invalid results:
  - contamination or cross-contamination.

Reduced function of equipment

Lack of proper maintenance can lead to decreased lifespan of equipment. That is why second-hand cars sold with a 'full service history' are considered better buys. As well as this, equipment being out of service for repair or because it has not been properly maintained is likely to increase costs and cause delays in getting the job done.

For all these reasons, it is quite common for regular maintenance (sometimes called **preventative maintenance**) to be included in various SOPs.

Similarly, there might be SOPs for regular maintenance of some or all key equipment. These could include:

- regular checking that all connections are secure to make sure there are no leaks
- regular lubrication of moving parts
- replacement of batteries to ensure they do not cause damage if they leak
- regular calibration of equipment, as described in the next section.

> **Research**
>
> Endoscopes are used to view the inside of the body, typically the gut. An endoscope can be introduced via the nose or mouth to examine the oesophagus, stomach and upper part of the small intestine. Alternatively, it can be inserted via the anus to examine the bowel. Because of the way it is used, the endoscope can become heavily contaminated with pathogens during use and so must be cleaned, disinfected and sterilised between patients.
>
> More healthcare-associated outbreaks of infectious disease have been linked to contaminated endoscopes than to any other medical device. Source: www.cdc.gov/infectioncontrol/guidelines/disinfection/healthcare-equipment.html
>
> Some endoscopes are heat-sensitive, so they cannot be steam sterilised (which is the preferred method). Chemical sterilisation or high-level disinfection must be used instead.
>
> Endoscopes use delicate fibre-optics to provide a view deep inside the body, so they can be easily damaged. Care must be taken in handling, cleaning and sterilising endoscopes to prevent damage.
>
> The NHS provides extensive advice on endoscope decontamination. The Medicines and Healthcare products Regulatory Agency (MHRA) publishes an information sheet on this: (https://assets.publishing.service.gov.uk/government/uploads/system/uploads/attachment_data/file/372220/Endoscope_decontramination.pdf or search the gov.uk website for 'endoscope decontamination').
>
> - Why are endoscopes at higher risk of microbial contamination than other types of medical device?
> - What are the aspects of good scientific and clinical practice covered in this chapter that are included in the MHRA information sheet?
> - Can you think of examples from your own practice where these principles would apply?

A9.7 Why it is important to calibrate and test equipment to ensure it is fit for use

The **true value** of a measurement is the ideal or perfect value. Except for some of the physical constants used as the basis of SI units (see section B1.62, page 277), we can never determine the true value because of the inherent **uncertainty** in any measurement.

The uncertainty in any measurement reflects the difference between the actual measurement and the true value as a result of the level of **accuracy** of the measuring equipment or apparatus.

> **Key terms**
>
> **Accuracy:** measurements that are close to the true value.
>
> **Precise:** measurements that are close to each other, but they may be inaccurate.
>
> **Calibration:** the process of comparing measurements, usually against a reference standard.
>
> **Reference standard:** something of known size, mass, concentration, etc. that we can use to calibrate equipment or methods.

Ensuring accuracy of measurements

Accuracy and **precision** are terms that are not always used correctly. Figure 9.1 illustrates this using the analogy of shooting at a target.

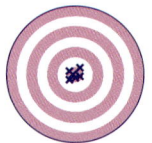 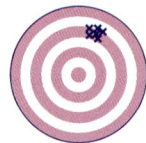 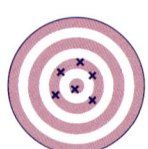 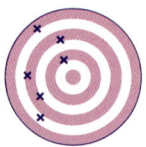

High accuracy Low accuracy High accuracy Low accuracy
High precision High precision Low precision Low precision

▲ Figure 9.1 The target analogy of accuracy and precision

Accuracy in measurement depends on the quality of the apparatus used for measurement, the skill of the person using it and how well the apparatus has been **calibrated**. The degree of precision of a piece of equipment is related to the number and size of **random errors** that it generates. The accuracy will depend on whether and how well it has been calibrated.

Calibration methods will depend on the equipment being used, but they usually involve use of a standard. Calibration is essentially the process of comparing measurements. One measurement is of a known size or correctness, e.g. a **reference standard**. The other is on the device or instrument being calibrated.

Calibration is required for:
- any instrument that has moving parts, such as an analogue ammeter or voltmeter, because movement can upset the balance of the instrument
- anything that can be affected by temperature change
- electronic equipment, as the performance of various electronic components can change over time, for example, the glass membrane in a pH electrode can be affected by deposits (dirt, oils and grease, protein, inorganic materials) and should be calibrated before each use.

However, calibration is only as good as the reference standard used, so it is important to take care of standards, for example, by preventing cross-contamination of standard solutions, corrosion of standard masses, etc.

Prolonging the life of equipment

As well as ensuring the accuracy of measurements, calibration and testing equipment will form an important part of any programme of preventative maintenance. This will help to extend the useful life of the equipment.

Meeting legal requirements

It is not so common to buy loose produce in a grocery store these days. It takes a lot longer to weigh out 1 kg of rice than it does to simply pick a packet off the shelf. However, you also have to consider the time and expense in maintaining and calibrating the scales used. There is a legal requirement for all measuring equipment used in trade to be certified to meet certain standards. This ensures that consumers are not cheated and that they can be confident in their purchases.

Now imagine you are not simply buying 1 kg of rice in the supermarket. If you buy a medicine, you need to have confidence that the dosage shown on the packaging is correct. For this reason, all equipment used in every stage in the manufacture of the raw materials and finished products has to be certified so that it meets the necessary standards of accuracy.

A9: Good scientific and clinical practice

> **Research**
>
> Think about your workplace and the types of measuring equipment that are used. Research the types of measuring equipment used and the legal requirements covering the certification and calibration of the equipment. What records have to be kept? One or more of the following pieces of legislation might be relevant:
> - Ionising Radiation Regulations (2017)
> - Weights and Measures Act 1985
> - National or International Standards such as BSI or ISO
> - Control of Substances Hazardous to Health (COSHH) Regulations 2002
> - Environmental Protection Act 1990.

> **Test yourself**
>
> 1. Give two consequences of not keeping up with a regular cleaning programme of both work areas and equipment.
> 2. What is meant by an **accurate** measurement?
> 3. Explain how proper calibration reduces the risk of error.

A9.8 How to escalate concerns if equipment is not correctly calibrated/unsuitable for intended use

The details of the procedures to follow will vary according to the workplace. However, the principles to follow if any equipment is not fit for purpose remain the same. For some critical pieces of equipment, the course of action might be covered in the SOP.

Taking the equipment out of action

This should be obvious, for the reasons discussed in the previous sections. If a pH meter or thermometer is found to be out of calibration or specification, it should be simple to stop using it and find another one. However, it is not always possible to simply throw a switch. Whenever you encounter new equipment or a new task, give some thought to what you would need to do if that equipment had to be taken out of action.

Labelling the equipment as being out of use, if appropriate

It is not enough to simply stop using the equipment yourself, you need to let other people know that the equipment should not be used. Ideally, there should be signs or stickers available that can be used – if not, perhaps you should suggest some. It is important that any sign or label is prominent so it cannot be overlooked. Also, make sure that it cannot simply fall off or be removed too easily.

Reporting concerns to the relevant person, in line with organisational policies and procedures

You might have to report any concerns to your line manager. Alternatively, there may be someone, such as a safety officer, who should be informed of any issues that could have an impact on safety.

You need to make sure that some action is taken, even if you do not need the equipment right away. Repairs or re-calibration may take time. It may not be your responsibility to actually do that, or arrange for it to be done. However, you should certainly take responsibility for informing the appropriate person so that they can take the necessary action.

Recording concerns according to organisational procedures

Reporting concerns is important, but so is making a record of those concerns. We saw in section A9.3 that you need to be able to demonstrate that an SOP has been followed for audit purposes. The same is true about documenting concerns about equipment being fit for purpose. This might look like 'covering your back' in case there are any repercussions. That may be a benefit, of course, but it is not the real reason that you need to document everything related to equipment – particularly if it has a safety implication.

Key equipment will often have an associated log, either on paper or electronically. This might cover:
- who used the equipment
- when it was used
- what it was used for
- any routine calibration or maintenance carried out.

A log of this sort might be the appropriate place to record concerns about the equipment so that everyone using the equipment is aware of any issues, either current or historical.

Healthcare Science T Level: Core

Research

Think about any pieces of equipment that are used in your workplace. Which of these require regular calibration? How often are the different pieces of equipment calibrated? Some types of equipment might require calibration before each use (do you know which these are in your workplace?) while others might need calibration at regular intervals, such as weekly, monthly, quarterly or annually. Are there SOPs covering this? Is there a record or log of what was calibrated, when it was calibrated and what the outcome was? Do you know whether each piece of equipment that you use will be fit for purpose?

If you feel that any equipment is not fit for purpose, what are the procedures for escalating your concerns? For example, should you report it to your supervisor or line manager? Is there an individual or department that is responsible for maintenance and/or calibration of equipment? Is there a procedure for reporting issues with equipment? Do you feel confident that you could handle this? If not, what steps can you take, such as asking for training or other form of support?

Case study

In August 2021, Becton Dickinson, a company that makes consumables for the NHS, announced that there was a global shortage of blood collection tubes. This was due to record demand for these tubes, partly because of the increased need for tests for COVID-19 patients. An additional factor affecting the UK was transport and import issues related to Brexit.

As a result of this, the NHS in England and Wales told GP surgeries and hospitals to temporarily stop some blood testing. Patients would only be able to get tests if they were urgent. The tests that were suspended included those for fertility, allergy, and pre-diabetes.

Doctors and nurses in GP surgeries were asked to:
- only request blood tests where they were clinically urgent, or time-critical (such as in pregnancy)
- when taking blood samples, not send an extra tube 'just in case'
- not duplicate tests that may have already been carried out in hospital.

Source: www.hey.nhs.uk/wp/wp-content/uploads/2021/08/bloodTubeShortageCCGs.pdf

In addition, practice managers in GP surgeries were asked to:
- review their local stocks to ensure they had a maximum of 3–7 days' supply
- not over-order tubes so that the central Pathology stores teams could manage stocks based on expiry dates and availability
- return any short-dated blood tubes that would not be used before the expiry date to the central stores.

Source: NHS blood test tube shortage: Doctors 'facing difficult choices' - BBC News www.bbc.co.uk/news/health-58374553

This was an exceptional situation, based on the combination of worldwide and local factors. Nonetheless, can you see aspects of how normal stock control was managed?

What are the lessons for proper ordering and managing of stock?

A9.9 Why it is important to order and manage stock

Ensuring sufficient supply of required consumables and materials

Clearly, it is important that you have access to sufficient stocks of all the items you need to carry out your work. You may not be responsible for the purchase or ordering of **consumables** or **materials**, but you will almost certainly be responsible for ensuring that you have access to everything you need. That may mean knowing how to get them from stores or ensuring you have your own stock in your work area.

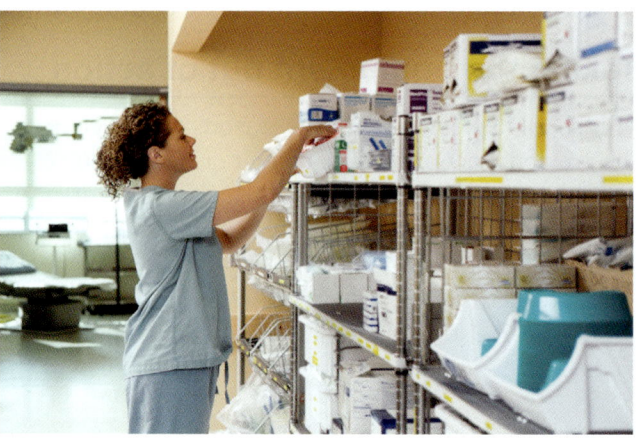

▲ Figure 9.2 Make sure you always have the right amount of stock

A9: Good scientific and clinical practice

> **Reflect**
>
> Think about the things you use every day in the workplace, such as gloves, paper towels, cleaning materials, etc. What impact would it have on your work if supplies of any of these ran out? Have you been in a situation where shortage of consumables has prevented you from doing a job, or having to do the job in a less-than-ideal way?

> **Key terms**
>
> *Consumables:* items that are used and then disposed of. They are mostly single-use but might be re-used in some circumstances.
>
> *Materials:* include items such as ingredients or components used in the manufacture of a product.

Ensuring that materials are used before their expiry date

We are used to seeing 'use by' or 'best before' dates on most of the items we buy in the supermarket. Do you know what they mean? In general, they mean what they say. Some products might become harmful if kept beyond the 'use by' date. On the other hand, something eaten after the 'best before' date may not be as tasty but it is unlikely to cause you harm.

In a science or healthcare environment you are more likely to come across products with expiry dates. Some of these will be more important than others.

If the expiry date on a pack of self-adhesive envelopes has passed, the adhesive may not be fully effective and you might have to resort to sticky tape to seal the envelope. That is inconvenient but is not dangerous and is therefore minor in the overall scheme of things.

However, most of the items that you encounter in a healthcare or clinical setting are likely to have expiry dates that must be respected, including:
- medicines that may no longer be sufficiently effective, meaning the patient does not receive the effect of a full dose
- packs of fluids, swabs, dressings, etc. that may no longer be sterile and could cause harm to the patient if used.

Reducing the costs of excess stock

Sometimes it is necessary to maintain high levels of stock, such as:
- items for which there is a long lead time, meaning we need to order them well in advance
- items that are critical to patient care, where running out might harm the patient.

However, in your working environment it is possible that excess stock will be wasted for no good reason. That puts a drain on resources and means there will be less budget available for essentials. Implementing robust stock control procedures can save huge amounts of money.

Improving efficiency and productivity

Efficiency and productivity are linked. Whether you measure productivity in the amount of work you get done in a given time or how much product goes out of the door every day, if you can work more efficiently, you will be more productive. However, being productive does not necessarily mean being quick. If you rush things and make a mistake, you may find that everything takes longer and costs more than if you had worked at a more steady, methodical pace. Efficiency and productivity also mean being careful.

> **Reflect**
>
> Think of the ways in which your work could be adversely affected if you do not have the consumables or materials you need. Have you ever had to delay doing something because you did not have all the necessary consumables? Have materials been wasted because they could not be used in time when key items were not available?
>
> Think about all the ways in which poor stock control can reduce efficiency. Think about ways in which your own work could be made more efficient.

Ensure safety of stock

We have considered the importance of good stock control. It should be obvious that stocks need to be looked after, which we will cover in the next section.

Ensuring stock is safely looked after might mean keeping it under the correct conditions, for example, in a fridge or freezer. It might also mean ensuring the security of stock. That might be to prevent unauthorised use or to prevent access to hazardous or controlled substances. For example, the Misuse of Drugs Act 1971

and Misuse of Drugs Regulations 2001 apply strict procedures to storage of **controlled drugs**, including:
- ensuring safe and secure storage, including restricting personnel access (for example, by use of locked storage cabinets, keycard access, etc.)
- undertaking inventory record-keeping
- following sign-in/sign-out protocols.

A9.10 The potential consequences of incorrectly storing products, materials and equipment

Are you the sort of person who reads the small print on jars of jam or bottles of tomato sauce? If so, you may notice that they nearly always have the instruction 'refrigerate after opening'. This is increasingly common, as food manufacturers reduce the amount of artificial preservatives added to foodstuffs. The consequence is that something that may have been kept in a cupboard many years ago should now be stored in the fridge. It probably explains why large fridges are becoming more popular, but it also illustrates the importance of proper storage.

Cross-contamination

Keeping with the domestic theme, we are told that cooked foods should never be stored in the fridge on a shelf below raw meat. Raw meat may be contaminated with harmful bacteria. Although these are destroyed by cooking, fluids from the raw meat may drip down onto the cooked food. The benefits of cooking are lost if cooked foods become contaminated. You will encounter many similar situations in your workplace, so pay attention to procedures for safe storage of any items that might be at risk of cross-contamination.

Breakdown of limited stability products

Many products that you will encounter in a healthcare setting are sensitive to heat or light and need to be stored accordingly.

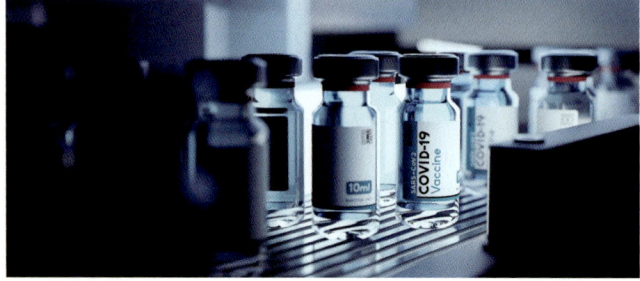

▲ Figure 9.3 COVID-19 vaccine vials in refrigerated storage

Consider the recent example of two COVID-19 vaccines (see Figure 9.3):
- The Pfizer vaccine needs to be stored and transported at −70°C.
- The Oxford/AstraZeneca vaccine can be stored at up to +4°C.

It is clear from this that the Oxford/AstraZeneca vaccine is easier to handle, particularly outside of hospitals or in developing countries that may not have access to ultra-cold storage.

Light-sensitive products are often stored in brown glass bottles (see Figure 9.4), so take care if you need to transfer such liquids to other containers.

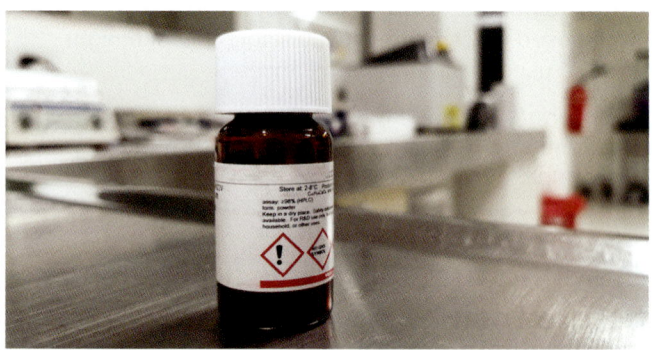

▲ Figure 9.4 A light-sensitive laboratory reagent packed in a brown glass bottle

Products exceeding expiry dates

Stock rotation is a term you are likely to encounter. It means always using the oldest batch first, providing the oldest has not passed its expiry date. Stock should always be kept in a way that makes proper stock rotation possible, rather than in such a way that items are left for months or years at the back of a cupboard. Physically arranging stocks of materials with the oldest batches at the front of a shelf can help, for example.

Loss of samples or degradation of reagents not stored at the correct temperature (−20°C, −4°C, 4°C or room temperature)

NHS guidance to GP surgeries is that blood samples and urine samples should be sent to the lab the same day (see Figure 9.5). If this is not possible, they must be stored refrigerated at 4–8°C and analysed within 24 hours. Cells in the blood can start to break down and release substances that mean the results may not be valid. It is not just high temperatures that can be damaging.

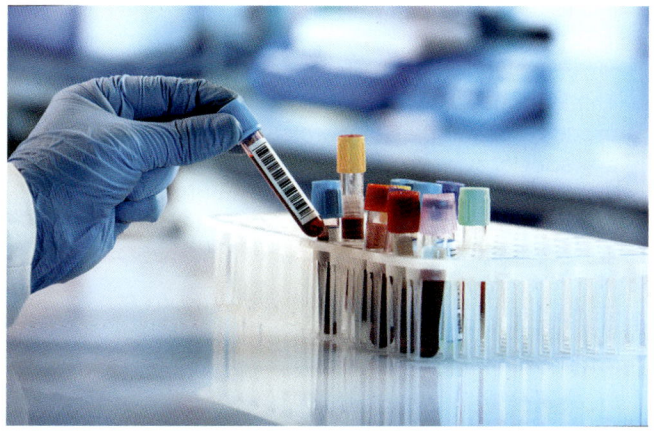

▲ Figure 9.5 Blood samples ready for analysis

In general, blood samples should not be frozen before analysis as this can also lead to damage to cells.

The World Health Organization (WHO) has strict guidelines for transport and storage of water samples. Microbiological analysis should ideally be performed within 6 hours or no later than 24 hours after sample collection. Failure to do this means that the results may not be valid.

Correct storage of reagents is equally important. Here are some examples:
- Antibodies and proteins usually need to be stored at −20 °C or −80 °C, but conjugated antibodies (antibodies with enzymes attached) must not be frozen and so should be stored at 4 °C.
- Antibodies and other reagents that have a fluorescent dye attached must be kept dark to prevent photobleaching of the fluorescent dye, which will make it useless.
- Many solids are **hygroscopic**, meaning that they will absorb moisture from the air. When they do so, they are more likely to degrade by **hydrolysis**. This is when a compound is broken down by water – see section B1.7 for examples of hydrolysis. Also, if the solid has absorbed moisture, you cannot weigh it accurately.

So far, we have described the need for low-temperature storage. What about storage at room temperature? Obviously, it can be expensive to maintain large fridges or freezers, particularly ultra-cold freezers at −80 °C. Therefore, it makes sense to store materials at room temperature where possible. However, there is another reason why it can be better to store at room temperature. Whenever a bottle of solid is removed from a fridge or particularly a freezer, there is a risk of condensation forming on the powder when the bottle is opened. This can also cause damage to the material by hydrolysis. For that reason, it is important that you leave a bottle to reach room temperature before opening. This could take several hours, so if there is no need to store the product at low temperature, it would be better to keep it at room temperature.

> ### Practice point
>
> One useful tip when handling products that require storage at low temperature is to **aliquot**. This means sub-dividing a larger amount into single-use quantities. This will avoid many freeze–thaw cycles that can be damaging to temperature-sensitive materials.
>
> If you do this, you need to make sure that the process of aliquoting does not introduce contamination.

Risks to health and safety

Incorrect storage can have serious, sometimes life-threatening, consequences.
- Cultures or samples containing pathogens could be released and that could lead to spread of infection.
- Toxic, corrosive or other dangerous chemicals could be released into the lab or into the environment.
- Heavy items stored above a safe height could fall and cause injury or could injure someone trying to reach or lift them.

Stock is difficult to locate

What happens when one member of staff goes on holiday and they are the only person who knows that the spare toner cartridges are kept in a particular cupboard in an obscure location? Storage of stocks of consumables and materials should follow a logical pattern so that things can be found easily (see Figure 9.6).

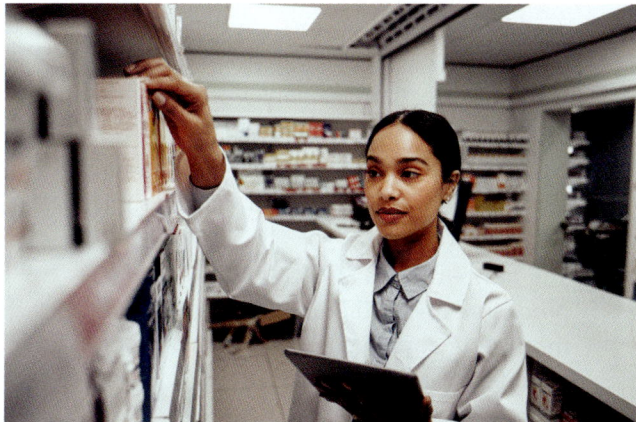

▲ Figure 9.6 Computerised stock control has many advantages

Financial loss

We have focused mainly on the health and safety consequences, but incorrect storage that leads to loss of or writing off stock has a financial implication as well. Think about the high cost of medicines and other clinical supplies and consider how much money could be saved if you reduced losses from incorrect storage.

> **Research**
>
> Think about your workplace and the materials, products or samples that are stored. Do they require any special storage conditions? Is it always clear what these conditions are? For example, are the containers marked or is there information about correct storage conditions in any relevant SOPs?
>
> What would be the consequence of incorrect storage of any of these items?

> **Project practice**
>
> You have been asked to review the way in which SOPs are used in your organisation (you can base this on your own workplace or an organisation you are familiar with). The results of the review will be considered by the management and used as the basis for future action.
>
> You need to complete the following steps:
> 1 Research a strategy.
>   a Carry out a review of the legislation and regulations that affect your organisation.
>   b Gather information about clients, customers, stakeholders of different types and how they are affected by your organisation's performance.
> 2 Plan a project based on the information that you have gathered.
>   a Identify who is responsible for production and maintenance of SOPs.
>   b How and where are SOPs kept, issued or referred to and by whom?
>   c What procedures are in place for documenting and auditing adherence to SOPs?
>   d How are SOPs incorporated into induction and training?
> 3 Present your findings in the form of a written report or PowerPoint presentation. You should include the following:
>   a What weaknesses are there in the existing SOPs?
>   b Who is responsible for maintaining SOPs and do they have the relevant training and experience?
>   c Are all members of staff familiar with the SOPs that affect them?
>   d Recommendations for improved systems.
> 4 Discuss the following questions:
>   a How should members of staff be made aware of the importance of following SOPs?
>   b Is the culture of the organisation to impose or to encourage the following of SOPs?
>   c What are the risk factors if SOPs are not followed correctly?
> 5 Write a reflective evaluation of your work.

> **Assessment practice**
>
> 1 What are the main principles of good practice in scientific and clinical settings?
> 2 Give two advantages and one disadvantage of keeping all SOPs on an organisation's intranet/computer network.
> 3 You notice that an SOP does not include a procedure for calibrating an important piece of measuring equipment. Justify why it should be included in a revised SOP.
> 4 Which of the following is the correct course of action if you find a piece of equipment is not performing correctly?
>   a Put a note on the door of the room containing the equipment.
>   b Unplug the equipment, stick a label on the front saying 'Do not use' and inform your line manager.
>   c Inform the safety officer when you next meet them.
>   d Put a note in the equipment log to say that it is not working correctly.

A9: Good scientific and clinical practice

5. Amir and Sofia are arguing about the terms 'precision' and 'accuracy'. Amir says that calibrating a piece of equipment makes the results more **precise**, but Sofia says this makes the results more **accurate**. Who is correct? Explain why.
6. A package arrives by next-day courier containing several bottles of a therapeutic enzyme. Explain what should happen to the package.
7. A healthcare practitioner is supporting a patient with reduced immunity during chemotherapy. The patient has complained of feeling unwell and the practitioner is taking the patient's temperature and blood pressure. Give two reasons why it is important to ensure that the information is accurate, and for each, explain a possible impact of not doing so.
8. What precautions would you take when preparing blood samples for transfer to an analytical laboratory?
9. You have been asked to review the way in which stocks of consumables are handled in a large care home. Each floor has a supervisor who is responsible for ordering and maintaining stocks of cleaning materials, hygiene products and some patient medications such as insulin. Identify two weaknesses in the current approach.
10. Explain the importance of proper stock control.

A10: Good scientific practice

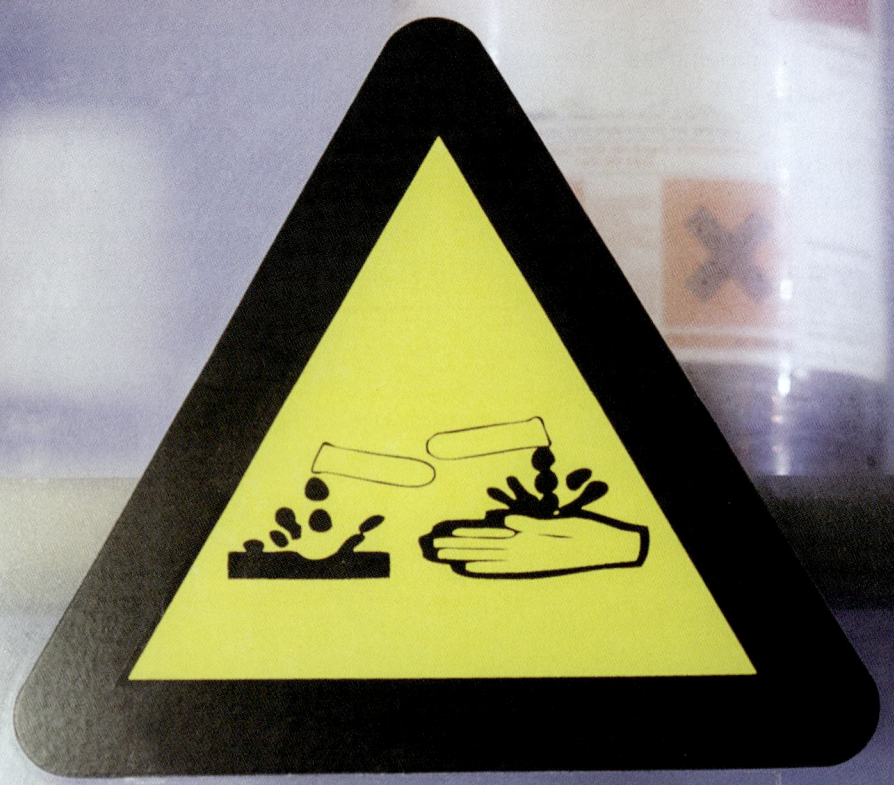

Introduction

Good scientific practice describes the basis on which we work and the standards to which we are held as healthcare professionals. This chapter examines this as well as covering how this is applied in the context of laboratory and manufacturing practice. This is linked to quality management and, finally, we will look at some specific aspects of health and safety that you will encounter in healthcare science.

Learning outcomes

The core knowledge outcomes that you must understand and learn:

- **A10.1** the five domains of good scientific practice (GSP)
- **A10.2** the importance of good laboratory practice (GLP)
- **A10.3** the importance of following good manufacturing practice (GMP) and basic requirements for the production of medical products
- **A10.4** how application of quality management policies and procedures facilitates continuous service improvement
- **A10.5** the requirements within GSP for the handling of hazardous materials and substances.

A10.1 The five domains of good scientific practice (GSP)

Good scientific practice (GSP) sets out the professional standards on which safe and good working practice is based, and applies to everyone in the healthcare science workforce. GSP also indicates the standards of behaviour and practice that employers should help their employees to achieve and maintain. The five domains of GSP were drawn up by the Academy for Healthcare Science (AHCS), which was set up as a joint initiative between the Department of Health and Social Care and professional bodies across healthcare science.

Professional practice

As healthcare science workers, we should always provide patients and service users with good standards of professional practice and probity. To maintain fitness to practice, we must observe professional codes of conduct and ethics, much of which follows the principles of person-centred care outlined in Chapter A5.

Probity means conducting ourselves in a way that justifies the trust of patients, carers and colleagues, and maintains the public's trust in the scientific profession. Therefore, we must be open and honest in our work and act with integrity in everything we do. We must also work within the standards of conduct, performance and ethics set by whatever professional body we belong to.

Working with colleagues means that we must work with other professionals, support staff, service users, carers and relatives in a way that best serves the patients' interests. This often involves working effectively as a member of a multidisciplinary team – a group of people with different skills and backgrounds working together. We should respect the skills and contributions of our colleagues, and consult them and take advice when appropriate. It is important that team performance is reviewed on a regular basis and we should always participate openly and honestly in these.

Training and developing others means that, if we are in a position to supervise and support others, we should do this diligently so that they can develop their professional skills and practice.

Scientific practice

It is essential to keep scientific and technical knowledge and skills up to date if we are to work effectively in healthcare science. Scientific practice involves developing investigative skills as well as an understanding of methodology and how to apply experimental methods to screening, diagnostics and monitoring or treatment. We also need to be able to produce good, clear reports of our work with full and appropriate analysis, as well as being able to critically evaluate data with proper conclusions and recommendations for further investigation, where appropriate.

Technical practice means knowledge and understanding of the skills needed to be able to take scientific ideas and make them work in an experimental setting. This requires knowledge of experimental methods, instruments and their capabilities and limitations, and how these should be used. It also requires an ability to understand and manage risk in all its forms and to apply the principles of good practice in health and safety to the workplace. Having the knowledge and skills needed to carry out investigations and deliver services is not enough – we also need the complementary skills and experience to be able to use information and communications technology (ICT) to provide and share the results of that work.

> **Practice point**
>
> You will need to undertake the experimental methods covered in this book during your study and in your work placement. Technical practice will ensure that you are competent in undertaking the methods and using the relevant instruments. This is just the beginning – you will build on your skills and experience throughout your professional life.

Quality must be central to any work in healthcare science. Quality standards are essential, and these must be applied across all clinical, scientific and technological activities. However, we need to be thoughtful and critical – we must always assess the effectiveness of any processes and procedures we are responsible for. This underlines the importance of quality assurance (QA) programmes (see section A5.2) and the need to maintain an effective audit trail in all our work (see section A9.4).

Documenting our work is central to good scientific practice. Anything that is not documented may as well not exist. This is likely to be part of any standard operating procedure (SOP) that we follow and will certainly be required for audit purposes.

Clinical practice

This embodies many of the principles that were covered in Chapter A5. You will need to apply these principles both

to your own work and that of any staff that you supervise during investigation and reporting. For example:
- The need to obtain consent; this could apply to a patient consenting to a particular procedure or course of treatment, or it could apply to obtaining consent to record and use patient data or personal information.
- Maintaining confidentiality of patient information and records.
- Demonstrating expertise in the wider clinical situation that applies to patients you interact with.
- Planing the clinical or scientific investigations required to meet the needs of patients.
- Ensuring that detailed clinical assessments are undertaken and recorded, and that the outcomes are reviewed regularly with service users.
- Ensuring expert interpretation of complex and/or specialist data.
- Undertaking and recording detailed clinical assessment and providing specialised clinical investigation and/or analysis.
- Prioritising the delivery of investigations, services or treatment on the basis of the clinical needs of patients.
- Ensuring regular and systematic clinical audit is undertaken.

Research, development and innovation

Research, development and innovation are central to the role of workers in the healthcare sciences. This is essential in assisting the NHS to address the challenges posed by an ageing population, often with complex and chronic disease, as well as health inequalities and increasing public expectations.

Some of the things that you will need to do, both in the course of the ESP and throughout your professional life, are:
- search and appraise published scientific literature and other information sources
- engage in evidence-based practice, including the use of audit procedures
- apply a range of research methodologies
- develop, evaluate, validate and verify new procedures and, if supported by evidence, incorporate them into routine practice
- evaluate research and other evidence to inform your own practice to ensure it remains at the cutting edge of innovation
- carry out experimental work, and produce and present results to colleagues
- support the wider healthcare team in the spread and adoption of innovative technologies and practice.

Clinical leadership

As you move into positions with managerial responsibility, you will need to ensure that the services you provide are managed efficiently and effectively. This will include:
- maintaining responsibility when delegating activities, providing support where needed
- respecting the skills and contributions of your colleagues
- ensuring cover for absence and effective handover to competent colleagues
- ensuring that everyone understands the role and responsibility of each team member
- reviewing team performance, taking steps to develop and strengthen the team and remedy any deficiencies.

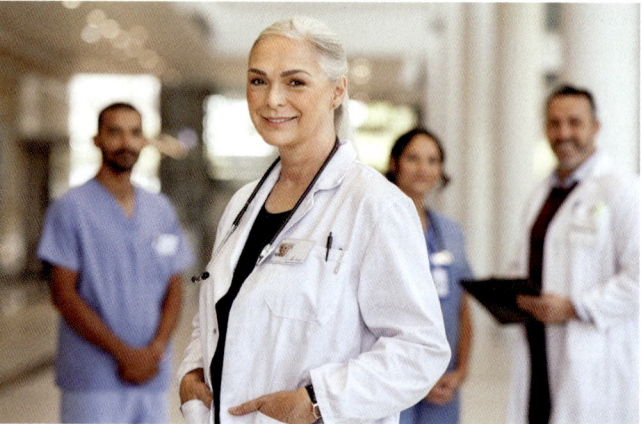

▲ Figure 10.1 Clinical leadership includes managing a team effectively

Research

The Academy for Healthcare Science (AHCS) website (www.ahcs.ac.uk) contains a lot of useful information about the healthcare science sector. Find out more about the work they do and how it relates to your own field.

You can also download a PDF copy of the 2021 edition of the AHCS publication Good Scientific Practice from www.ahcs.ac.uk/download/263/general/5214/ahcs-good-scientific-practise.pdf

Think about how some or all of these principles are likely to apply to you in your professional life.

Test yourself

1. What are the five domains of good scientific practice (GSP)?
2. Define the following terms:
   a probity
   b technical practice.

A10.2 The importance of good laboratory practice (GLP)

Good laboratory practice (GLP) is used most often in academic environments and non-clinical laboratories, but it is particularly important in laboratories that are subject to additional regulation. GLP helps to ensure that everyone can have confidence in the results of your laboratory work. GLP is a set of principles providing a framework for planning, performing, monitoring, recording, reporting and archiving.

> **Practice point**
>
> GLP only applies to non-clinical laboratories. Clinical laboratories and clinical trials are covered by good clinical practice (GCP) and other regulations intended to protect the safety of human participants in clinical studies.
>
> It is important not to confuse GLP with standards for laboratory safety.

GLP is particularly important in laboratories involved in testing (Figure 10.2). According to the Medicines and Healthcare products Regulatory Agency (MHRA) any test facility must comply with GLP when carrying out tests on:

- pharmaceuticals
- agrochemicals
- veterinary medicines
- industrial chemicals
- cosmetics
- additives for human food and animal feed
- biocides.

To ensure compliance, the test facility must belong to the UK GLP compliance monitoring programme that is run by the UK GLP Monitoring Authority.

A key aspect of GLP is following SOPs (see section 7.2), but these need to have been drawn up to incorporate the principles of GLP.

By following GLP, organisations can ensure:

- the quality, reliability and integrity of studies that they undertake, meaning that the results will be valid and the work carried out to the correct standards
- they are able to report verifiable conclusions that can be accepted by customers or collaborators
- there is full traceability of data, for example by using proper laboratory notebooks or **laboratory information management systems (LIMSs)**. A LIMS is like an electronic filing cabinet in the sense that it contains lots of different types of data and information in dedicated files. It is a software system that supports almost the entire operations of a modern laboratory.

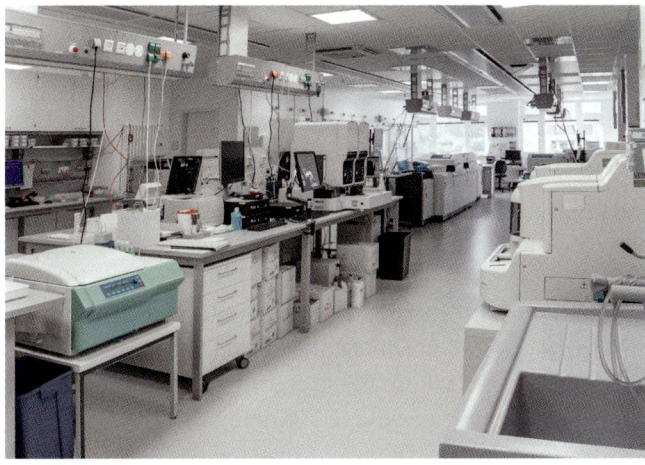

▲ Figure 10.2 A modern testing laboratory

> **Case study**
>
> **Industrial Bio-Test Laboratories (IBT Labs)**
>
> IBT Labs was an American company responsible for the safety testing of pharmaceuticals, pesticides and food additives, supporting registration approval of these products by the US Food and Drug Administration (FDA). The company was founded in 1953 by an American professor and quickly gained a reputation for producing high-quality work at a reasonable price.
>
> However, in 1966 IBT Labs was bought by another company and this led to rapid expansion of the business. In 1976, an investigator from the FDA questioned the work being done by IBT Labs. Further investigation showed irregularities and discrepancies in the data and suspected scientific misconduct in the work of IBT Labs. Eventually, the company and three former officials were convicted of making up or altering the results of key product safety tests used to obtain approval for two popular pesticides and two commonly used drugs. The company was fined, and senior personnel were imprisoned.

> Further investigation by the FDA showed that the problems were not restricted to this one company. There were other cases of fraud, but there was a more widespread problem of poor organisation and management.
>
> The FDA decided that the problem could only be dealt with by imposing regulations – the US GLP regulations. Soon after, everyone realised that there was a need for international agreement on GLP and this led the Organisation for Economic Co-operation and Development (OECD) to publish its 'Principles of Good Laboratory Practice' in 1982 based on the US GLP regulations. These became the international standard for GLP.
>
> ▶ Does this make you feel that GLP came about because companies could not be trusted to work to high ethical standards without being forced to follow regulations?
> ▶ Or do you think that organisations view GLP as a framework to follow to ensure that they always operate to the highest standards?

In essence, GLP:
▶ outlines the requirements for quality assurance of process and conditions
▶ sets minimum standards of suitability of facilities and equipment
▶ sets requirements for recording and reporting results.

The main principles of GLP are covered in what are known as the ten sub-divisions of GLP. These are outlined in the following sections.

Organisational and personnel

The structure and responsibilities of the organisation should be clearly defined and staffing levels should be sufficient to perform the required tests. Qualifications and training of staff should be documented.

Quality assurance programme

The organisation should have a documented quality assurance (QA) programme (see section A5.2) to ensure that the work carried out complies with the principles of GLP. This work should be undertaken by someone who is not involved in the work that is subject to the QA programme, to ensure impartiality. QA means that there will be a separate team of people who can assure the management that the laboratory has complied with GLP.

Facilities

Facilities and equipment should be sufficient and in working order. This is achieved by having a strict programme of qualification (ensuring it is fit for purpose), calibration and maintenance of all equipment (this was covered in section A9.7). Different activities should be segregated adequately to ensure that each is undertaken properly. For example:
▶ Waste should be stored in an area where it cannot be a potential hazard or source of cross-contamination.
▶ Stocks of products, materials and equipment should be stored in a way that maintains quality and integrity, prevents cross-contamination and reduces any risk to health and safety – this was covered in sections A9.9 and A9.10.

Equipment, reagents and materials

As well as being in good working order and fit for purpose, these should all meet agreed specifications. Chemicals, reagents and solutions should be labelled to show:
▶ identity (including concentration, where appropriate)
▶ expiry date
▶ specific storage instructions.

Information about the source, preparation date and stability of all reagents should be available. This might be in the form of a Material Safety Data Sheet (MSDS) supplied with all chemical products. Records should also be kept of all products and reagents produced in-house. How and where these records are kept will vary, but this will often be covered in an applicable SOP.

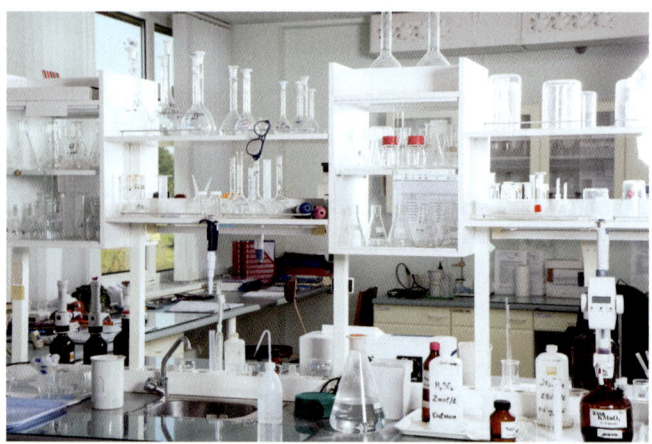

▲ Figure 10.3 Laboratory reagents: note how all the containers are labelled, even if it is with hand-written labels

Test systems

As well as apparatus for the generation of physical or chemical data, test systems may also be biological, for example animals or plants used in experiments or testing. Steps must be taken to ensure these are free from disease and are maintained in good health throughout. Full records must be kept.

Test and reference items

Test items are materials, samples, etc. that have been submitted for analysis or testing. **Reference items** are materials or reagents that are used as **standards** (for comparison or calibration) in any analysis or testing. Records must be kept showing the test item and reference item characterisation, date of receipt, expiry date, and quantities received and used in any studies. Items must be handled and stored in a way that does not risk contamination or mix-up. As much as possible should be known about the materials used (identity, purity, etc.) and the test systems (usually the animal or plant) to which the materials are administered.

Standard operating procedures (SOPs)

These are covered in sections A9.2–A9.4. SOPs must be available for all of the following:
- test and reference items
- apparatus, materials and reagents
- record keeping, reporting, storage and retrieval
- test system(s)
- QA procedures.

Performance of study

Research studies will usually have a study plan or protocol showing how the study is to be performed. Within this plan, routine procedures will be described in written SOPs. All raw data must be documented (written down).

Reporting of results

A final report should be prepared, which must describe the study accurately and interpret the results correctly. The final report should be signed and dated by each of the principal investigators or scientists involved. A QA programme statement should be included to confirm that the final report reflects the raw data. The report should include all of the information and data required by the study plan as well as:
- statistical analysis
- evaluation and discussion of results
- conclusions, where appropriate.

Archival – storage of records and reports

Records must be stored (archived) for many years so that they can be consulted in future if necessary. This might be required for audit purposes (to show that procedures were correctly followed, for example) or in case of mishap or potential harm (to patients, employees or clinical trial subjects, for example).

How long records and reports are stored may be specified by legislation, such as Control of Substances Hazardous to Health (COSHH) and RIDDOR (see section A3.1). Research records, such as those relating to clinical trials and other medical research should be kept for between 3 and 30 years depending on the type of trial. Individual organisations may also have their own rules about the length of time that records should be stored for.

Legislation may also specify how and where records are stored, and individual organisations may have their own policies about storage. This will often involve a central archive where all records are stored. This means that information is more likely to be kept secure and available for access; this might not be the case if records are dispersed throughout an organisation.

> **Test yourself**
>
> 1 What labels should be shown on chemicals, reagents and solutions?
> 2 Who should carry out the quality assurance (QA) programme?
> 3 According to GLP, what should be included in a final report besides information and data?

A10.3 The importance of following GMP and basic requirements for the production of medical products

GLP, which was covered in the previous section, is particularly important in research, development and testing. However, once a product has been developed and is manufactured on a large scale, the principles of **good manufacturing practice (GMP)** are used instead, particularly in pharmaceutical companies and diagnostic test kit manufacturers.

The aim of GMP is to ensure that:
- products are of consistent high quality

- products and constituent materials are appropriate for their intended use
- products meet the requirements of the product specification.

One way to ensure the product meets the required specification is to analyse or test it (quality control – see section A5.2). However, testing of the final product does not always identify or eliminate possible risks. GMP is designed to minimise the risks involved in any food, cosmetic or pharmaceutical production that cannot be eliminated by testing of the final product.

GMP is the minimum standard that a medicines manufacturer must meet in their production processes.

There are 11 sub-divisions of GMP.

Clean and hygienic manufacturing area

Maintain those facilities and equipment so that they go on performing as designed or expected. This also helps to prevent contamination of the product.

Controlled environment (protect against cross-contamination)

Facilities and equipment should be designed and constructed to provide a controlled environment to eliminate (as far as possible) any risk of contamination or cross-contamination. Protect against contamination, for example by incorporating cleaning, disinfection and decontamination processes into the workflow.

Clearly defined and controlled process

This means writing step-by-step SOPs and ensuring that they are followed; over time, operators (people carrying out the process) sometimes find their own ways of working or cut corners for convenience in ways that could harm the product or process. It is important to control components and processes; this might mean monitoring storage temperatures to ensure that they are sufficiently low or that heat-treatment of a product is carried out at the correct temperature – neither too high nor too low.

Good documentation practices

This means, for example, that the process is clearly recorded. You should document all work; if it is not written down, assume it is not done! An organisation cannot afford to look back at production records and find blank spaces.

Any proposed process changes require evaluation

This means that we should validate all work; does the proposed change to the process or procedure do what we intend it to do?

Records must be maintained (manual or electronic)

This means records of everything, including:
- processes and procedures
- any departure from SOPs.

Carry out periodic audits to a planned schedule as a way of ensuring that GMP is being followed correctly. Any areas for improvement can be addressed before they can cause a problem with the product.

Training

All personnel should have appropriate job training so as to define, develop and demonstrate the competence of those employees involved in the process.

Production and distribution records

These must be retained as evidence that SOPs were followed and as part of the overall QA process.

Distribution means and channels

The way in which products are distributed must minimise risk to product quality. This might include the need for specialised packaging or controlled temperature storage and distribution.

Recall system must be in place

If a problem is identified with a product, possibly because of a customer complaint or testing of retained samples, it must be possible to recall the affected batch. This illustrates the importance of batch control so that only affected batches can be recalled, rather than the whole production.

Proper complaints procedure

A well-designed complaints procedure should be established and carried out in full. The organisation must make sure that complaints procedures are effective and taken seriously by everyone in the organisation. This will ensure that customers or service users have confidence that their complaint will be handled properly and any necessary action taken.

A10: Good scientific practice

This might include recall of a batch, replacement of affected materials or even compensation for consequential losses if this is included in the contract.

A proper complaints procedure also means that an organisation is able to learn from its mistakes and should be seen as part of a process of continuous improvement (see section A10.4).

> **Research**
>
> In addition to GMP, good distribution practice (GDP) requires that medicines are obtained from the licensed supply chain and are stored, transported and handled under suitable conditions.
>
> In the UK, the MHRA is responsible for carrying out inspections to check if manufacturing and distribution sites comply with GMP and/or GDP.
>
> You can learn more about this process, if it might be relevant to your own area of work, from the following website:
>
> www.gov.uk/guidance/good-manufacturing-practice-and-good-distribution-practice

> **Test yourself**
>
> 1. What are the three aims of GMP?
> 2. How can you protect against contamination?
> 3. Why is it important to have a proper complaints procedure?

A10.4 How application of quality management policies and procedures facilitates continuous service improvement

Just as quality assurance (QA) is intended to ensure the production of a high-quality product and to avoid errors or failures in production processes, quality management means embedding quality in the whole of an organisation. The intention is to always provide the highest level of service and to avoid problems rather than trying to fix them later.

The NHS Long Term Plan for science in healthcare has four priorities to maximise the potential of emerging technologies in improving patient outcomes:

- to deliver transformation in scientifically led services by taking advances in technology and using them to transform service models in healthcare science to improve all aspects of patient care
- to attract and support research and innovation in healthcare science
- to provide scientific leadership for transformational change
- to partner with academics, industry, charities, the health and social care system and government departments to improve and integrate information and knowledge.

You can download a copy of the NHS Long Term Plan from the following link:

www.longtermplan.nhs.uk/publication/nhs-long-term-plan

Use of a mission statement

A mission statement is a short statement of an organisation's goal or purpose. A good mission statement can provide direction so that the organisation does not lose track of its objectives. It can also give an organisation a clear purpose and act as a motivational tool within the organisation. This means that employees can all work towards a common goal that benefits the organisation and themselves.

> **Research**
>
> For some examples of mission statements, visit
> https://tomislavhorvat.com/mission-statement-examples
> This website has a list of the mission statements of the 500 largest companies in the USA (the 'Fortune 500', published annually by *Fortune* magazine). It is interesting to see which words occur most commonly in mission statements.
>
> Does your organisation have a mission statement? Could you write a better mission statement, or even a mission statement for your own professional life?

Standard operating procedures (SOPs)

We have already seen in this chapter how SOPs are an important part of GSP and GMP. The clue is in the name: 'standard' implies that the process or procedure should always be carried out in the same way. This is important in achieving high-quality service. Of course, quality must be built into the SOP. Consistency on its own is not enough – there is no advantage in delivering a consistently poor service.

Establishing an evidence base for practice

Evidence-based practice is the idea that healthcare science practice should be based on scientific evidence. The approach involves making decisions and providing the best standard of care by considering all the available research, knowledge and data, and then using this information as the basis for decision-making in practice. Evidence-based medicine has been widely accepted since the 1990s and the approach has spread to other areas of healthcare and healthcare sciences.

Clearly, evidence-based practice requires a body of evidence to use in decision-making. Therefore, it is necessary to monitor our work and identify performance indicators so that we can judge whether what we are doing is effective. Doing things in a certain way because that is the way they have always been done may not give the best outcomes for patients or service users. By reviewing how we work and measuring performance, it is possible to accumulate a body of evidence that can be used as the basis of our practice.

> **Case study**
>
> Earlier detection of breast cancer can lead to better patient outcomes. However, accurate detection and diagnosis earlier using **mammography** (X-ray examination of the breast) is challenging. If a mammograph shows any signs that a tumour may be present, the woman is referred for a **biopsy** – removal of a small pieces of tissue for laboratory analysis. Thousands of cases are missed each year and 90 per cent of women referred for biopsy do not have the disease.
>
> To tackle this, healthcare scientists at the Royal Surrey NHS Foundation Trust have partnered with artificial intelligence (AI) specialists from Google Deep Mind. Together they are developing an innovative 'virtual clinical trial' to evaluate commercial breast cancer screening technologies using an AI-powered computer model.
>
> Early indications suggest that this new technology improves the accuracy of mammogram screening analysis, which improves early breast cancer detection while reducing the number of unnecessary invasive biopsies.
> ▶ Why is it desirable to reduce invasive biopsies?
> ▶ What other applications of AI are you aware of?

> **Reflect**
>
> Have you encountered evidence-based practice in your work or placement?
>
> How could you monitor your own performance to provide evidence on which to base improvements in your own practice?

Planning and monitoring service provision

A famous management theorist is often quoted as saying 'what can be measured can be managed'. Delivery of a quality service begins with planning, but effective management of the quality the service provided requires measurement, i.e. monitoring.

This includes:
▶ managing quality as a key factor in service provision
▶ analysing quality-based information (measurement)
▶ carrying out an **audit cycle**: a systematic and independent examination of the service provided in order to determine whether the required level of service was actually delivered
▶ verifying compliance with the quality plan.

> **Practice point**
>
> The famous management theorist never actually said what is attributed to them! What they did say was more complex. The problem with managing what can be measured is that we risk managing only what can be measured easily rather than measuring what is actually important. So, it is essential that we monitor the quality of the service that we provide, but we must always ensure that we are measuring the important aspects of delivering that quality service.

Regular service quality improvement meetings

There is always a risk that our working lives become one long round of meetings without ever being able to deliver our primary objective. Nevertheless, quality improvement meetings are a valuable tool for reviewing the quality of the service we provide, looking for opportunities for improvement, and planning and implementing those improvements.

The corrective and preventative action (CAPA) process

This is a method of evaluating, identifying and implementing improvements.

Corrective action involves finding the root cause – the event or error that preceded and led to the problem. This can involve a lot of 'why did…?' questions before identifying the root cause and then being in a position to implement an improvement.

> **Key terms**
>
> *Corrective action:* putting right something that has gone wrong.
>
> *Preventative action:* taking action to ensure that nothing goes wrong.

Case study

A hospital pharmacy was preparing an experimental medicine in a liquid formulation for a small research project. Several batches were produced, but only one passed the quality control testing. A root cause analysis was carried out:
- Why did the batches fail? Because they contained too much of ingredient X.
- Why did they contain too much of ingredient X? Because the quantity weighed out was variable.
- Why was the quantity variable? Because the technician doing the weighing used different balances each time.
- Why did they use different balances? Because others were sometimes using the preferred balance, so the technician used a less-accurate balance instead.

In this case, corrective action meant adding more ingredient X to those batches that contained too little, but the batches that contained too much had to be discarded.

The pharmacy then introduced preventative measures to ensure future batches were always within specification:
- Staff training was improved so that the importance of using the correct equipment was understood by everyone.
- A detailed SOP was prepared that made clear the equipment to be used at each stage and the action to be taken if that equipment was not available.
- Batch sheets were introduced so that a second person had to check all measurements to ensure that they were done correctly.

Do you think the technician should have been blamed for the failure of the batches? Can you see why it is better to design preventative action into a process rather than relying on corrective action?

Practice point

Six Sigma

This is a system of statistical tools and techniques that are focused on eliminating defects and reducing process variability. The 'sigma' refers to the Greek letter used as a symbol for standard deviation, so Six Sigma means plus or minus three standard deviations from the mean (i.e. 99.73 per cent will be within this limit). In a 'process designed for Six Sigma' a product should be outside of specification only 0.27 per cent of the time. This approach has been used widely in the electronics, aerospace and automotive industries.

However, applying this approach to pharmaceutical manufacturing is not always easy. Licensed pharmaceuticals must be manufactured according to approved processes. This means that changing a process can be costly and time consuming because of the need to obtain regulatory approval for the modifications.

> **Reflect**
>
> Think about CAPA and how it relates to the principles of QA and GMP.
>
> Think about how the CAPA process is an essential part of a quality management system. Can you identify any examples in your own practice?

Enforcing legislative requirements

Various aspects of healthcare science are regulated, sometimes by professional bodies but also by legislation.

For example, legislation and regulations cover health and safety in the workplace as well as environmental regulations – this was covered in Chapter A3. Chapter A4 covered legislation and regulations specific to healthcare science, such as the Health and Social Care Act 2012, the Misuse of Drugs Act 1971 and the role of the Medicines and Healthcare Products Regulatory Agency (MHRA).

The Academy for Healthcare Science (AHCS, www.ahcs.ac.uk) is a joint initiative of the UK Health Departments and various professional bodies across the Healthcare Sciences. The AHCS develops regulation, for example by establishing voluntary registers, as well as carrying out quality assurance of education and training and developing common standards for healthcare science practice.

Organisations that have oversight of aspects of healthcare science that is based upon legislation include:
- The Care Quality Commission (CQC)
- The Medicines and Healthcare products Regulatory Agency (MHRA)
- The Health Research Authority
- The Human Tissue Authority (HTA)
- The Human Fertilisation and Embryology Authority.

For example, the HTA was set up by the Human Tissue Act 2004 following events in the 1990s that found a culture in hospitals of removing and retaining human organs and tissue without consent. The HTA regulates organisations that remove, store and use human tissue for research, medical treatment, post-mortem examination, education and training, and display in public. The HTA also gives approval for organ and bone marrow donations from living people.

Central to the legislation is the principle of consent and the Act lists the purposes for which consent is required - these are called **Scheduled Purposes**.

> **Practice point**
>
> If you are working in a laboratory that deals with human tissue, either from the deceased or the living, you need to be aware of these key points of the Human Tissue Act 2004 as well as the offences that have been established under the Act:
> - Removing, storing or using human tissue for Scheduled Purposes without appropriate consent.
> - Storing or using human tissue donated for a Scheduled Purpose for another purpose (for example, using tissue from a donated organ for experimental purposes).
> - Trafficking in human tissue for transplantation purposes.
> - Carrying out licensable activities without holding a licence from the HTA.
> - Having human tissue, including hair, nail and gametes, with the intention of its DNA being analysed without the consent of the person from whom the tissue came or of those close to them if they have died. This is sometimes known as 'DNA theft'.
>
> A HTA Licence is required for the following (known as 'licensable activities'):
> - Carrying out an anatomical examination.
> - Making a post-mortem examination.
> - Removing relevant material from a deceased person.
> - Storing relevant material from a deceased person (other than for a specific ethically approved project).
> - Storing anatomical specimens.
> - Storing relevant material from a living person for research (other than for a specific ethically approved project).
> - Public display of a body or material from a deceased person.
> - Procurement, testing, processing, storage, distribution, import and export of tissues and cells for human application.

> **Test yourself**
>
> 1 What is a mission statement?
> 2 What are the principles of evidence-based practice?
> 3 Explain the difference between corrective and preventative action.

A10.5 The requirements within GSP for the handling of hazardous materials and substances

Handling of hazardous materials and substances has been covered in previous chapters (Chapters A3 and A6, particularly). In this section, we will look at some specific aspects relevant to GSP in healthcare sciences.

Identifying and managing sources of workplace risk

The procedures involved in identifying and managing sources of risk in the workplace were covered in section A3.2. In some healthcare science situations, you might be exposed to risks from **biohazards**. A biohazard, also called a **biological agent**, is a micro-organism, cell culture or human endoparasite that may cause infection, allergy, toxicity or otherwise create a hazard to human health. You might encounter these when dealing with specimens or clinical waste. If so, you need to be aware of the specific precautions that must be taken, including disinfection of work surfaces and the need to sterilise any waste before disposal.

Application of health and safety practice to all areas of the workplace

This was covered in Chapters A3 and A4.

Refer to and adhere to Control of Substances Hazardous to Health (COSHH) assessment and/or SOPs

For more information about COSHH, look back at section A3.1. SOPs were covered in sections A9.2–A9.4.

Application of correct methods of disinfection, sterilisation and decontamination when dealing with waste and/or spillage

As well as complying with waste disposal regulations that apply to all laboratories (described in section A3.1), there are specific requirements for laboratories handling biohazards.

There should be a system for identification and separation of infectious materials (and their containers). Categories should include:

▶ non-contaminated (non-infectious) waste that can be reused or recycled or treated as controlled waste (Figures 10.4 and 10.5)
▶ contaminated (infectious) sharps – hypodermic needles, scalpels, knives and broken glass; these should be collected in biohazard-labelled, puncture-proof containers fitted with covers and treated as infectious (Figure 3.2 in Chapter A3)
▶ contaminated material that can be decontaminated by chemical treatment or by autoclaving and then washed for reuse or recycling
▶ contaminated material for autoclaving (see Chapter A6) and disposal
▶ contaminated material for direct incineration
▶ clinical waste (Figure 10.6) and biohazard waste (Figure 10.7) could be either of the last three categories.

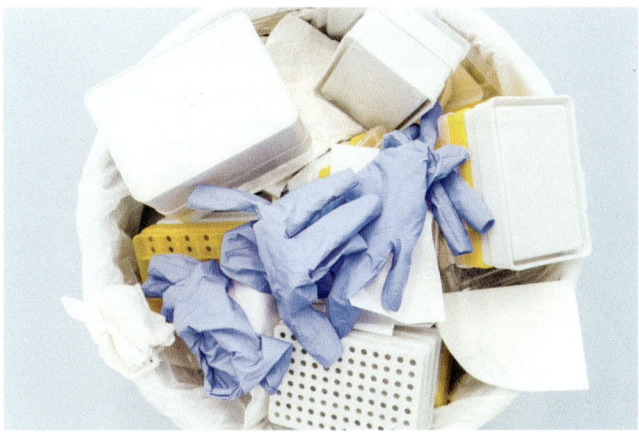

▲ Figure 10.4 General laboratory waste can be treated as controlled waste

Healthcare Science T Level: Core

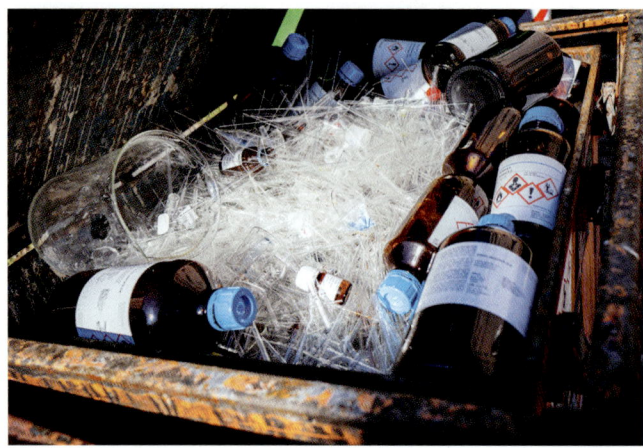

▲ Figure 10.5 Collection bins for broken glassware for recycling

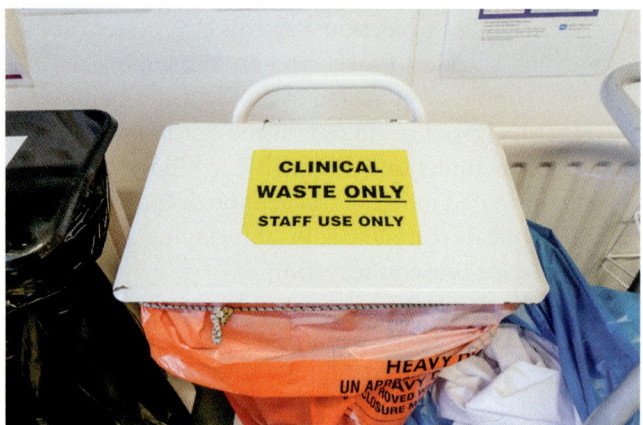

▲ Figure 10.6 Clinical waste bin

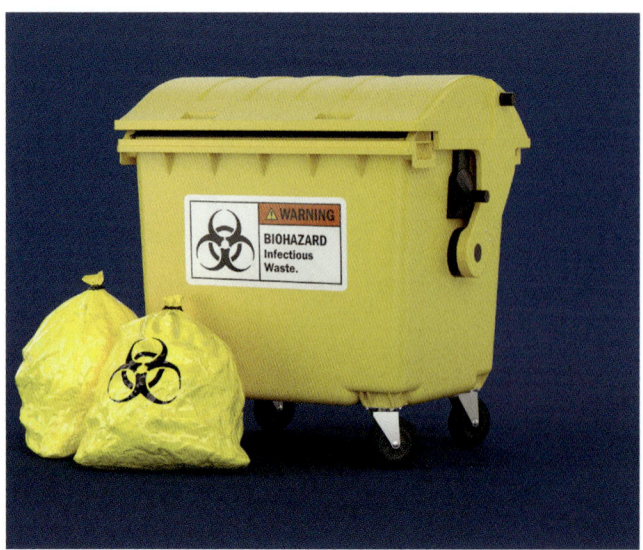

▲ Figure 10.7 Biohazard waste bagged for disposal

All infectious materials should be decontaminated, autoclaved or incinerated within the laboratory wherever possible to remove the need for transport of biohazard waste. Steam autoclaving is the preferred method for all decontamination processes unless an incinerator is available on site.

Sharps disposal containers (see previously) should never be filled more than three-quarters full. They should then be placed in infectious waste containers. Other contaminated materials should be incinerated. If there is no incinerator on site, all contaminated materials should be autoclaved in leakproof containers before transfer to the incinerator.

Once decontaminated, all materials should be incinerated following local regulations.

Maintain and apply quality standards across all clinical, scientific and technological activities

This means applying what you have learned in this and previous chapters to everything that you do in a healthcare science environment.

Remember:

Quality control indicates that the work that you do, or the service that you provide, is fit for purpose and produces the required results or outcomes that can be trusted. This happens when the work has been done. For example, a product is tested to ensure that it meets the required standards before being released for use.

Quality assurance means that you have taken all necessary steps (before you start work) to ensure that your work will be carried out to a high standard and that all possible steps have been taken to incorporate high quality into all aspects of your work. For example, a process is designed to ensure that a product, when tested, will meet the required standards and will be fit for purpose.

You must also protect patients from risk or harm at all times, as described in section A1.3 (the key principles of ethical practice) where we looked at:
- autonomy and informed consent
- truthfulness and confidentiality (for example, ensuring validity of outcomes)
- beneficence
- nonmaleficence
- justice (for example, fairness, equality and respect for all).

Test yourself

1. What is defined as a biohazard?
2. In what situation might you encounter biohazards?
3. What must be done with infectious materials before disposal?

Project practice

Thinking about your workplace, prepare a report or infographic that covers the following aspects of GSP:

1. The five domains and how they relate to your workplace.
2. The importance of GLP:
   - examples of QA programmes
   - SOPs that are used
   - how facilities contribute to GLP.
3. Whether there is a mission statement.
   - how SOPs are used
   - the role of evidence-based practice.
4. Present your work to the rest of the group and lead a discussion of your findings.
5. Carry out a reflective evaluation of your work.

Assessment practice

1. What is meant by good scientific practice?
2. Why is it important to maintain an archive of results?
3. In the context of GLP, what is meant by the following terms?
   a. Test systems.
   b. Test and reference items.
4. The director of a laboratory carrying out PCR testing of nasal swab samples for the presence of the SARS-CoV-2 virus stated that: 'Standard operating procedures must be developed and followed for all procedures used in the laboratory.'
   a. Define the term 'standard operating procedure' (SOP).
   b. Evaluate the importance of SOPs in this setting.
5. Explain the importance of regular service quality improvement meetings in a healthcare science laboratory.

B1.1–B1.32: Core science concepts: Biology

Introduction

Biology is the study of living organisms, which makes it an enormous subject! In this chapter we will cover some important basics, such as the structure of cells and the way in which they are organised. We cannot really understand how organisms work without understanding cells, and we cannot understand how cells work without learning about the main types of biological molecules: proteins, carbohydrates and lipids. Exchange and transport mechanisms – the ways in which substances enter or leave – are essential for the working of individual cells and multicellular organisms. Genetics helps us understand how characteristics are inherited and introduces the fourth main type of biological molecules – the nucleic acids – as well as providing a basis for our understanding of evolution. Microbiology is not just the study of very small organisms; it helps us to understand infectious diseases. Finally, immunology helps to explain how our bodies protect themselves against infection.

Learning outcomes

The core knowledge outcomes that you must understand and learn:

Cells and tissues
- **B1.1** the three principles of cell theory
- **B1.2** the different types of cells that make up living organisms
- **B1.3** the structure and function of the organelles found within eukaryotic cells
- **B1.4** the similarities and differences between plant and animal cells in relation to the presence of specific organelles and their function
- **B1.5** how eukaryotic cells become specialised in complex multicellular organisms
- **B1.6** how prokaryotic cells differ from eukaryotic cells

Proteins, carbohydrates and lipids
- **B1.7** the relationship between the structure, properties and functions of proteins
- **B1.8** the relationship between the structure, properties and functions of carbohydrates
- **B1.9** the relationship between the structure, properties and functions of lipids

Exchange and transport mechanisms
- **B1.10** how the surface area to volume ratio affects the process of exchange and gives rise to specialised systems
- **B1.11** the principles of cellular exchange and the transport mechanisms which exist to facilitate this exchange
- **B1.12** the advantages of having specialised cells in relation to the rate of transport across internal and external membranes

Genetics
- **B1.13** the purpose of deoxyribonucleic acid (DNA) and ribonucleic acid (RNA) as the carrying molecules of genetic information and the role they play in the mechanism of inheritance
- **B1.14** the relationship between the structure of DNA and RNA and their role in the mechanism of inheritance
- **B1.15** the function of complementary base pairing in forming the helical structure of DNA
- **B1.16** the process and stages of semi-conservative replication of DNA
- **B1.17** how this semi-conservative replication process ensures genetic continuity between generations of cells
- **B1.18** the link between the semi-conservative replication process and variation
- **B1.19** the difference between genetics and genomics

Microbiology
- **B1.20** the classification and characteristics (size of cell, type of cell, presence of organelles) of the following micro-organisms
- **B1.21** the benefits of using light and electron microscopes when investigating micro-organisms.
- **B1.22** how to calculate magnification from the size of the image and the size of the object
- **B1.23** the uses of differential staining techniques

Immunology
- **B1.24** the nature of infection
- **B1.25** causative agents of infection and examples of resulting diseases

B1.26 the different ways in which causative agents may enter the body
B1.27 how infectious diseases can spread among populations and communities
B1.28 the definition of an antigen and an antibody
B1.29 the link between antigens and the initiation of the body's response to invasion by a foreign substance
B1.30 the stages and cells involved in the body's response to an antigen
B1.31 the differences between cell-mediated immunity and antibody-mediated immunity
B1.32 the role of T and B memory cells in the secondary immune response.

Cells and tissues

We can study and understand biology at different levels of organisation. Starting with the whole **organism**, we can move upwards to study the ways in which organisms interact in populations and ecosystems. Alternatively, we can look at the way in which organisms work in increasing levels of detail. The cell is the basic unit of all organisms. We need to learn the structure and organisation of the cell to get a proper understanding of how cells work together and also understand the environment in which the chemical reactions of the cell take place.

Key terms

Organism: an individual plant, animal or single-celled lifeform.

Membrane: all membranes consist of a **phospholipid** bilayer together with proteins and other components. They are selectively permeable (meaning they let some things through and not others) and can control movement of substances across the membrane as well as being the sites of many important processes in the cell.

Phospholipid: a large molecule formed from a glycerol molecule covalently bound to two fatty acid molecules and a phosphate group. It has a hydrophilic (can interact with water) head group (because of the phosphate) and a hydrophobic (repels water) tail (because of the fatty acids).

Cytoplasm: the fluid component of the cell, enclosed by the cell membrane and surrounding the organelles.

Organelles: specialised structures within plant and animal cells that have specific functions. Some types of organelle are also found within bacterial cells.

B1.1 The 3 principles of cell theory

Robert Hooke (1635–1703) was the first person to recognise cells, although the 'cells' in cork that he saw using his microscope were the empty spaces between the cell walls of the cork. Hooke laid the foundations for what we now know as the three principles of cell theory. This states that:

▶ All living things are made up of one or more cells. This means that living things can be **unicellular** (single cells) or **multicellular** (made up of more than one cell).
▶ Cells are the most basic unit of structure and function in all living things. Cells contain many components (nuclei, mitochondria, etc.) but these cannot exist or reproduce on their own.
▶ All cells are created by pre-existing cells, i.e. cells cannot just appear from nowhere. New cells are created from pre-existing cells in the process of **mitosis** (cell division).

B1.2 The different types of cells that make up living organisms

There are two types of cell: **prokaryotic** cells and **eukaryotic** cells. Eukaryotic cells are complex and include all animal and plant cells as well as yeasts, other fungi and algae. Prokaryotic cells are simpler and smaller and include the bacteria. Both types of cell have **membranes**, **cytoplasm** and DNA. However, eukaryotic cells have membrane-bound **organelles**, such as mitochondria or chloroplasts. Also, the DNA is contained within the nucleus. The DNA is bound to proteins known as histones and together they form a complex known as chromatin (see below). In prokaryotic cells, the DNA just floats freely in the cytoplasm, or is found as small circular molecules known as plasmids, and is not associated with proteins.

B1.3 The structure and function of the organelles found within eukaryotic cells

Plasma membrane

Also called the **cell surface membrane**, this is found around the outside of the cell and consists of a **phospholipid bilayer** together with proteins and other components. The **plasma membrane** controls entry and exit of substances into and out of the cell.

> ### Key terms
>
> *Phospholipid bilayer:* a double layer of phospholipids with the hydrophobic tails arranged towards the middle and the hydrophilic head groups on the outside. It forms the basis of all biological membranes.
>
> *Plasma membrane:* sometimes called the cell-surface membrane, it is the membrane that surrounds all types of cell; animal, plant and bacterial. Like all membranes, the plasma membrane consists of a phospholipid bilayer together with proteins and other components.

Nucleus (containing chromosomes)

The nucleus is the largest organelle and is surrounded by the **nuclear envelope**. This is a double membrane that has many gaps or **pores**.

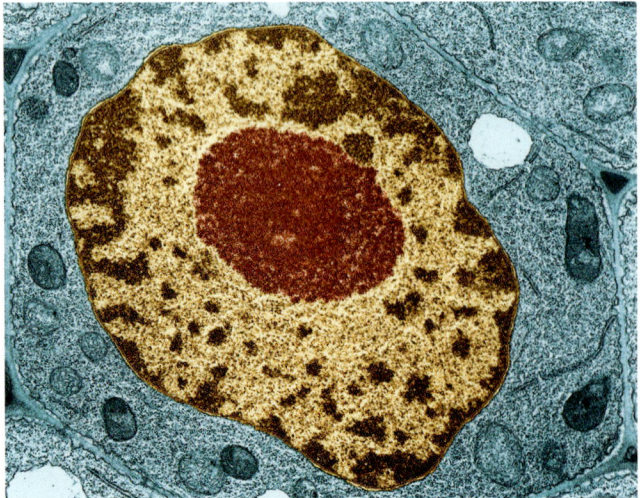

▲ Figure 11.1a An electron micrograph (x 25 000) showing a nucleus

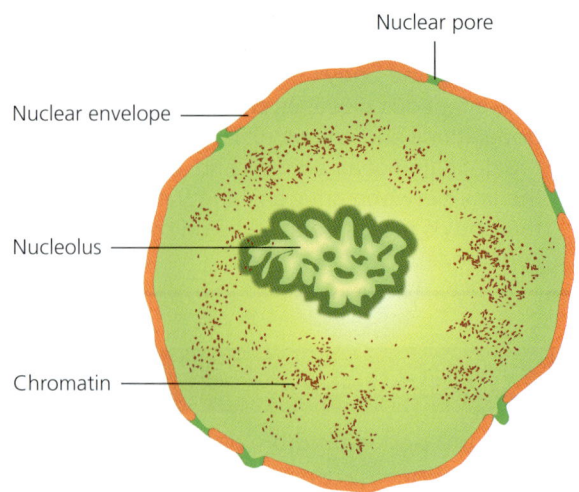

▲ Figure 11.1b A diagram showing the structure of the nucleus

The nucleus contains the genetic information, in the form of DNA. The DNA is combined with proteins known as histones; this forms the complex known as **chromatin**. The chromatin is coiled and super-coiled to form the chromosomes.

Mitochondria

Mitochondria (the singular is mitochondrion) are the site of **aerobic respiration** and therefore the site of adenosine triphosphate (ATP) production. Aerobic respiration is the process where glucose is reacted with oxygen to produce carbon dioxide and water. As this reaction is exothermic, the energy transferred from this reaction is used to produce ATP, the 'energy currency' of the cell. Almost all processes in the cell that require energy obtain it from ATP.

Like nuclei and chloroplasts, mitochondria are enclosed by a double membrane (envelope). The inner membrane is folded into structures called **cristae**.

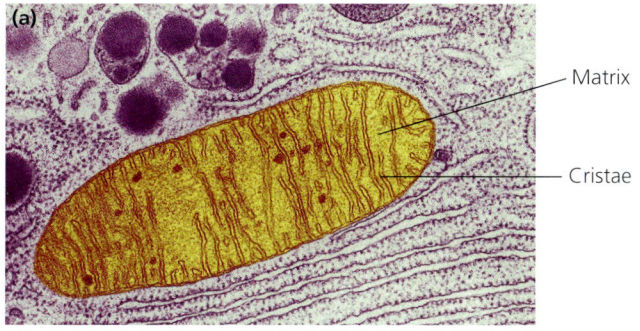

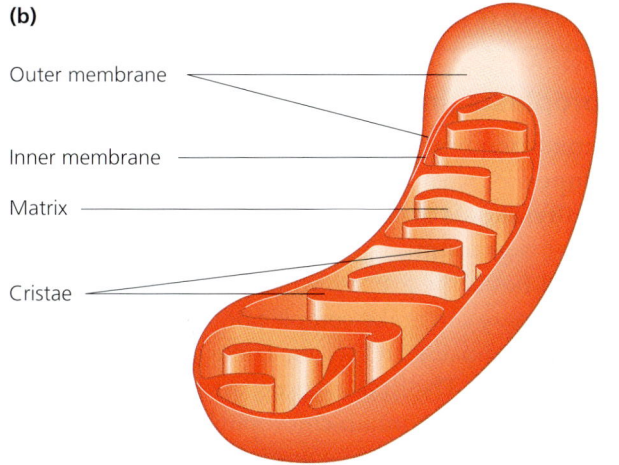

▲ Figure 11.2 A mitochondrion: (a) an electron micrograph (× 1100) and (b) a diagram

Ribosomes

Ribosomes are the smallest of the organelles and are the site of protein synthesis. Some float free in the cytoplasm and make the proteins needed within the cell, whereas others are attached to the rough endoplasmic reticulum. Ribosomes use the information coded in an mRNA molecule to assemble the correct order of amino acids in the protein.

Rough and smooth endoplasmic reticulum

The **endoplasmic reticulum (ER)** is a system of membrane-bound flattened sacs that fills a large part of the cytoplasm. The **rough ER (RER)** has ribosomes attached to its outer surface. Proteins that will be released from the cell or incorporated into the plasma membrane are made on these attached ribosomes and then folded and transported in the RER to the Golgi apparatus.

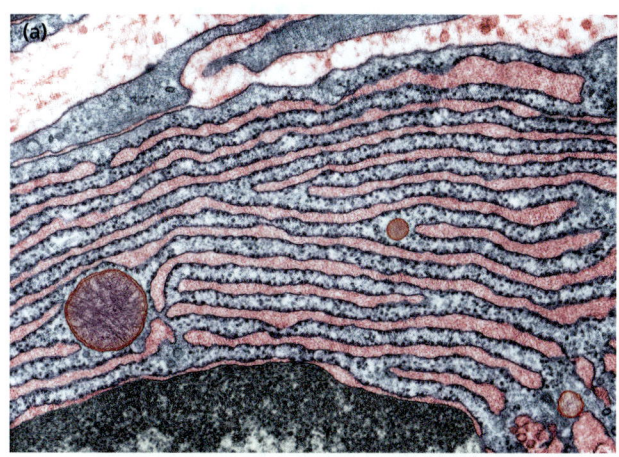

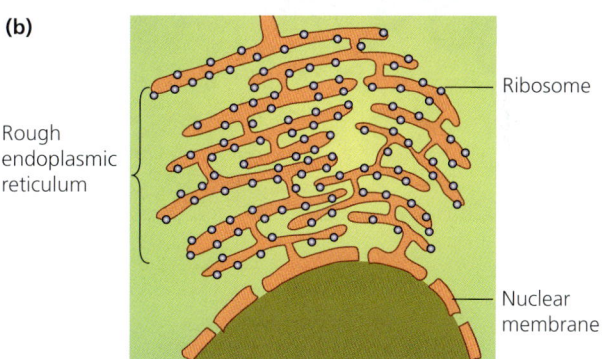

▲ Figure 11.3 Rough endoplasmic reticulum: (a) an electron micrograph (× 18 000) and (b) a diagram

The **smooth ER** does not have attached ribosomes and is responsible for synthesising, storing and transporting lipids and some carbohydrates.

Golgi apparatus and Golgi vesicles

The Golgi apparatus is a stack of flattened sacs, known as cisternae (singular is cisterna). Each cisterna is surrounded by a single membrane and filled with fluid. The Golgi modifies proteins that have been transported from the RER, for example by adding carbohydrates to them. These modified proteins are then transported by **Golgi vesicles** that form when the ends of the cisternae are pinched off. These vesicles can form **lysosomes** (see below). Others, called **secretory vesicles**, carry their contents to the plasma membrane where they can be released to the outside of the cell.

Healthcare Science T Level: Core

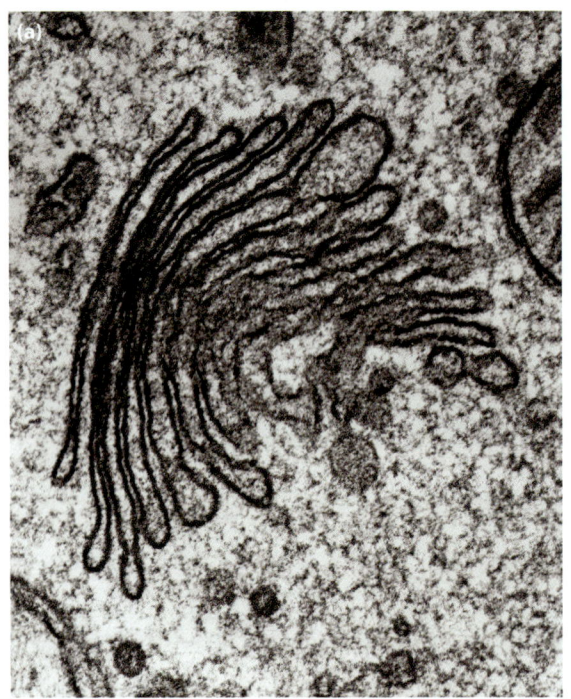

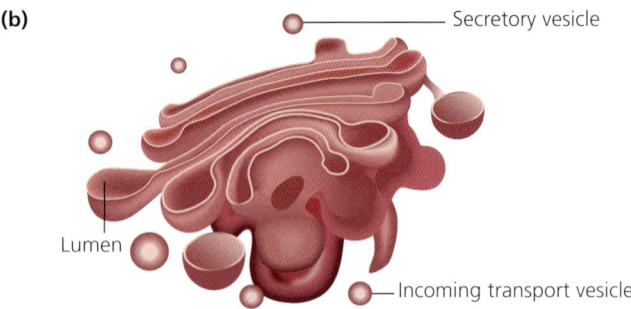

▲ Figure 11.4 The Golgi apparatus: (a) an electron micrograph (x 50 000) and (b) a diagram showing the Golgi vesicles and secretory vesicles

Lysosomes

These are the cell's recycling facility. When proteins and other cell components get worn out, they are moved into lysosomes. Digestive enzymes break these down into their constituents, e.g. amino acids that can be re-used to make new proteins. It is important that these enzymes are kept separate from the rest of the cytoplasm because of the damage they could do. Lysosomes are also involved in digestion of invading **pathogens** (bacteria and viruses) that are taken into the cell by the process of **phagocytosis** (see page 237 later in this chapter).

Centrioles

Centrioles are structures made of a tubular protein called tubulin. They are involved in the formation of the spindle in **mitosis** as well as formation of **cilia** and **flagella**. They are not present in many types of plant cells.

> ### Key terms
>
> **Pathogen:** a micro-organism that causes illness or disease by damaging host tissues and/or by producing toxins.
>
> **Cilia:** (singular **cilium**) are hair-like structures found on the plasma membrane of some types of cell, particularly in the lungs.
>
> **Flagella:** (singular **flagellum**) are similar in structure to cilia but are much longer and are involved in propulsion of the cell.

Chloroplasts (in plants)

Like mitochondria, chloroplasts are enclosed by an **envelope** (double membrane) and contain membranes called **thylakoids** arranged in stacks called **grana** (singular is **granum**). The chloroplast is the site of photosynthesis, the process whereby plants and algae use light energy to make complex organic molecules from carbon dioxide and water. There are two stages to photosynthesis. The first stage occurs in the thylakoid membranes which contain chlorophyll and other pigments that absorb light energy as well as proteins involved in the production of ATP. The rest of the chloroplast consists of a fluid called the **stroma**, which is where the second stage of photosynthesis take place.

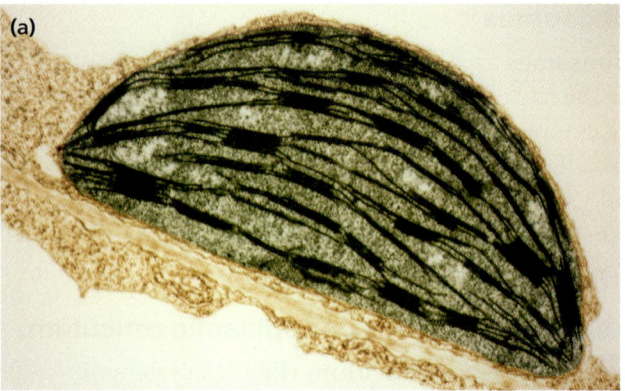

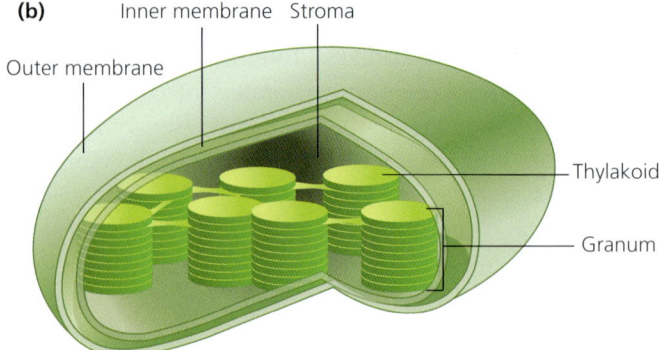

▲ Figure 11.5 A chloroplast: (a) an electron micrograph (x 13 750) and (b) a diagram

Cell wall (in plants)

Plant cell walls consist mainly of the carbohydrate **cellulose**. Cell walls provide strength and rigidity for protection and support. If animal cells take up too much water they burst, whereas in plants the cell wall prevents this.

Cell vacuole (in plants)

Cell vacuoles are fluid-filled sacs surrounded by a single membrane. Their size varies; in some cells the vacuole almost fills the cell. The fluid is a dilute solution of molecules and ions. The vacuole can be used to store mineral salts, amino acids, sugars and waste products. Vacuoles are also involved in maintaining the water balance of the cell.

B1.4 The similarities and differences between plant and animal cells in relation to the presence of specific organelles and their function

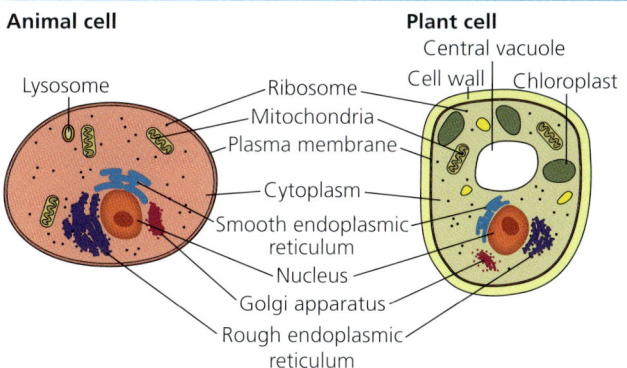

▲ Figure 11.6 Components of plant and animal cells

If you compare the animal and plant cells shown in Figure 11.6 you will see that there are many similarities. In fact, the main difference between the two types is that plant cells have structures such as the cell wall, chloroplasts and vacuoles that are not found in animal cells.

The cell wall provides support to plant cells and helps to keep them rigid. This also means that they have similar shapes. There are some types of highly specialised plant cells, but there is a much greater variety of types of animal cells. Animal cells also have a larger variety of shapes as they do not have a cell wall to keep them rigid and hence the need for skeletons in larger organisms.

B1.5 How eukaryotic cells become specialised in complex multicellular organisms

In multicellular organisms, different cells are specialised to fulfil different functions. This is controlled by which genes are expressed (i.e. genes that are switched on and therefore have an effect). Every **somatic** cell (i.e. all cells excluding gametes) contains in its nucleus the whole **genome** (all the genes) of the organism. How the cell functions is determined by which of the many genes are expressed and which are not.

The process by which a cell changes from one cell type to another is known as **cell differentiation.** To understand this, consider how a **zygote** (fertilised egg cell) develops into an embryo and how one single cell gives rise to not just many cells, but many different types of cell.

Stem cells can differentiate to form specialised cells. The human embryo contains stem cells that can give rise to the more than 200 cell types of the adult human body. By the time a baby is born, most cells have already differentiated. This is why the term 'adult cells' applies to cells in babies and children as well as in adults. However, adult stem cells persist and are responsible for cell turnover, e.g. production of red blood cells from bone marrow cells (see Figure 11.7). These bone marrow cells also differentiate to form the various types of lymphocytes involved in the immune response (see section B1.30). Most epithelial cells (see section B1.12) need to be replaced throughout the life of an organism. Examples include cells in the skin, lungs, cornea and intestine. In each case, stem cells are responsible for replacement of worn-out cells.

> **Key term**
>
> **Stem cells:** undifferentiated (non-specialised) cells that can give rise to one or more types of differentiated (specialised) cell.

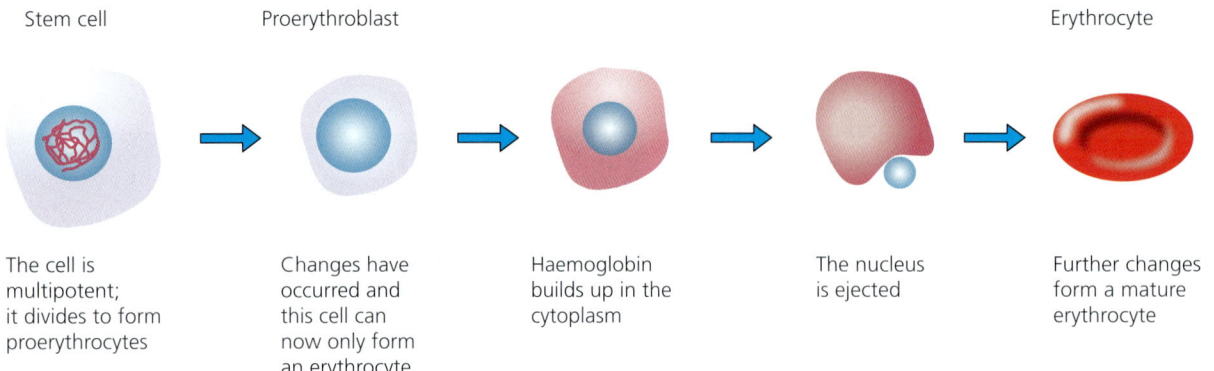

▲ Figure 11.7 Differentiation of red blood cells (erythrocytes)

B1.6 How prokaryotic cells differ from eukaryotic cells

You need to be able to distinguish between prokaryotic and eukaryotic cells based on drawings. Differences can also be identified on electron micrographs.

Figure 11.8 shows a diagram of a typical prokaryotic cell. The table summarises the differences between prokaryotic and eukaryotic cells.

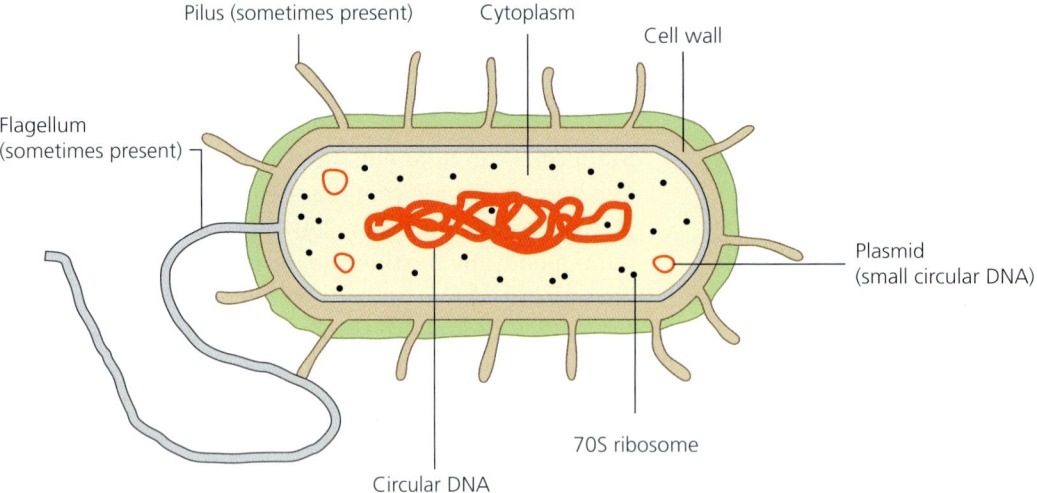

▲ Figure 11.8 A typical prokaryotic cell: some features are not present in all prokaryotic cells

Prokaryotic cells	Eukaryotic cells
They have cytoplasm that lacks membrane-bound organelles.	They have cytoplasm containing membrane-bound organelles.
They have smaller ribosomes.	They have larger ribosomes.
They have no nucleus; instead, they have a single circular DNA molecule that is free in the cytoplasm and is not associated with proteins.	Chromosomes are linear and contained within the nucleus. The DNA is associated with proteins called histones.
They have a cell wall that contains murein/peptidoglycan, a glycoprotein.	Plant cells have a cellulose cell wall while fungi have a cell wall made of chitin.
They may have one or more plasmids.	There are no plasmids.
They may have a capsule surrounding the cell.	There is no capsule, even in plant cells. Some fungal cells can form a carbohydrate capsule.
They may have one or more simple flagella.	Flagella, where present, are more complex.

> **B1.1–B1.32:** Core science concepts: Biology

> **Test yourself**
>
> 1. What are the three principles of cell theory?
> 2. State two differences between prokaryotic and eukaryotic cells.
> 3. State two differences between plant and animal cells.

> **Key terms**
>
> **Peptide:** a compound containing two or more amino acids joined together by **peptide bonds**. A **dipeptide** contains two amino acids bonded together.
>
> **Amino acid:** a molecule with both an amino group and a carboxyl group. Amino acids are the small molecules (monomers) from which all **proteins** are made. There are 20 naturally occurring amino acids found in proteins and all have the amino and carboxyl groups attached to the same carbon. This carbon also has a hydrogen and another substituent – the side chain, or R-group – which is different in each different amino acid; see Figure 11.9. Amino acids are the monomers from which all proteins are made.
>
> **Protein:** a **polypeptide** with a recognisable three-dimensional structure. It may contain more than one polypeptide chain.
>
> **Condensation reaction:** a reaction between two small molecules to produce a larger molecule and water; most large biological molecules are formed by condensation reactions.
>
> **Polypeptide:** a **polymer** of amino acids joined together by peptide bonds.
>
> **Polymer:** a long molecule made from many small molecules called **monomers**.

Proteins, carbohydrates and lipids

Proteins, carbohydrates and lipids are three of the main classes of large biological molecules. We will encounter the fourth class in section B1.14 (page 226).

B1.7 The relationship between the structure, properties and functions of proteins

Dipeptides are formed by joining two **amino acids** in a **condensation reaction** (Figure 11.10). **Polypeptides** are formed by the condensation of many amino acids, joined by **peptide bonds**.

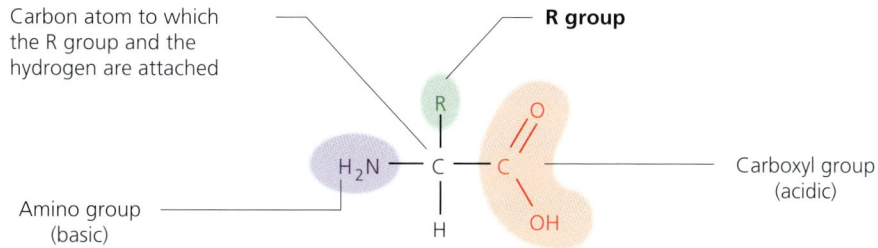

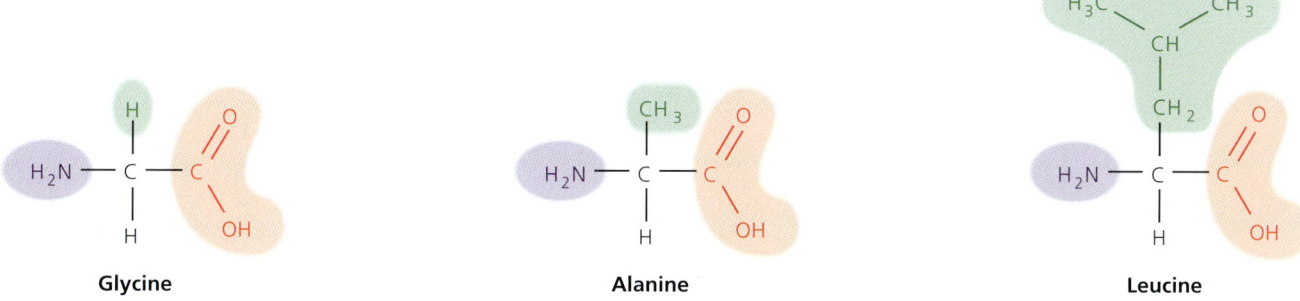

▲ Figure 11.9 The basic structure of an amino acid and three examples of different amino acids

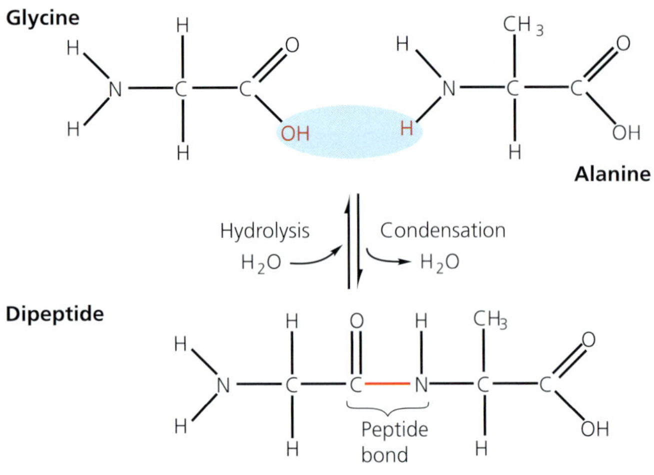

▲ Figure 11.10 The formation of a peptide bond between two amino acids in a condensation reaction produces a dipeptide; the reverse reaction is a hydrolysis

Functional proteins, such as fibrous proteins or globular proteins, contain one or more polypeptide chains. The sequence of amino acids is different in each different protein. It is the amino acid sequence which will determine how the polypeptide chain folds up. This, in turn, determines the 3D shape of the protein.

B1.8 The relationship between the structure, properties and functions of carbohydrates

Carbohydrates are important energy sources, for example, sucrose ('sugar', refined from sugar cane), lactose (found in milk) or maltose (used as an energy source for yeast in the brewing industry). Polysaccharides are polymers formed by condensation reactions of many monosaccharide molecules (monomers). As they are such large molecules, they are usually insoluble. This makes them suitable to carry out storage functions (glycogen and starch) and support functions (cellulose).

Type of carbohydrate	Examples	Notes
Monosaccharides	Glucose 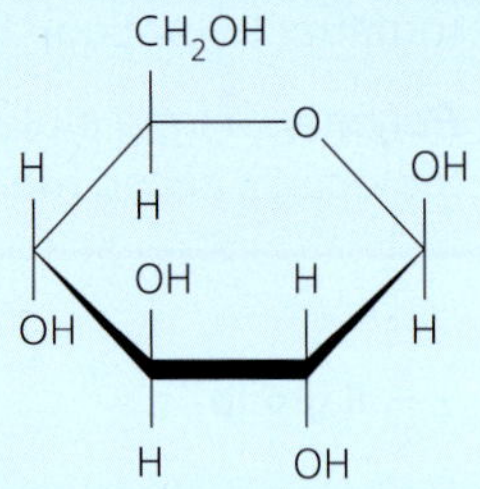	Monosaccharides contain just one sugar molecule and include glucose, fructose and galactose.
Disaccharides	Maltose 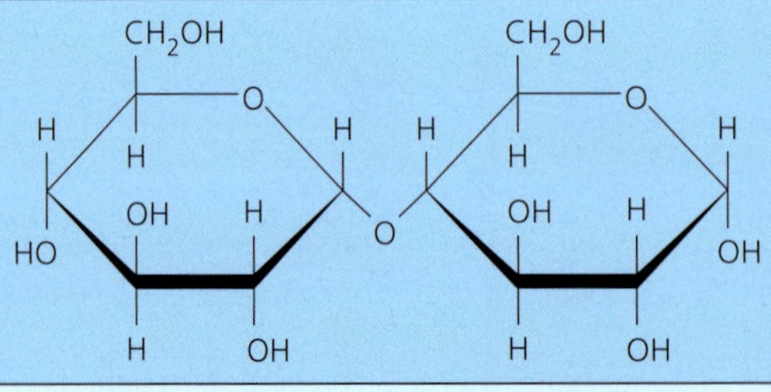	Disaccharides are formed by condensation reactions between two monosaccharides – the bond formed is known as a glycosidic bond. Common disaccharides include maltose (containing two glucose molecules), sucrose (containing glucose and fructose) and lactose (containing glucose and galactose).
Polysaccharides	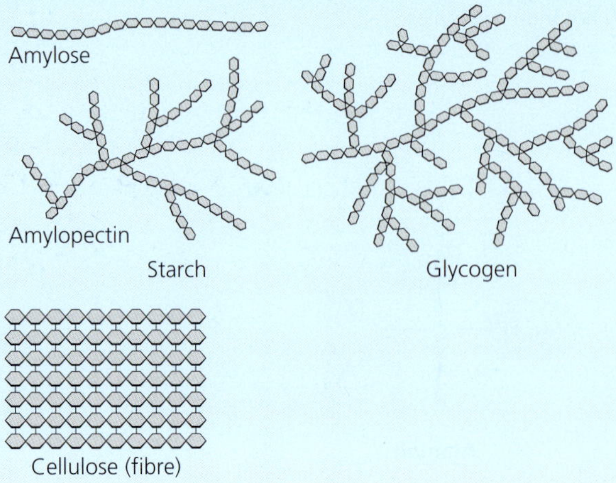 Amylose, Amylopectin, Starch, Glycogen, Cellulose (fibre)	Polysaccharides are polymers of monosaccharide monomers. The most common are starch (straight chain amylose or branched chain amylopectin), glycogen and cellulose, all of which are polymers of glucose.

> **Test yourself**
>
> 1. What are the monomers in:
>   a proteins
>   b polysaccharides?
> 2. Name the type of reaction in which polypeptides or polysaccharides are formed.
> 3. What property of polysaccharides makes them good for storage and support?

> **Key term**
>
> **Diffusion:** is the movement of a substance from a high concentration to a low concentration. For instance, if you drop a crystal of copper sulfate into a beaker of water and watch the blue colour spread then you can see diffusion occur.

Single-celled organism (*Paramecium caudatum*)
Maximum distance for diffusion = 50 μm
Time taken = 8 seconds

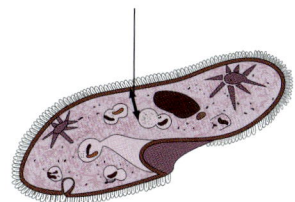

Maximum distance for diffusion = 15 cm
Time taken = 7 hours

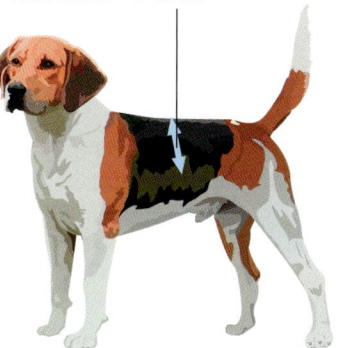

▲ Figure 11.11 The problem of increasing size on the rate of diffusion

B1.9 The relationship between the structure, properties and functions of lipids

Lipids are the only group of large biological molecules that are not polymers. They all contain carbon, hydrogen and oxygen and are usually insoluble in water. More complex lipids can also contain phosphorous and nitrogen.

Lipids consist of two or three fatty acids, which are joined to a molecule of glycerol in condensation reactions. The fatty acids have long hydrocarbon chains, which explains why lipids are generally insoluble.

The main groups of lipids are:
- **triglycerides** (for example, fats and oils). These are used mostly as energy stores as well as for insulation (under the skin) and protection (around delicate organs such as the kidneys)
- **phospholipids**. These are found in plasma membranes and provide flexibility and help control what can move into and out of cells.

The role of phospholipids in membranes was covered in section B1.2.

Exchange and transport mechanisms

All organisms exchange substances with their surroundings. Single-cell organisms that respire aerobically need to absorb oxygen and get rid of carbon dioxide. They also need to absorb nutrients and get rid of waste products. This happens by the process of simple **diffusion**.

Large multicellular organisms cannot rely on simple diffusion. The distances are too great and it would take too long, as illustrated in Figure 11.11.

B1.10 How the surface area to volume ratio affects the process of exchange and gives rise to specialised systems

Efficient exchange (of gases, nutrients or waste products) requires three things:
- a large surface area for exchange
- a short diffusion distance
- a high concentration gradient.

The dog in Figure 11.11 has a much longer diffusion distance than the *Paramecium*, although it does have a much larger surface area. However, for efficient exchange the surface area must be large in comparison to the volume. We describe this as having a large surface area to volume ratio. This is illustrated in Figure 11.12. To make it simpler we have used a cube, but the principle is the same for animals with more complex shapes.

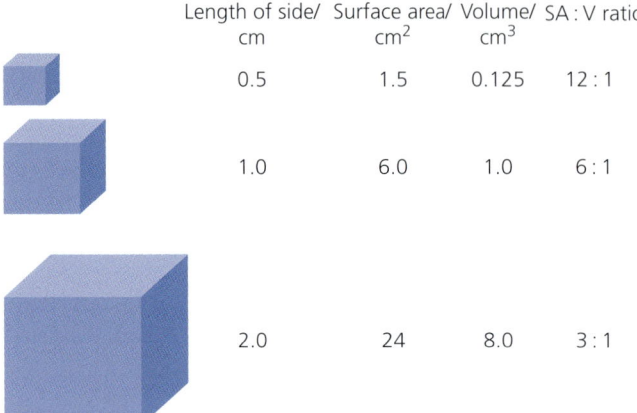

▲ Figure 11.12 Decrease of surface area: volume ratio in cubes of increasing size

Where the surface area is small compared to the volume (i.e. a low surface area to volume ratio), organisms cannot rely on simple diffusion across the whole body area like in *Paramecium*. Specialised exchange and transport mechanisms are required to maximise the rate of diffusion, such as lungs or gills and the heart and circulatory system.

Gills and lungs are adapted to make the diffusion distance as short as possible; between the air or water and the blood. For example, the walls of the alveoli in the lungs are only a single cell thick. There are also mechanisms, such as breathing, that maintain a high concentration gradient. Breathing brings air into the lungs that has a higher concentration of oxygen than within the blood. This ensures that oxygen diffuses into the blood.

Reflect

Temperature and the rate of the chemical reactions needed to support life (**metabolic rate**) also play a part. The heart rate of a mouse is about 500–600 beats per minute, whereas an elephant's heart rate is about 25–30 beats per minute. Why is this?

Think about the following:
▶ Heat loss also depends on surface area to volume ratio.
▶ Mammals, such as mice and elephants, generate body heat from respiration.

More active animals have a higher metabolic rate and therefore require more substances such as glucose for aerobic respiration. This increases their need for specialised exchange and transport mechanisms. In terms of heat loss, the mouse has a larger surface area to volume ratio and therefore has an increased rate of heat loss. Because of this, they need to generate more heat from respiration, increasing their need for glucose and oxygen within their cells, explaining their higher heart rate.

B1.11 The principles of cellular exchange and the transport mechanisms which exist to facilitate this exchange

The lipid component of cell membranes consists of a double layer known as the phospholipid bilayer. As discussed in section B1.2, phospholipids consist of a **hydrophilic** head group and a **hydrophobic** tail. This is shown in Figure 11.13 and is a very stable structure. Either side of the membrane is in an aqueous medium (meaning the main solvent is water). This means the tails arrange themselves on the centre, due to being hydrophobic. As a result, the hydrophilic heads arrange themselves on the outside, creating the phospholipid bilayer.

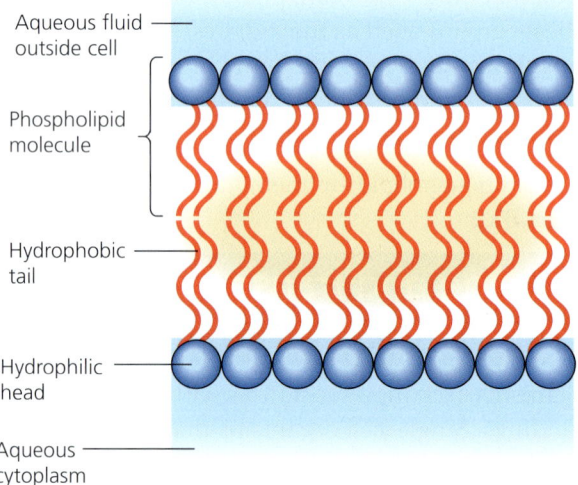

▲ Figure 11.13 Structure of the phospholipid bilayer

The phospholipid bilayer acts as a barrier to diffusion of many substances and only allows small, non-polar molecules through. Polar substances (see section B1.42, page 253) such as water, glucose, amino acids or inorganic ions (e.g. Na^+, K^+ or Cl^-) cannot diffuse through the hydrophobic core of the bilayer.

This means that they require specialised transport systems involving proteins and glycoproteins (proteins with sugar molecules attached) embedded in the phospholipid bilayer. We can see an example of an adaptation to increase the efficiency of exchange if we look at the small intestine. The intestine is effectively a tube, and the central space (where digestion occurs) is called the lumen. The epithelial cells that line the small intestine are specialised cells; the plasma membrane facing the lumen is folded into many tiny finger-like projections called microvilli. This greatly increases the surface area for absorption of the products of digestion. Figure 11.14 illustrates the **fluid mosaic model** of the plasma membrane.

> **Key term**
>
> *Fluid mosaic model:* describes the structure of the plasma membrane and how its components are arranged. The proteins, lipids and carbohydrates that are found in the plasma membrane vary in shape, size and location which creates the mosaic pattern. Due to the relatively weak forces between phospholipids, the membrane can be considered to be fluid as these components can move throughout the membrane.

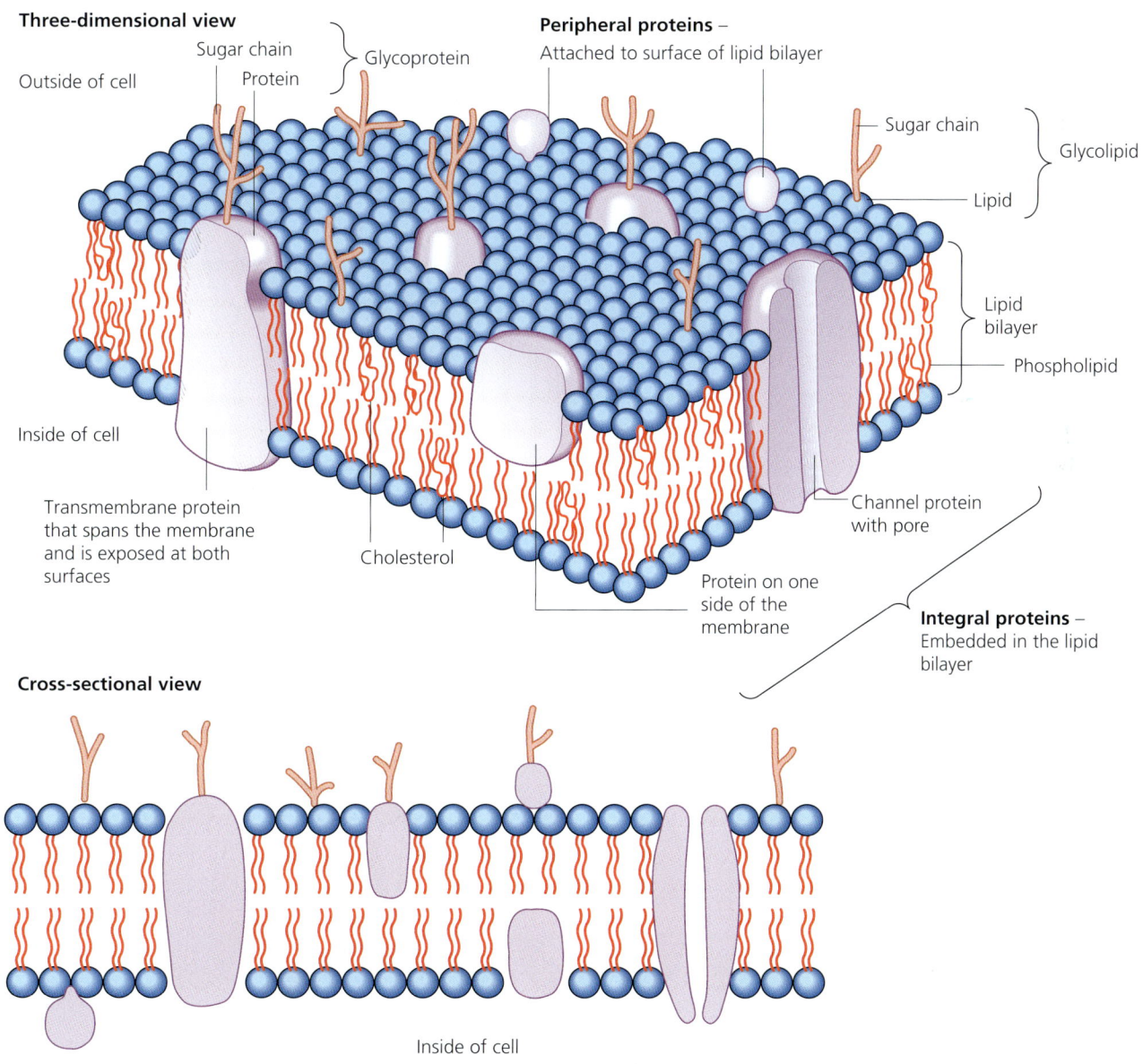

▲ Figure 11.14 The fluid mosaic model of the eukaryotic plasma membrane

Mechanisms: passive, active and co-transport

Simple diffusion, facilitated diffusion and osmosis are all passive processes, meaning that they do not require energy. Therefore, movement is always from high concentration to low concentration, sometimes described as down a diffusion gradient.

Simple diffusion

The phospholipid bilayer with its hydrophobic core can be a barrier to diffusion of polar substances; we say that it is *partially permeable*. So, small, non-polar molecules (e.g. carbon dioxide, oxygen, steroid hormones, lipids or fat-soluble vitamins) can move into the phospholipid bilayer and diffuse across the membrane.

Facilitated diffusion

Polar molecules, such as water, glucose and ions such as Na^+ or Cl^- cannot diffuse across the membrane, so they rely on **facilitated diffusion**. This is where diffusion is assisted by proteins in the membrane. Ions and small polar molecules (including water) are transported by **channel proteins** (Figure 11.15) that act like pores in the membrane. Some of these can open and close, and these are called **gated channels**. Ion channels are usually specific for particular ions such as Na^+ or Ca^{2+}.

Larger polar molecules, such as glucose or amino acids, use **carrier proteins** (Figure 11.16). They are specific to the substance being transported which binds to the carrier protein in a similar way to a substrate binding to an enzyme (see section B2.5, page 301). The carrier protein then changes shape, which transfers the substance to the other side of the membrane.

The rules of diffusion still apply to both channel proteins and carrier proteins. Substances move only from a high concentration to low concentration.

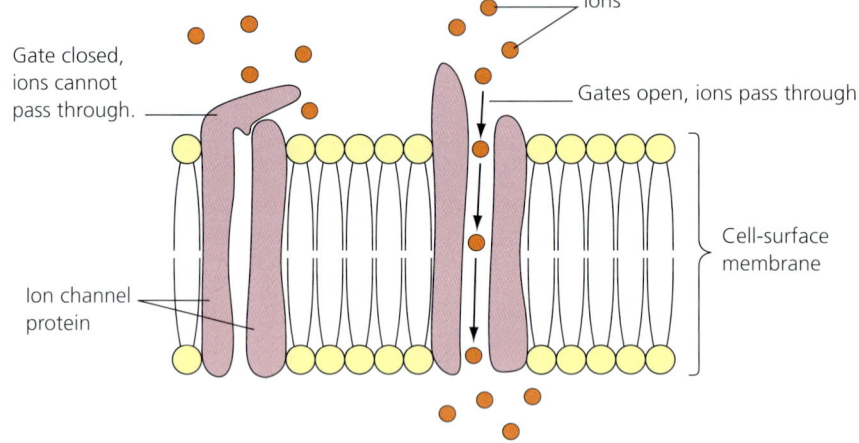

Channel proteins help the diffusion of ions. Some ion channels have gates that open and close.

▲ Figure 11.15 Facilitated diffusion through a channel protein. The ones shown here are gated (they can open and close) while others are open all the time

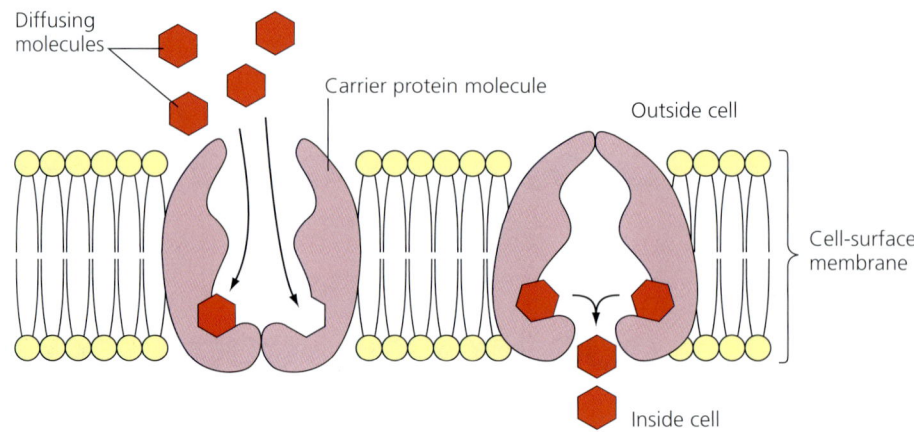

Diffusing molecules bind to a carrier protein. The protein changes shape and takes the molecules through the membrane.

▲ Figure 11.16 Facilitated diffusion by a carrier protein

Osmosis

This is a particular type of facilitated diffusion where water moves across a partially permeable membrane from a high concentration of water molecules to a low concentration of water molecules. Do not be confused by this – a dilute solution (or pure water) will have a high concentration of water molecules, whereas a concentrated solution (e.g. a high concentration of glucose) will have a low concentration of water molecules. Therefore, water moves by osmosis from pure water or a dilute solution to a more concentrated solution.

Active transport

Substances do not move by themselves from low to high concentration (i.e. up a concentration gradient). However, **active transport** is a process that uses energy to move substances against a concentration gradient. This involves carrier proteins that use ATP as a source of energy. The mechanism is like that shown in Figure 11.16 with the addition of ATP as an energy source. These types of active transport proteins are often called pumps.

Co-transport mechanisms

The absorption of glucose from the gut is an example of a co-transport mechanism. Epithelial cells lining the small intestine have carrier proteins that only transport a glucose molecule together with a sodium ion. A sodium ion pump in the plasma membrane pumps sodium ions out of the epithelial cells into the blood capillaries which lowers the concentration of sodium ions inside the epithelial cells. This creates a sodium ion concentration gradient from the inside of the small intestine into the epithelial cells. It is this concentration gradient that causes sodium ions to diffuse into epithelial cells via a co-transport protein which brings with them glucose molecules. This helps ensure all the glucose is absorbed from the small intestine and is known as co-transport. Once inside the epithelial cell, the glucose diffuses down a concentration gradient into the blood. However, as glucose is a polar molecule, this requires a carrier protein too. The process is illustrated in Figure 11.17.

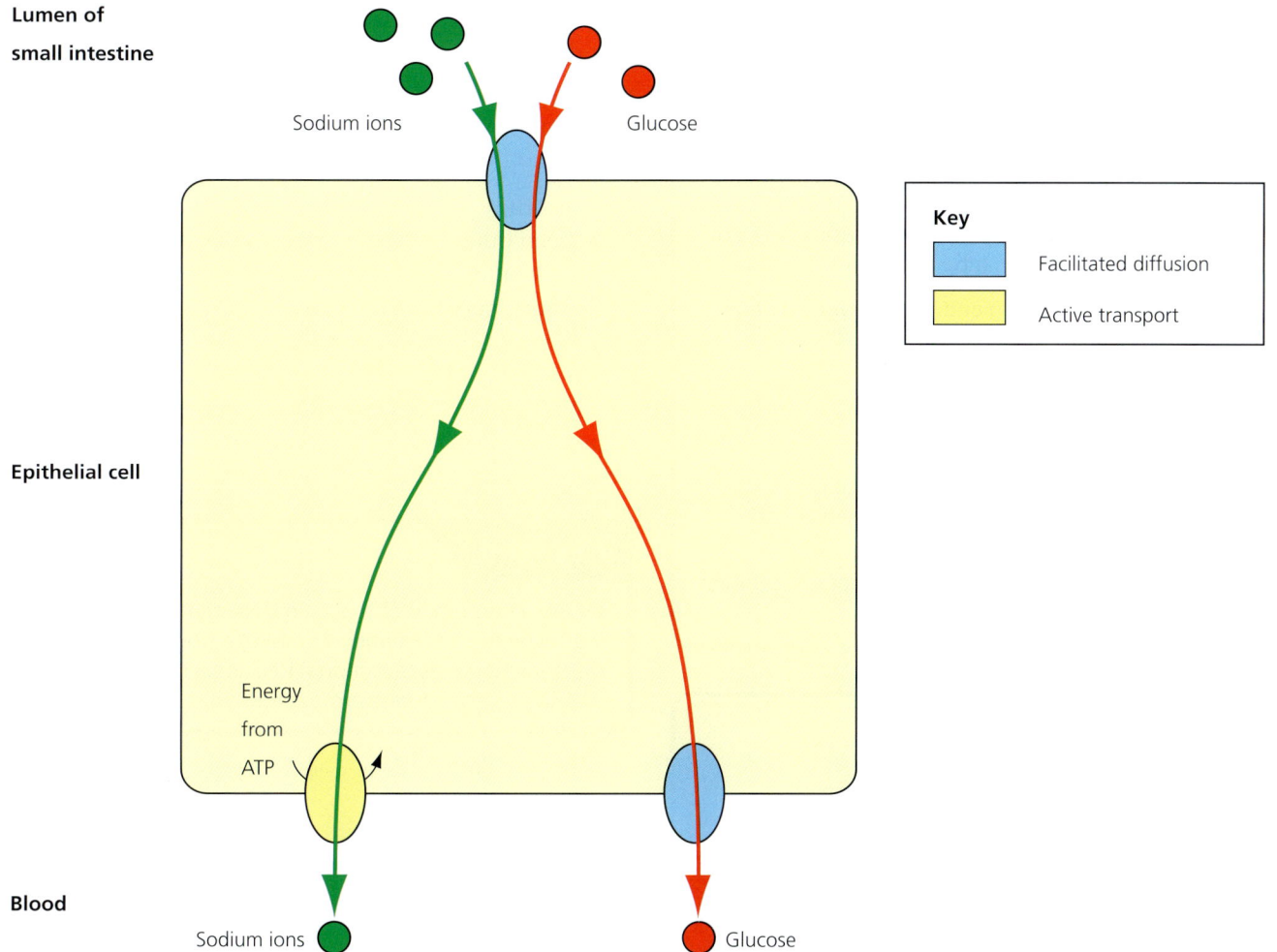

▲ Figure 11.17 Co-transport of glucose and sodium ions in the gut

B1.12 The advantages of having specialised cells in relation to the rate of transport across internal and external membranes

We saw in section B1.10 that multicellular organisms above a certain size can no longer rely on diffusion for exchange of substances with their environments. This usually means that specialised exchange organs have evolved, such as:

- gills or lungs for gas exchange
- the gut for absorption of nutrients
- kidneys for excretion of nitrogenous waste (urea).

Each of these organs have specialised cells adapted to maximise the efficiency of transfer of specific substances. Many of these cells are described as **epithelial** or **endothelial** and they are well adapted to their function.

> **Reflect**
>
> Epithelial and endothelial tissues are usually single layers of cells that line or coat organs. The easiest way to decide whether a particular cell or tissue is epithelial or endothelial is to consider if it is in contact with the outside world. Of course, the place where it interacts with the 'outside world' can be contained within the body – just think about the gut, which is really just a long tube from mouth to anus.
>
> Think about the following and decide whether they are examples of epithelial or endothelial:
> - skin cells
> - cells lining the mouth
> - cells lining the trachea and lungs
> - cells lining the gut
> - cells lining the kidney tubules and bladder
> - cells lining blood vessels (arteries, veins and capillaries).
>
> Hint: only one of these is an example of endothelial cells!

> **Research**
>
> Choose an organ from the following list and research ways in which specialised cells in that organ are adapted to maximise the rate of transport across membranes:
> - blood vessels
> - lungs
> - gut.

> **Test yourself**
>
> 1. Explain why large multicellular organisms require specialised exchange and transport mechanisms.
> 2. What are the three features of a good exchange surface?
> 3. Describe the fluid mosaic model of cell membranes.
> 4. Explain why polar molecules require special transport mechanisms to cross cell membranes.
> 5. State two differences between active transport and facilitated diffusion.

Genetics

Genetics is the study of inheritance. We resemble our parents, but do not look exactly like either of them. **Genes** are passed from parent to offspring and these interactions control the appearance of those offspring.

The laws of genetics were worked out in the nineteenth century by Gregor Mendel. However, the role of DNA as the genetic material was only established for certain in the middle of the twentieth century.

We can study genetics using Mendel's laws that have been built on by subsequent researchers. We can work out the rules and how to apply them, and in this way, genetics is a type of logic puzzle. More recent approaches involve trying to work out what is happening at the molecular level. That requires an understanding of DNA, RNA and the synthesis of proteins. This section will help you gain a good understanding of this modern approach to genetics.

> **Key term**
>
> *Gene:* a sequence of bases in DNA that codes for (contains the information to make) a polypeptide, or, in some cases, functional RNA (this is involved in regulating how genes are expressed).

B1.13 The purpose of DNA and RNA as the carrying molecules of genetic information and the role they play in the mechanism of inheritance

Our understanding of genetics is based on some key points. We now know:
- Genes consist of **DNA** (deoxyribonucleic acid) and so we can say that DNA holds the genetic information.
- Genes control production of proteins by transferring the genetic information from DNA via **RNA** (ribonucleic acid) to the ribosomes where proteins are synthesised.
- Proteins are what determine the characteristics of an organism.

To fully understand genetics, we need to understand:
- how DNA stores the genetic information
- how DNA is replicated to pass on that genetic information to future generations
- how DNA and RNA are involved in the production of proteins.

B1.14 The relationship between the structure of DNA and RNA and their role in the mechanism of inheritance

As with all biological molecules, there is a strong relationship between the structure of nucleic acids (DNA and RNA) and their function. Both molecules are polynucleotides – that is polymers of nucleotides – in the same way that a polypeptide is a polymer of amino acids.

Each nucleotide contains a **pentose** (5-carbon sugar), a nitrogen-containing **organic base** and a phosphate group.
- In RNA (ribonucleic acid) the pentose is ribose, in DNA (deoxyribonucleic acid) the pentose is deoxyribose.
- In RNA the organic bases are adenine (A), cytosine (C), guanine (G) or uracil (U), while in DNA the organic bases are adenine (A), cytosine (C), guanine (G) or thymine (T).

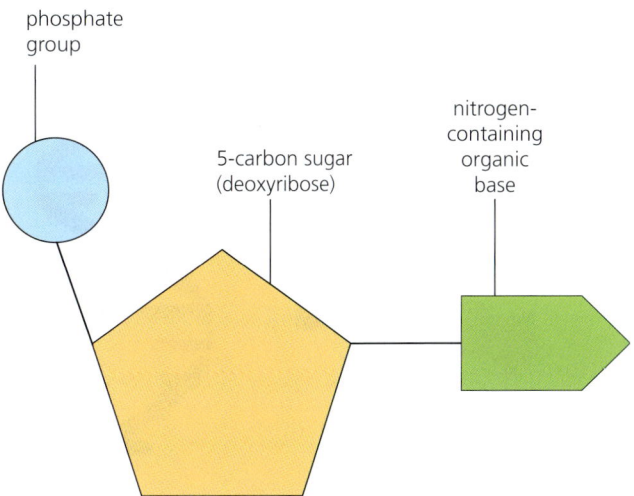

▲ Figure 11.18 General structure of a DNA nucleotide

The nucleotides are joined together in long chains by phosphodiester bonds between the pentose sugars; this is often described as a **sugar-phosphate** backbone. Phosphodiester bonds are formed in a condensation reaction like the one that forms peptide bonds (see Figure 11.10 in section B1.7).

The DNA molecule is a double helix where two very long polynucleotide chains are wound around each other and held together by hydrogen bonds between **complementary** base pairs: A pairs with T and C pairs with G. Complementary base pairing is central to how DNA stores and passes on genetic information, as well as to how genes control the synthesis of proteins.

RNA is a much shorter single-stranded polynucleotide chain.

The structure of DNA and RNA is shown in Figure 11.19.

The sequence of bases (sometimes called the **base sequence**) of DNA is how the genetic information is stored and passed on to future generations.

Healthcare Science T Level: Core

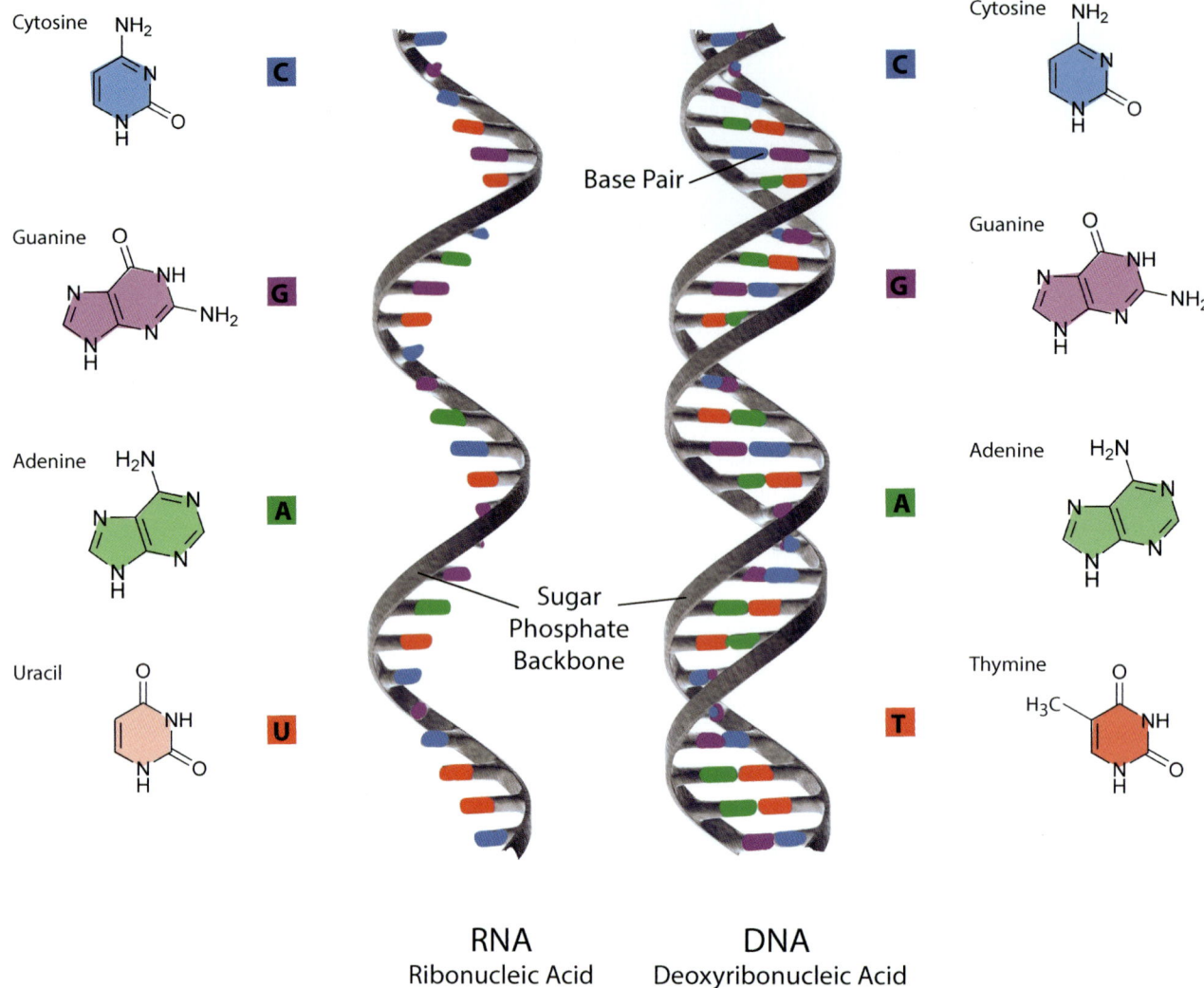

▲ Figure 11.19 The structure of DNA and RNA

B1.15 The function of complementary base pairing in forming the helical structure of DNA

Complementary base pairing holds the two strands of DNA together in the double helix structure. This makes the DNA molecule very stable, which is important for the molecule that contains and passes on the genetic information. Complementary base pairing is also the basis for how DNA is replicated.

B1.16 The process and stages of semi-conservative replication of DNA

The stages of DNA replication are as follows:
▶ The DNA double helix is progressively unwound. This involves an enzyme (**helicase**) that breaks the hydrogen bonds between the bases, allowing the strands to separate.
▶ Each strand now has unpaired bases.
▶ The strands each act as templates to assemble new strands. DNA nucleotides bind to the unpaired bases through complementary base-pairing.
▶ The enzyme **DNA polymerase** catalyses (speeds up) the formation of the phosphodiester bonds between the nucleotides.

This process is shown in Figure 11.20.

B1.1–B1.32: Core science concepts: Biology

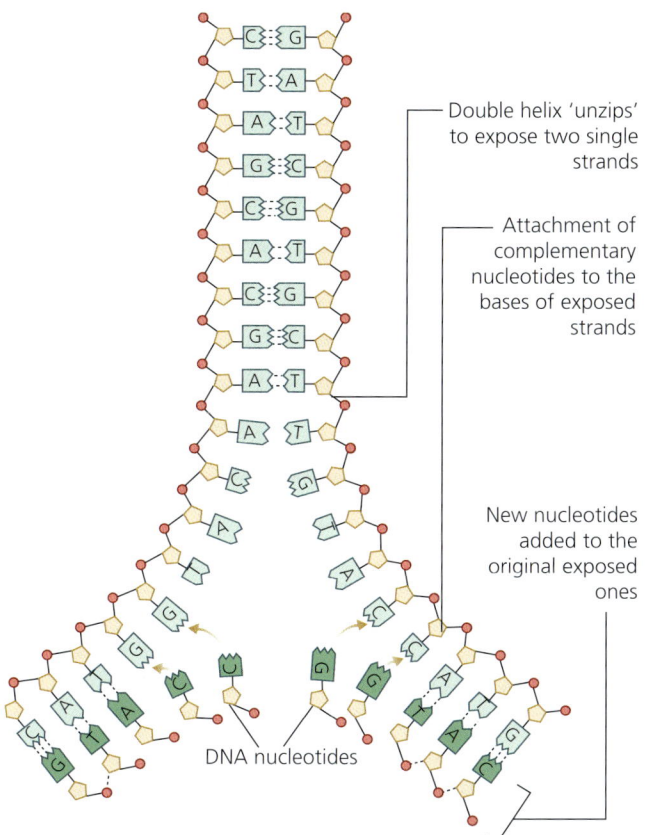

▲ Figure 11.20 Semi-conservative replication of DNA

> **Key terms**
>
> **Semi-conservative replication:** when DNA replicates two new double helix molecules are formed, but each one consists of one of the original strands and one newly synthesised strand.
>
> **Mutation:** a change in the sequence of bases in DNA. This can occur in a number of ways. When a mutation occurs within a coding region of DNA a new **allele** can be formed.
>
> **Allele:** a variant of a gene.
>
> **Genetics:** the study of how single genes, or a small group of genes, function and how they affect the appearance and functioning of the organism.
>
> **Genomics:** the study of how all the genes in an organism interact, as well as the role of non-coding sequences of DNA.
>
> **Genome:** the entire genetic material of an organism. This includes DNA that does not code for proteins as well as the coding DNA (genes).

B1.17 How this semi-conservative replication process ensures genetic continuity between generations of cells

The product of **semi-conservative replication** of DNA is two molecules of DNA, both identical to the original. This is how the genetic information, contained in the DNA, can be passed from one generation of cells to the next. Because the two new molecules are identical to each other and to the original, the new generation of cells will be identical to the previous generation.

B1.18 The link between the semi-conservative replication process and variation

We saw in section B1.17 how semi-conservative replication ensures genetic continuity between generations of cells. However, the process is not always 100 per cent accurate. Sometimes the 'wrong' base is inserted by DNA polymerase. This random event is one source of **mutation**. A mutation is a change in the sequence of bases in DNA, although this very rarely results in the formation of new **alleles**, partly because a lot of the DNA does not code for proteins. However, when a mutation occurs within the coding region of a gene, a new allele can sometimes be formed leading to the formation of a new characteristic. This is the source of genetic variation.

Genetic variation is the reason that we do not all look the same and is the basis of natural selection and evolution.

B1.19 The difference between genetics and genomics

We saw at the start of this section how the laws of **genetics** were worked out by a nineteenth-century monk working with pea plants. In contrast, **genomics** requires a great deal of technology to analyse and understand the **genomes**, particularly DNA sequencing and bioinformatics.

Both genetics and genomics are important in medicine. Genetics allows us to understand how inherited disorders like haemophilia, sickle cell anaemia or Huntingdon's disease are passed on.

This understanding helps us assess the risk of children inheriting such conditions from their parents. Genomics is being used to investigate the link between all the genes we carry and the development of a wide range of diseases and conditions, from obesity and diabetes to heart disease and cancer.

> **Practice point**
>
> The terms 'genetics' and 'genomics' are similar and easily confused. Use of precise language is essential in science, so it is a good idea to develop good practice at an early stage that will stand you in good stead throughout your career.

> **Test yourself**
>
> 1 What is a gene?
> 2 State two differences between DNA and RNA.
> 3 What is meant by 'complementary base pairing'?
> 4 Give the names of two enzymes involved in DNA replication.

Microbiology

B1.20 The classification and characteristics (size of cell, type of cell, presence of organelles) of the following micro-organisms

Micro-organisms are often thought of simply as pathogens. This may be because that is how we see them having the greatest impact on our lives. However, that is only part of the story.

> **Reflect**
>
> Think of all the ways in which micro-organisms are of benefit or even essential. You could include:
> ▶ foods and food production
> ▶ production of medicines, such as antibiotics
> ▶ agriculture
> ▶ production of chemicals and clean-up of chemical contamination.

> **Practice point**
>
> See sections B1.62 and B1.63 (pages 277 and 278) for more about SI units and conversion between units. These are two units that you will encounter when studying micro-organisms.
>
> **Micrometre** (μm) is the most commonly used measure of size when studying micro-organisms and is 10^{-6} m (one millionth of a metre) or 10^{-3} mm (one thousandth of a millimetre).
>
> **Nanometre** (nm) is 10^{-9} m (one billionth of a metre), 10^{-6} mm (one millionth of a millimetre) or 10^{-3} μm (one thousandth of a micrometre).

Bacteria

Bacteria are typically 1–2 μm (micrometres) long (i.e. about 1/1000 to 2/1000 of a millimetre) and usually roughly cylindrical, although other shapes, such as rods and spirals, do occur. They do not have membrane-bound organelles (see sections B1.3 and B1.6) and so are prokaryotes. See Figure 11.8 for a diagram of a typical bacterium.

Fungi

As well as the more familiar mushrooms and toadstools, many fungi are microscopic – the yeasts, including those used in fermentation to produce ethanol, are single cell organisms. Yeast cells are bigger than bacteria – in the range of 4–12 μm.

Fungi are eukaryotes, meaning they have chromosomes contained within a nucleus and other membrane-bound organelles. Multicellular fungi are composed of microscopic threads or hyphae that grow over or through their food source. Figure 11.21 shows a diagram of the mould fungus, *Penicillium chrysogenum* (the original source of the antibiotic penicillin.

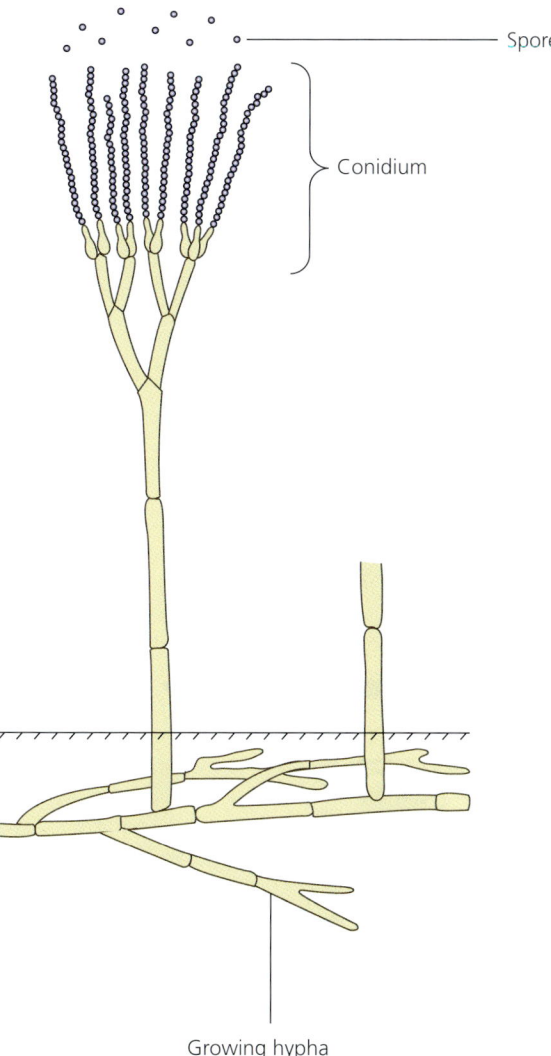

▲ Figure 11.21 Structure of the mould fungus, *Penicillium chrysogenum*

A honey fungus measuring 2.4 miles (3.8 km) across in the Blue Mountains in Oregon, USA is thought to be the largest living organism on Earth. That is certainly not microscopic! The structures that we recognise as mushrooms or toadstools are actually fruiting bodies, formed from very compact hyphae, that release spores.

Parasites

A parasite is an organism that lives on or in another organism at the expense of that organism. This includes multicellular organisms such as parasitic plants (e.g. mistletoe) and flatworms (e.g. tapeworms). Microscopic parasites are single-celled eukaryotic organisms such as *Plasmodium* (Figure 11.22), the parasite that causes malaria, or *Phytophthora infestans*, a parasite of plants that causes potato blight. Microscopic parasites can be different sizes, but usually in the range 1–10 μm.

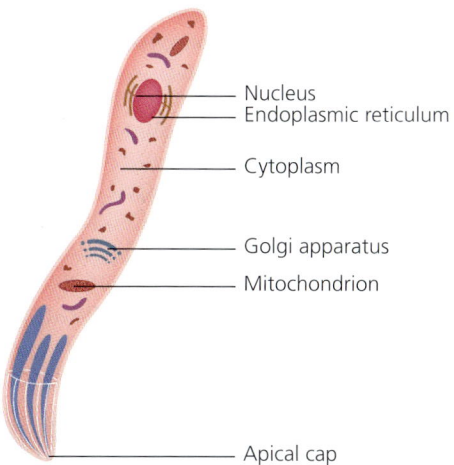

▲ Figure 11.22 Diagram of *Plasmodium*, a microscopic eukaryotic parasite

Viruses

As we saw in section B1.1, viruses are acellular (they are not made of cells) and do not contain organelles in the way that prokaryotes and eukaryotes do. They consist of genetic material (DNA or RNA) surrounded by a protein coat. Sometimes, the protein coat is itself surrounded by an envelope of lipid bilayer and glycoproteins that originated from the cell in which the virus replicated. Most viruses are very small – in the range 20–200 nm, although some giant viruses are as large as 1 μm – about the size of a bacterium and come in many shapes as well as sizes (Figure 11.23).

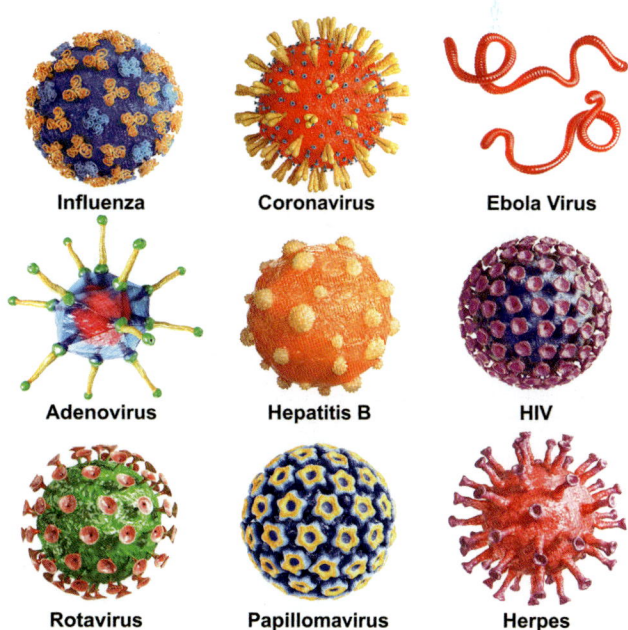

▲ Figure 11.23 A small selection of different virus structures

Healthcare Science T Level: Core

> **Reflect**
>
> Are viruses alive? It is a question that has been asked many times and there is no simple answer. What we *can* say is that viruses are **acellular** – they are not made up of cells – and need to infect other cells to reproduce. Think about whether the first principle of cell theory (section B1.1) means that viruses cannot be classed as living organisms. If we consider viruses as alive, is the first principle wrong? Nothing in biology is ever simple!

B1.21 The benefits of using light and electron microscopes when investigating micro-organisms

As the name suggests, micro-organisms cannot be seen with the naked eye. Therefore, we need to use some form of microscope to view and study them. The type of microscope used will depend on the size of the micro-organism we want to study – and, as some microscopes are more expensive, what we have access to.

> **Key terms**
>
> **Magnification:** how much bigger the image is than the actual object we are viewing. It should not be confused with **resolution**.
>
> **Resolution:** the ability of a microscope to distinguish between two adjacent points. The resolution of a microscope is the smallest distance between two points that can be seen as separate. A high-resolution microscope can show a clearer image.
>
> You have probably encountered resolution when using a camera phone. An old phone will probably have quite a low resolution. If you take a photo you may be able to enlarge the image to the same size as one taken with the latest high-resolution camera phone, but the modern phone will give a much clearer, sharper image.

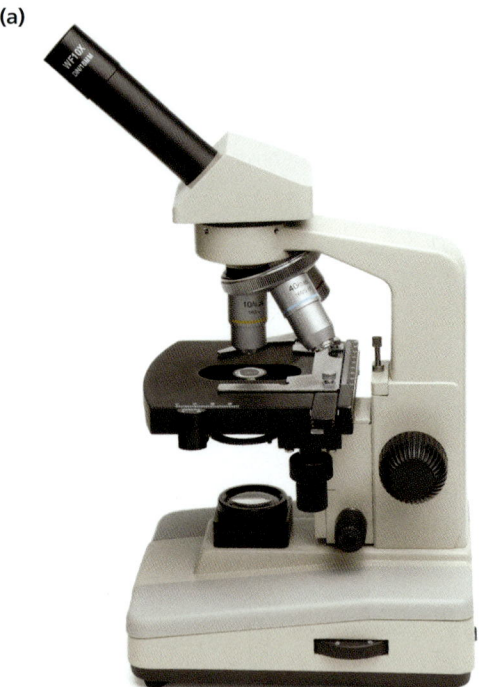

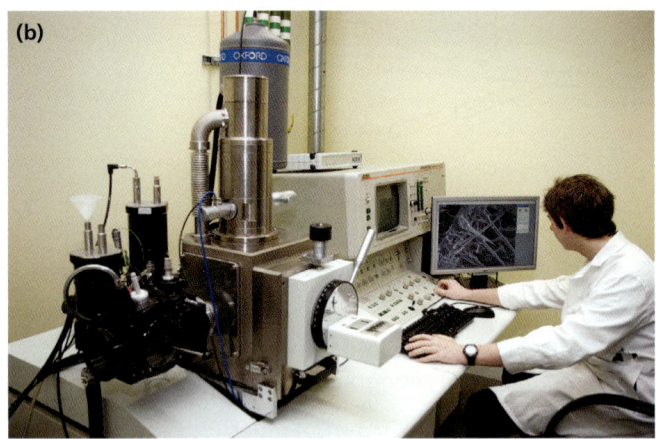

▲ Figure 11.24 (a) A light microscope and (b) an electron microscope

The principle of light and electron microscopes is the same: lenses are used to magnify the image. The difference is that, unlike light microscopes, electron microscopes use a beam of electrons to obtain an image. Whereas light microscopes use glass lenses for **magnification**, electron microscopes use magnets as lenses.

Light microscopes

The good news about light microscopes is that they are relatively inexpensive. They are also relatively easy to use, although they must be used with care to avoid damage. Thin sections of plant and animal tissues are usually prepared, but light microscopes can also be used to examine living micro-organisms as long as they are not too small, like most viruses. Electron microscopes cannot use living material as they have to operate in a vacuum.

> ### Health and safety
>
> Modern light microscopes usually contain a built-in light source. Halogen bulbs are likely to become very hot during use, so make sure you do not touch the bulb or try to disassemble the microscope.
>
> When using a high power objective lens it is easy to drive the lens through the slide as you focus. This is likely to damage the lens as well as creating a hazard from the broken glass of the microscope slide. To avoid this, always lower the stage when changing lens. Ensure the stage is lowered and raised carefully when using the highest power lens. Once in view, only adjust the focus using the fine focus knob to prevent damage to the lens or slide.

Scanning electron microscopes

In a **scanning electron microscope** (**SEM**), the beam of electrons is scanned across the surface of the sample. The electrons bounce off the surface and a computer is used to build up a 3D image of the surface of the sample, showing more surface detail than is possible with a light microscope.

Transmission electron microscopes

In a **transmission electron microscope** (**TEM**), the electrons pass through the sample in the same way as light rays pass through a sample in the light microscope. This means a TEM shows a 2D image of the sample. Very thin sections are required as electrons cannot penetrate materials very deeply. This allows a TEM to reveal details of virus particles or cell organelles that would not be visible with the light microscope. A series of thin sections can be used to take multiple 2D images that can be assembled into a 3D image.

The table compares the approximate magnification and **resolution** of these three types of microscope.

Instrument	Maximum magnification	Maximum resolution
Light microscope	x 1500	200 nm
SEM	x 100 000	10 nm
TEM	x 500 000–1 000 000	0.2 nm

Figure 11.25 illustrates what can be seen with the human eye, a good quality light microscope and a transmission electron microscope.

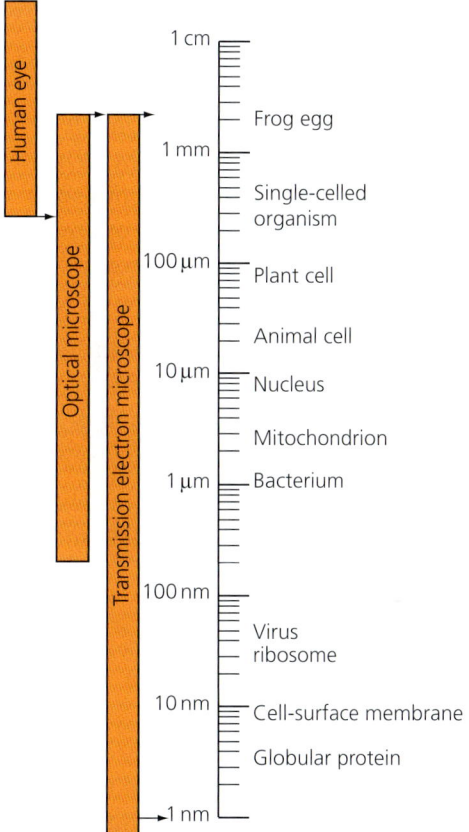

▲ Figure 11.25 A scale from 1 nm to 1 cm showing what can be seen with the naked eye, a light microscope and a transmission electron microscope. A log scale has been used because of the large range of measurements

> ### Practice point
>
> **Units**
>
> The following units are commonly used in microscopy:
>
> μm (micrometre) = 10^{-6} m
>
> nm (nanometre) = 10^{-9} m

Healthcare Science T Level: Core

B1.22 How to calculate magnification from the size of the image and the size of the object

Magnification is simply how much bigger the image is than the object. We can express that mathematically as:

$$magnification = \frac{size\ of\ image}{size\ of\ object}$$

It looks simple – and it is – but it can cause confusion. When calculating magnification, make sure you use the same units for the size of the image and the size of the object. We would normally measure the size of an image (e.g. a photomicrograph) in cm or mm, but microscopic objects are usually measured in μm. It is better to measure the size of the image in mm. When you calculate the magnification, make sure both sizes are expressed in the same units – either mm or μm, as shown in the example. There is more about converting between units in section B1.63.

A photomicrograph of a cell shows a mitochondrion that you know to be 1.5 μm long. You measure the image of the mitochondrion and find that it is 112.5 mm long. What is the magnification?

Method 1: convert the measurement of the image from mm to μm = 112 500 μm by multiplying by 1000 so 112.5 mm.

Now divide the size of the image by the size of the object to calculate the magnification:

$$magnification = \frac{112\,500}{1.5} = \times 75\,000$$

Method 2: convert the size of the object from μm to mm by dividing by 1000 so 1.5 μm = 0.0015 mm

Now, divide the size of the image by the size of the object to calculate the magnification:

$$magnification = \frac{112.5}{0.0015} = \times 75\,000$$

As you see, both methods give the same result. Remember that magnification should be quite a large number and always greater than one. If your answer is not, then you have made a mistake!

B1.23 The uses of differential staining techniques

Staining uses dyes to help make objects clearer under the light microscope by increasing contrast and making it easier to see cells. Unstained cells are almost transparent, which makes it very difficult to see them. Staining makes micro-organisms stand out against the background.

Differential staining adds another dimension by allowing us to distinguish different cell types, including specific types of bacteria or even parasites. There are a number of common ways this is done.

> **Health and safety**
>
> If you are involved in preparing stained sections, make sure that you are aware of any hazards associated with the chemicals used.

Gram staining

The **Gram stain** differentiates bacteria by detecting the peptidoglycan present in the cell wall of Gram-positive bacteria. Crystal violet is used to stain the peptidoglycan and then iodine is added to fix the stain permanently to the peptidoglycan molecules. Stained bacteria appear dark blue or violet. Gram-negative bacteria only have a very thin peptidoglycan layer – they have an outer membrane of lipopolysaccharides – and so the stain can be washed out of the cells. A counterstain of fuchsin or safranin is then used to stain all bacteria red/pink. As Gram-positive bacteria have already been stained dark blue/violet, only the Gram-negative bacteria appear red/pink.

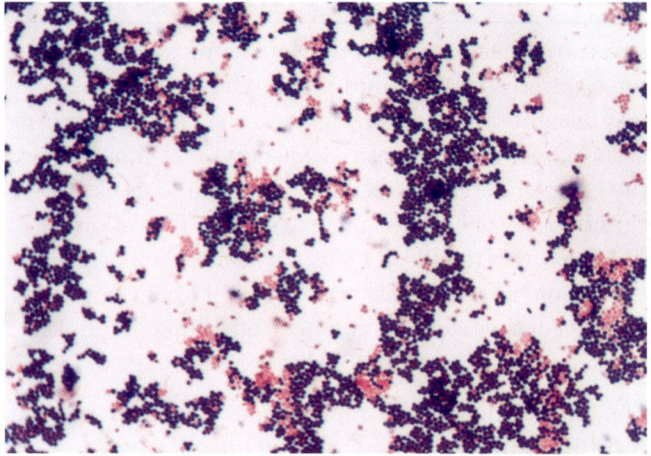

▲ Figure 11.26 Gram staining showing Gram-positive (purple) and Gram-negative (pink) bacteria

Giemsa staining

The Giemsa stain contains a mixture of Azure B, methylene blue and eosin stains. The methylene blue stains the chromosomes and nucleus dark purple while Azure B and eosin stain the cytoplasm pale blue or pink.

Giemsa stain can be used for:

▶ identification of specific bacteria such as *Chlamydia trachomatis*; these are stained blue-mauve to dark purple
▶ identification of *Plasmodium vivax* and *Plasmodium falciparum*, the malarial parasites; these are stained with a red or pink nucleus and blue cytoplasm
▶ identification of blood diseases such as anaemia and leukaemia; the different blood cells stain differently with Giemsa stain and any abnormalities can be identified (Figure 11.27).

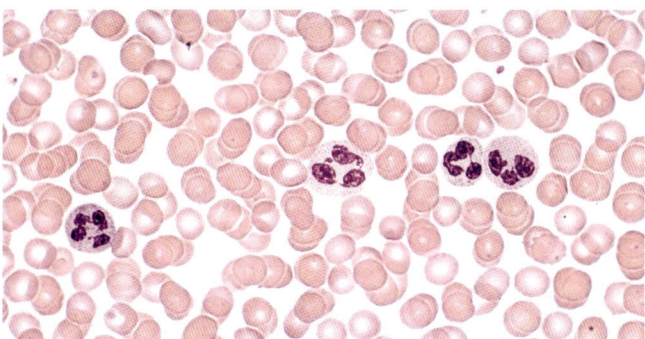

▲ Figure 11.27 A peripheral blood smear stained with Giemsa stain. Red blood cells do not have nuclei and so are stained pink, while the white blood cells have prominent nuclei that stain purple. This allows the different types of blood cell to be identified

Haematoxylin and eosin staining

Also known as H&E staining, this is the most widely used stain in medical diagnosis. The haematoxylin stains cell nuclei blue while the eosin stains the cytoplasm pink.

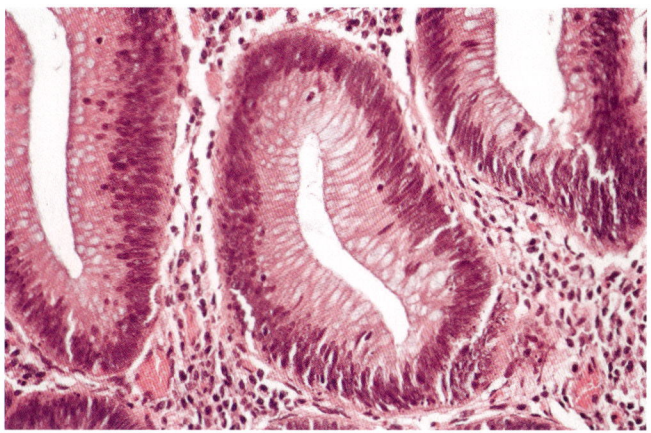

▲ Figure 11.28 Human breast cancer tissue section stained with H&E

> **Test yourself**
>
> 1. What is meant by the term pathogen?
> 2. For each the following pathogens, state whether they are prokaryotes or eukaryotes:
>   a. The *Plasmodium* parasite that causes malaria.
>   b. The tuberculosis bacterium.
>   c. The yeast that causes athlete's foot.
> 3. Explain the difference between the terms 'magnification' and 'resolution'.
> 4. Explain why light microscopes usually require thin sections of tissue.
> 5. Explain why electron microscopes cannot be used to examine living tissue.
> 6. Give two differences between transmission and scanning electron microscopes.
> 7. What type of stain would you use for the following:
>   a. Diagnosis of leukaemia, where there are abnormally large numbers of white blood cells
>   b. Examination of a food sample to detect food poisoning bacteria
>   c. Diagnosis of skin cancer from a skin biopsy
>   d. Diagnosis of a blood-borne parasitic infection.

Immunology

Immunology is the study of the immune system, which is an important part of the body's response to infection. We will see in section B1.30 that the immune system is just one way in which the body defends itself against disease. First, we need to consider the causes of infectious diseases.

B1.24 The nature of infection

Infection describes an organism replicating inside the body, resulting in disease. Some organisms, including all viruses, some bacteria and some parasites, infect body cells. Others replicate in organs such as the gut, in the blood or the spaces between cells.

B1.25 Causative agents of infection and examples of resulting diseases

Pathogen	Example of disease	Notes
Bacteria	• chlamydia • gonorrhoea • tuberculosis	Bacterial infections are treated by antibiotics, but bacteria are becoming increasingly resistant to antibiotics.
Viruses	• common cold • mumps • measles	SARS-CoV-2, the coronavirus that causes COVID-19, has recently become the best-known virus.
Fungi	• yeast infection (thrush)	Other fungal skin infections include toenail fungus and athlete's foot.
Prions	• Creutzfeldt-Jakob disease (CJD)	Prions are non-living pathogenic proteins. The mutant form of prion protein, when ingested, can cause normal prion proteins to change shape. This causes damage to the nervous system and eventual death.
Protoctists	• malaria	Don't confuse the pathogen (*Plasmodium*, a protoctist) with the *Anopheles* mosquito that transmits the pathogen.
Parasites	• toxoplasmosis	Toxoplasmosis is caused by *Toxoplasma gondii*, a parasitic protoctist. Many multicellular parasites can also cause infections, particularly in developing countries.

You may notice that there is an overlap between protoctists and parasites; malaria and toxoplasmosis are both caused by parasitic protoctists. However, some parasite diseases are due to infection by multicellular parasites, such as tapeworms.

> **Key term**
>
> **STI** or **sexually transmitted infection:** caused by a pathogen that is passed from person to person during sexual contact.

B1.26 The different ways in which causative agents may enter the body

During the COVID-19 pandemic everyone paid much greater attention to hand hygiene, mask wearing, social distancing and improved ventilation of indoor spaces. Although many people died from COVID-19, one effect of these precautions was that there were far fewer deaths from seasonal flu. This illustrates the importance of understanding the ways in which infections are transmitted.

Direct transmission

▶ Physical contact with an infected person (for example, skin-to-skin contact) or contaminated surface (for example, door handles and other hard surfaces).
▶ Sharing of needles can result in transmission of blood-borne pathogens.
▶ Pathogens such as HIV or hepatitis C virus can be spread by transfusion with contaminated blood or blood products. Unprotected sexual contact can lead to **STIs**.

Airborne transmission

The pathogen is carried by dust or droplets in the air. Some droplets (aerosols) can exist in the air for many hours and inhaling infected droplets can lead to infection. COVID-19 and tuberculosis are spread in this way.

Indirect transmission

Vehicle transmission occurs when infected food or water are ingested (eaten or drunk). Faecal-oral transmission is the result of poor hand hygiene and is a significant cause of food poisoning. Another example of vehicle transmission is from infected blood on inanimate objects such as clothing or bedding.

Another form of indirect transmission is being bitten by an infected **vector** (the organism that transfers the pathogen from host to host). Insect bites can introduce pathogens into the body. The best-known example is the malaria protoctist (*Plasmodium*), for which the vector is the *Anopheles* mosquito. There are many others, including Lyme disease (caused by a bacterium) and Zika fever (caused by a virus).

B1.27 How infectious diseases can spread among populations and communities

Understanding how infection spreads from person to person helps our understanding of how infectious diseases spread among populations. Once we understand that, we can consider ways in which the spread can be prevented, or at least minimised.

Inadequate sanitation includes:
- a lack of access to clean water for washing. Clean water is also unlikely to carry water-borne diseases
- inadequate sewage disposal, which increases the risk of faecal-oral transmission of a wide range of pathogens, including parasites that have evolved alongside human populations.

Dense populations lead to overcrowding in households as well as a lack of social distancing outside the home. These will both increase the rate of transmission by direct, airborne and indirect routes.

Inadequate healthcare infrastructure, such as inadequate hospitals or clinics, or a lack of doctors or nurses, increases the risk of disease spreading unnoticed as well as making it harder to treat and prevent further spread.

Ignorance can be deadly. Lack of accessible health promotion information means that people are less likely to take necessary precautions to prevent spread of infection. They may also be more resistant to prevention measures, such as vaccination.

It is worth noting that while all these factors are more prevalent in countries with developing economies, they are associated with areas of deprivation worldwide.

Case study

Between 1846 and 1860, a worldwide pandemic of cholera was responsible for over a million deaths worldwide. Cholera was thought to be caused by particles of decaying matter in the air ('miasma'). During 1854 there was a severe outbreak near Broad Street in the Soho district of London. A physician, John Snow, had been studying cholera for several years by this time. He mapped all the outbreaks of cholera in the district and showed that they were concentrated around a public water pump on Broad Street. Snow did not understand that cholera was caused by a bacterium, but the evidence he collected showed that in this outbreak it was transmitted by infected water from the Broad Street pump and not miasma. The authorities were unwilling to accept the results of Snow's work, although the pump handle was temporarily removed to prevent its use.

Snow also investigated the quality of water provided by different water companies. Individual houses in the same area received their water supply from different companies. Snow showed that there was a higher incidence of cholera in those households receiving their water from two large companies who extracted it directly from the River Thames. At that time, the river was heavily contaminated with raw sewage. Other households obtained their water from smaller companies who provided cleaner, better filtered water. These households had much lower incidence of cholera.

John Snow's work was a good example of the scientific method, including his use of statistical analysis. His work led, eventually, to great improvement in sanitation through the installation of more efficient sewage handling and provision of clean water.

- Think about the nineteenth-century cholera outbreak. Can you see any parallels with the COVID-19 pandemic?
- John Snow investigated a range of different factors in order to see a pattern. Can you think of factors that should be considered when studying the COVID-19 pandemic?
- Do you think that we have learned the lessons of John Snow's work?

B1.28 The definition of an antigen and an antibody

> **Key terms**
>
> **Antigen:** a substance that is recognised by the immune system as self (the body's own cells) or non-self (foreign cells and pathogens) and stimulates an immune response. Antigens are found on pathogens but also on the surfaces of all body cells.
>
> **Antibody:** a blood protein that is produced in response to a specific antigen. An antibody binds specifically to an antigen in a similar way to an enzyme binding specifically to its substrate.

B1.29 The link between antigens and the initiation of the body's response to invasion by a foreign substance

We can think of **antigens** as chemical markers rather like ID cards. They are usually proteins or **glycoproteins** (proteins with sugar molecules attached) on the surface of pathogens or body cells.

Some antigens on the surface of body cells allow the immune system to distinguish between the body's own cells ('self' antigens) and foreign cells, including pathogens ('non-self' antigens).

The response to invasion by a foreign substance involves several stages that we can think of as defence mechanisms. The immune response is part of that process but is not the only part.

B1.30 The stages and cells involved in the body's response to an antigen

The stages of defence against non-self antigens, for example, on pathogens, is shown in Figure 11.29.

Physical and chemical barriers

The first line of defence is to keep pathogens out. The skin plays a significant part as an external barrier. Mucous membranes are also important. These line the gut, airways and reproductive system. Goblet cells produce thick, sticky mucous that helps to trap bacteria and other pathogens. Antimicrobial proteins and peptides also help to destroy pathogens and can also be involved in stimulation of the immune system.

Lysozyme is an enzyme that hydrolyses bonds in the cell wall components of some bacteria. This weakens the cell walls, meaning that the bacteria swell and burst. Lysozyme is present in tears, helping to protect the surface of the eyes, as well as in breast milk providing protection to infants while their immune systems are developing.

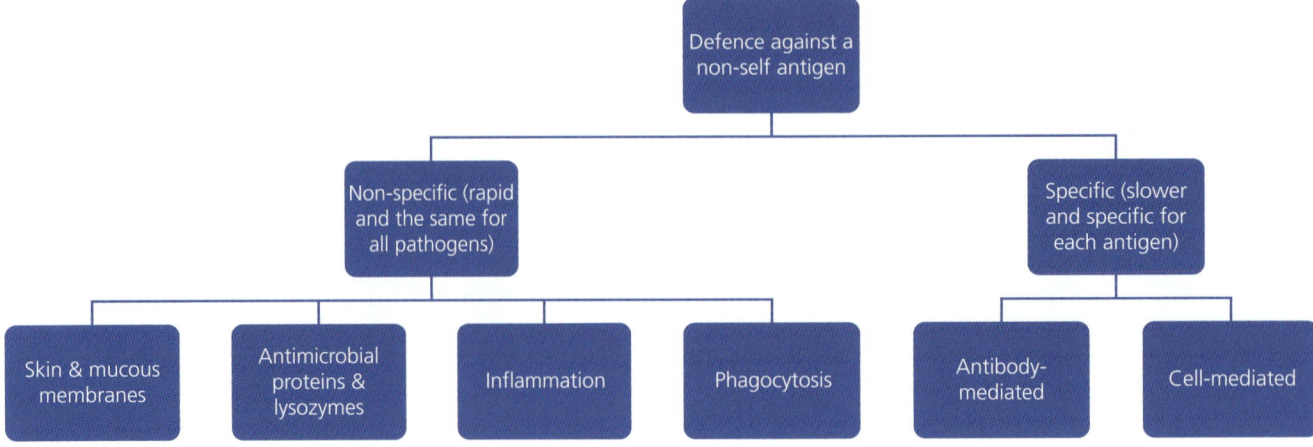

▲ Figure 11.29 Defence mechanisms

Inflammation

Inflammation is a response to injury or infection where the area becomes hot, red and swollen as a result of increased blood flow. Mast cells respond to tissue damage (caused by injury or infection) by secreting histamine. This **cell-signalling** compound stimulates a range of responses, including:

- increased blood flow in capillaries;
- capillaries begin to leak more, allowing fluid to enter the tissues resulting in swelling;
- **phagocytes** leave the blood and enter the tissues where they can engulf foreign material.

Histamine also stimulates cells to release cytokines, including interleukins that lead to more inflammation. Cytokines also lead to the promotion of **phagocytosis**.

> ### Key terms
>
> *Inflammation:* a local response to injury and infection.
>
> *Cell-signalling:* the process by which cells communicate with each other, usually by release of chemicals such as histamine, cytokines and interleukins.
>
> *Phagocytes:* produced in the bone marrow and circulate in the blood. Some leave the blood and are present in the tissues.
>
> *Phagocytosis:* the process of a phagocyte engulfing a pathogen or other foreign material.
>
> *Lymphocytes:* small white blood cells. B lymphocytes, or B cells, are responsible for antibody production. Different types of T lymphocytes, or T cells, play different roles in the immune response.

Phagocytosis

Chemicals released by pathogens into the blood attract phagocytes. Receptors on the surface of phagocytes bind to antigens that are present on the surface of most pathogens, and this leads to the phagocyte engulfing and digesting the pathogen (Figure 11.30).

Some types of phagocyte known as macrophages do not completely digest the pathogen. Instead, antigens from the partially digested pathogen are processed and then appear on the plasma membrane of the macrophage. These are then known as antigen-presenting cells (APCs), as they 'present' the antigens to **lymphocytes** (T cells). This process of antigen presentation initiates the immune response. This is the slower, more specific and more effective stage of defence against infection.

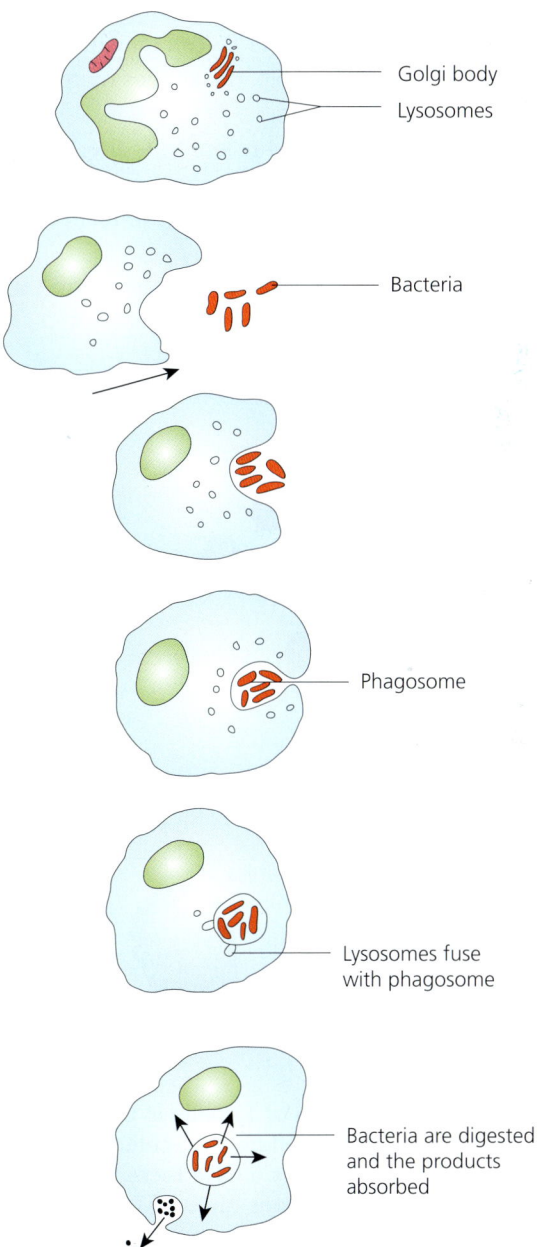

▲ Figure 11.30 The stages in phagocytosis

Healthcare Science T Level: Core

The role of T cells

The two main groups of T cells are T helper cells (T_H cells) and cytotoxic T cells (T_C cells) also known as T killer cells (T_K cells).

T_H cells have a type of cell-surface receptor known as CD4. There are many different shapes of CD4 receptor corresponding to the millions of antigen shapes that we might encounter. When a T_H cell encounters an APC, the CD4 receptors on the T_H cell may be complementary to the antigen, i.e. the shapes match. If so, the following events happen:

▶ The T_H cell binds, via its CD4 receptor, to the APC.
▶ This activates the T_H cell.
▶ The activated T_H cells divide by mitosis to form a clone of active T_H cells and memory cells.
▶ Activated T_H cells are then able to activate T_w and B cells.

This is shown in Figure 11.31.

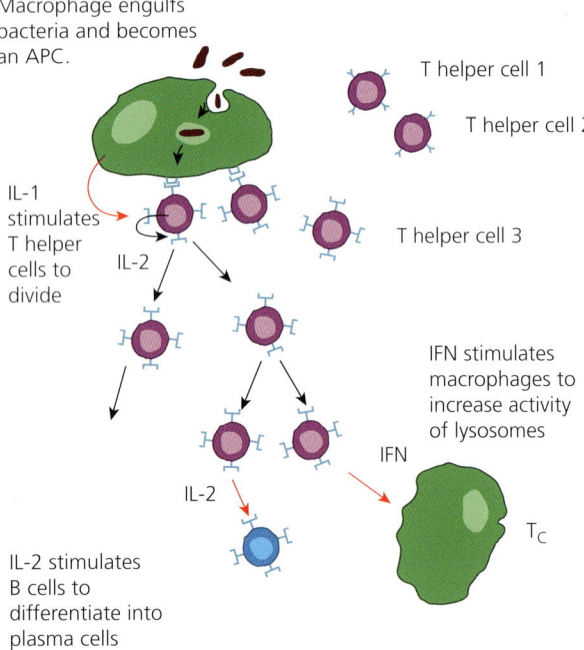

▲ Figure 11.31 The activation of T_H cells in the immune response. Three different T_H cells are shown, but only T_H cell 3 has a CD4 receptor complementary to the antigens on the APC

When body cells are infected by pathogens such as viruses, they also process pathogen antigens and present them on their cell surfaces, becoming APCs. T_C cells also have cell-surface receptors known as TCRs. Like CD4 receptors on T_H cells, there are many different shapes of TCR, complementary to different antigens. If a T_C cell encounters an APC with complementary antigens the following series of events occurs:

▶ The T_C cell becomes activated. This process also involves T_H cells.
▶ Once activated, the T_C cells will divide by mitosis to form a clone of activated T_C cells and memory cells.
▶ The T_C cells will bind to the surface of other infected cells and destroy them.

It might seem drastic to destroy the body's own cells, but infected cells will usually end up dead anyway and the action of T_C cells prevents pathogens such as viruses replicating inside the infected cells. This process is shown in Figure 11.32.

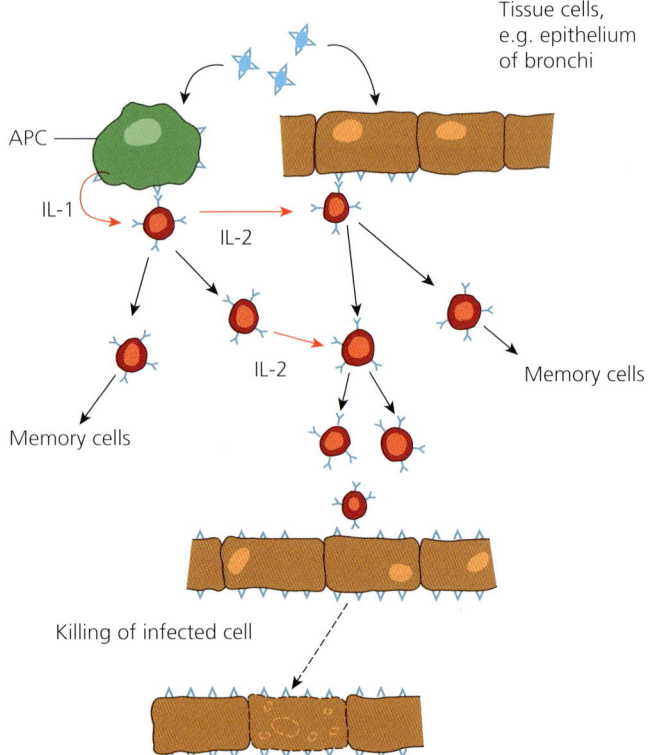

▲ Figure 11.32 Activation of T_C cells by infected host cells leads to killing of other infected cells

The role of B cells

B cells also have cell surface receptors, the B cell receptor or BCR. Again, there are many different shapes of BCR. When a B cell encounters antigens complementary to (i.e. which match) its BCR, the following events take place:

▶ The antigen binds to the BCR.
▶ B cell takes in the BCR and antigen.
▶ The B cell processes the antigen and so becomes an APC.

At this stage, activated T_H cells become involved.
- Any activated T_H cells with complementary CD4 receptors will then bind to the antigens on the APC.
- The T_H cell then secretes cytokines (such as IL-1 and IL-2).
- The cytokines activate the B cell.
- The activated B cell divides to form a clone of activated B cells and memory cells.
- The activated B cells differentiate to form plasma cells that produce large quantities of antibodies.

This process is shown in Figure 11.33.

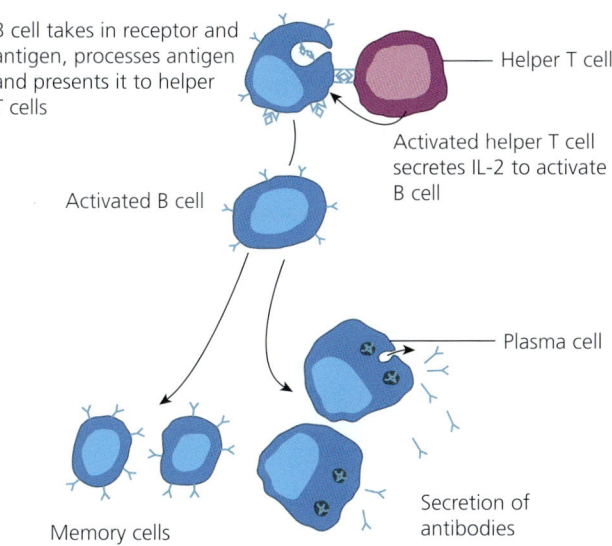

▲ Figure 11.33 Selection and activation of B cells with a BCR complementary to pathogen antigens

Antibodies bind to antigens on the surface of pathogens. Antibodies protect against pathogens in several ways, including:
- binding to toxins produced by bacteria and making them harmless;
- cross-linking pathogens so that they are too large to spread or infect cells;
- signalling to phagocytes to engulf the pathogens;
- binding to pathogen proteins that the pathogens use to enter body cells, for example, the spike protein on the surface of the SARS-CoV-2 virus.

B1.31 The differences between cell-mediated immunity and antibody-mediated immunity

In the previous section, we looked at the parts that T cells and B cells play in the immune response. It is useful to separate the two parts of the immune response. T_H cells play a key role in both of these parts, but there are important differences between the way in which the immune system protects the body from pathogens.

In the **cell-mediated response**, T cells destroy pathogens by destroying infected body cells. This means the pathogens cannot replicate and infect more body cells. Antibodies are not involved in the cell-mediated immune response.

In the **antibody-mediated** response, B cells produce antibodies, and it is the antibodies that lead to destruction of pathogens. Some antibodies are known as antitoxins, because they bind to and neutralise toxins produced by pathogens.

B1.32 The role of T and B memory cells in the secondary immune response

If we are infected by a pathogen, it takes the body about 10–17 days to produce antibodies. This process, known as the primary response, was described in section B1.31 and explains why we get ill with an infection. Once antibodies (and active T_C cells) are produced, the pathogen is removed and we get better. Plasma cells do not live long in the blood and the antibodies they produce are gradually broken down.

If, after some time, we are infected with the same pathogen, then antibodies are produced more rapidly and in much larger quantities. This is known as the **secondary immune response** and is illustrated in Figure 11.34.

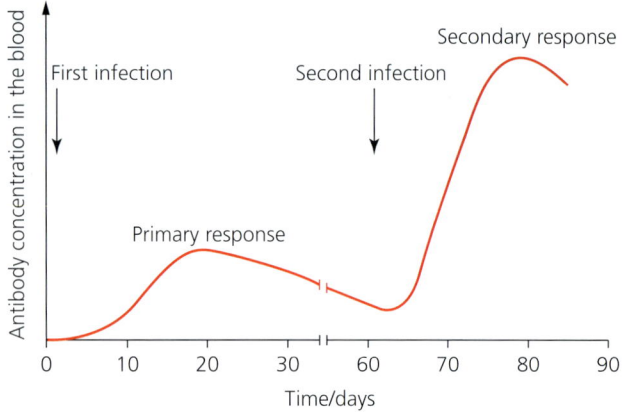

▲ Figure 11.34 The change in the concentration of antibodies during the primary and secondary immune responses

We saw how memory T cells and memory B cells were produced during the primary immune response. These remain in the body for a long time. When they encounter the pathogen for a second time, they multiply much more rapidly to form clones of plasma cells and T_C cells. The plasma cells produce high concentrations of antibodies in just a few days. In this way, the secondary immune response can clear pathogens from the body before we even show symptoms of the disease.

The secondary immune response is the basis of how vaccines work. A vaccine will stimulate the primary immune response without needing exposure to the pathogen, so the body is ready when it is exposed to the same pathogen later.

> **Test yourself**
>
> 1 Give two examples of diseases caused by each of the following types of pathogen:
>   a Bacteria   b Viruses
> 2 Explain the difference between a pathogen and a vector.
> 3 Give two examples of each of the following methods of disease transmission:
>   a Direct   b Airborne   c Indirect
> 4 Describe two factors that cause infections to spread within populations.
> 5 What is an antigen?
> 6 Give two differences between the specific and non-specific immune responses.
> 7 What is meant by an antigen presenting cell (APC)?
> 8 Give two differences between the primary and secondary immune responses.

> **Project practice**
>
> You are working in a lab that analyses ingredients for use in food manufacture. It is important that these meet required standards of identity, purity and safety. Choose one of the following areas.
> ▶ DNA analysis of meat to confirm species (lamb, beef, pork, etc.)
> ▶ Microbiological analysis of ingredients for contamination with pathogens.
> ▶ Immunological techniques for confirming identity and purity of ingredients.
>
> You then need to carry out the following:
> 1 Research a strategy.
>   a Carry out a literature review.
>   b Justify why you have chosen specific sources and not others.
> 2 Plan a project using the sources that you selected in your literature review.
>   a Set out the techniques you would use in your chosen form of analysis.
>   b Include all appropriate risk assessments.
>   c Identify the data that you would need to collect and how you would record the data.
> 3 Analyse the data.
>   a You will normally be presented with the data you need, as there will not be time to actually carry out the investigation.
>   b Produce a report of your analysis; think about what statistical tests you might need to apply.
> 4 Present your outcomes and conclusions in the form of a scientific poster showing:
>   a the techniques being used
>   b the strengths and weaknesses of your chosen technique
>   c your conclusions about the technique you have chosen.
> 5 Group discussion covering topics such as:
>   a the need for food analysis
>   b the practicality of different techniques
>   c do these techniques help to reassure consumers?
> 6 Reflection – write a reflective evaluation of your work.

Assessment practice

1. For each of the following organelles, state whether they are found in eukaryotes, prokaryotes, or both:
   a. Nuclei
   b. Plasma membrane
   c. Ribosomes
   d. DNA associated with proteins
   e. Plasmids

2. Which of the following statements is true?
   A. Lipids are polymers of fatty acids and glycerol.
   B. Polysaccharides are highly soluble molecules which makes them suitable as energy stores.
   C. Proteins are used as a form of storage molecule.
   D. Proteins, polysaccharides and lipids are all formed by condensation reactions.

3. A short section of DNA has the following base sequence.

   A G C T T A G C T

   Give the base sequence of the complementary strand of DNA.

4. Explain how semi-conservative replication ensures genetic continuity from one generation of cells to the next.

5. A student was using a light microscope to study a stained section of animal tissue. Explain what type of stain is likely to have been used in preparing the section.

6. A class was studying micrographs of animal cells.
   a. One micrograph showed a mitochondrion that was labelled as being $1.5\,\mu m$ long. A student measured the micrograph and found that the image of the mitochondrion was $11.3\,cm$ long. Calculate the magnification of the microscope.
   b. Another micrograph was labelled 'x 500 000'. The student measured the thickness of the plasma membrane on the micrograph and found it was $2\,mm$ wide. Calculate the actual width of the plasma membrane in nm.
   c. Explain what type of microscope will have been used to create the micrographs.

7. Antibiotics can be used to treat bacterial infections because they do not harm eukaryotic cells.
   a. Explain why antibiotics cannot be used to treat malaria.
   b. Explain why malaria can be controlled using insecticides.

8. During the COVID-19 pandemic, the UK government's advice was built around the slogan 'Hands, face, space'. This was later amended, adding 'fresh air'. Evaluate the use of this slogan.

9. Which of the following are involved in antibody-mediated immunity?
   A. B cells, T helper cells, plasma cells, phagocytes
   B. B cells, T killer cells, plasma cells
   C. Phagocytes, T killer cells, plasma cells
   D. Phagocytes, T killer cells, T helper cells

10. During the early stages of development of a COVID-19 vaccine, the concentration of antibodies in the blood of volunteers was measured in the weeks after vaccination. One vaccine produced significantly more antibodies than another type of vaccine. However, both were found to be similarly effective in preventing COVID-19 infection. Suggest an explanation for this finding.

B1.33–B1.44: Core science concepts: Chemistry

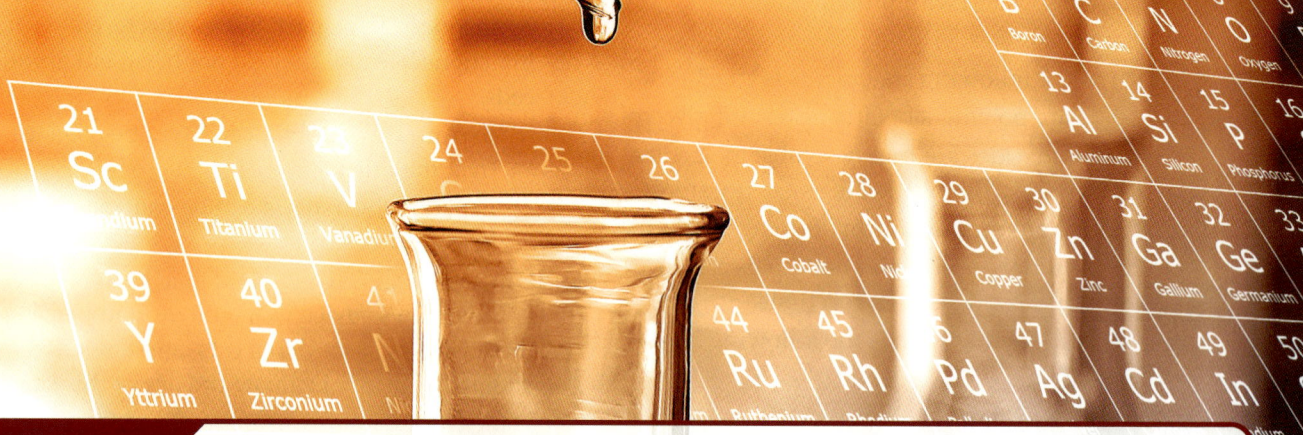

Introduction

Chemistry is the study of substances, their properties and how they combine to make other substances. All substances are made up of atoms, so we need to understand the structure of atoms and the arrangement of electrons within atoms. This is important because electrons are responsible for the bonds between atoms and chemical reactions involve making and breaking bonds.

This chapter also covers basic concepts of acids and bases, the factors that affect the rates of chemical reactions and some methods we can use to analyse substances.

Learning outcomes

The core knowledge outcomes that you must understand and learn:

Materials and chemical properties
B1.33 the relationship between the atomic structure and physical and chemical properties of metals
B1.34 how the arrangement of electrons is linked to the way in which elements are situated within groups in the periodic table
B1.35 the correct names for subatomic particles and their position in an atom – protons, electrons and neutrons

Acids/bases and chemical change
B1.36 the physical properties of acids
B1.37 the concept of strong and weak acids (as distinct from dilute and concentrated solutions)
B1.38 how to determine the name of the salt produced in acid–base reactions

Rates of reaction and energy changes
B1.39 the principles of collision theory
B1.40 the effect of temperature on rates of reaction
B1.41 the definition of a catalyst and the role of catalysts in a reaction

Chemical analysis of substances
B1.42 the principles of tests and techniques that are used to separate, detect and identify chemical composition
B1.43 the tests that could be used to quantify components in a mixture
B1.44 the principle of titration.

B1.33–B1.44: Core science concepts: Chemistry

> **Practice point**
>
> **Standard form**
>
> Throughout the coming chapters, and elsewhere in this book, you will see numbers written in what is known as **standard form**.
>
> For example, the number 3200 can be written as 3.2×10^3.
>
> 10^3 is one thousand ($10 \times 10 \times 10$; try it on your calculator). So we are writing a number which we might say as three thousand two hundred as 3.2 thousands, hence 3.2×10^3.
>
> 3200 is not a very large number, so you might ask, 'why bother?' But what about the following number?
>
> 3 200 000 000 000 000 000 000
>
> That takes too much space to write. But it also has the complication of working out millions, billions and so on. It is much easier to write it as 3.2×10^{21}.
>
> The same is true of very small numbers:
>
> 5.5×10^{-11} is much easier to work with than 0.000000000055. Can you be sure to keep track of all those zeroes?
>
> Numbers in standard form always have two parts. The number before the '×' sign is always greater than or equal to 1 but less than 10. The number after the '×' sign is always a power of 10. Here are some examples:
>
> $1.25 \times 10^3 = 1250$
>
> $3.5 \times 10^{-4} = 0.00035$
>
> You can count decimal places to convert between standard form and 'ordinary' numbers. 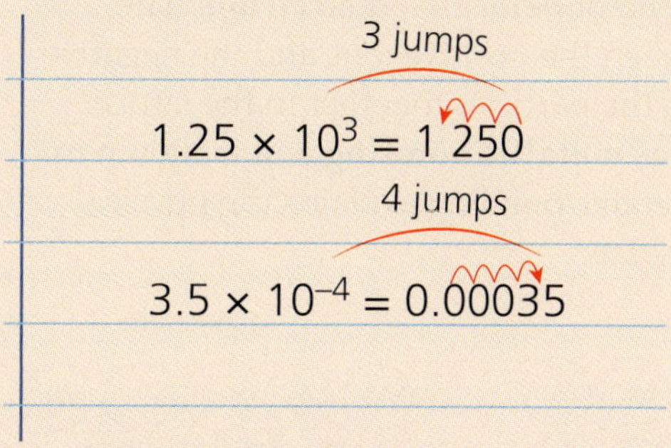
>
> 3 jumps
> $1.25 \times 10^3 = 1\,250$
> 4 jumps
> $3.5 \times 10^{-4} = 0.00035$
>
> ▲ Figure 12.1 Converting between standard form and 'ordinary' numbers
>
> There are two ways to work out if the power of 10 is positive or negative:
> ▶ If the decimal point jumps to the left, it is a positive power of 10. If it jumps to the right, it is a negative power of 10.
> ▶ If the number is greater than 10, then the power is positive. If the number is less than 1, the power is negative.
>
> You will find more detail about this topic with further examples in section B1.64.

Materials and chemical properties

Materials science is the study of the properties of solid materials and how they are determined by the chemical and physical composition of the material. Materials science is of great importance in the modern world. It inhabits the space between chemistry, physics, biology and engineering. Therefore, in chemistry, we must study both the physical and chemical properties of substances and understand how they are related to get a full understanding of the substances we are studying.

B1.33 The relationship between the atomic structure and physical and chemical properties of metals

> **Key terms**
>
> **Ions:** atoms that have lost electrons (positive ions) or gained electrons (negative ions).
>
> **Delocalised electrons:** 'free' electrons that are not associated with any single atom.

Physical properties

Metals are usually solids at room temperature (mercury is the only metal that is liquid at room temperature), with particles packed closely together in a repeating 3D grid arrangement called a lattice. The atoms in the lattice have lost their outer shell electrons, so the structure consists of metal **ions** and a sea or cloud of **delocalised electrons**. The attraction between the positive ions and the negative electrons holds the particles together in the lattice. This is known as **metallic bonding** and is shown in Figure 12.2. Metallic bonding explains the physical properties of metals.

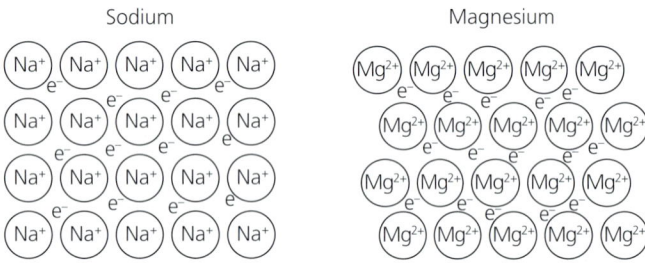

▲ Figure 12.2 A 2D diagram of metallic bonding in sodium and magnesium

Conductivity (electrical and thermal)

The delocalised electrons are free to move throughout the lattice. This means that they can carry an electric current (a flow of charge), so metals are good electrical conductors.

The delocalised electrons can move and vibrate and so transfer thermal energy from one to another through the metal, making metals good conductors of heat.

Malleability/ductility

Metals are **malleable** (they can be hammered into shape) and **ductile** (they can be drawn into wires). This is because of the layered structure. As you can see in Figure 12.3, if a force is applied to a metal, the layers can slide without disrupting the bonding.

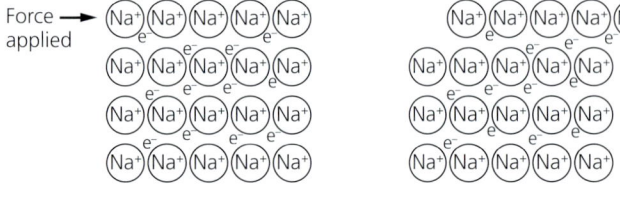

▲ Figure 12.3 Applying a force to part of a metal causes the layers to slide over each other without disrupting the bonding

Strength

The close packing of the particles in a metal explains their high density. You can see from Figure 12.3 that the Mg^{2+} ions have twice the charge of the Na^+ ions and there are also twice as many delocalised electrons. This is because magnesium has two electrons in its outer shell, so forms 2+ ions, whereas sodium has only one electron in its outer shell, so forms 1+ ions (see section B1.34). This means that magnesium has 2+ ions and twice as many delocalised electrons compared with the 1+ ions and fewer delocalised electrons in sodium. Therefore, there is a greater electrostatic attraction between the positive ions and delocalised electrons in magnesium. As a result, more energy is needed to overcome these forces in magnesium and so magnesium is stronger and has a higher melting point than sodium. The transition metals have even more delocalised electrons, which explains their greater strength and density – for instance, iron or tungsten. These are very hard compared with sodium which is soft enough to be cut with a knife and spread with a spatula.

Chemical properties

See section B1.34 for more information about how elements are divided into groups and blocks.

Group 1

Group 1 metals are all highly reactive. They react with water to form hydrogen gas and the metal hydroxide, for example, sodium:

$$2Na(s) + 2H_2O(l) \rightarrow 2NaOH(aq) + H_2(g)$$

They react with oxygen to form solid white oxides, for example:

$$4Na(s) + O_2 \rightarrow 2Na_2O(s)$$

Group 1 metals all have a single electron in their outer shells and so they form ionic compounds containing 1+ ions (Na^+, K^+, etc.). The outer electrons are further from the nucleus as you move down the group, from lithium to rubidium. This means there is a weaker force of attraction between the negative outer shell electron and the positive nucleus (because of the increased distance and increased shielding from the other electron shells). That means the outer electron is lost more easily in rubidium, making it more reactive.

The reactivity of group 1 metals increases down the group from lithium (least reactive) to rubidium (most reactive).

Transition metals

Transition metals are much less reactive with oxygen and acids compared with either group 1 or group 2 metals. Iron will rust (in other words, form iron oxide), but only when in contact with air containing water vapour – there is no reaction with dry air or oxygen-free water. Other transition metals react even more slowly, which makes them resistant to **corrosion**.

> **Key term**
>
> **Corrosion:** the process where metals react with substances in the air to form oxides, carbonates, hydroxides or other compounds.

The reaction of transition metals with acids is variable – it depends on the metal and the acid.

For example, iron will react with hydrochloric acid to produce iron chloride and with sulfuric acid to produce iron sulfate. In both cases hydrogen is also produced and the iron forms Fe^{2+} ions.

The reaction with nitric acid is a little different because concentrated nitric acid is a stronger oxidising agent than either sulfuric, hydrochloric, or dilute nitric acids. This means that the Fe is oxidised to Fe^{3+} rather than Fe^{2+}. Also, the nitrate (NO_3^-) in nitric acid is reduced to nitrogen monoxide (NO).

Copper is one of the least reactive transition metals and does not react with dilute hydrochloric or sulfuric acids. However, nitric acid and concentrated sulfuric acids are strong oxidising agents, and will both react with copper:

- Dilute nitric acid reacts to form copper nitrate and nitrogen monoxide.
- Concentrated sulfuric acid reacts to form copper sulfate and sulfur dioxide.

Notice that hydrogen is not produced in either case.

The table compares some properties of transition metals with group 1 metals.

Property	Group 1 metals	Transition metals
Melting points	Low	High
Density	Low – lithium, sodium and potassium are less dense than water	High
Hardness and strength	Soft and weak (can be cut with a knife)	Hard and strong
Reactivity with:		
Oxygen	High to very high (need to be stored under a protective layer of oil)	Slow to very slow
Chlorine	React vigorously to produce solid metal chlorides	Less reactive. Iron wool heated strongly will react with chlorine to produce iron (II) chloride
Water	Vigorous to very vigorous	Relatively unreactive

> **Reflect**
>
> Think about metallic bonding – positive ions surrounded by a sea of delocalised electrons.
>
> Can you use this to explain the difference in physical properties between the group 1 metals and the transition metals?

The relationship between the structure and properties of the following materials

Composite materials

As the name suggests, composite materials are made from two or more materials that have different properties. Reinforcing fibres or particles are embedded in a softer matrix that helps to bind the material together. Some common examples include concrete, fibreglass and carbon fibre.

- Concrete, used since Roman times, consists of small stones embedded in a matrix of sand and cement.
- Fibreglass has the strength of glass but is not brittle. Relatively rigid glass fibres act as reinforcement in a flexible resin matrix. Fibreglass can be created in a mould to produce a strong but lightweight material.
- Carbon fibre consists of carbon nanotubes embedded in a polymer matrix. It can combine great strength in a lightweight material. Although it is more expensive than metals such as iron and steel, carbon fibre is used increasingly in engineering applications (automotive and aircraft), sports equipment (golf clubs and tennis racquets) and many others.

Ceramics

Ceramics are made from materials such as clay, sand and other minerals that are moulded and then baked to form strong bonds between the atoms in the structure. This makes them hard, strong under compression and chemically unreactive.
- Clay ceramics have been made for thousands of years by moulding clay and heating in a furnace to produce decorative items and tableware.
- Glass is made from sand (a silicate) with either sodium carbonate and limestone to make soda-lime glass or with boron trioxide to make the stronger, heat-resistant borosilicate glass.

Polymers

Polymers are long chain molecules made from repeating monomer units. For example, poly(ethene) is a polymer with many thousands of repeating units based on ethene.

Some polymers have weak forces between the chains – this makes them softer and more flexible – while others have strong bonds holding the chains in a stronger and more rigid structure.

Polymers are chemically unreactive and electrical insulators (as they do not have any delocalised electrons to carry a current). This makes them very useful for storing and packaging items to keep them from changing.

Poly(ethene) is known commonly as **polythene**. Low density poly(ethene) (LDPE) and high density poly(ethene) (HDPE) are examples of **thermosoftening** polymers. Weak forces between the molecules allow the chains to slide over each other. This means they can be heated to soften them, allowing them to be moulded and reformed. Recycling thermosoftening polymers is therefore relatively easy and it is used in various consumer products to take advantage of this fact.
- HDPE is stronger and more rigid because it has a higher density. This is because it contains unbranched chains that can pack together more tightly. HDPE is used for bottles and other containers.
- LDPE is weaker and more flexible because it has a low density. This is because the chains are branched and therefore cannot pack together as easily. LDPE is used for bags, sheets and films.

Thermosetting polymers use heat to create cross-links between the chains. This makes the polymer stronger and less flexible. However, thermosetting polymers cannot be heated and reformed, which means they are less easily recycled.

> **Research**
>
> Make a list of the different types of material covered in this section. Choose at least one of each type.
>
> Then make a list of the different uses of the materials. For each example, try to show how the properties are related to the use.

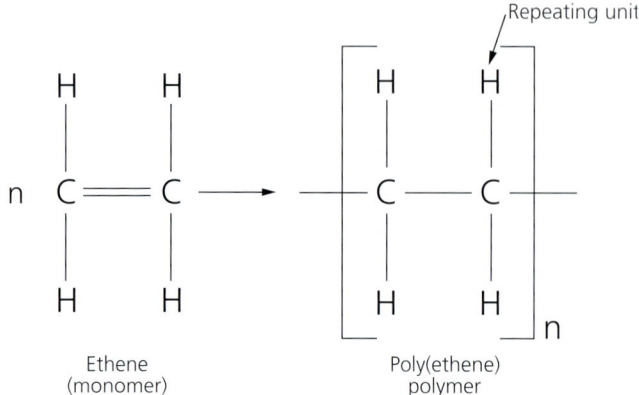

▲ Figure 12.4 Formation of poly(ethene) from ethene. The square brackets with n indicates that the repeating unit is repeated n times (i.e. many times)

B1.34 How the arrangement of electrons is linked to the way in which elements are situated within groups in the periodic table

The simplest definition of an **atom** is a **nucleus** surrounded by a cloud of **electrons**. The atom is more complex than this, but this model of the atom can be useful in some circumstances.

The **nucleus** is at the centre of the atom. It consists of **protons** and **neutrons** and contains most of the mass.

Elements consist of only one type of atom. **Compounds** consist of two or more types of atoms.

Electrons do not orbit the nucleus like planets orbiting the sun. Instead, they are located in **shells**, numbered from 1 to 7. Each shell is higher energy than the previous.

We can think of each shell being further from the nucleus than the last, and you will often see shells represented like this in diagrams. However, this can be misleading, making it look as if the electrons really are orbiting the nucleus. It is better to think of these 7 shells as being the 7 principal energy levels.

Electrons within each shell are located in various orbitals – s, p, d and f. The **orbitals** are found in different shells as follows:
- Each shell has only one s orbital.
- In shell 2 and above, there are also p orbitals.
- In shell 3, there are also d orbitals.
- In the highest shells, there are also f orbitals.

The modern periodic table is arranged in increasing order of **atomic number**, but the elements are also arranged according to their electronic structure into the s, p, d and f blocks (Figure 12.5).

The periodic table is also organised into **groups** – the columns in the table. Elements in the same group have similar chemical properties. This is because they have the same number of electrons in the outer shell.

The periodic table can be divided into blocks depending on which type of orbital the outer electrons are located in (Figure 12.6):
- Group 1 (the 'alkali metals') have one electron in the outer shell. It is in an s orbital, so these are all in the s block.
- Group 2 (the 'alkaline earths') have two electrons in the outer shell, both in the s sub-shell, so these are also in the s block.
- Groups 3 through 0 have from three to eight electrons in the outer shell. These are all in p orbitals, so these are in the p block.
- The d block includes the transition metals.

> **Key terms**
>
> **Orbitals:** are where electrons are located. Each orbital can be empty or can contain one or two electrons.
>
> **Atomic number:** refers to the number of protons in the nucleus.
>
> **Group:** refers to the columns in the periodic table. Elements in each group have the same number of outer shell electrons. Period refers to the rows in the periodic table. Elements in each period have the same number of shells.

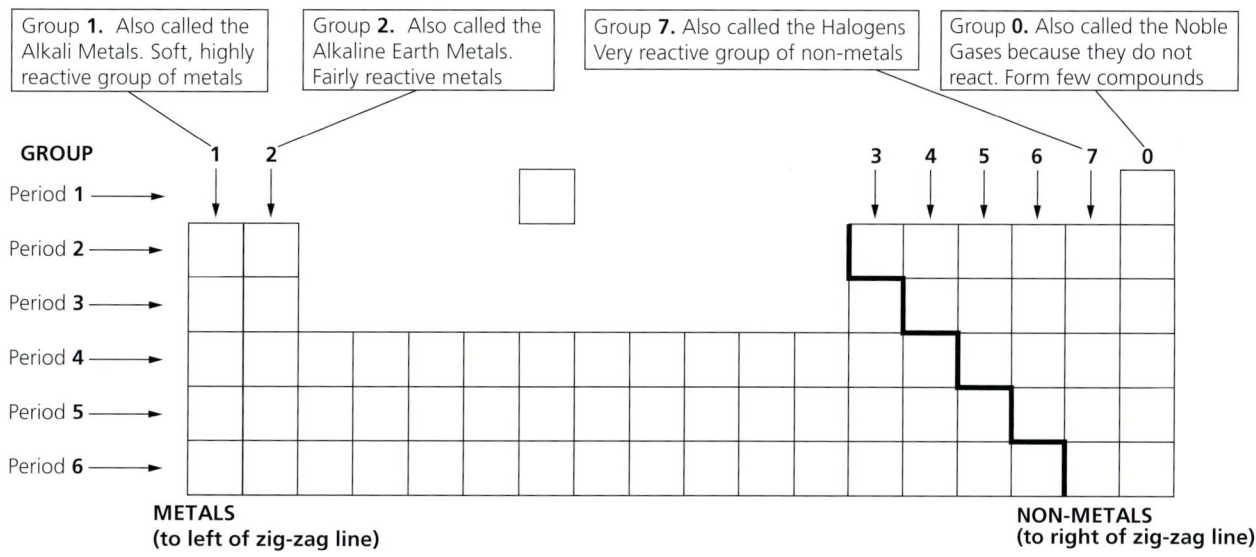

▲ Figure 12.5 The periodic table showing the groups and periods

Healthcare Science T Level: Core

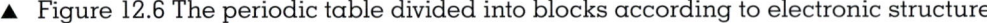

▲ Figure 12.6 The periodic table divided into blocks according to electronic structure

B1.35 Subatomic particles – protons, electrons and neutrons

An atom was originally thought of as being the smallest particle that an element could be broken down into. We now know that is not the case. Nuclear physics studies the many types of subatomic particle, but in chemistry we are only concerned with three types:

▶ Protons are found in the nucleus and have a charge of +1 and a relative mass of 1.
▶ Neutrons are also found in the nucleus. They have no charge but also have a relative mass of 1.
▶ Electrons are found in orbitals around the nucleus and have a charge of −1. The relative mass of electrons is approximately 1/2000th that of a proton or neutron.

From this, you can see that the majority of the mass of an atom is in the nucleus.

B1.33–B1.44: Core science concepts: Chemistry

Test yourself

1. Explain the terms 'malleable' and 'ductile'.
2. Explain how the structure of metals means that they are good conductors of electricity.
3. Explain, with examples, the difference between a composite and a ceramic.
4. State what is meant by the following:
   a. an atom
   b. an element
   c. a compound.
5. Explain the difference between a shell and an orbital.
6. Complete the following table:

Particle	Location	Charge	Relative mass
Proton			
	Nucleus	0	
			approx. 1/2000

Acids/bases and chemical change

pH is a measure of the hydrogen ion concentration. It is a **logarithmic scale**, usually from 0 to 14, although pH values can go above or below this range. Because it is a logarithmic scale, a change of one pH unit means the hydrogen ion concentration changes by a factor of 10. At room temperature, pure water has a pH of 7, which is considered the neutral point. Below pH 7 the solution is **acidic** and above pH 7 the solution is **alkaline**. **Neutralisation** occurs when acid and **base** react to form water and a salt.

Acid–base reactions are particularly important in chemistry. As well as being used to determine concentrations in titration (see section B1.44), they are used for preparation of a wide range of salts.

Key terms

Acid: a proton (H^+ ion) donor. An **acidic** solution contains H^+ ions.

Alkali: a water-soluble base, such as sodium hydroxide. An **alkaline** solution contains hydroxide (OH^-) ions.

Base: a proton (H^+ ion) acceptor. Examples include hydroxides as well as ammonia and amines. (See B1.38.)

B1.36 The physical properties of acids

Acids release hydrogen (H^+) ions – we say that they are H^+ **donors**. This explains the properties of acids:

- They are an irritant (cause inflammation of the skin) and often corrosive.
- They react with bases in a neutralisation reaction to produce a salt and water (see section B1.38).
- They react with most metals to form hydrogen gas (H_2).
- Because they have a high concentration of H^+ ions, they have a pH value less than 7.

Health and safety

The fact that acids are irritant or corrosive and highly reactive means they need to be treated with caution. Make sure you have carried out a risk assessment and are using adequate PPE (see Chapter A3, page 53) before working with acids.

B1.37 The concept of strong and weak acids

It will be useful to look at sections B1.62 and B1.63 on units before going further if you are at all unsure about use of the different units used for concentration in this section. Anyone who has tried drinking orange squash without diluting it will be familiar with the idea of concentrated and dilute solutions. To use a more chemical example, if we prepare a solution containing 0.1 mol hydrochloric acid in 1 dm^3 water, the hydrochloric acid will dissociate completely into its ions:

$$HCl(aq) \rightarrow H^+(aq) + Cl^-(aq)$$

In this equation, '(aq)' means **aqueous**, a solution in water. The concentration of H^+ will be 0.1 mol/dm^3 and the solution will have a pH = 1.00. This process is usually described as **dissociation** of the acid (into its constituent ions), but you will also come across the term **ionisation** (see page 273) to describe the same thing.

We can do the same with nitric acid or sulfuric acid:

$$HNO_3(aq) \rightarrow H^+(aq) + NO_3^-(aq)$$

$$H_2SO_4(aq) \rightarrow 2H^+(aq) + SO_4^{2-}(aq)$$

The only difference with sulfuric acid is that the concentration of H⁺ will be 2 mol/dm³ because 1 mol of sulfuric acid releases 2 mol of H⁺.

In contrast, if we have a 1 mol/dm³ solution of ethanoic acid and measure the pH, it will be 2.88 because the H⁺ concentration is only 0.0013 mol/dm³. This is because ethanoic acid is a weak acid, which means that it only partially **dissociates** in aqueous solution. We can represent this as the following reversible reaction:

$$CH_3COOH(aq) \rightleftharpoons H^+(aq) + CH_3COO^-(aq)$$

A **reversible reaction**, also known as an equilibrium reaction, is represented by the double arrow ⇌ and can move in either direction. In any **equilibrium**, there will be a mixture of all the components (reactants and products) in varying proportions. In the case of weak acids, such as ethanoic acid, the position of the equilibrium lies well to the left, i.e. only a small amount will dissociate – most will remain as CH_3COOH.

Once we understand the difference between strong/weak and concentrated/dilute, it should be clear that we can have a dilute solution of a strong acid and a concentrated solution of a weak acid.

You will also see from the above that when we have solutions of the same concentration, e.g. 0.1 mol/dm³, the pH of the strong acid (pH = 1.00) will be lower than that of the weak acid (pH = 2.88). If you consider the H⁺ concentration you will see that ethanoic acid (the weak acid) has a H⁺ concentration almost one thousand times lower than the hydrochloric acid.

This illustrates another important feature of pH. For each one unit decrease in pH, the H⁺ concentration increases by a factor of 10.

B1.38 How to determine the name of the salt produced in acid–base reactions

Bases, such as sodium or potassium hydroxide, react with acids, such as hydrochloric acid, in a neutralisation reaction to produce a salt plus water. For example, with hydrochloric acid and sodium hydroxide:

$$NaOH(aq) + HCl(aq) \rightarrow NaCl(aq) + H_2O(l)$$

Group 2 hydroxides (hydroxides of group 2 elements) react in the same way. The salt formed always takes the name of the metal (positive ion) together with the name corresponding to the acid used. Ammonia solution (ammonium hydroxide) reacts in the same way to form ammonium salts.

The table shows the names of salts formed from some common acids.

Practice point

The table shows the modern (systematic) names of the chemicals. You will probably encounter older, non-systematic names as well, such as 'acetate' for 'ethanoate'. There are many other examples, although we will not be covering those chemicals here.

Acid	Formula of acid	Type of salt formed	Formula of anion	Example
Hydrochloric	HCl	Chlorides	Cl^-	Sodium chloride, NaCl
Sulfuric	H_2SO_4	Sulfates	SO_4^{2-}	Sodium sulfate, Na_2SO_4
Nitric	HNO3	Nitrates	NO_3^-	Sodium nitrate, $NaNO_3$
Phosphoric	H_3PO_4	Phosphates	PO_4^{3-}	Sodium phosphate, Na_3PO_4
Ethanoic	CH_3COOH	Ethanoates	CH_3COO^-	Sodium ethanoate, CH_3COONa

Test yourself

1. What is meant by:
    a. an acid
    b. a base?
2. Explain the difference between a concentrated solution of a weak acid and a dilute solution of a concentrated acid.
3. Name the salts produced in the following acid-base reactions:
    a. Potassium hydroxide and nitric acid.
    b. Calcium hydroxide and phosphoric acid.
    c. Ammonia solution and sulfuric acid.

Rates of reaction and energy changes

We need to understand the factors that affect the rate of chemical reactions. That understanding is important if we are running a chemical factory producing ammonia for use in artificial fertiliser or preparing a sample of a medicine such as aspirin in the laboratory.

B1.39 The principles of collision theory

Our understanding of rates of reaction and energy change in chemical reactions is based on **collision theory**. This was originally worked out for reactions between gases, but the principles also apply to reactions in solution. We can summarise this theory in three statements:

1 Molecules must collide in order to react.
2 Molecules must have sufficient energy when they collide. Chemical reactions involve breaking chemical bonds (which requires energy) before new bonds are made (which releases energy). The energy required to break bonds is known as the activation energy. If molecules that have less energy than the activation energy collide, they will just bounce off each other without reacting.
3 Molecules must be in the correct spatial orientation when they collide. The bonds being broken and reformed will be in specific positions in space. This means molecules must be aligned correctly when they collide – see Figure 12.7.

B1.40 The effect of temperature on rates of reaction

As temperature increases, the kinetic energy of the molecules increases. This means they move faster. If they move faster, they are more likely to collide.

So increasing temperature increases the rate of reaction in two ways:
- The probability of collision increases.
- The proportion of molecules with sufficient energy to react also increases.

On the other hand, decreasing temperature decreases the kinetic energy of molecules. Therefore, molecules move slower, decreasing the probability of successful collisions and hence decreases the rate of reaction.

B1.41 The definition of a catalyst and the role of catalysts in a reaction

Catalysts increase the rate of chemical reactions. They do this because they provide an alternative reaction pathway that has a lower activation energy. This means that more molecules will have sufficient energy to react and this will increase the rate of reaction. In short, more reactants will exceed the activation energy and so can successfully collide.

Transition metals are often used as catalysts. In some reactions between gases the solid transition metal catalyst provides a surface for the reaction to take place. In other cases, the transition metal takes part in the reaction. Acids are common catalysts in organic chemistry. In both cases, the catalyst will participate in the reaction but will be reformed at the end of the reaction. This means that the catalyst is not **permanently** changed. It is used, but not used up. In all cases, remember the catalyst provides an alternative reaction pathway that has a lower activation energy.

> **Test yourself**
>
> 1 What are the three statements of collision theory?
> 2 Explain why temperature increases the rate of reaction.
> 3 Explain how a catalyst increases the rate of reaction.

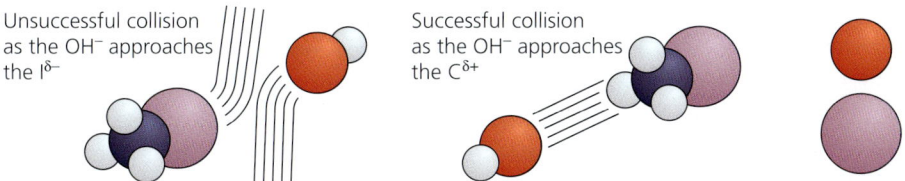

▲ Figure 12.7 Effect of orientation on reaction outcome

Chemical analysis of substances

Our knowledge of chemistry is built upon the ability to analyse substances. We need to understand the composition of substances and how this changes when they undergo chemical reactions.

B1.42 The principles of tests and techniques that are used to separate, detect and identify chemical composition

Separation is central to most forms of analysis. As well as separating the components of a mixture, we sometimes need to **quantify** them (work out how much of them there is).

Examples of analysis based on separation of the components of a mixture include:
- detecting additives in foodstuffs
- analysing urine samples to detect use of performance-enhancing drugs in sport (doping)
- determining the purity of pharmaceutical raw materials.

> **Reflect**
>
> List as many types of substance you might need to analyse as you can. For each one, decide whether it would be enough to know what is present (**qualitative analysis**) or whether you would need to know how much of each substance is present (**quantitative analysis**).

> **Key terms**
>
> *Chromatography:* the separation of the components of a mixture dissolved in a liquid or gas (the mobile phase) carrying it through a structure holding the stationary phase.
>
> *Adsorption:* when a substance (e.g. a gas, liquid or solute) binds to or attaches to another, usually solid.
>
> *Adsorbent:* often used to describe the stationary phase in chromatography because substances become adsorbed to it during separation.

In all types of **chromatography**, separation depends on substances in a mixture having a different **affinity** or attraction towards two phases. The **stationary phase** is fixed while the **mobile phase** (a liquid or gas) is able to move. It is important, in this context, that we use the term **adsorption** for the process of binding to a material in the stationary phase. (This is not the same as **absorption**, which is a term sometimes used, incorrectly, in this context. In absorption, one substance is taken in or **absorbed** by another, rather like a sponge absorbing water.)

Thin layer chromatography

Thin layer chromatography (TLC) is used to separate non-volatile mixtures such as amino acids, pharmaceuticals or dyestuffs. These are substances that cannot be easily vaporised. Separation is based on their solubility in the mobile phase (solvent) or affinity for (attraction to) the stationary phase (on a coated plate). The stationary phase is a thin layer of **adsorbent** such as silica gel, alumina or powdered cellulose on a flat, **inert** (non-reactive) support, such as glass or (more usually) plastic.

TLC can be used to detect the number of components in a mixture. The stages are:

1. A pencil line (the **origin**) is drawn about 1 cm from one short edge of the TLC plate.
2. The sample or samples are applied in solution at various points along the origin and left to dry.
3. The plate is placed vertically in a container with a shallow layer of solvent, so that the origin is above the level of the solvent (Figure 12.8).
4. The container is covered or sealed to prevent evaporation. The solvent will be drawn up the paper by **capillary action** (the process where a liquid is drawn into narrow spaces like those between the fibres in filter paper or a kitchen towel).
5. When the solvent reaches the origin, substances in the sample will dissolve and begin to move.
6. Substances with greater affinity for the stationary phase will move more slowly than substances with a greater affinity for the solvent and so the mixture will become separated.
7. After the solvent has moved far enough up the paper (usually almost to the top), the plate is removed from the container.
8. The position that the solvent has reached (the **solvent front**) is marked.

Efficient separation requires choice of solvent (mobile phase) so that the different components of the mixture will have different solubility in the mobile phase. If all components are equally soluble, they will all move the same distance. If they are insoluble, they will remain at the origin. Therefore, different solvents or mixtures of solvents with a range of **polarities** (ability to mix or dissolve) are used depending upon the substances being separated.

B1.33–B1.44: Core science concepts: Chemistry

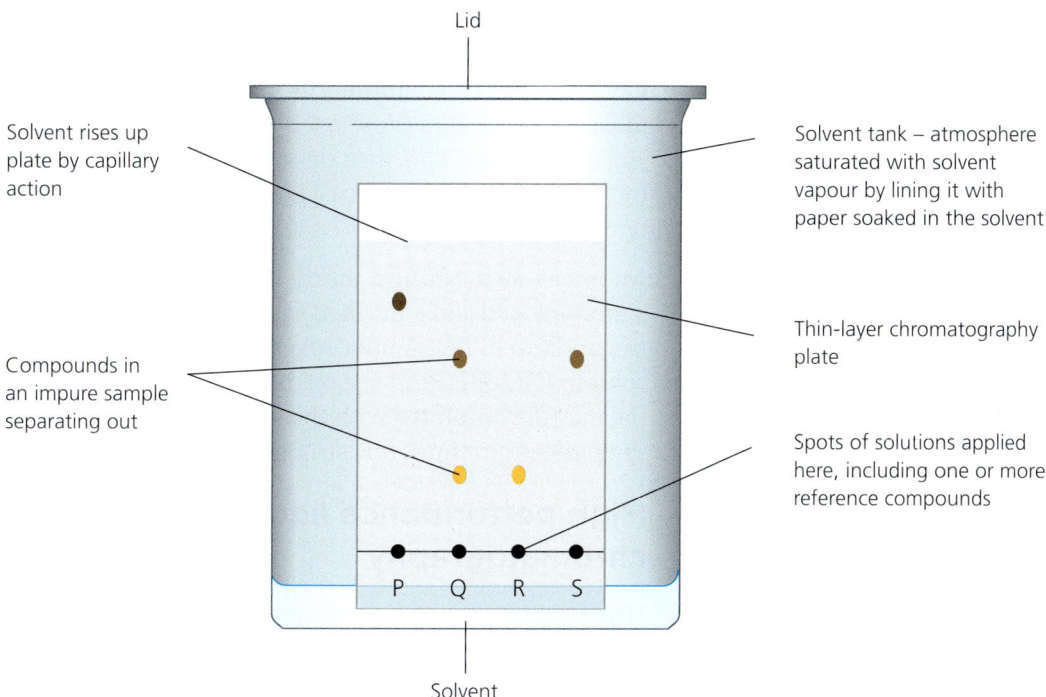

▲ Figure 12.8 Apparatus for TLC. Samples for analysis are spotted on the origin at P, Q, R and S

In the same way, the nature of the stationary phase will determine how far a particular substance moves. If a substance has a high affinity for the stationary phase, it will not move far up the plate. If it has a low affinity for the stationary phase, it will move further.

TLC is often used to separate the different coloured dyes in a mixture or to analyse the different coloured pigments in a plant extract. In other cases, the components of the mixture are colourless. This means we need to make the spots visible in some way. A common method is to use a dye that will bind to the chemicals in our mixture:
- Ninhydrin will stain amino acids purple. If a TLC plate is used to separate a mixture of amino acids, it can be dried and then sprayed with ninhydrin solution. The amino acids spots are then stained purple.
- Iodine vapour will stain many chemicals brown.

Another method to make the spots visible is to use a TLC plate that contains an inert fluorescent dye. After the separation is done and the plate is dried it can be illuminated with UV light. The spots will appear dark on a bright background.

If we analyse a substance by TLC and see just a single spot, it suggests the substance is pure. However, it is possible that two substances move the same distance. To be sure a sample is pure, we need to repeat the analysis in a different system, for example, with a different solvent mixture or different adsorbent.

As well as separating the components of a mixture, paper chromatography and TLC can be used to identify the components. One way is to run pure samples (**standards**) alongside the mixture. The distance travelled by a component of the mixture can then be compared to the distance travelled by one of the standards.

Another method is to calculate the **retention factor** or R_f **value**. R_f values can be used in TLC to identify unknowns based on standard published literature values.

Column chromatography

Column chromatography uses similar stationary phases to TLC but a much wider range is available, particularly those used in the separation of biologicals. In all cases, the sample is applied to the top of the column and **eluted** with a suitable mobile phase, the **eluent**. The stationary phase runs the entire length of the column. The substances then travel down the column based on their affinity for the eluent. Substances with a higher affinity for this mobile phase, will be separated and eluted earlier from the bottom of the column. The advantage of column chromatography is that the **eluate** can be collected in small amounts (**fractions**) as it emerges from the bottom of the column. Different substances will be in the different fractions because they elute from the column at different times. This allows column chromatography to be used for purification of a single chemical compound as well as for analysis.

> **Key terms**
>
> *Elution:* to wash out. In column chromatography this means 'washing out' a substance that has become adsorbed to the column (stationary phase).
>
> *Eluent:* the solvent (mobile phase) used to wash substances out of a column.
>
> *Eluate:* the mobile phase, containing dissolved substances, as it emerges from a column.

Gas chromatography

Gas chromatography (GC) is used to separate and analyse **volatile** compounds (ones that can be vaporised). GC uses an inert carrier gas as the mobile phase. The stationary phase can be a thin layer of high boiling point liquid on an inert solid support packed into a column. Substances that have a higher affinity for the stationary phase, will interact with it more, meaning it will take longer for it to emerge from the column. Substances with a lower affinity for the stationary phase, will then emerge sooner and be detected first. More recently, capillary GC uses a polymer lining a very fine capillary column as the stationary phase. The column will be coiled inside an oven to maintain the relatively high temperature needed (Figure 12.9).

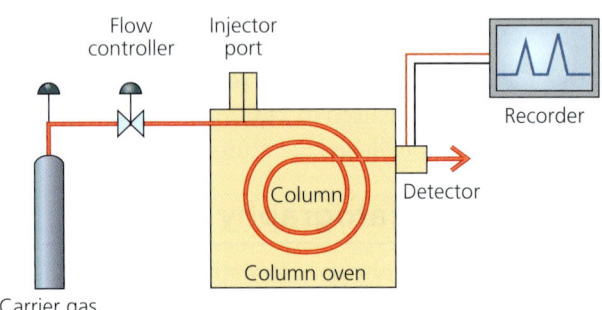

▲ Figure 12.9 Apparatus for GC

The sample is injected into the gas stream and the components of the mixture being separated will interact with the stationary phase to different degrees and so will emerge from the column at different times. The substances emerging from the column are detected, usually by a **flame ionisation detector (FID)** or a **thermal conductivity detector (TCD)**. These work with a wide range of substances, although other detection methods are available for specific applications.

The time taken between injection and detection of a particular component is known as the **retention time**. We saw how R_f values can be used in TLC to identify unknowns based on standard published literature values. The same is true of retention time in GC. However, conditions used for the analysis must be identical to those used when determining the standard values. This includes use of the same column (not just the same stationary phase), mobile phase, temperature, etc.

Another way to confirm the identity of a substance in a mixture is to add a purified sample of that substance (a standard) to the sample when it is injected onto the column (GC or HPLC, see below). If the substance in the mixture **co-elutes** with the standard (i.e. has the same retention time), it is strong evidence of identity.

High performance liquid chromatography

High performance liquid chromatography (HPLC) is a type of column chromatography that uses very small particles and high pressures to achieve better separation. The very fine particles make it difficult to force the solvent through and so HPLC requires powerful pumps and pressure-resistant columns to be fitted. The sample being analysed or purified cannot simply be applied to the top of the column – the system is sealed and under pressure – so the sample needs to be introduced by injection through a valve or port. The advantages of using HPLC for separation are much greater speed and higher resolution (ability to separate two very similar substances). HPLC has become one of the standard methods of separation in analytical laboratories. It can also be scaled up to operate as a purification method on a much larger scale, handling grams or even kilograms of substance.

A more recent development of HPLC, **ultra-high performance liquid chromatography** or **UPLC**, uses capillary columns to separate mixtures before analysis by mass spectrometry.

Mass spectrometry

Mass spectrometry (MS) can identify the amount and type of compound, which makes it very useful in identifying unknown compounds. The sample is ionised by removing electrons. The mass spectrometer then measures the ratio of mass to charge (m/z) of the positive ions produced. This can be done in various ways:

▶ By measuring how far the ions were deflected by a magnetic field; ions with greater mass are deflected less (Figure 12.10).

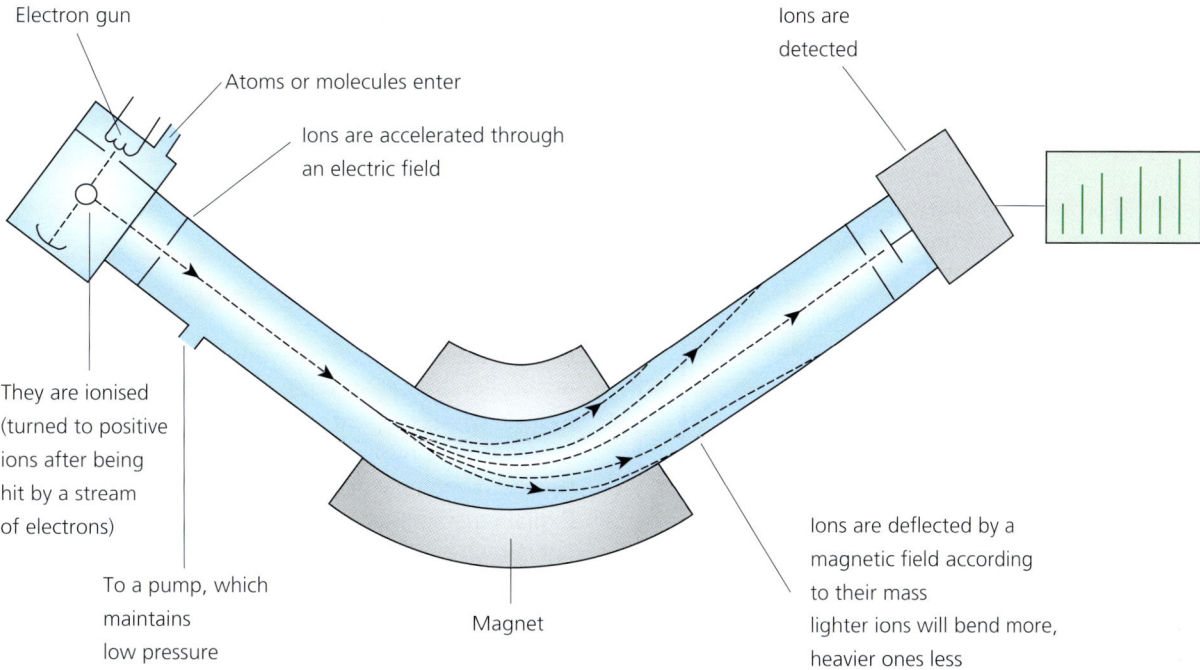
▲ Figure 12.10 Diagram of a mass spectrometer

▶ More recent methods such as **time of flight (TOF)** measure how long it takes for ions to reach the detector; ions with greater mass are slower and take longer.

MS provides the molar mass (M_r) of the compound, but additional information about the structure of the compound can be obtained from the way in which the ion breaks up (fragments) in the mass spectrometer.

By feeding the output of a GC column into a mass spectrometer, it is possible to identify the compounds being separated much more accurately than simply by retention time. This technique, known as GC-MS, is used widely because of the compact nature of the equipment, its speed and relatively low cost. Applications (uses in the real world) include airport screening for drugs and explosives, fire forensics (investigating the causes of a fire) and space exploration. Probes containing miniaturised GC-MS have been sent to Mars, Venus and Titan.

Research

A similar approach to GC-MS can be taken with liquid chromatography. In LC-MS, a very small capillary column is used for separation of complex mixtures such as proteins and peptides. Other applications involve analysis of drug metabolites in pharmacology and anti-doping laboratories. An internet search for 'applications of LC-MS' will help you learn more.

B1.43 The tests that could be used to quantify components in a mixture

GC, HPLC and MS are all powerful analytical techniques that separate the components of a mixture. This means they can be used to determine whether a sample is pure or is contaminated with other substances. To be really useful, we need to be able to calculate the percentage of each component, so that we can work out the percentage purity.

In both GC and HPLC, substances emerging from the column pass through a detector. The output from the detector gives a type of graph called a chromatography trace where the area under the peaks is proportional to the amount of the substance. This data is captured by a computer and analysed to show the percentage of each component.

It is also possible to use a standard of known content to convert the relative values we get from measuring peak area into absolute values, i.e. actual masses, in µg or mg.

In mass spectrometry, the output gives the relative abundance of each component. It is possible to determine the absolute quantity of each component using standards made with heavy isotopes.

B1.44 The principle of titration

Key terms

Mole: an amount of substance. This helps us to work out the reacting proportions in any reaction. We can also use the mole to work out reacting masses or volumes. The abbreviation is **mol**.

Indicator: a substance that changes from one colour to another or from coloured to colourless depending on whether it is in acidic or basic solution.

Analyte: the solution of unknown concentration in a titration.

Standard solution: the solution of known concentration in a titration.

Burette: a long glass tube that has a tap at the bottom and is marked in 0.1 cm^3 divisions. It is used to deliver an accurate volume of liquid (the **titre**) to reach the **end point**.

End point: the point in a titration where the indicator changes colour.

Equivalence point: the point of neutralisation where the number of moles of acid and base are equal. This should ideally be the same as the **end point**.

Titre: the volume of standard solution needed to neutralise the analyte (i.e. to reach the end point of the titration).

Neutralisation occurs when an equal number of **moles** of H^+ (from an acid) and OH^- (from a base) react together to form water. If a strong acid, such as hydrochloric acid, reacts with a strong base, such as sodium hydroxide, in exactly equal proportions, the mixture will be neither acid nor base but neutral (pH 7.0). At this point an **indicator** will change colour. We use this in the process of **titration** to calculate the concentration of a solution of acid or base.

In titration we have one unknown – the number of moles in the **analyte**. We titrate this against the **standard solution**. Titration involves adding the standard solution from a **burette** to a known volume of the analyte in a conical flask until we reach the **end point** – when the indicator changes colour. This should be the **equivalence point**, where we have equal moles of acid and base. Because we know the concentration of the standard solution, we can use the **titre** to calculate how many moles were required to reach the equivalence point. This will tell us the number of moles of analyte in the flask and therefore the concentration of the analyte.

Test yourself

1. Explain the difference between the terms adsorption and absorption.
2. Explain what is meant by the mobile phase in chromatography.
3. Give two examples of a stationary phase.
4. Explain the similarities and differences between column chromatography and HPLC.
5. State the meaning of the following terms:
   a. titre
   b. end point
   c. equivalence point.

Project practice

You have been asked to prepare visuals for a school outreach display that your company is supporting.

Choose one of the following themes and prepare a poster or PowerPoint illustrating how this is relevant to your workplace. Use resources from the internet where necessary.
- ▶ 'The right material for the job' – the ways in which different types of material are suited to particular applications in science or healthcare.
- ▶ 'Not just a corrosive liquid' – the importance of strong and weak acids in industry, foodstuffs and analysis.
- ▶ 'Time is money' – the importance of rates of reaction in industrial processes.
- ▶ 'What's in my lunch?' – the use of chemical analysis to test the quality and purity of the food and drink we consume.

Your presentation should include at least one graph, chart or diagram to help illustrate the relevance of your theme to your workplace.

Assessment practice

1. Explain the reasons for the properties and the uses of the following metals:
   a. Sodium is soft and low density, but iron is hard and high density.
   b. Sodium reacts vigorously with cold water, but iron only reacts very slowly with water.
   c. Copper is used to make electric wiring.
   d. Copper is used to make pipes in central heating systems.
2. The table shows a range of applications with the corresponding material. For each combination, select the appropriate explanation for why the material is suited to the application.
   A. Lightweight, can be formed into wires (ductile) good electrical conductor
   B. Lightweight, strong
   C. Strong, can be moulded into shape (malleable)
   D. Inert, strong and can be moulded into shape
   E. Transparent, inert, heat-resistant
   F. Strong, inert, very heat resistant
   G. Strong, can be formed into shape, non-conductor of electricity

Application	Material	Explanation (letter)
Body panel for budget-priced car	Steel	
Body panel for high performance sportscar	Carbon fibre composite	
Bottle for storage of corrosive liquids	High density polyethene (HDPE)	
Crucible for heating solids at high temperatures	Clay ceramic	
Flask for use in reflux where the contents are heated for a prolonged period	Borosilicate glass	
Insulator for use in high-voltage power lines	Clay ceramic	
Cable for use in high-voltage overhead power lines	Aluminium	

3. Use the periodic table to complete the following table.

Element	Group	Period
Sodium		
Magnesium		
Iron		
Nitrogen		
Neon		

4. Classify the following as to whether they are (i) strong or weak and (ii) concentrated or dilute:
   a. a 5 mol/dm^3 solution of ethanoic acid
   b. a 0.001 mol/dm^3 solution of hydrochloric acid
   c. a 10 mol/dm^3 solution of sulfuric acid.
5. Name the salts that would be produced by mixing each of the following pairs of acid and base:
   a. nitric acid and calcium hydroxide
   b. sulfuric acid and barium nitrate
   c. hydrochloric acid and ammonia
   d. ethanoic acid and potassium hydroxide.
6. One method of preparing a salt involves adding an excess of insoluble substance such as a metal, metal oxide, metal hydroxide or metal carbonate to an acid. Suggest how you could prepare a solution of copper sulfate from insoluble copper oxide and sulfuric acid. Explain the advantage of this method over mixing an acid and a soluble base.
7. Collision theory states that particles with sufficient energy must collide in order to react.
   a. Explain why increasing the concentration of reactants in solution will increase the rate of reaction.

b Suggest why increasing the temperature has a bigger effect on rate of reaction than increasing the concentration.

8 You have been asked to analyse the amino acids in a food supplement to show that it contains the amino acid lysine.

   a Outline how you would use TLC with ninhydrin spray and a pure sample of lysine to do this.

   b You find that the food supplement contains two spots. The impurity spot moves a shorter distance than lysine. What can you tell about the properties of this impurity?

   c Describe how you could use chromatography to obtain a sample of the impurity for further analysis.

9 You have been asked to analyse a sample of petrol to see if it is contaminated. You are provided with a pure sample of the potential contaminant.

   a Explain how you could use GC to show that the contaminant was present in the sample.

   b Explain how you could use MS coupled to GC to identify an unknown contaminant in the sample.

10 Describe how you would determine the percentage purity of the following:

   a crude pellets of sodium hydroxide

   b a volatile compound for use in food flavouring using gas chromatography.

B1.45–B1.64: Core science concepts: Physics

Introduction

Physics is the study of atoms, particles, energy, forces, mechanics and waves – in fact, the whole physical universe.

There is overlap with chemistry in places – atomic structure, for example. The overlap with biology is less obvious, but biophysics is an important part of modern biology. It uses physical methods to understand the interactions between biological molecules and within biological systems. Also, physics is based very firmly on a foundation of mathematics. In fact, mechanics is often an option in mathematics courses and the difference between theoretical physics and applied mathematics can be hard to spot! The field of medical physics is another important area of overlap, where physics contributes to treatment and diagnosis.

Whichever way you look at it, a good understanding of physics is important for work in many areas of science, healthcare and engineering.

Learning outcomes

The core knowledge outcomes that you must understand and learn:

Electricity
B1.45 the definitions of, and how to calculate, charge and current using $Q = It$
B1.46 the definitions of, and how to calculate, current, potential difference and resistance, using Ohm's law $V = IR$
B1.47 how to calculate total resistance of multiple fixed resistors in a series and parallel circuit
B1.48 the difference between alternating and direct current
B1.49 the properties of mains electricity in the UK

Magnetism and electromagnetism
B1.50 magnetism and magnetic poles
B1.51 magnetic fields
B1.52 the uses of electromagnetism and electromagnets

Waves
B1.53 the definition of a wave
B1.54 the relationship between frequency, wavelength and speed using the wave equation $v = f\lambda$
B1.55 the properties of longitudinal and transverse waves
B1.56 the uses of different types of waves

Particles and radiation
B1.57 the types and properties of ionising radiation
B1.58 the definitions of half-life and count-rate
B1.59 the main types of radioactive decay in relation to unstable nuclei
B1.60 how radiation interacts with matter
B1.61 the applications of radioactivity within the health and science sector

Units
B1.62 the use of the international system of units (SI)
B1.63 how to convert between units
B1.64 the importance of using significant figures and science notation.

Electricity

Electricity in the home, laboratory or industry is usually **alternating current (AC)**. However, low-voltage lighting circuits or anything that you plug into a 5 V USB power supply (like a phone charger) will use **direct current** or **DC**.

We now know that an electric **current** is caused by a flow of electrons, i.e. from negative to positive poles of a battery or power supply. However, electricity and electric currents were discovered long before electrons. Investigators realised that something was flowing – which they called **current** – but did not know what it was. They decided that it must flow from positive to negative.

Although we understand electricity better now, we still follow this convention. You will sometimes see this described as **conventional current**, to distinguish it from flow of electrons. There has been so much work done assuming that current flows from positive to negative that we would have to rewrite too many formulae and textbooks!

> **Reflect**
>
> Why are electrons negative and protons positive? What do we mean by positive and negative?
>
> Those are philosophical questions that we could spend hours thinking about. But what is important is the fact that electrons and protons have *opposite* charges, and we just call one 'negative' and the other 'positive'.

B1.45 The definitions of, and how to calculate, charge and current using Q = It

The size of the **current** is the rate of flow of **charge**. That means that when current (I) flows past a given point in a circuit for a length of time (t), we can calculate the charge (Q) that has flowed past this point using the formula:

$$Q = I \times t$$

Where Q is in **coulombs**, I is in amps and t is in seconds. This can be rearranged to give:

$$I = \frac{Q}{t}$$

In other words, current equals charge divided by time. This is the amount of coulombs of charge per second, which is the rate of flow of charge, which is the definition of current!.

To give an example, if a battery charger passes a current of 3.0 A through a rechargeable cell (battery) for a period of two hours, the total charge transferred to the cell can be calculated (don't forget to convert hours to seconds!):

$$Q = I \times t = 3.0 \times (2 \times 60 \times 60) = 21\,600\,C$$

> **Key terms**
>
> **Charge:** a fundamental property of many subatomic particles. Electrons, by convention, have a negative charge. The unit of charge is the **coulomb (C)** and the symbol is Q.
>
> **Coulomb (C):** the unit of charge. **Current** is the rate of flow of charge past a given point in a circuit, i.e. how fast it flows past. The unit of current is the ampere (A), often shortened to 'amp', and the symbol is I.

B1.46 The definitions of, and how to calculate, current, potential difference and resistance, using Ohm's law V = IR

The relationship between **current**, **potential difference** and **resistance** is one of the most useful concepts in electronics:

$$V = I \times R$$

Potential difference (**voltage**) is the driving force that causes charge to flow round a circuit. It is defined as the electrical work done per unit of charge flowing through components in the circuit. The unit of potential difference is the volt (V) and the symbol is also V. Potential difference is often abbreviated to 'p.d.'.

Resistance is the property of any component of a circuit that slows the flow of current. The unit of resistance is the ohm (Ω) and the symbol is R.

To calculate the current that is flowing in a circuit with resistance $3\,\Omega$ and a potential difference of 12 V, we simply rearrange the formula and substitute the values:

$$I = \frac{V}{R} = \frac{12}{3} = 4\,A$$

B1.47 How to calculate total resistance of multiple fixed resistors in a series and parallel circuit

For resistors connected in **series**, the total potential difference (p.d.) of the supply is shared between the components (see Figure 13.1) and the current through each component is the same (see Figure 13.2).

> **Key terms**
>
> **Series:** circuits where the components are connected in line, end to end between the positive and negative terminals of the power supply. See Figure 13.1 for an example of a series circuit.
>
> **Parallel circuits:** where the components are each connected separately to the positive and negative terminals of the power supply. See Figure 13.3 for an example of a parallel circuit.

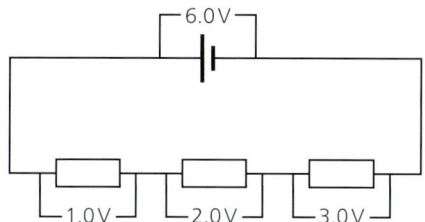

▲ Figure 13.1 Circuit diagram showing p.d. across resistors connected in series

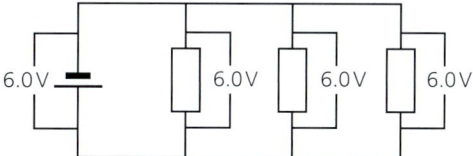

▲ Figure 13.2 Circuit diagram showing current in series circuits

When resistors are connected in series, the total resistance is equal to the sum of the individual resistors, so the total resistance of a circuit with n resistors is given by:

$$R_{total} = R_1 + R_2 + R_n$$

In **parallel circuits**, the p.d. across each route is the same (see Figure 13.3) and the total current through the whole circuit is the sum of the currents passing through each of these possible routes (see Figure 13.4).

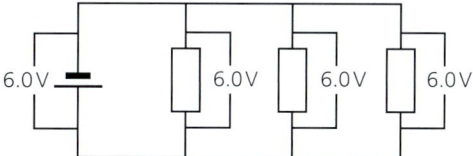

▲ Figure 13.3 Circuit diagram showing sharing of p.d.s in parallel circuits

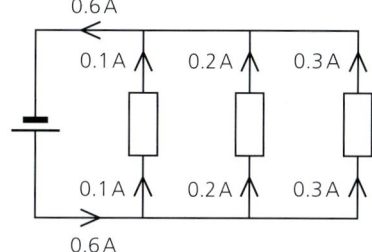

▲ Figure 13.4 Circuit diagram showing sharing of current in parallel circuits

When single resistors are connected in parallel, the potential difference across each will be the same, but the total resistance will be less than the sum of all the resistances. The total resistance is given by:

$$\frac{1}{R_{total}} = \frac{1}{R_1} + \frac{1}{R_2} + \frac{1}{R_n}$$

So, if three resistors of 5 Ω, 10 Ω and 15 Ω are connected in parallel to a power supply we can calculate the total resistance of the circuit by substituting the numbers in the equation:

$$\frac{1}{R_{total}} = \frac{1}{R_1} + \frac{1}{R_2} + \frac{1}{R_3} = \frac{1}{5} + \frac{1}{10} + \frac{1}{15} = 0.37$$

Therefore, rearrange this to find R_{total}:

$$R_{total} = \frac{1}{0.37} = 2.7\,\Omega$$

B1.48 The difference between alternating and direct current

In **direct current**, DC, the **conventional current** constantly flows in one direction from the positive terminal to the negative terminal – although we now know that it is electrons flowing from negative to positive.

Alternating current, AC, as used in the mains electric supply in the UK and most other countries, has current that constantly changes direction alternating potential difference where the positive and negative ends alternating.

B1.49 The properties of mains electricity in the UK

By using alternating current, it is possible to transmit electricity over long distances at high voltages – between 275 kV and 400 kV (1 kV = 1000 V). This reduces the current and so less electrical energy is **dissipated** (scientific term for wasted) as heat.

The high voltage used for transmission can then be transformed to a lower voltage of 230 V for supplying to residences and businesses, and higher voltages can be supplied to businesses with a greater demand for energy.

The frequency of mains electricity in Europe is 50 Hz (see page 281), which means there are 50 cycles per second. This is the frequency at which electricity is generated.

Test yourself

1. What do the following terms mean?
   a. current
   b. potential difference (voltage)
   c. resistance.
2. 1.2 C of charge flows through a light bulb in a time of 30 s. Calculate the current flowing through the bulb.
3. A 9 V battery is connected to a 4 Ω resistor. Calculate the current flowing through the resistor.
4. Two more resistors of 5 Ω and 6 Ω are added in parallel with the 4 Ω resistor.
   a. Calculate the total resistance.
   b. What voltage battery would you need to use to maintain the same current as in question 3?

Magnetism and electromagnetism

We are all familiar with **magnets** and **magnetism**. The earth's **magnetic field** causes a compass needle to point towards the (magnetic) north pole. Magnetic fields are invisible, but we can see their effects all around us. A fridge magnet holds notes, family photos or children's artwork on a fridge door. Magnetic clasps are used on handbags and briefcases. Magnets have many other uses and **electromagnets** are particularly useful in science and engineering.

Key terms

Magnet: a material or object that produces a magnetic field.

Magnetism: the force experienced by some types of metals in the earth's magnetic field or in a magnetic field of a magnet. It is also defined as the attractive or repulsive force produced by a moving electric charge.

Magnetic field: a region where magnetic materials experience a force.

Electromagnet: produced when a current flows through a coil of wire.

B1.50 Magnetism and magnetic poles

All magnets have two **poles**, **north** (or north-seeking) and **south** (or south-seeking). These are determined by whether the pole points towards the earth's magnetic north pole (north-seeking) or south pole (south-seeking). For this reason, we call magnets **dipoles**. However, if you cut a magnet in half, you produce two smaller dipoles – you cannot produce a magnetic **monopole** (just a north or south pole).

The north and south poles of a magnet are where the magnetic forces are strongest because the **magnetic field** is strongest. When magnets are placed close together, they will **attract** or **repel** each other, even if they are not touching. For this reason, we say that magnetism is a **non-contact force**. Other types of non-contact force include:

- electrostatic force – opposite charges attract, even if they are not in contact
- weight – objects with mass attract each other and the greater the mass, the greater the attraction. A satellite falling out of orbit does not have to be in contact with the earth to feel the attractive force of the earth's gravity.

If we place two north poles or two south poles close together, they will repel each other. If we place north and south poles together, they will attract each other.

There are two types of magnet: **permanent** and **induced**. A permanent magnet produces its own magnetic field. If we bring a **magnetic material** close to a permanent magnet, the magnetic material becomes an induced magnet. It has its own induced poles and magnetic field (Figure 13.5).

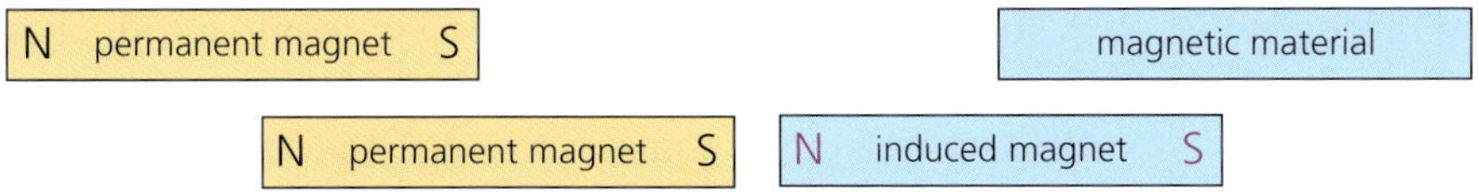

▲ Figure 13.5 A permanent magnet causes magnetic material to become an induced magnet when they are placed close together. **N** and **S** are induced poles

> **Key terms**
>
> *Permanent magnet:* produces its own magnetic field.
>
> *Induced magnet:* an object that can become a magnet when it is placed in a magnetic field.
>
> *Magnetic materials:* such as iron, steel, nickel and cobalt will experience an attractive force when placed in a magnetic field.
>
> *Lines of magnetic flux:* indicate the direction and strength of a **magnetic field**.

If the induced magnet is removed from the magnetic field of the permanent magnet, it will quickly lose most or all of its magnetism.

B1.51 Magnetic fields

We cannot see a magnetic field, but we can see its effect using iron filings (Figure 13.6). The small pieces of iron act as temporary magnets and line up along the magnetic field lines, also called **lines of magnetic flux**. This means that we can see the shape of the magnetic field.

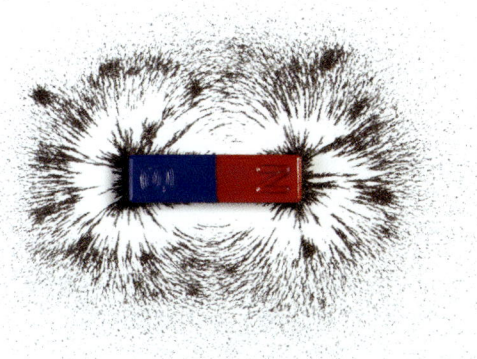

▲ Figure 13.6 Iron filings reveal the invisible lines of flux around a bar magnet

The iron filings allow us to see the shape of the field, but they do not show the direction of the lines of flux. We can plot the magnetic field lines around a bar magnet using a **compass needle**. The north pole of the magnet in the compass needle will always point towards the south pole of the bar magnet and away from the north pole. We can use this to plot the flux lines of the field around a bar magnet (Figure 13.7). If we move the compass far enough away from the bar magnet, it will point to the earth's north pole.

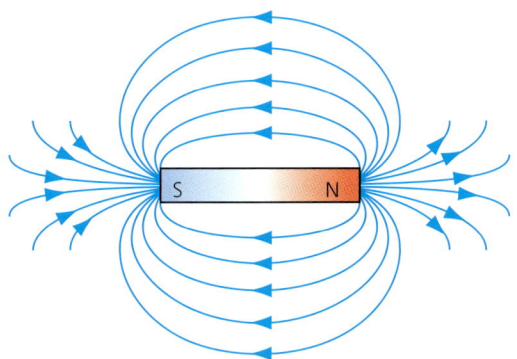

Field lines around a bar magnet

▲ Figure 13.7 Flux lines for a bar magnet. The lines are closest together near the poles, showing where the field is strongest

We follow the convention that the flux lines always go from north to south, indicated by the arrows on the lines in Figure 13.7. You can see how the flux lines are closest together near the two poles. This is where the magnetic field is strongest. Another way to describe the strength of the magnetic field is the **magnetic flux density**, which is defined as the number of magnetic flux lines that pass through an area of $1\,m^2$.

> **Reflect**
>
> The north pole of the magnet in a compass needle points towards the south pole of a bar magnet. But the north pole of the compass needle points towards the geographic north pole of the earth.
>
> Does this mean that the earth generates its own magnetic field? If so, does it mean that the south pole of this 'magnet' is at the geographic north pole?

If you place a compass next to a wire carrying an electric current, you will see the compass needle move as you move the compass around the wire.

This must mean that the current flowing through the wire is generating a magnetic field; you are using the compass needle to trace the magnetic flux lines around the wire.

If you reverse the flow of current in the wire you will notice that the compass needle now points in the opposite direction. We can therefore tell that the direction of the magnetic field has reversed (Figure 13.8).

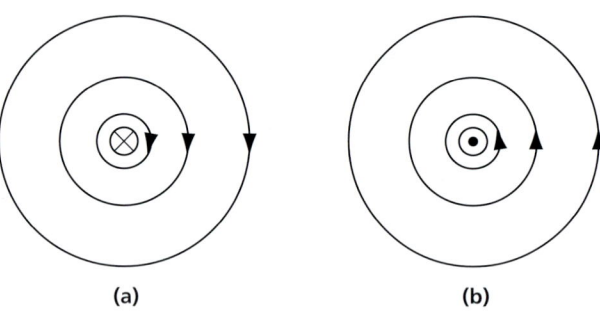

▲ Figure 13.8 The magnetic flux lines of a wire carrying a current. Symbols inside the wire indicate the direction of the current. In (a) the current is flowing into the page – away from you – and in (b) the current is flowing out of the page – towards you

From this we can conclude that moving charges (the electric current) generate a magnetic field. This phenomenon is of great importance in physics, engineering, electronics and many areas of our everyday lives.

Notice that the magnetic flux lines get further apart as the distance from the wire increases. This must mean that the strength of the field decreases as distance from the wire increases.

If we increase the size of the current flowing through the wire, we will see that the magnetic flux lines get closer together. Therefore, the greater the current, the stronger the magnetic field.

B1.52 The uses of electromagnetism and electromagnets

The magnetic field generated by a current flowing through a wire can be used to make magnets that can be switched on or off – these are **electromagnets**.

A **solenoid** is created by wrapping wire into a coil. This increases the strength (flux density) of the magnetic field when a current passes through the coil of wire (Figure 13.9). All the magnetic flux lines around each loop of wire line up with each other. This results in lots of flux lines all pointing in the same direction, very close to each other.

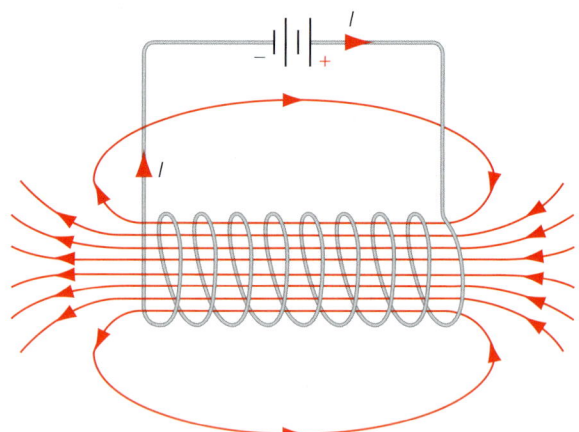

▲ Figure 13.9 The magnetic field generated by a solenoid

Note how close together the magnetic flux lines are in the centre of the solenoid. This means that this is where the magnetic field is strongest. Outside the coil, the magnetic field is just like the one around a bar magnet (Figure 13.7).

You can increase the strength of the magnetic field of the solenoid even more by placing an iron bar in the centre of the coil. This iron core becomes an induced magnet when the current flows – we have made an electromagnet. When the current is switched off, the magnetic field disappears.

A **portative** electromagnet is designed to hold material in place. An example is the type of electromagnet used for lifting materials made of iron or steel in a scrapyard.

A **tractive** electromagnet is one that applies a force and moves another object. An example is a simple solenoid where the coil surrounds a plunger. When the current is switched on, the solenoid applies a force to the plunger making it move. This can be used in many different ways, such as in valves or switches.

B1.45–B1.64: Core science concepts: Physics

Electromagnetic induction

> ### Key terms
>
> **Ammeter:** measures the flow of current; always connected in series. **Voltmeters** measure the potential difference in a circuit and are always connected in parallel.
>
> **Electromotive force (emf):** like **potential difference**, except that it refers to power supplies such as cells (batteries), generators or mains power supplies. These transfer other forms of energy, such as light energy or kinetic energy, into electrical energy. The unit of emf is also the volt (V).
>
> **Generator effect:** when a **potential difference** (voltage) is induced in a wire that experiences a change in magnetic field.

Electromagnetic induction can be demonstrated using the apparatus shown in Figures 13.10 and 13.11.

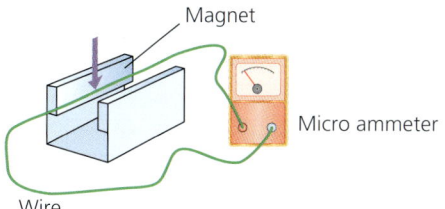

▲ Figure 13.11 Moving a wire into a magnetic field induces a potential difference

Figure 13.11 shows that, as the length of wire moves between the two magnets, the micro ammeter will flick in one direction when the wire moves down and in the opposite direction when the wire moves up. In this case, a potential difference is induced in the wire because there is a moving electric charge (the electrons in the wire) **perpendicular** (at a 90-degree angle) to the magnetic field and they experience a force. This causes them to move towards one end of the wire, creating a potential difference across the wire.

The principle of electromagnetic induction is the basis of the **generator effect** and is used in dynamos and alternators to generate an electric current (Figure 13.12).

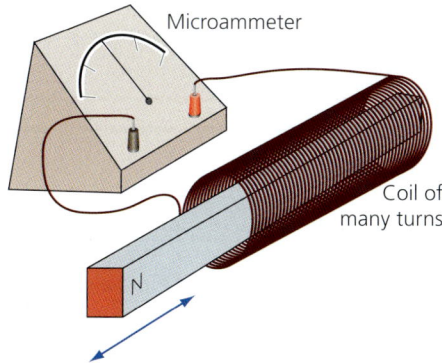

▲ Figure 13.10 Using a moving magnet to produce a potential difference

Figure 13.10 shows that if you move the bar magnet into the coil, you will see the needle on the micro **ammeter** flick in one direction and then in the opposite direction when the magnet is pulled out. The reading will be zero when the magnet is stationary. As the magnet moves, lines of magnetic flux are being crossed by the wires in the coil. Therefore, moving the magnet into the coil induces a potential difference. Providing the circuit is complete, this induces a current resulting in the reading on the microammeter. Moving the magnet back out causes the induced potential difference to change direction and therefore the current flow changes direction. The effect is the same if you move the coil and keep the magnet still.

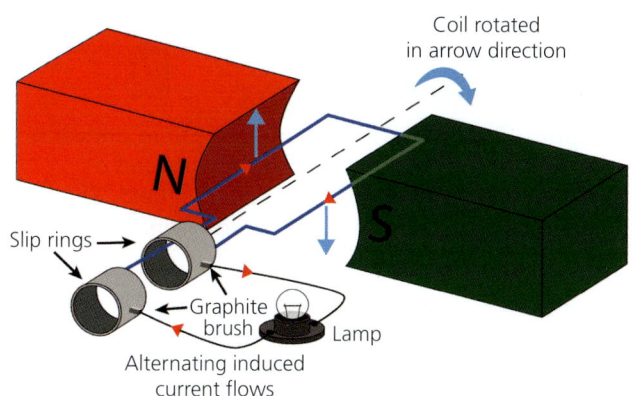

▲ Figure 13.12 A simple alternator

The motor effect

When a current passes through a wire placed in a magnetic field, it moves because a force acts on it. When a current passes through a wire, we know it induces a magnetic field. This results in the wire exerting a magnetic force onto the permanent magnet. When the current-carrying wire is placed in between the two poles of the magnet the magnetic fluxes combine to form what is known as a **catapult field**. This field exerts a force on the wire causing it to move. Figure 13.13 (a) shows the lines of magnetic flux between the poles of two magnets and Figure 13.13 (b) shows the lines of magnetic flux around the current-carrying wire.

265

Healthcare Science T Level: Core

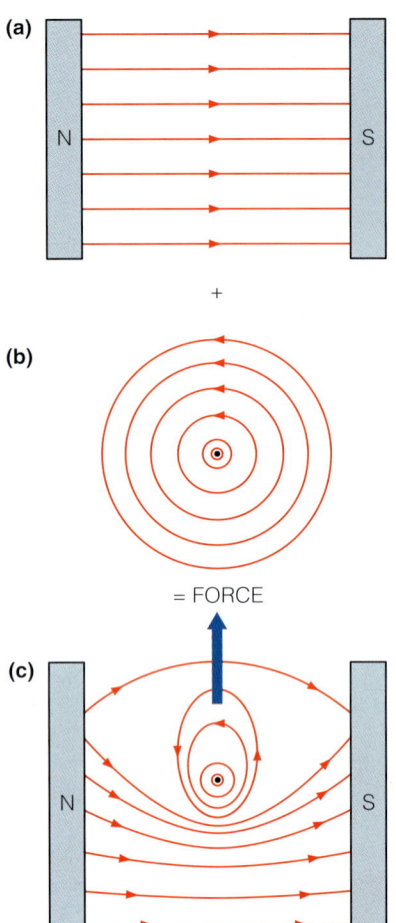

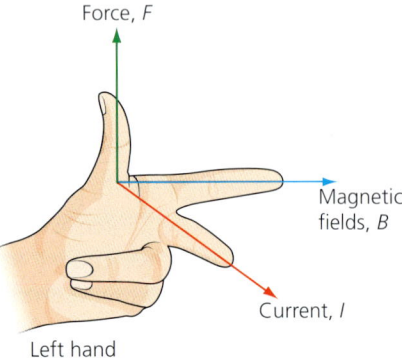

▲ Figure 13.13 (a) A uniform magnetic field between two poles of a magnet; (b) the field around a current-carrying wire; (c) the catapult field. The force is from the strong field (greater flux density) to the weak field (lower flux density)

You can use Fleming's left-hand rule (Figure 13.14) to work out the direction of the force on the wire.

▲ Figure 13.14 Fleming's left-hand rule. Using your left hand, point your first finger in the direction of the field, your second finger in the direction of the current and your thumb will point in the direction of the force (motion)

As the name suggests, the **motor effect** is the basis of electric motors (Figure 13.15).

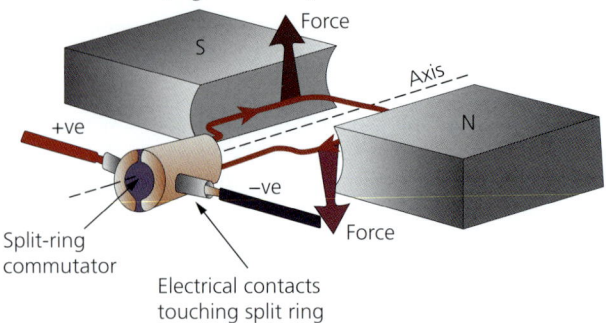

▲ Figure 13.15 A DC electric motor. The current flowing in the wires means they experience a force perpendicular to the magnetic field. The split-ring commutator reverses the current every half turn to ensure the motor keeps turning in the same direction

Key term

Motor effect: when a current-carrying wire is placed between magnetic poles. The magnetic field around the wire interacts with the magnetic field it is placed in. This causes the wire and magnet to exert a force on each other and can cause the wire to move.

Reflect

Look at Figure 13.14 and use Fleming's left-hand rule to work out the direction of the magnetic field. Is that the direction you expect? It is always worth checking your answer!

Induction heating

Induction heating has many applications. Perhaps the most familiar is the 'induction hob' used to heat saucepans in domestic and commercial kitchens. An electronic oscillator passes a high-frequency alternating current through an electromagnet. This generates a rapidly alternating magnetic field. If a pan made of iron or steel is on the hob then currents, known as **eddy currents**, are generated inside the conductor (the pan). These currents generate heat which will then heat the contents of the pan.

Induction heating has the advantage that the heat is generated inside the object itself, so it is rapid. Also, it does not rely on conduction from an external heat source, such as a naked flame in a gas hob or a hot element in a traditional electric hob. This means that the hob becomes hot only because of being in contact with the hot pan and cools quickly once the pan is removed. It is therefore safer in many ways than using naked flame or a traditional electric hob, since heating does not occur without the conductor.

There are many other applications of induction heating, particularly in manufacturing, including:
- welding and brazing
- induction furnaces to produce molten metals
- cap sealing of containers in food and pharmaceutical industries
- heat treatment (e.g. hardening) of metals.

Research

There are many uses for permanent and temporary magnetic materials such as iron, steel, cobalt and nickel.

There are also many applications of electromagnets in electric and electromechanical devices:
- transformers
- motors, generators, alternators
- loudspeakers and microphones
- induction heating
- MRI machines
- cranes and sorting or separation equipment used in recycling
- relays.

Select a number of these applications and see if you can find others. For each, research the application and how our understanding of the topics covered in this section has allowed advances in technology. In particular, think about:
- the type of magnetic material used – permanent or temporary
- how the type of material relates to its function
- is this an example of the generator effect, motor effect or magnetic induction?
- for electromagnets:
  - does the material affect the properties of the electromagnet?
  - is the electromagnet tractive, portative or neither?

Test yourself

1. Explain the difference between a permanent magnet and an induced magnet.
2. What is the convention for drawing flux lines of a magnetic field?
3. How do flux lines indicate the strength of a magnetic field?
4. Describe how you would make an electromagnet.
5. Explain the difference between portative and tractive electromagnets.

Waves

We learn about waves from an early age – a toddler dropping a pebble into a still pond and watching the ripples is observing waves. Studying waves in water can help us understand a lot about how waves behave. However, watching waves crashing onto a shore, or even just watching the tide come in on the beach, can give us a misleading impression of what a wave is.

Key terms

Amplitude: the maximum displacement of any point from the equilibrium position (Figure 13.16).

Frequency: in Hz, the number of complete waves that pass a given point in one second (Figure 13.17). One complete wave is a **cycle**, so a frequency of 1 Hz corresponds to one cycle per second. This is a very low frequency, so you will often see frequency measured in kHz (kilohertz, 10^3 Hz), MHz (megahertz, 10^6 Hz) or GHz (gigahertz, 10^9 Hz).

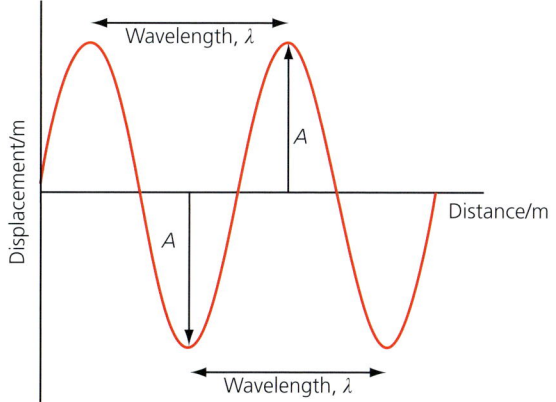

▲ Figure 13.16 Wave terminology. A represents the amplitude. This is an example of a transverse wave

Healthcare Science T Level: Core

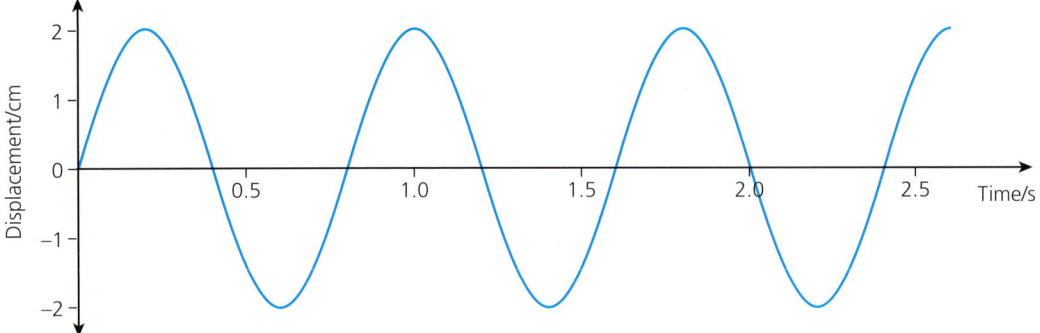

▲ Figure 13.17 If you measure from one peak to the next peak you can calculate that the **frequency** is 1.25 Hz. You will get the same answer if you measure from trough to trough

B1.53 The definition of a wave

Waves transfer **energy** from one energy store to another, they do not transfer **matter** (e.g. objects or water, for example). For example, electromagnetic waves transfer energy from the nuclear store of energy in the Sun to the thermal store of energy on Earth. This is why waves crashing onto the shore can be misleading. When waves travel through a medium (e.g. the ocean) the particles in the medium (i.e. water molecules) **oscillate** (move up and down). However, the particles stay in the same place, only the energy is transferred. When the wave hits the beach, things change, because now the particles of water are interacting with the particles of sand, and the wave is changed into a movement of the water – and anything floating in it, which is why things get washed up on the beach by the waves.

B1.54 The relationship between frequency, wavelength and speed using the wave equation $v = f\lambda$

The speed of a wave is a measure of how fast energy is transferred. More simply, it is the speed the wave is moving at. The relationship between wave speed, frequency and **wavelength** is the same for all types of wave and is given by the wave equation:

$$v = f\lambda$$

where:

v = wave speed in m/s

f = frequency in Hz

λ = wavelength in m.

For example, radio waves travel at the speed of light (approx. 3.0×10^8 m/s). A radio station transmits at a frequency of 92.3 MHz, calculate the wavelength of the radio waves.

$92.3 \text{ MHz} = 92.3 \times 10^6 \text{ Hz} = 9.23 \times 10^7 \text{ Hz}$

Rearrange the equation above to give:

$$\lambda = \frac{v}{f}$$

So

$$\lambda = \frac{30 \times 10^8}{9.23^7} = 3.25 \text{ m}$$

Key term

Wavelength: the distance between the same point in successive cycles. For example, the distance from the peak of one wave to the peak of the next wave (Figure 13.16). The standard unit of wavelength is the metre, m. However, **electromagnetic** waves can have wavelengths from 10^4 m to 10^{-15} m, so you will often see wavelengths expressed in units such as **nanometres**, nm. (1nm = 1×10^{-9} m – see section B1.63, page 277 for more about units.)

B1.55 The properties of longitudinal and transverse waves

There are two types of wave, **transverse** and **longitudinal**.

Most waves are **transverse**, where the waves transfer energy in a direction at right angles to the direction in which the particles are vibrating. This means the oscillations are **perpendicular** (at right angles) to the direction of energy transfer (Figure 13.16). The particles move away from and towards the horizontal line – this is represented by the arrow 'A' (for amplitude) – so the energy transfer is in the forward direction even though the particles just move from side to side, or up and down, depending on how you look at the wave.

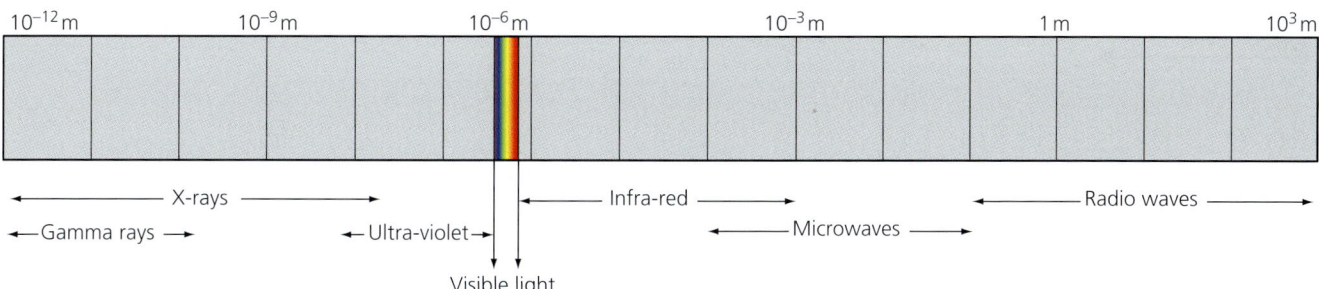

▲ Figure 13.18 The **electromagnetic spectrum**

> **Key terms**
>
> *Electromagnetic spectrum:* describes all the different types of electromagnetic waves. The properties of the different types of waves vary considerably, so we usually consider the spectrum as seven groups, with slight overlaps (Figure 13.18).
>
> *Electromagnetic waves:* include gamma rays, X-rays, visible light, microwaves and radio waves. Their energy is carried by oscillating electric and magnetic fields.

Examples of transverse waves include:
- all **electromagnetic waves**, e.g. light, radio waves, X-rays (Figure 13.18)
- ripples in a pond or waves in the ocean
- a wave on a string, e.g. a violin or guitar string that is made to vibrate when it is bowed or plucked.

Electromagnetic waves are a little more complicated because the wave represents changes in the electric and magnetic fields, but the principles are the same.

Longitudinal waves transfer energy in the same direction in which the particles are vibrating. This means that the oscillations are **parallel** to the direction of energy transfer. These oscillations create **compressions** (where the particles get closer together) and **rarefactions** (where the particles move further apart) (Figure 13.19).

Examples of longitudinal waves include:
- sound waves moving in air
- **ultrasound** (very high-frequency sound waves) that move through materials, for example:
  – metals, when used to detect cracks in components or structures
  – the body, when used in medical imaging such as scans in pregnancy
- **shock waves**, such as some types of **seismic** waves (produced by earthquakes).

> **Reflect**
>
> You can use a metal spring such as a Slinky to demonstrate both transverse and longitudinal waves (Figure 13.20).
> - If you lay the spring out on a surface, hold it at one end and wiggle it from side to side, you will see a transverse wave move along the length of the spring.
> - If you push the end of the spring quickly back and forward, you will see a longitudinal wave move along the length of the Slinky.
>
> Does a longitudinal wave in the Slinky explain why, when you speak, the sound waves travel through the air, but they do not create a vacuum in your mouth?

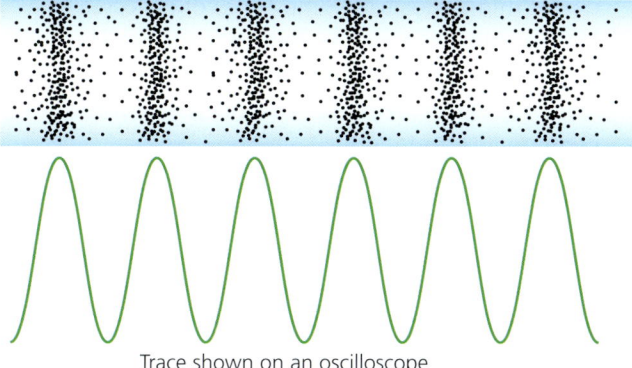

Trace shown on an oscilloscope

▲ Figure 13.19 Changes in air pressure at a microphone diaphragm, measured over a period of time

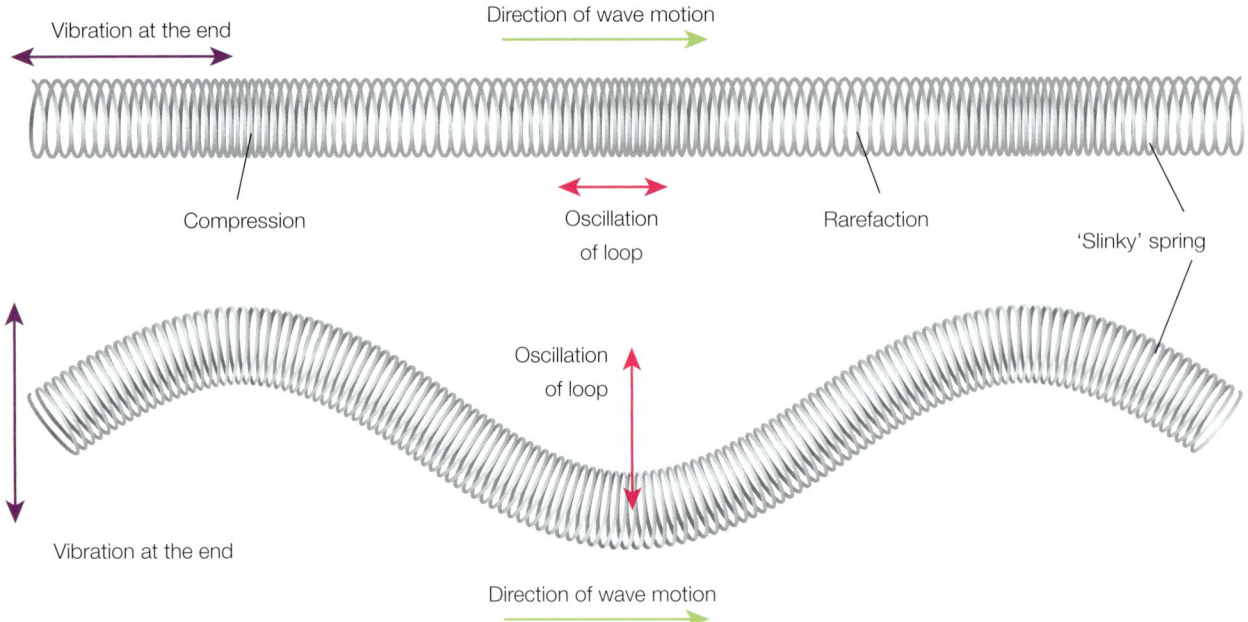

▲ Figure 13.20 Longitudinal (top) and transverse (bottom) waves in a Slinky spring

B1.56 The uses of different types of waves

Waves transfer energy, but they can also transfer information. The simplest example is signalling, using beacon fires to send warnings or flashlights to send signals using Morse code – light waves are being used to transfer information.

Communication

Radio waves are probably a better example of the use of waves in communication. Since the pioneering experiments of Marconi, we now use radio waves for many different types of communication. You can probably think of many more examples than these:
▶ TV and radio broadcasts (although not satellite TV – see below)
▶ wireless broadband (WiFi).
▶ Bluetooth® and other wireless technologies used in computing and control systems.

Microwaves have a slightly shorter wavelength/higher frequency than radio waves but can also be used for short-range radio communication. A major use of microwaves now is in satellite communication, including satellite TV. This uses microwaves of a wavelength that is not absorbed by water molecules in the atmosphere.

Medical uses

There are numerous examples of the use of waves of different types in science and medicine:
▶ X-rays are used in different types of imaging from a simple X-ray taken to show a broken bone to the much more complex CT (computerised tomography or CAT) scan. A CT scan can build up a three-dimensional image of the whole body or part of the body.
▶ Gamma rays are used for cancer treatment, to kill cancer cells.
▶ Gamma rays can also be used to sterilise medical instruments and equipment.
▶ Ultrasound is used in scanning, particularly to create images of soft tissues that don't show up well on X-rays such as the heart, liver, kidneys, gallbladder and major blood vessels. This can be useful in diagnosis of some types of cancer.
▶ Ultrasound can also be used for cleaning. The high-frequency sound waves help to dislodge dirt from objects as diverse as jewellery, electronic components and medical equipment.

Food processing

We saw in section B1.52 how magnetic induction can be used for heating in both domestic and commercial food processing. Waves are also important in food processing:

- Infrared heating uses electromagnetic radiation with a longer wavelength than visible light:
  - Heat lamps to keep food hot before serving, for instance, in canteens.
  - Infrared ovens, particularly small ones, heat up more rapidly than conventional electric or gas ovens.
- Microwave heating can be used for cooking and reheating food. This uses microwaves of a different wavelength to satellite communication. In microwave heating, energy from the microwaves is absorbed by water molecules in the food. This transfers the energy to the water molecules, causing them to heat up. The energy is then transferred to the rest of the food by heating, which quickly cooks the food.
- Gamma radiation can be used in food preservation (see section B1.61).

Reflect

You are at a festival listening to a band and realise that the lead guitar produces high-frequency sounds, while the bass guitar produces low-frequency sounds. Also, you can tell that the drum kit is similar – the hi-hat cymbals produce high-frequency sounds and the bass drum produces low-frequency sounds. In spite of that, you hear all the different sounds at the right times – this band has rehearsed!

What does that tell you about the relationship between frequency and speed of sound?

Could you devise an experiment to test your hypothesis?

Test yourself

1. What is meant by the frequency of a wave?
2. What are the units of frequency used for waves?
3. A student was studying waves in a swimming pool of 25 m in length. They created a wave that had a frequency of 5 Hz and wavelength of 0.05 m. Calculate how long, in seconds, the wave would take to travel the length of the pool.
4. Give two examples of transverse waves and one example of longitudinal waves.
5. Give two examples of the use of microwaves.

Particles and radiation

This is an area where chemistry and physics overlap. You will have learnt about the structure of the atom in section B1.33 and about subatomic particles in section B1.35 in the chapter on chemistry. Knowledge of these subatomic particles helps us understand the basis of radiation and radioactive decay.

B1.57 The types and properties of ionising radiation

Key term

Ionising radiation: any form of radiation that interacts with matter, resulting in **ionisation** of that matter.

There are three types of ionising radiation that you need to know about: alpha (α), beta (β) and gamma (γ). The first two are types of particle, whereas gamma radiation is a form of electromagnetic radiation, mentioned in sections B1.55 and B1.56. It helps us understand the properties of these types of radiation if we understand their nature and origin.

Alpha radiation

Alpha particles are helium **nuclei** (plural of nucleus), meaning that they consist of two **protons** and two **neutrons** which give them a positive charge (+2). On the atomic scale, alpha particles are relatively large compared to beta particles (they have a relatively large mass). This means that they can easily remove electrons from atoms when they collide with them. This makes alpha radiation highly ionising.

However, because of their size, alpha particles do not penetrate materials very far – they are more likely to collide with atoms or nuclei of atoms. Alpha radiation can travel just 1–2 cm in air and can be absorbed by a sheet of paper.

Beta radiation

A beta particle is a fast-moving **electron**, therefore they have almost no mass (about 1800 times less than a proton) and a negative charge (−1). Beta particles are less ionising than alpha particles and can penetrate materials a moderate amount.

Beta radiation can travel approximately 15 cm in air and can be absorbed by a sheet of aluminium about 5 mm thick.

Gamma radiation

Unlike alpha and beta radiation, gamma radiation is a form of electromagnetic radiation – like X-rays or radio waves (see section B1.55). Gamma rays tend to pass through atoms rather than be absorbed by them. This makes them only weakly ionising, but with high penetrating power. Gamma rays have a range of many kilometres of air but can be absorbed by thick sheets of lead or several metres of concrete.

B1.58 The definitions of half-life and count-rate

Key terms

Radioactive decay: the random process that occurs when an unstable nucleus (see B1.34, page 247) loses energy by giving out **alpha** or **beta** particles or **gamma** radiation.

Ionisation: the formation of charged particles from neutral molecules or atoms by adding or removing electrons.

Activity: the rate at which a radioactive source decays. The unit of activity is the **becquerel** (Bq) where 1Bq = 1 decay per second. **Count-rate** is the number of radioactive decays recorded each second. You can see that activity and count-rate can be used interchangeably.

Half-life: the time taken for half the unstable nuclei in a sample to decay.

Radioactive decay is detected and measured by using a **Geiger-Muller tube** and counter – usually referred to as a **GM tube** or **Geiger counter**. This measures the radiation such as alpha particles, beta particles or gamma rays that are emitted when a radioactive source decays.

The rate at which a radioactive source decays can be plotted in a graph of activity against time or number of nuclei against time (Figure 13.21).

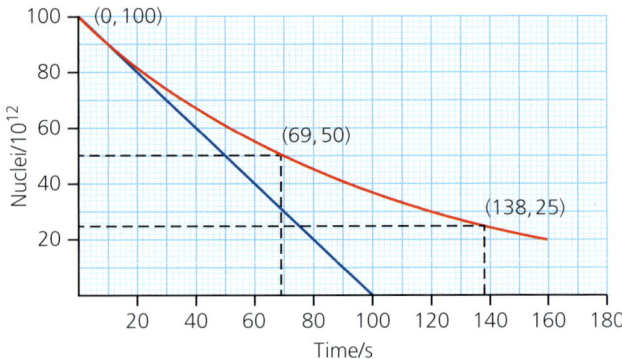

▲ Figure 13.21 A graph of radioactive decay showing how the number of nuclei decrease with time

There is a lot of useful information in Figure 13.21. First, we can see that the rate of radioactive decay (the **activity**) decreases with time. The tangent (blue line) is drawn at time = 0. If we measure the slope, we can calculate the rate of decay. Try drawing tangents at other times, such as 60s and 120s. You will see that the slope of the line is a maximum at time = 0 and then decreases. This shows that the rate of decay is decreasing. This is called an **exponential decay**.

Look at how the number of nuclei change with time. We start with 100×10^{12} nuclei but after 69s there are 50×10^{12} nuclei remaining – the number has reduced by half. After another 69s (at 138s) the number has reduced by half again to 25×10^{12} nuclei. This is characteristic of exponential decay: the time it takes for the number of nuclei to halve is constant. We call this the **half-life**, sometimes written as $T_{1/2}$.

We can make the same calculation from a graph where the y-axis (vertical axis) is **activity** rather than number of nuclei.

B1.59 The main types of radioactive decay in relation to unstable nuclei

There are two important facts about radioactive decay that you need to know:
1 Radioactive decay is **spontaneous**. Radioactive nuclei are **unstable**, which is why they decay. However, there is nothing that triggers decay.
2 Radioactive decay is **random**. We cannot predict which nucleus in a radioactive source will decay nor can we predict when it will decay.

As we saw in section B1.58, we can measure the half-life of a radioactive source and then use this to make predictions about the behaviour of the radioactive source, even though the decay is a random process.

Alpha decay

We saw in section B1.57 that an alpha particle consists of two neutrons and two protons and is equivalent to a helium nucleus. It is represented by the symbol $^{4}_{2}\text{He}$ in nuclear equations. The top number represents the mass number – the sum of the protons and the neutrons. The bottom number represents the atomic number (see section B1.34), i.e. the number of protons. You generally will not see atomic and mass numbers featured in chemical equations as they do not change in a chemical reaction. However, because nuclear equations can involve transformation of one element into another, it is useful to include these to show the changes that have taken place.

An alpha particle is formed when an unstable nucleus loses two neutrons and two protons and becomes more stable in the process. An example is the decay of uranium-238 into thorium-234, represented by the nuclear equation:

$$^{238}_{92}\text{U} \rightarrow {}^{234}_{90}\text{Th} + {}^{4}_{2}\text{He}$$

In this case, the uranium-238 has lost 2 neutrons and 2 protons, so the atomic number (number of protons) decreases by 2, forming thorium and the mass number decreases by 4, so the isotope of thorium is thorium-234. We can see that the mass and atomic numbers all balance, because the alpha particle (helium nucleus) has 2 protons and 2 neutrons, giving it an atomic number of 2 and a mass number of 4.

Beta decay

A beta particle is a high-speed electron. It is represented in nuclear equations by the symbol $^{0}_{-1}\text{e}$. This electron is formed and then ejected at high speed from the nucleus when a neutron turns into a proton. This means that the number of protons increases by 1, therefore the atomic number increases by 1 although the mass of the nucleus remains the same. An example is the decay of carbon-14 into nitrogen-14, represented by the nuclear equation:

$$^{14}_{6}\text{C} \rightarrow {}^{14}_{7}\text{N} + {}^{0}_{-1}\text{e}$$

Note that in both alpha and beta decay, a new element will be formed as the nucleus produced will always have a different number of protons. The atomic number determines which element it is, so this means the atomic number changes and therefore the element changes.

Gamma radiation

Gamma radiation is a form of electromagnetic radiation from the nucleus produced when excess energy is lost from the nucleus. When a nucleus decays by alpha, beta or other types of emission, the protons and neutrons in the nucleus are often left in an excited state. The protons and neutrons then return to a lower energy level and the difference in energy is emitted as gamma radiation. Unlike alpha and beta decay, there is no change to the atomic structure and so no new elements are formed.

> ### Health and safety
>
> Some radioactive sources have a short half-life and others have a long half-life. A source with a short half-life will usually decay rapidly – i.e. the nuclei will be very unstable and the source will have a high activity. This means it will emit a high level of radioactivity, which could be dangerous. However, it will become safe relatively quickly as the unstable nuclei decay quickly.
>
> A long half-life means that the source will have a low activity and will emit a relatively low level of radioactivity. However, it could still be dangerous because it will go on emitting radiation for a long time – even for millions of years.
>
> We also need to consider the type of radiation emitted. For example, an alpha source is the most dangerous via contamination; an alpha source absorbed into the body will do damage to any tissues it is in contact with. On the other hand, a beta source is more dangerous by irradiation as beta particles are more penetrating.

B1.60 How radiation interacts with matter

Radiation interacts with matter in two ways: **ionisation** and **excitation**.

Ionisation

Ionisation occurs when electrons are removed from atoms or molecules to produce positive ions. All forms of radioactive decay produce radiation that can cause ionisation – hence the term **ionising radiation**.

We saw in section B1.57 that alpha radiation is the mostly highly ionising while gamma radiation is the least ionising. Beta radiation is in between the two in its ability to cause ionisation.

Excitation

Excitation occurs when radiation transfers energy to atoms or molecules. Excitation involves moving an electron to a higher energy level (**shell** or **orbital**). If enough energy is transferred to the electron, it will be removed from the atom and ionisation will have occurred. Gamma radiation can cause excitation. In fact, other types of electromagnetic radiation such as X-rays and visible light can cause excitation of electrons. This is why some types of ultraviolet (UV) light can cause sunburn or, in the worst cases, skin cancer. The UV light causes excitation of electrons in the DNA molecules found in skin cells, leading to ionisation which can result in cancer-causing mutations.

B1.61 The applications of radioactivity within the health and science sector

Health and safety

Before we look at applications of radioactivity, it is worth considering the biological effects of radiation – how radiation interacts with biological materials, including the human body.

The human body is made up of many complex molecules. Removal or addition of an electron changes a molecule chemically – this means that it may behave differently in any interaction with other molecules. As you have learned from Biology, interaction between molecules is central to how the body works.

UV light has sufficient energy to ionise biological molecules. Alpha, beta and gamma radiation all have energy millions of times greater than that of UV light. This means that these types of ionising radiation can be highly dangerous because they can change the chemistry of the body. The function of enzymes can be changed, cells can be damaged and the DNA in cells can be damaged, which can lead to cancer.

Case study

Because radiation can be so damaging, we must exercise great care when handling radioactive sources.

Hasini is working as a technician in a college science laboratory. She is responsible for the safe storage and demonstration of radioactive sources.

Hasini decides that, for each source, she must consider the following:
▶ the activity of the source
▶ the type of radiation (see section B1.57).

Based on these two considerations, Hasini can decide what protection is required.
▶ Alpha radiation is highly damaging but has low penetration, so can be relatively easily screened. This makes it relatively harmless outside the body, but if a source emitting alpha radiation enters the body, it can be highly damaging.
▶ Beta and gamma radiation are less ionising, but they have much greater penetration and may require screening with thick sheets of lead.

The table shows the radioactive sources kept in the college laboratory. For each source, the type of radiation emitted is shown.

Source	Radiation emitted
cobalt-60	pure gamma
strontium-90	pure beta
americium-241	alpha and some gamma

There are strict regulations covering working with radioactive sources, including those described in Chapter A3 (page 50).
▶ What precautions should Hasini use for storing each source?
▶ What precautions should she take when using each source?

Using 'l' as the abbreviation for litre can be confusing – it can look like the number 1. That is why the SI symbol for litre is 'L' and so 1 millilitre is 1 mL. You may see 'l' used as the symbol for litre, as in 1 ml (1 cm^3) but it is likely to be printed in italics, as in 1 *l*. Because of this, particularly in chemistry, you are more likely to use 1 dm^3 instead of 1 litre.

> **Practice point**
>
> Another unit you will see used quite often is the cubic decimetre or dm^3. This is the same volume as one litre and is preferred now in chemistry. You will often see concentrations expressed in mol/dm^3 or mol dm^{-3}, for example. This is replacing the older method of mol/L or M (molar), but you will still encounter these units sometimes.
>
> In fact, you might encounter other unfamiliar units in the workplace. Different industries are moving at different rates towards using SI units.

B1.64 The importance of using significant figures and science notation

Powers of 10

You will have encountered several numbers in this chapter and elsewhere using powers of 10. This is very convenient in science (see **Standard form** below) because it allows us to write very large or very small numbers more easily. There is another advantage: when we multiply two numbers shown as powers of 10 we **add** the powers. This is illustrated in the following example:

$100 \times 1000 = 100\,000$

Using powers of 10, 100 becomes 10^2 and 1000 becomes 10^3. This means that we can rewrite the calculation as follows:

$10^2 \times 10^3 = 10^5$

Notice that when we multiply the numbers shown as powers of 10, we simply add the powers to get the answer. This makes life so much easier!

If you look at the table of prefixes in section B1.63 you will see a range of values from 10^{-12} (pico) all the way up to 10^{12} (tera). These are examples of scientific notation where we use powers of 10 rather than writing the number out in full.

For example:

1 million can be written as $1\,000\,000$ or 10^6

1 nm is equal to $0.000\,000\,001$ m or 10^{-9} m

It is not difficult to see that using powers of 10 makes it much easier to write (and understand) very large or very small numbers.

Standard form

When we use scientific notation, using powers of 10, we follow a convention known as **standard form**. A number in standard form has two parts. For example, 2 650 000 would be written as:

2.65×10^6

The first part is a number between 1 and 10. The second part is a power of 10. So we should not write that number as 26.5×10^5.

By using numbers in standard form, calculations become less cumbersome. Also, with a little practice, it is easier to write down and understand very large or very small numbers using standard form.

Significant figures

> **Reflect**
>
> Measure the line below with a ruler. What answer do you get?
>
> _____
>
> If the printing process has worked correctly, that line should be 75.405 mm long. Can you measure it that accurately with a ruler?
>
> If the smallest division on your ruler is 1 mm, it is possible that you could estimate between the smallest divisions. But how reliable would your measurement be?

Because there is **uncertainty** in any measurement, we must take care not to imply a greater accuracy than is possible. In the case of the measurement of the line (75.405 mm), we would probably round it down to 75.4 mm, but is that the **true value**? We cannot estimate 0.4 of the smallest division.

Therefore, we use **significant figures**. These are the digits in a number that we believe are reliable. In the example, the first two digits (7 and 5) are reliable, but the third digit, after the decimal point, is not. We can be confident that the **true value** is closer to 75 mm than to 76 mm.

There are seven SI base units, as shown in the table.

Unit name	Unit symbol	Quantity name
ampere	A	electric current
candela	cd	luminous intensity
kelvin	K	temperature
kilogram	kg	mass
metre	m	length
mole	mol	amount of substance
second	s	time

There are many other SI units that are derived from these base units. Some that you may have come across include:

- hertz (Hz) for frequency
- volt (v) for electrical potential difference
- coulomb (C) for electric charge
- joule (J) for energy, work or heat
- watt (W) for power.

B1.63 How to convert between units

The metre and kilogram are both SI base units. That does not make them useful for measuring very short lengths or small masses. If you look at a ruler, the smallest division is usually the **millimetre** (mm). Paracetamol tablets are usually 500 **milligrams** (mg). The **prefix** 'milli' represents one thousandth, so we can work out the following conversions:

Length – metres (m) and millimetres (mm)

$1\,m = 1000\,mm$ or $10^3\,mm$

$1\,mm = 0.001\,m$ or $10^{-3}\,m$

Mass – grams (g) and milligrams (mg)

$1\,g = 1000\,mg$ or $10^3\,mg$

$1\,mg = 0.001\,g$ or $10^{-3}\,g$

Prefixes

You can see that millimetres use the prefix 'milli' to represent one thousandth. There are other prefixes used in SI units, as shown in the table.

Prefix name	Prefix symbol	Base 10
Tera	T	10^{12}
Giga	G	10^{9}
Mega	M	10^{6}
Kilo	K	10^{3}
Hecto	H	10^{2}
Deca	Da	10^{1}
Deci	d	10^{-1}
Centi	c	10^{-2}
Milli	m	10^{-3}
Micro	μ	10^{-6}
Nano	n	10^{-9}
Pico	p	10^{-12}

Many of these prefixes will be familiar, although not all of these examples are SI units:

- centimetre (cm) is common in everyday measurement
- micrometre (μm) is common in microscopy
- nanometre (nm) is commonly used to measure wavelength of visible light
- megabytes (MB), gigabytes (GB) and terabytes (TB) are used in computing for capacity of hard drives, memory modules and data transmission speeds. Unfortunately, these can be misleading because they can be calculated in **binary** as well as in **decimal**. This is the reason that a 400 GB hard drive (decimal) is shown by Microsoft Windows as only 372 GB (binary).

Notice that the base unit of mass is the kilogram, which is named as if the base unit is the gram.

Volume

The SI unit of volume is the cubic metre (m^3). This is too large to be useful in many situations – particularly in biology, chemistry and everyday life – it is much easier to ask for 1 litre of orange juice than asking for '0.001 m^3 please'.

In chemistry, the most common units of volume are the litre (L) and millilitre (mL):

$1\,L = 1000\,mL$

$1\,mL = 10^{-3}\,L$

Healthcare Science T Level: Core

Dating deceased organisms

Radiocarbon dating measures the age of any object that contains organic material. This includes dead organisms as well as anything made from dead organisms – such as a wooden table or pair of leather shoes.

Carbon-14 (^{14}C) is the radioactive isotope of carbon. The isotope is constantly made in the atmosphere from nitrogen using energy absorbed from **cosmic radiation**. This is the reverse of the reaction shown in section B1.59 illustrating beta-decay.

The carbon-14 then combines with atmospheric oxygen to produce carbon dioxide. This is taken up by plants and used in **photosynthesis** to produce sugars and other organic compounds. Plants are eaten by animals and so the carbon-14-containing organic compounds are incorporated into animal tissues as well. Both plants and animals respire and emit carbon dioxide. This means that the level of carbon-14 remains constant while the organism is alive.

Once the organism dies, it no longer exchanges carbon-14 with the environment and the carbon-14 undergoes radioactive decay. We can calculate how long ago the organism died by measuring the proportion of carbon-14 in a sample of bone, skin, fur, wood, etc.

The half-life of carbon-14 is about 5730 years. That means we can only date samples from organisms that died less than about 50 000 years ago. After that long, there will not be enough carbon-14 left to measure accurately.

Key terms

Radiocarbon dating: the process that uses a radioactive isotope of carbon, **carbon-14**, to determine the age of an object containing organic material.

Cosmic radiation: (also called cosmic rays) originates from the sun as well as from outside the solar system. It is a mixture of high energy protons (hydrogen nuclei), alpha particles (helium nuclei) and beta particles (electrons).

Photosynthesis: the process that plants use to make complex organic compounds such as sugars from carbon dioxide and water using light energy.

Test yourself

1. Explain how gamma radiation is different to alpha or beta radiation.
2. Nobelium-254, $^{254}_{102}No$, undergoes radioactive alpha decay to form an isotope of the element fermium, Fm.
   a. What is meant by isotopes of an element?
   b. Write a balanced equation to show the radioactive (alpha) decay of nobelium-254.
3. A radioactive source had an activity of 500 000 Bq and a half-life of 2.5 years. Calculate the activity remaining after 10 years.
4. The only foods that can be legally irradiated for sale in the UK are dried herbs and spices. Explain what type of radiation would be most appropriate for irradiation of herbs and spices.

Units

You will have encountered units already in this chapter – for length (e.g. wavelength) as well as various electrical measurements (charge, current, voltage). There have been many different types of unit used over the years. The **imperial** system uses fluid ounces, pints and gallons for volume and feet, inches and miles for distance. The **metric** system uses millilitres and litres for volume and millimetres, metres and kilometres for distance. Getting measurements from these two systems mixed up can be confusing or worse. In 1999, NASA lost the $125 million Mars orbiter because of confusion between imperial and metric units.

B1.62 The use of the international system of units (SI)

The international system of units is known as SI, from the French *Système international*. It is a modern form of the metric system but extends to units used for all kinds of measurement, particularly in science and engineering.

The metric system originally used **standards** for several units, such as the standard **kilogram** and standard **metre**, both of which were made of platinum–iridium alloy and kept in Paris. These are no longer sufficiently accurate for modern measurements and have been replaced by definitions based on **defining constants**, such as the speed of light, the Planck constant and the Avogadro constant.

Radioactive tracers

A major use of radioactive tracers is in medical diagnosis (next section).

In industry, radioactive tracers can be used to detect the presence of materials such as dust, cellulose fibres, glass fragments or organic materials as these all adsorb radioactive tracers from solution.

Another use of radioactive tracers is in monitoring hydraulic fracturing ('fracking') used to extract oil and gas from rocks.

Medical diagnostic applications

Radioactive **isotopes** (**radioisotopes**) can be injected or swallowed and their course around the body followed using an external detector. One example is iodine-123. This is taken up by the thyroid gland, just like the non-radioactive isotope (iodine-127). The radiation given out can be detected and used to show whether the thyroid gland is absorbing iodine correctly.

Radioactive tracers are usually gamma emitters as these are weakly ionising but highly penetrating. This means that they are less likely to cause damage to the body but can be easily detected from outside the body. Radioisotopes used as tracers also need to have short half-lives so that their activity disappears soon after the procedure is completed.

Computerised tomography uses X-rays to build up a 3D image of the body – known as a CT scan. More recently, gamma radiation detectors have been used to detect gamma emission of a radioactive tracer from many angles. A computer can then build up an image from the points of emission. This technique, known as **single photon emission computerised tomography (SPECT)** is now the main scanning technology used to diagnose a range of medical conditions.

Iodine-123 is an example of a **diagnostic radiopharmaceutical**. Various radioisotopes can be attached to biologically active substances, such as amino acids, hormones, therapeutic drugs, etc. These can be used together with SPECT to examine a wide range of processes:
- blood flow to the brain
- functioning of the liver, lungs, heart or kidneys
- assess bone growth.

Food preservation

Sufficiently high doses of radiation will kill micro-organisms in food. Some of these may be harmful (**pathogens**), so **irradiation** can kill the organisms that cause food poisoning, for example.

Other micro-organisms cause food to 'go off' – these are known as **spoilage** micro-organisms. Because irradiation will kill these spoilage micro-organisms as well, it can help to preserve food or extend the shelf-life of fresh or prepared foods.

> **Key terms**
>
> *Isotopes:* atoms of the same element (they have the same number of protons) but with different number of neutrons.
>
> *Radioisotopes:* unstable isotopes that undergo radioactive decay emitting radioactivity as they do so.
>
> *Radiopharmaceuticals:* therapeutic drugs (medicines) that incorporate radioisotopes. Some radiopharmaceuticals are used to treat disease whereas **diagnostic radiopharmaceuticals** are used to help in diagnosis of disease.

> **Research**
>
> The Food Standards Agency is responsible for ensuring the safety of the food that we buy and eat. Its website has a lot of information about the use of irradiation to preserve food.
>
> Visit the website: www.food.gov.uk
>
> Search for 'irradiated food', then research the following:
> - Is irradiated food safe to consume?
> - How does irradiation change food?
> - What types of food can be irradiated and sold?
> - How can you tell that a food has been irradiated?

This value of 75 mm is quoted to two **significant figures**, the number of digits that we believe are reliable.

If the smallest division on the ruler was only 10 mm, we would have to give a value of 70 mm – this is **one** significant figure.

Here are some more examples of a different measurement (1257.59) to various numbers of significant figures.

Number	Significant figures
1257.59	6
1258	4
1300	2
1000	1

From this example, you can see that **trailing zeros** do not count as significant figures – we call them **placeholders** as they stand for the 1s and 10s.

Similarly, **leading zeros** (usually after the decimal point) do not count towards the number of significant figures – so 0.075 m has two significant figures. We could write it as 75 mm and it would be the same length with the same uncertainty.

Trailing zeros in a **decimal** do count as significant figures. So, a concentration of 0.0500 mol/dm^3 is to **three** significant figures.

One important feature of significant figures is that they help us to reduce the chances of data errors:
▶ making sure data is not recorded to more digits than the measurement allows (e.g. ruler, balance, burette)
▶ in calculations, ensuring that we report the same number of digits as the original measurements allow.

As a rule in **calculations**, we look at the number of significant figures in the items of data. A calculator may give an answer to 10 digits, but using all of them would give **spurious** digits – they would not all be reliable. We should not report the answer to more significant figures than are in the item of data with the **lowest** number of significant figures.

In a titration (see section B1.44) we might have a standard solution that is 0.0500 mol/dm^3 (three significant figures) and a titre of 24.5 cm^3 (three significant figures). This means that we can calculate the number of mol:

mol = concentration × volume

mol = 0.0500 × 0.0245 = 1.225 × 10^{-3} or 0.001225 mol

However, we should only report this answer to three significant figures, or 1.23 × 10^{-3} mol.

There are some exceptions to this rule. For example, if we have a set of data and calculate a mean, it can be acceptable to quote the mean to one more significant figure than the values in the data. This is justified because calculating a mean allows us to get closer to the **true value** than any individual data point would be.

> **Test yourself**
>
> 1 Give the SI unit for the following measurements:
>   a mass
>   b length
>   c temperature.
> 2 Which of the following is not an SI unit?
>   a candlepower
>   b coulomb
>   c joule
>   d watt.
> 3 Complete the following table of conversions.
>
> | Convert from | Convert to | Answer |
> |---|---|---|
> | 1250 mm | m | |
> | 0.0005 kg | g | |
> | 1 250 000 J | kJ | |
> | 0.005 W | mW | |
> | 2.5 MHz | Hz | |
>
> 4 Convert the following to numbers in standard form to three significant figures:
>   a 1 256 000
>   b 0.000 000 135 023

Healthcare Science T Level: Core

Project practice

You are working for a company that provides components for use in lateral flow diagnostic test kits, like those used for COVID-19 testing in schools. The kits include swabs used to collect a sample from the nose and throat. These are currently sterilised with ethylene oxide gas. People have been concerned that ethylene oxide is dangerous and that children should not be exposed to the risk.

Exposure to ethylene oxide in large quantities can have serious health consequences. However, you know that there is no ethylene oxide remaining on the swabs after sterilisation and ethylene oxide has been used safely for decades to sterilise medical equipment and devices, including swabs and dressings. There has never been any evidence of harm caused to patients or users.

You have been asked to investigate other sterilisation methods and prepare a report with recommendations for alternatives to ethylene oxide.

You will need to carry out the following:
1 Research the options:
   a Carry out a literature review of sterilisation methods.
   b Investigate sources of safety information.
2 Prepare a plan:
   a Make a shortlist of possible methods.
   b Justify your choice of methods.
   c Prepare risk assessments of the different methods.
3 Analyse the data in comparison with the current method (ethylene oxide) and reach conclusions:
   a comparison of effectiveness of different methods
   b relative costs, including any specialist equipment needed and consumable items, e.g. chemicals
   c possible damage to components caused by the different methods
   d risk factors associated with the different methods, either to people carrying out the tests or to end users/patients.
4 Present your analysis and conclusions in the form of a PowerPoint presentation.
5 Group discussion covering:
   a the relative effectiveness and safety of the different methods
   b would they be more or less effective than the existing method
   c the perception of risk by members of the general public.
6 Write a reflective evaluation of your work.

Assessment practice

1 Karen has an iPhone XR. She has found out that it has a battery with a capacity of approximately 2900 mAh. A charge of 1 mAh is transferred when a current of 1 mA flows for 1 hour.
   a Calculate the total electric charge, in coulombs, in the iPhone XR battery.
   b Karen sees that the charger supplied with the iPhone XR is marked '5 V, 1000 mA'. She also has a charger for an iPad mini that is marked '5 V, 2100 mA'. Karen believes that the iPad charger will charge the iPhone more quickly. Is Karen correct? Calculate the time taken to charge the iPhone using each type of charger. Give your answers in hours, minutes and seconds.
2 The figure shows a circuit with a 9.0 V battery and three resistors.

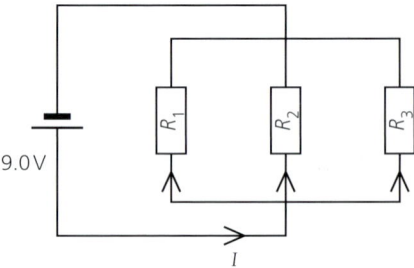

   a Is this an example of a series or parallel circuit?
   b The resistors are marked as follows: $R_1 = 10\,\Omega$, $R_2 = 22\,\Omega$, $R_3 = 47\,\Omega$. Calculate the total resistance in the circuit. Give your answer to an appropriate number of significant figures.
   c Based on your answer to part b, calculate the current flowing from the battery. Give your answer to an appropriate number of significant figures.

3. Describe two ways you could use to make a piece of iron magnetic.
4. Electromagnets are used in the recycling industry.
   a. What type of electromagnet would be found in a crane used for lifting scrap iron in a scrapyard?
   b. Explain how electromagnets can be used to separate scrap iron from scrap copper.
   c. A strong magnet will not attract aluminium. However, if a mixture of scrap aluminium and scrap plastic moves along a conveyor belt, eddy currents are created in the aluminium. These eddy currents cause the aluminium to be attracted to the magnet so it can be separated from the plastic. Explain how a current is formed in the aluminium.
5. Which of the following statements about waves is true?
   a. Gamma radiation is a type of transverse wave.
   b. Light waves transfer energy but sound waves transfer matter.
   c. The displacement of particles in a longitudinal wave is perpendicular to the direction of travel.
   d. The displacement of particles in a transverse wave is parallel to the direction of travel.
6. Make sketch graphs of transverse waves travelling along a Slinky. The y-axis should show the transverse displacement of the waves and the x-axis should show the distance along the Slinky.
   a. Two waves with the same frequency but one wave has double the amplitude of the other.
   b. Two waves with the same amplitude. One wave has double the frequency of the other wave.
7. Two radioactive sources were contained in glass bottles stored inside lead-lined containers. Both sources had approximately the same activity marked on the container. The bottles were removed from their containers and the following measurements taken using a Geiger counter:
   – Source A gave a very low reading.
   – Source B gave a very high reading.
   – When a sheet of aluminium was placed between source B and the Geiger counter, the reading fell by 75 per cent.
   – When a sheet of lead was placed between source B and the Geiger counter, the reading fell by 95 per cent.
   Explain what type of radiation was emitted by each source. Justify your answer.
8. A sample of radioactive material has been spilled. Discuss the options that you would consider in order to deal with the situation. You should include consideration of type and level of radiation emitted, half-life, and level or intensity of the radiation.
9. You are investigating sound waves moving in air or in water.
   a. In air, the wavelength of the sound is 250 cm and its frequency is 131 Hz. Calculate the speed of the wave. Give your answer in the correct SI units to an appropriate number of significant figures.
   b. Sound from the same source travels in water at 1480 m/s but the frequency remains the same. Calculate the new wavelength to the appropriate number of significant figures.
10. You have been asked to produce a wallchart showing the electromagnetic spectrum. You have been given the following table of values for the wavelength of the different types of electromagnetic radiation. Convert these values to metres (m) expressed in standard form so that they can be plotted more easily on the wallchart.

Type of radiation	Wavelength	Wavelength in standard form (m)
Gamma rays	1 pm to 10 pm	
X-rays	5 pm to 10 nm	
Ultra-violet	5 nm to 380 nm	
Visible light	380 nm to 750 nm	
Infra-red	750 nm to 1 mm	
Microwaves	0.1 mm to 10 cm	
Radio waves	10 cm to 2000 m	

B2: Further science concepts

Introduction

This chapter will build on the basic science concepts in biology that were discussed in Chapter B1. We will explore human physiology – the study of the normal functioning of the body and its component systems – as well as how this relates to the diseases and disorders that you are likely to encounter in your work.

Learning outcomes

The core knowledge outcomes that you must understand and learn:

B2.1 the components of the endocrine system; where they are located, their function and structure, including how they are organised

B2.2 the components of the respiratory system; where they are located, their function and structure, including how they are organised

B2.3 the components of the nervous system; where they are located, their function and structure, including how they are organised

B2.4 the components of the musculoskeletal system; where they are located, their function and structure, including how they are organised

B2.5 the components of the digestive system; where they are located, their function and structure, including how they are organised

B2.6 the components of the cardiovascular system; where they are located, their function and structure, including how they are organised

B2.7 the components of the reproductive system in males and females; where they are located, their function and structure including how they are organised

B2.8 the components of the renal system; where they are located, their function and structure, including how they are organised

B2.9 the components of the integumentary system; where they are located, their function and structure, including how they are organised

B2.10 the basic function of the eye and visual system

B2.11 the use of physiological measurement tools and techniques in monitoring the action of physiological systems

B2.12 the normal expected ranges for physiological measurements and how to identify when physiological measurements fall outside the normal expected ranges, including factors that can contribute to measurement outside of usual parameters

B2.13 the principles of homeostasis and how this links to maintaining the functions within the physiological systems and contributes to preserving a healthy body

B2.14 how failure of homeostasis mechanisms can impact the body and the subsequent development of disorders

B2.15 different classification systems and their purpose

B2.16 specific diseases and disorders and their relationship to the classification systems, including the possible causes and symptoms

B2.17 injury and trauma and how the body reacts systematically as a response.

B2.18 what is meant by epidemiology and how its objectives provide information to plan and evaluate strategies to prevent illness, including how this has contributed to the prevention of the spread of specific diseases

B2.19 how health promotion helps to prevent the spread and control of disease and disorders

B2.20 the concepts of genome and genomics and why these are different to the concept of genetics

B2.21 the characteristics of the different study areas within genomics

B2.22 how techniques in genomics are used to investigate, diagnose and treat disorders

B2.23 the applications of genomics within healthcare science

B2.24 the importance of bioinformatics within the area of genomics

B2.25 how physics principles are applied in the field of medical physics to support prevention, diagnosis and treatment of disease.

B2.1 The endocrine system

The **endocrine system** involves a series of **endocrine glands** (Figure 14.1) that secrete **hormones** into the blood. These act as chemical messengers because they are transported around the body in the blood and act on specific target cells or organs.

The endocrine system is involved in:
- regulation of growth and development
- regulation of the reproductive system
- **homeostasis** – the regulation of the internal environment of the body.

The reproductive system will be covered in more detail in section B2.7 and homeostasis in section B2.12.

There are two types of hormone, based on their chemical structure:
- **steroid hormones** are based on cholesterol and include:
  - the sex hormones, which regulate the reproductive system
  - the corticosteroid hormones that help regulate carbohydrate metabolism and mineral ions
- other hormones are amino acid derivatives, peptides or proteins.

> ### Key terms
>
> **Endocrine system:** a system of **hormones** that control many aspects of physiology (the normal functioning of the body).
>
> **Endocrine glands: secrete** (release) their products directly into the blood. Examples are the alpha (α) and beta (β) cells in the pancreas, which secrete the hormones glucagon and insulin, respectively.
>
> **Gland:** a group of cells that make chemicals such as hormones or enzymes.
>
> **Hormone:** a chemical messenger released into the blood by an **endocrine gland** that acts on target tissues elsewhere in the body.

The components and organisation of the endocrine system

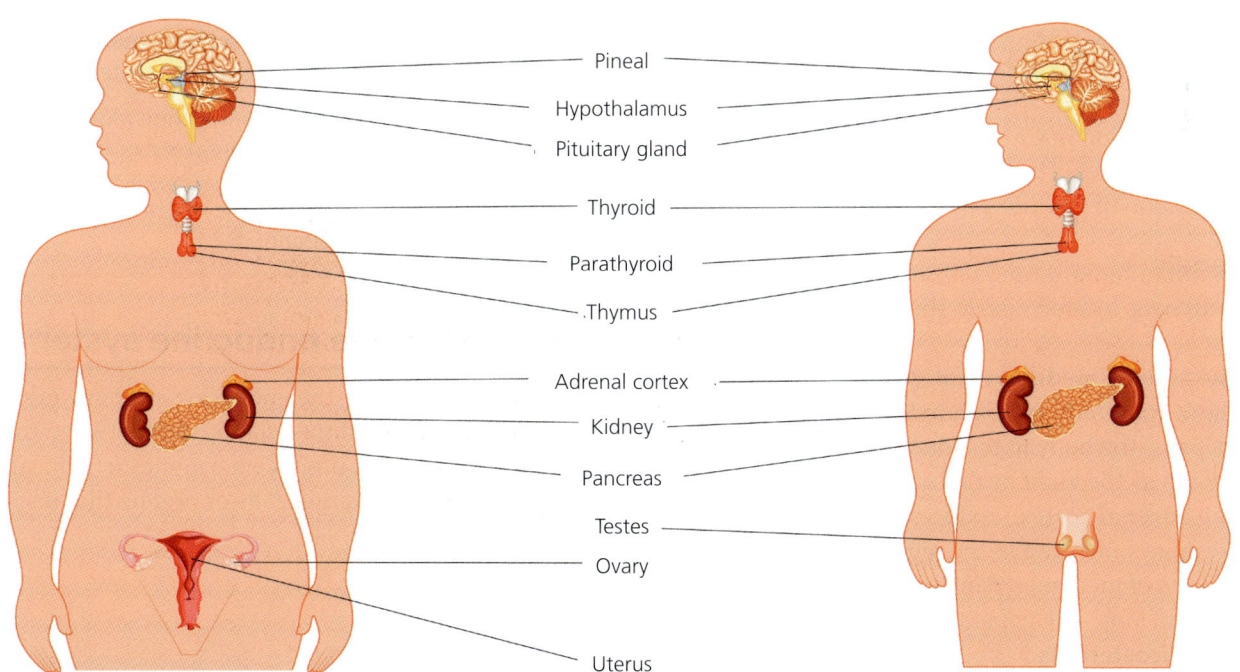

▲ Figure 14.1 The human endocrine system showing the endocrine glands in females (left) and males (right)

Hypothalamus

The hypothalamus is located in the brain and is responsible for control of body temperature, water balance (**osmoregulation**) and secretion of hormones via the **pituitary gland**. The hypothalamus is responsible for controlling most of the **homeostatic mechanisms** that regulate the internal environment of the body – with the exception of blood glucose concentration – either directly or by controlling other endocrine glands, such as the **thyroid** gland.

Pituitary

The pituitary is divided into **anterior** and **posterior** parts or lobes. Hormones produced in the hypothalamus are stored in the posterior lobe before secretion. The hypothalamus also produces releasing factors that stimulate the anterior lobe to secrete various hormones.

Thyroid and parathyroid

The thyroid is responsible for the regulation of **metabolic rate**. **Metabolism** is the term that describes all the chemical reactions that take place in the body. Metabolic rate is the rate at which the energy stored in our food is transferred by all the **metabolic reactions** that take place in the body. The thyroid is controlled by the releasing factor **TRH**, secreted by the hypothalamus.

The parathyroid works with the thyroid to control the levels of calcium in the body. **Parathyroid hormone (PTH)** is secreted by the parathyroid and increases the concentration of Ca^{2+} ions in the blood while **calcitonin**, secreted by the thyroid, reduces the concentration of Ca^{2+} ions in the blood.

Adrenals

The adrenals, located next to the kidneys, have two parts:
- ▶ The adrenal **medulla** is the central part of the gland and produces the hormone **adrenaline** that prepares the body to respond to threat or danger – known as the 'fight or flight' response.
- ▶ The **adrenal cortex** produces several steroid hormones involved in the regulation of different aspects of metabolism including carbohydrates and mineral ions. The general name for these hormones is **corticosteroids**.

There are two classes of corticosteroids:
- **glucocorticoids** (e.g. **cortisol**), which help regulate carbohydrate metabolism
- **mineralocorticoids**, which help regulate the balance of mineral ions such as Na^+ (sodium) and K^+ (potassium).

Ovaries

As well as their function in releasing egg cells (see section B2.7), the ovaries produce the female **sex hormones**, including **oestrogen** and progesterone, that are involved in the regulation of the **menstrual cycle**.

Testes

Like the ovaries, the testes have a dual function: production of **sperm cells** (see section B2.7) and secretion of the male sex hormones such as **testosterone**.

Pancreas

The pancreas has an important **exocrine** function producing digestive enzymes. The **endocrine** function of the pancreas is carried out by the **Islets of Langerhans**, which produce the hormones **insulin** and **glucagon**. These hormones are responsible for the regulation of blood glucose concentration.

> ### Key terms
>
> **Exocrine:** glands that release (secrete) their products into **ducts** or on to the body surface.
>
> **Ducts:** tubes that lead from an exocrine gland to the place where the products are used or needed. Examples include tear ducts in the eye (see section B2.10), or salivary and pancreatic ducts in the digestive system (see section B2.5).

Functions of the endocrine system

To understand the way the endocrine system works we need to understand the relationship between the endocrine glands that produce hormones (chemical messengers) and the target cells or organs that respond to those hormones.

Hormone	Secreted by	Acts on
Thyroxine	Thyroid	Most body cells, to regulate metabolic rate.
Cortisol	Adrenal cortex	**Cortisol** is produced in response to stress. It acts on liver and muscle cells and increases blood glucose concentration.
Adrenaline	Adrenal medulla	Heart (increases heart rate) and liver (increases conversion of glycogen to glucose); it also acts on blood vessels and lungs to prepare the body for action in the 'fight or flight' response.
Oestrogen	Ovaries	Pituitary and uterus. Oestrogen is involved in regulation of the menstrual cycle.
Testosterone	Testes	Muscle and bone cells. The **anabolic** action of testosterone increases muscle mass and bone density. Sex organs. The **androgenic** action of testosterone stimulates the development of the male sex organs and secondary sexual characteristics, such as facial hair. Testosterone is also required for the production of sperm cells.
Gastrin	Stomach	Gastrin has several actions in digestion involving the stomach and small intestine.
Growth hormone (GH)	Pituitary	Most body cells respond to GH, which is responsible for normal growth during infancy and childhood.
Follicle-stimulating hormone (FSH)	Pituitary	Ovaries. FSH stimulates the growth and development of the egg follicle during the first half of the **menstrual cycle**. Egg follicles are located in the ovaries and contain the developing egg cell.

▲ Table 14.1 The production and activity of specific hormones

Practice point

The term **cortisone** is often misused to describe either any corticosteroid or specifically **hydrocortisone**, which is the name given to cortisol when it is used as a medication.

Try to always use the correct terminology.

The specificity of hormones in relation to target cells/organs

Hormones are transported throughout the body in the blood. However, only specific target cells have **receptors** on their cell surface membranes. Each receptor is specific to a single hormone. Therefore, only cells with **insulin receptors** (e.g. muscle and liver cells) will respond to **insulin**, and only cells with **ADH receptors** (kidney cells) will respond to **ADH (anti-diuretic hormone)**.

This represents an important difference between the two systems involved in controlling many body functions. The signal or message carried by a hormone is 'broadcast' throughout the body but only picked up by cells that carry the correct receptors. In contrast, the nervous system (see section B2.3) uses nerve cells to deliver impulses only to specific target cells or tissues.

The endocrine system is like satellite TV. The signals are broadcast over the whole of a geographical area and can be picked up anywhere within that area, but only if you have a satellite dish. Unlike satellite TV, cable TV is carried over copper wires or fibre-optic cables to individual homes. If you do not live in an area supplied by cable, you cannot watch cable TV.

Reflect

Can you think of other examples that you could use to explain to someone how the endocrine system works? When you have covered the nervous system in section B2.3, think about the similarities between cable TV and the nervous system.

The role of the pancreas in the regulation of blood glucose

The pancreas produces two hormones, insulin and glucagon, that are involved in the regulation of blood glucose concentration (Figure 14.2).

The actions of insulin and glucagon are **antagonistic** – they work in opposition to each other. They are also examples of **negative feedback** (we will cover this in more detail in section B2.12). Both are features of how other hormones help to regulate systems in the body.

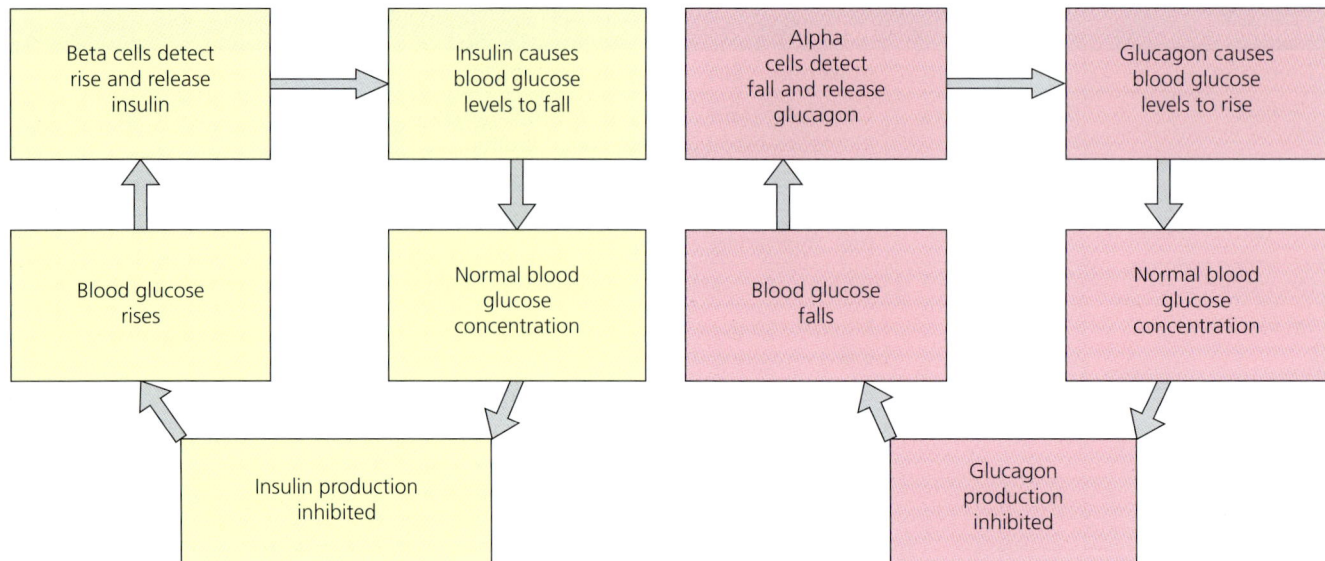

▲ Figure 14.2 Regulation of blood glucose concentration by insulin (left) and glucagon (right); These are both examples of negative feedback

The action of the anti-diuretic hormone (ADH) in urine production

The renal system is covered in more detail in section B2.8. The **kidney** produces urine, but this has two main functions:

- **excretion** of nitrogenous waste in the form of **urea**
- **osmoregulation** – the regulation of the water balance in the body.

The process of **ultrafiltration** in the kidney produces a **filtrate** (filtered substance) that contains all the components of the blood except for cells and large proteins. The process of converting the filtrate into urine involves the reabsorption of useful substances, such as glucose and amino acids, leaving a dilute solution of urea, which we call urine in everyday speech. Some water must also be reabsorbed, depending on the **water balance** of the body. When we drink a lot of water, the blood has a high **water potential**. When we are dehydrated, the blood has a low water potential. The water potential of the blood is detected by osmoreceptors in the hypothalamus that control release of ADH by the posterior pituitary. This is illustrated in Figure 14.3 and is another example of a mechanism involving negative feedback.

Digestion

Gastrin is produced by cells in the stomach and its main target is also the stomach, where it stimulates release of hydrochloric acid (see section B2.5). Gastrin has other actions on the stomach, including:

- stimulates secretion of digestive enzymes
- stimulates contraction of stomach muscles, which helps mix the food with acid and digestive enzymes
- stimulates emptying of the stomach into the **duodenum** (small intestine).

Gastrin also stimulates the release of pancreatic secretions involved in digestion.

Growth

The pituitary gland controls growth through the secretion of growth hormone (GH). GH stimulates muscle and bone cells to divide and stimulates the intestines to absorb calcium, required for bone development. Lack of GH in childhood can lead to someone having reduced stature (i.e. being unusually short), while over-production leads to **pituitary giantism**.

Testosterone and oestrogen both stimulate the pituitary to secrete growth hormone. Increased production of these sex hormones during **puberty** explains the increase in growth rate around that time.

B2: Further science concepts

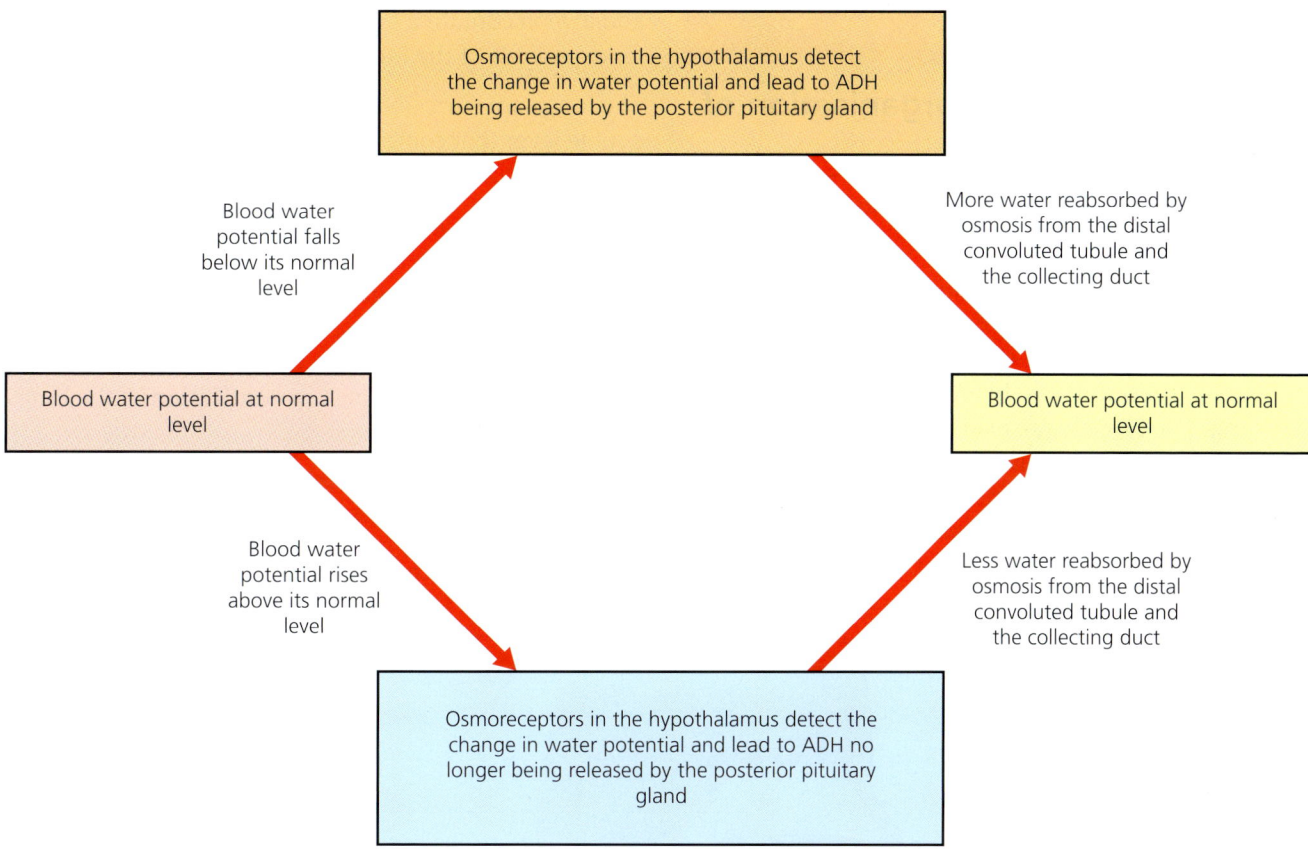

▲ Figure 14.3 Control of the water potential of the blood by ADH

Effects of adrenaline

Adrenaline, together with the nervous system, is responsible for preparing the body to deal with danger or emergency situations by taking drastic action – the 'fight or flight' response. The actions of adrenaline include:
- increased heart rate
- stimulation of liver cells to convert glycogen to glucose, which increases blood glucose concentration
- increased blood flow to the muscles and brain
- decreased blood flow to the gut and skin
- increase in diameter of bronchioles (see section B2.2) to increase air flow into the lungs
- dilation of the pupils.

> **Test yourself**
>
> 1 Most endocrine glands are the same in males and females. Name two endocrine glands that are present only in females and one that is present only in males.
> 2 Explain why hormones are carried throughout the body in the bloodstream but each hormone will only act on some types of cells.
> 3 Name two hormones involved in the regulation of blood glucose concentration.
> 4 For the hormone ADH, state:
>   a where it is produced
>   b where it acts
>   c its effect.

Healthcare Science T Level: Core

B2.2 The respiratory system

The components and organisation of the respiratory system

The respiratory system is contained largely within the **thorax** or chest cavity (Figure 14.4).

The two **lungs** almost fill the thorax. The mouth and nose lead to the **trachea** or windpipe, which is a wide tube kept open by C-shaped rings of cartilage. The trachea splits into two **bronchi**, one leading to each lung. The bronchi are also supported by rings of cartilage. The bronchi divide into many branches called **bronchioles**. The bronchioles lead to blind ends called **alveoli**. These are small air-filled sacs that have a wall consisting of a single layer of thin **epithelial cells**. The alveoli are the site of gas exchange (see section B1.10, page 220). The walls of the bronchioles and alveoli contain a lot of **elastic tissue**, which allows for expansion of the lungs during breathing.

The lungs are surrounded by **pleural membranes**, a double layer that contains the lungs and also allows for expansion during breathing.

The chest cavity is enclosed by the **ribs**, which are connected to each other by two layers of **intercostal muscles**. The **diaphragm** is a sheet of muscle that forms the floor of the chest cavity. The diaphragm separates the chest cavity from the abdominal cavity and plays an important part in **ventilation** of the lungs (breathing).

> **Key term**
>
> **Epithelial cells:** Cells that line structures in the body, usually in thin, single layers.

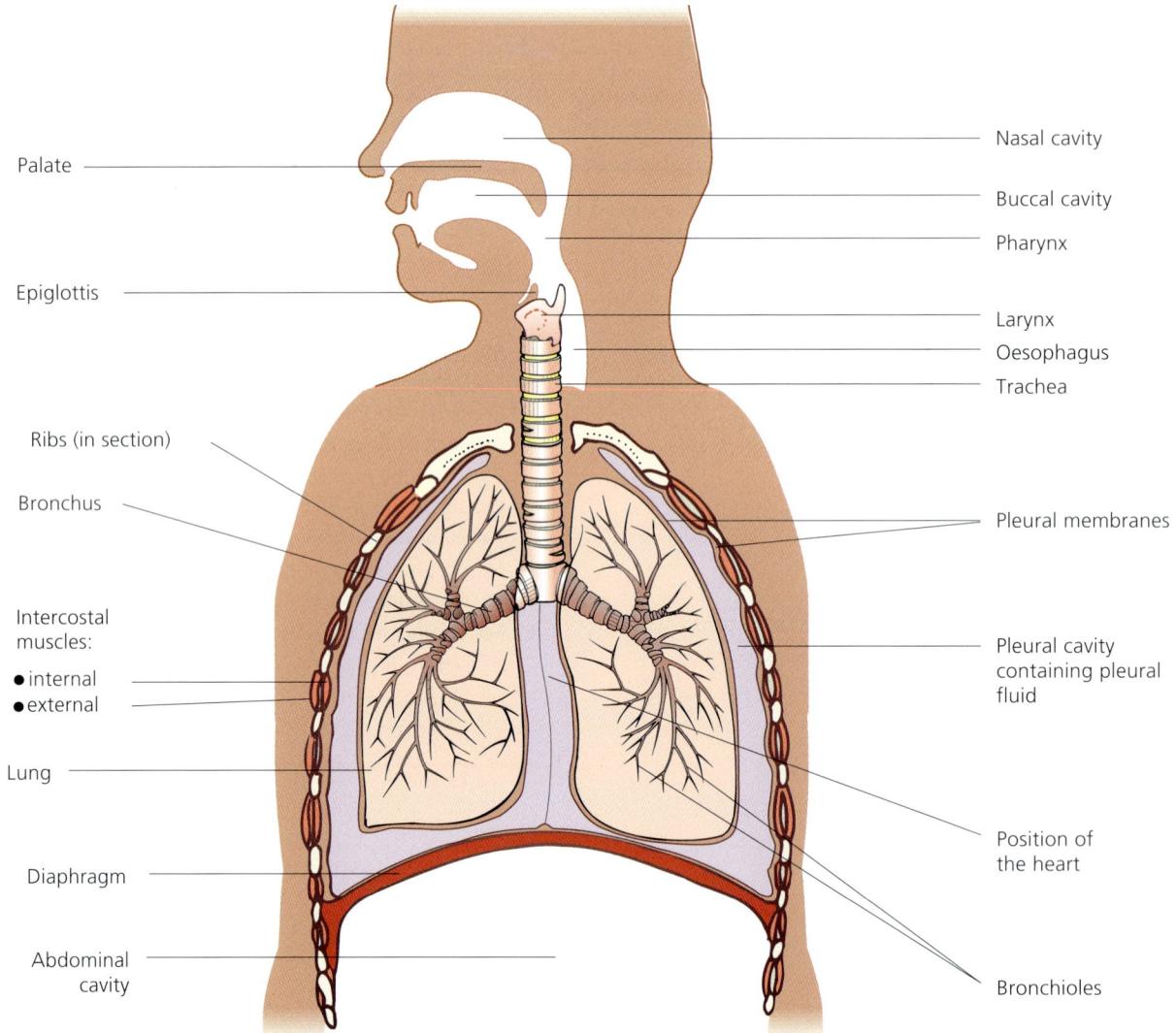

▲ Figure 14.4 The human respiratory system

Functions of the respiratory system:

The properties of an efficient gas exchange surface were covered in Chapter B1, section B1.10. In this section, we will discuss the ways in which the lungs are adapted for efficient gas exchange.

How gaseous exchange occurs by the process of ventilation

An important part of this is to maintain a high concentration gradient. The process of **ventilation** involves:

- **inspiration** or breathing in
- **expiration** or breathing out.

Ventilation of the lungs (Figure 14.5) ensures that fresh air high in oxygen is brought into the alveoli when we breathe in, and carbon dioxide is removed when we breathe out.

Inspiration (breathing in) involves the contraction of two sets of muscles:

- the **diaphragm** contracts, which causes it to move down
- the **external intercostal** muscles contract, which causes the rib cage to move up and outwards.

As a result, the volume of the chest cavity increases and so the pressure in the lungs is reduced below the pressure of the air outside the body (atmospheric pressure). Air moves down the pressure gradient into the lungs, causing them to expand. This is assisted by the elastic tissue in the walls of the bronchioles and alveoli expanding.

Expiration (breathing out) when we are breathing at rest usually just involves relaxation of these two sets of muscles. As a result, the chest moves in and down and the diaphragm moves up. Therefore, the volume of the chest cavity decreases, the pressure increases and air is forced out down a concentration gradient. As well as this, the elastic tissue *recoils*, which also increases the pressure in the lungs, helping to force air out.

The **internal intercostal** muscles are involved in **forced expiration**, which is what happens when you blow out candles, for instance. Contraction of the internal intercostal muscles causes the rib cage to be pulled in and down more forcefully, expelling air more rapidly from the lungs.

> **Key term**
>
> *Recoil:* the process by which elastic tissues or fibres return to their original length after having been stretched or expanded. This is what happens to an elastic band when you stretch it and then let go. Be careful not to use the term **contraction** to describe this process. Contraction is what muscles do, whereas elastic tissues recoil.

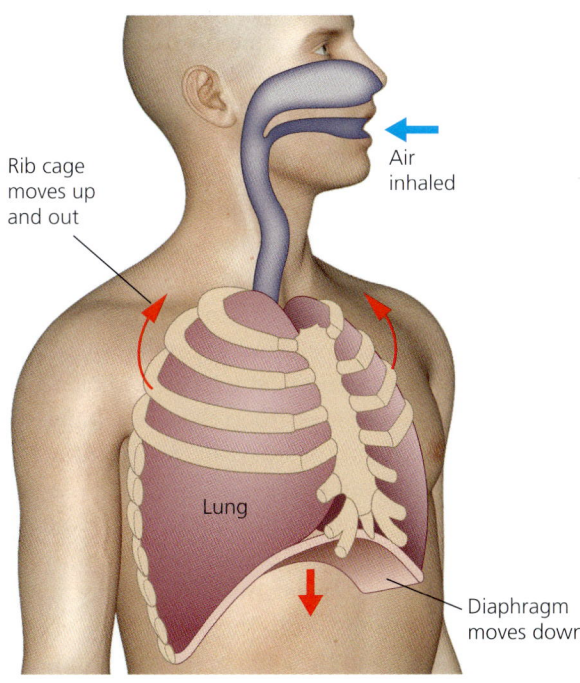
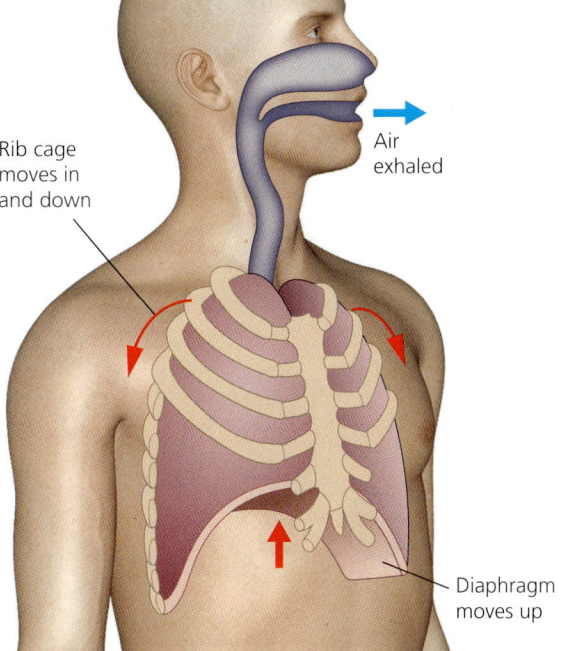

▲ Figure 14.5 Ventilation of the lungs

The role of ciliated epithelial tissue and pulmonary surfactant

The walls of the trachea and bronchi are covered with **ciliated epithelial cells** as well as **goblet cells** that produce mucus (Figure 14.6). The cilia contain proteins that can contract, causing them to move in a wave-like motion. The mucus traps dirt and bacteria, and the beating of the cilia moves the mucus up the trachea to the throat where it is swallowed so that any bacteria are destroyed by the acid in the stomach.

Pulmonary surfactant is produced by some cells in the wall of the alveoli and consists of a mixture of phospholipids and some protein. Surfactant acts like a detergent (for example, washing-up liquid). It coats the epithelial cells, reducing the **surface tension** of water. This makes it easier to inflate the lungs and stops the surfaces of the alveoli sticking together.

Proteins in the surfactant also help to protect against lung inflammation and infection.

How and where gaseous exchange takes place

So far, we have looked at the structure of the lungs and how the various parts are adapted to their function. We have also considered how ventilation of the lungs maintains a high concentration gradient of both oxygen and carbon dioxide in the alveolus. We now need to look at the detail of gas exchange in the alveolus (Figure 14.7).

The pulmonary artery brings deoxygenated blood from the heart (see section B2.6) and the pulmonary vein returns oxygenated blood to the heart. In between, there is a network of capillaries surrounding the alveoli.

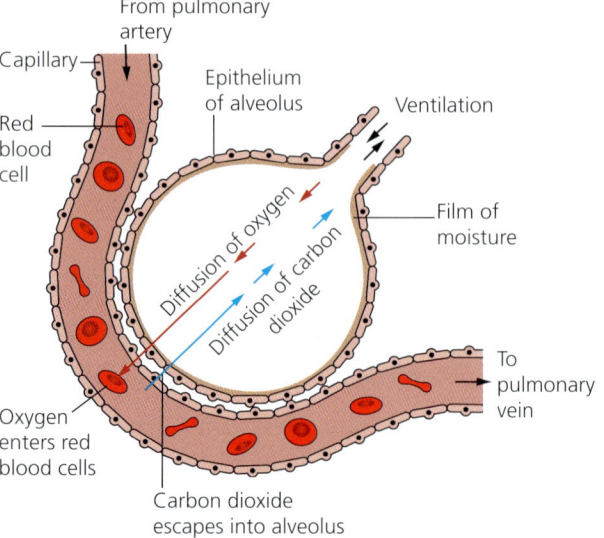

▲ Figure 14.7 Gas exchange in the alveolus

If you look back at Exchange and transport mechanisms, in Chapter B1 (page 220) you will see how the lungs have the three characteristics of an ideal exchange surface:
- ▶ The wall of an alveolus is a single layer of epithelial cells. The wall of a capillary is a single layer of endothelial cells. This means that there is a short diffusion pathway for oxygen from the air in the alveoli to the red blood cells in the capillary – i.e. it makes it easy for oxygen to get into the red blood cells. The same is true for carbon dioxide dissolved in the blood moving in the opposite direction.
- ▶ The many alveoli mean there is a large surface area for gas exchange – about 75 m² in an adult human.
- ▶ Ventilation of the lungs (i.e. breathing) maintains a high concentration of oxygen and low concentration of carbon dioxide in the air in the alveoli. In addition, blood flow in the capillaries is continually bringing carbon dioxide to the lungs and removing oxygen, which also helps maintain the high concentration gradient.

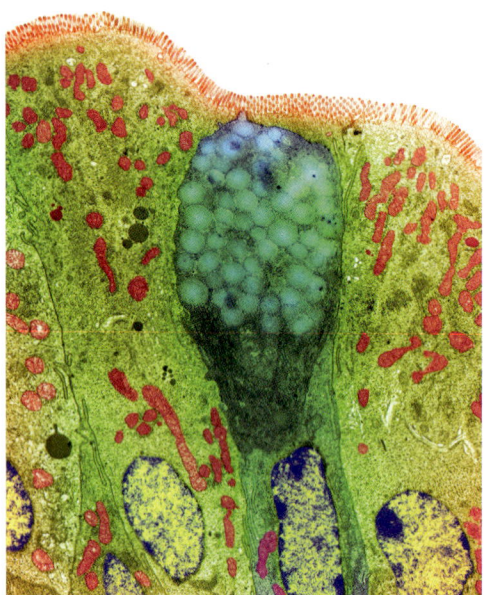

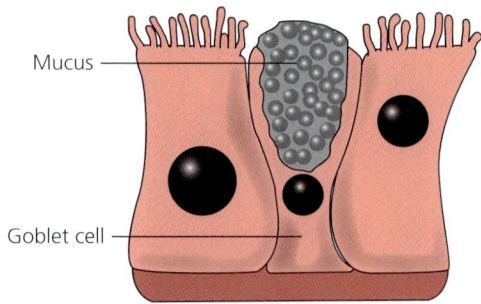

▲ Figure 14.6 A transmission electron micrograph (TEM) of a goblet cell with ciliated epithelial cells on either side (top); a diagram based on the TEM (bottom)

How breathing rate can be increased or decreased

Regulation of the breathing rate is performed by the **medulla oblongata** (often just referred to as the **medulla**), which is located at the base of the brain where it joins the spinal cord (see section B2.3). Carbon dioxide increases the acidity of the blood, which is detected by **chemoreceptors** in arteries in the neck and in the **medulla**. As the acidity of the blood increases, the **respiratory centre** in the medulla sends nerve impulses to the muscles that control breathing to increase the breathing rate. As the acidity of the blood decreases, this is also detected and other nerves send impulses to slow down the rate of breathing.

A similar mechanism controls the heart rate (see section B2.6) so that the two systems work together. For example, when we exercise the tissues produce more carbon dioxide and require more oxygen, so the heart rate increases. This increases blood flow to the tissues, which delivers more oxygen to the tissues and removes more carbon dioxide. At the same time, an increase in breathing rate means that more oxygen can diffuse into the blood in the lungs and more carbon dioxide can be removed.

The nose and nasal passages

The nose and nasal passages represent much more than just an alternative to the mouth for air entering the lungs, as you can see from Figure 14.8.

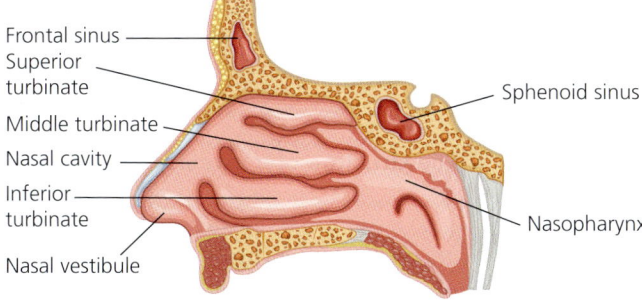

▲ Figure 14.8 The nose and nasal passages

The nasal passage allows air to flow into the throat and then to the lungs. As it flows through, the air is warmed, filtered and humidified.

Nasal turbinates are located on the outer walls of the nasal passage and consist of a network of bones, vessels and tissues. They are primarily responsible for warming, filtering and humidifying the incoming air. The turbinates swell and shrink to regulate airflow through the nose. Infections such as the common cold or allergies such as hay fever can lead to inflammation and congestion of the turbinates.

Nasal sinuses are air pockets in the bones surrounding the nose. They drain into the nasal passage and deliver clear mucus that also helps to humidify the air and trap dust and dirt. Inflammation of the sinuses (**sinusitis**) can occur when the drainage pathway becomes blocked. This can lead to infection of the sinuses.

Swallowing

If you look again at Figure 14.4, you will see the two remaining structures in the respiratory system that we need to consider. In fact, these are relevant more to the process of swallowing food than breathing.

The **oropharyngeal passage** connects the back of the mouth, or **buccal cavity**, with the lower part of the **pharynx** leading to the throat. The pharynx connects the nasal cavity and buccal cavity with the **trachea** (towards the lungs) and **oesophagus** (towards the stomach).

The **epiglottis** is a flap of cartilage covered with a membrane. The epiglottis remains open during breathing to allow air into the larynx so that it can pass into the trachea towards the lungs. When we swallow, the epiglottis closes, shutting off the larynx and forcing food to pass into the oesophagus and on towards the stomach.

Mucociliary transport

Also known as **mucociliary clearance**, the term mucociliary transport describes the process whereby dust particles and pathogens are trapped in the upper respiratory tract and cleared by the wave-like motion of the cilia described earlier. This protects the delicate tissues of the lungs.

> **Test yourself**
>
> 1. State the two groups of muscles involved in breathing (ventilation).
> 2. Describe three ways in which the human lungs show the properties of an ideal exchange surface.
> 3. Describe the function of:
>   a ciliated epithelia
>   b pulmonary surfactant
>   c nasal turbinates
>   d nasal sinuses.
> 4. Explain why breathing out at rest is sometimes described as a passive process compared to forced expiration.

Healthcare Science T Level: Core

B2.3 The nervous system

The nervous system controls and co-ordinates our movement. It also allows us to interact with our surroundings by use of **receptors** and **effectors** (such as muscles). It also controls many of the **autonomic** functions of the body – those over which we have no conscious control. These include the movement of food along the gut in digestion (section B2.5), regulation of breathing rate (section B2.2) and regulation of heart rate (section B2.6).

Components and organisation of the nervous system

The main distinction in the nervous system is between the **central** and **peripheral nervous systems** – the **CNS** and **PNS** (Figure 14.9).

> **Key terms**
>
> **Neurone:** a nerve cell.
>
> **Nerve:** a bundle of neurones.

Central nervous system

The CNS consists of the **brain** and **spinal cord**. The brain is where sensory inputs (hearing, touch, vision, etc.) are processed and responses (such as movement) are initiated. The spinal cord is important in reflex actions, for example moving your hand away from a hot plate.

Peripheral nervous system

The PNS consists of all the **sensory neurones** that connect receptors with the CNS as well as the **motor neurones** that connect to muscles or glands and bring about responses such as movement.

Figure 14.10 illustrates the structure of a motor neurone seen in mammals.

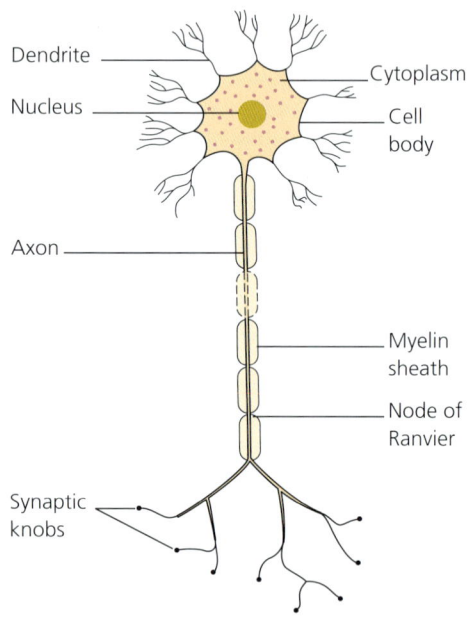

▲ Figure 14.10 The structure of a myelinated motor neurone

Motor neurones transmit **nerve impulses** in only one direction (away from the cell body) and have the following features:
- **Dendrites** make connections with other neurones, mostly within the CNS.
- The **cell body** contains the **nucleus** and other **organelles**.
- The **axon** carries the nerve impulse from the cell body.
- The **myelin sheath** consists of Schwann cells, a specialised type of cell wrapped around the axon (see Figure 14.11) that acts in a similar way to the insulation on an electric cable.

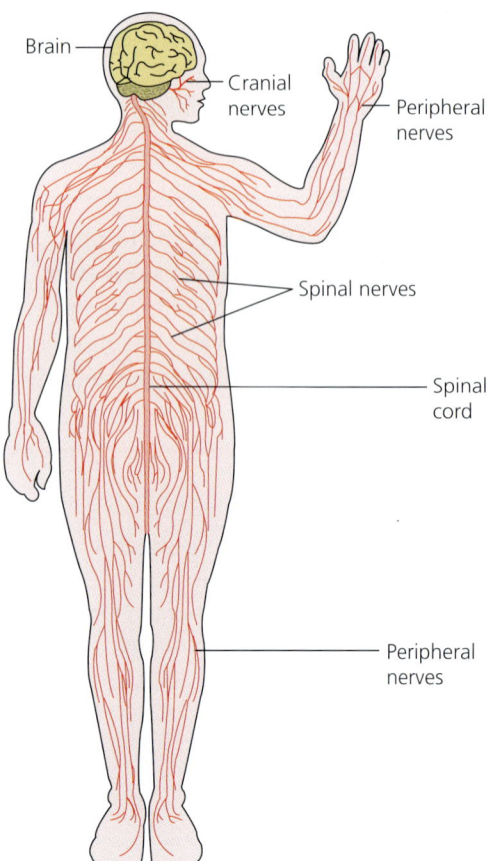

▲ Figure 14.9 The structure of the human nervous system

There are small gaps between the Schwann cells called **nodes of Ranvier**. The combination of the myelin sheath and nodes of Ranvier helps to significantly increase the rate at which the nerve impulse is carried along the axon.

At the end furthest from the cell body the axon branches to form **axon endings** or **terminals** that make connections, usually with muscle cells. These are called **synaptic ends** or **synaptic knobs**.

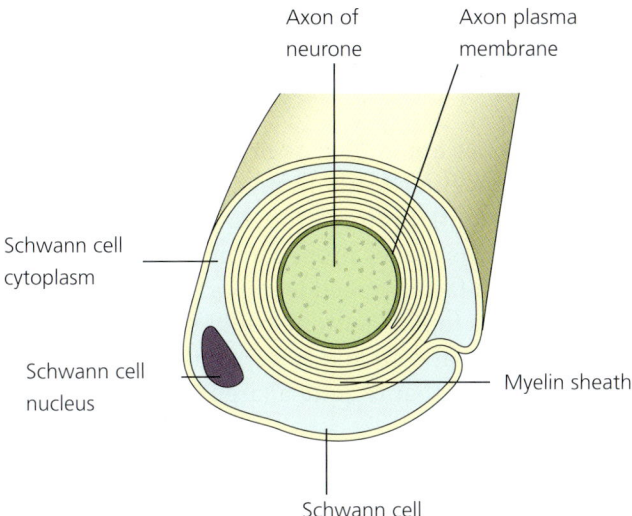

▲ Figure 14.11 A section across an axon showing the structure of the myelin sheath

Functions of the nervous system

The role of the PNS

The PNS carries nerve impulses from **receptors** that act as the body's **sensors** towards the CNS along sensory neurones. This is similar to the way in which a cable carries a message from a microphone to a loudspeaker. However, we should really refer to nerves carrying **impulses** and not messages.

Reflex actions are protective or survival responses and occur rapidly and without any conscious thought. The simplest reflex action is the knee-jerk reflex (Figure 14.12) where you sit with your legs crossed and a doctor or nurse hits a ligament just below your knee cap. This causes an involuntary straightening of the leg, like a kick. This reflex involves a receptor, a sensory neurone, a motor neurone and the quadriceps muscle (the effector).

If you look at Figure 14.12, you will see that there is also a connection, via the spinal cord, to the brain. This is how you become aware that you have been hit on the knee, but this will only be after your leg has responded automatically.

Other reflex actions are more complex. For example, if you touch a hot surface, you will pull your hand away. This reflex is similar to the knee-jerk reflex but includes an additional relay neurone in the spinal cord between the sensory and motor neurones.

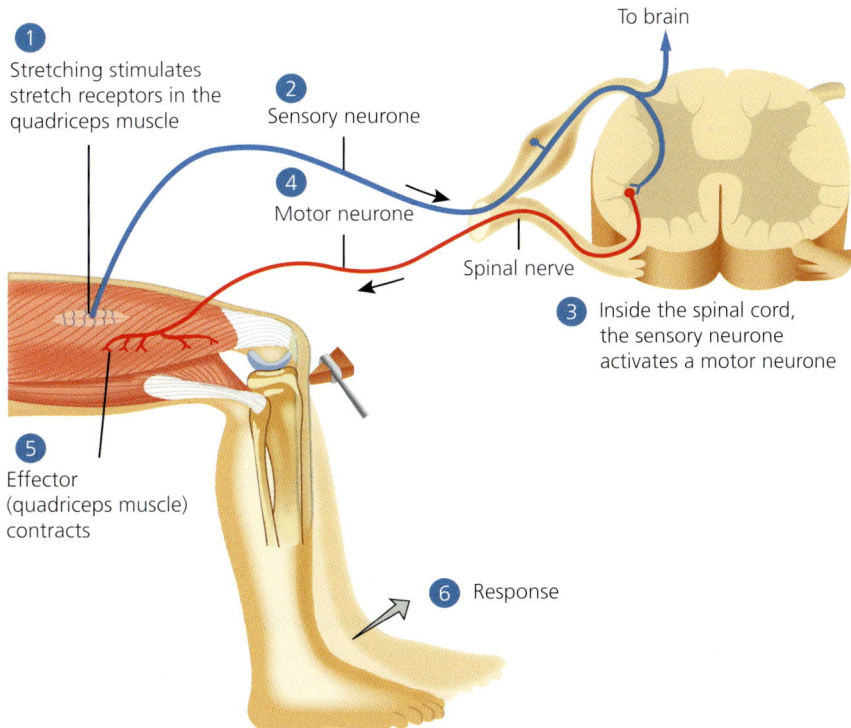

▲ Figure 14.12 The nervous pathway of the knee-jerk reflex

The blink reflex is even more complex, because several muscles are required to close the eyelids and different types of stimuli can initiate the reflex.

The role of the CNS

The CNS takes all the information contained in inputs from sensory neurones and processes it. It then sends impulses via **motor neurones** to **effector organs**. Effector organs are usually muscles, but they can also be **glands** (see section B2.1).

As well as this co-ordinating function, the brain is also where we store memories, feel emotion and generally experience what we call **consciousness**.

Motor neurones and synaptic transmission

> **Key terms**
>
> **Polarisation:** the different electrical charges on either side of the plasma membrane caused by the active transport of ions.
>
> **Depolarisation:** the reversal of the charge difference.
>
> **Repolarisation:** the restoration of the original charge difference.

Nerve impulses are electrical signals transmitted from the cell body towards the axon terminals. When a neurone is 'at rest' there is a small potential difference across the plasma membrane of about −60 mV.

In other words, the inside of the neurone is slightly more negative that the outside due to positive Na+ ions being pumped out of the neurone. This is described as the **resting potential**.

A nerve impulse involves a rapid change in the membrane potential so that the membrane is **depolarised** – the inside is now slightly positive compared to the outside. This process is rapidly reversed, within a few milliseconds, and the membrane becomes **repolarised**. This is known as an **action potential**. An action potential is **propagated** or transmitted along the axon – this represents a nerve impulse.

Motor neurones are known as **myelinated** because they have a myelin sheath. In myelinated neurones, the action potential **jumps** from one node of Ranvier to the next. This makes propagation of the nerve impulse much faster. Speed is important when you consider that a motor neurone could start at the base of the spinal cord and travel all the way down to your big toe – that is quite a large distance for a single cell!

Connections between neurones are known as **synapses**. Electrical transmission of the nerve impulse across the synapse is not possible because there is a physical gap between the cells. Instead, the nerve impulse is carried across the synapse by chemicals known as **neurotransmitters**.

Figure 14.13 illustrates the structure of a synapse.

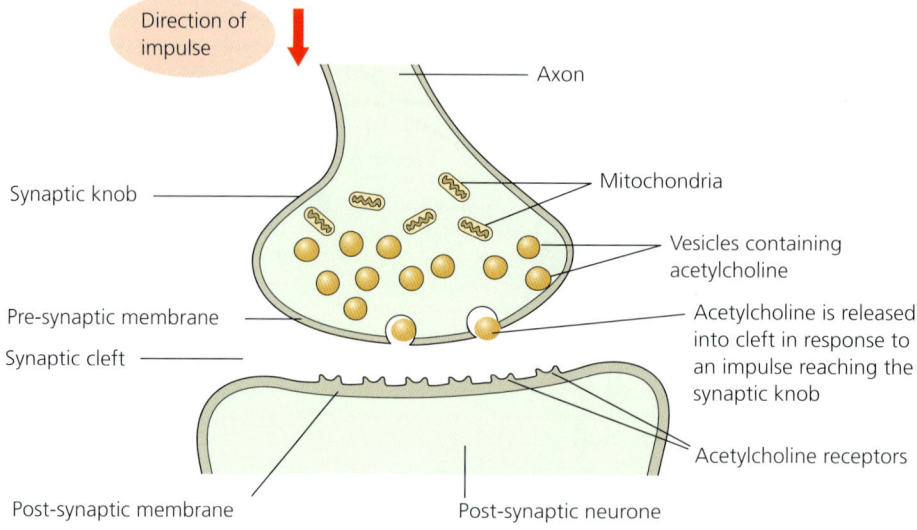

▲ Figure 14.13 The structure of a synapse

The synaptic knob makes a connection with a muscle or another neurone. When the nerve impulse arrives at the synaptic knob it causes release of neurotransmitter from membrane-bound **vesicles**. The most common neurotransmitter is **acetylcholine**. This diffuses across the synaptic cleft (see Figure 14.13) and then binds to **receptors** on the membrane of the muscle cell or the next neurone. If enough neurotransmitters bind, then the **post-synaptic** membrane will become depolarised and a new nerve impulse will be generated in the next neurone. The process is similar in muscle cells, except that the result is muscle contraction and not a new nerve impulse.

Different sensors in the body

We rely on our senses to tell us what is happening in the world around us. These work in different ways, depending on type, but they all have receptors connected to **nerve endings** of sensory neurones.

Pressure receptors detect, among other things, changes in blood pressure.

Temperature receptors are located in the skin, where they detect the external temperature, and in the CNS where they detect the core body temperature.

Sound receptors in the inner ear detect sound waves and so allow us to hear.

Light receptors are located in the retina of the eye and are involved in vision.

Touch receptors are a type of pressure receptor located in the skin and allow us to experience a range of sensations, from a gentle caress to a sharp slap, or to explore our surroundings using touch.

Pain receptors are located throughout the body. Their function is to signal to the CNS when injury has occurred. The ability to feel pain gives us an important survival advantage, particularly if it means that we can avoid more serious injury. Interestingly, there are no pain receptors in the brain – which is why some types of brain surgery can be performed just using a local anaesthetic.

Taste receptors fall in to two types:
- receptors on the tongue (taste buds) can detect the five main types of taste:
  - sweet
  - sour
  - bitter
  - salt
  - umami (this is the savoury taste we get from fried foods, fish sauce or mushrooms)
- **olfactory** receptors, located in the nasal passage, which detect smells or scents. Most of what we experience when we 'taste' food depends on our sense of smell rather than just taste.

> **Test yourself**
>
> 1 Describe the components of:
>   a the central nervous system
>   b the peripheral nervous system.
> 2 Describe the structure of the myelin sheath and explain why nerve impulses are transmitted faster in myelinated neurones.
> 3 Explain the difference in the way that a nerve impulse is transmitted along a nerve cell and the way it is transmitted between nerve cells.
> 4 Describe the location of temperature receptors.

B2.4 The musculoskeletal system

The term **musculoskeletal** refers to the skeleton and the muscles attached to the skeleton. The musculoskeletal system is involved in the support of the body and in movement. The adult human skeleton is made up of 206 bones connected by various types of **joints**.

Skeletal (striated) muscle is the type of muscle attached to the skeleton and involved in movement. The name striated refers to its striped appearance when viewed with a microscope (see Figure 14.19). Another name you might see is **voluntary** muscle because, when we move, we have conscious or voluntary control over the muscle.

> **Key terms**
>
> *Joint:* the area where two or more bones connect.
>
> *Skeletal muscle:* the main type of muscle involved in movement, because it is attached to the skeleton.

There are two other types of muscle.
- **smooth** or **involuntary** muscle (see page 302 for more), which is found in the gut (section B2.5) and blood vessels (section B2.6) and, as the name suggests, is involved in all the processes over which we have no conscious control, such as the movement of food along the gut or constriction or dilation of blood vessels
- **Cardiac** muscle, which is found in the heart (section B2.6).

The components and organisation of the musculoskeletal system

Figure 14.14 shows the main types of bone in the human skeleton.

Joints can be classified according to their **structure**.
- **Fibrous** joints (also called immovable joints) are where bones are fused together, usually to create a structure. A good example is the **skull**, which consists of a number of bones fused together.
- **Cartilaginous** joints have bones connected by relatively flexible cartilage that allows some degree of movement. An example is the rib cage (see section B2.2) where the ribs are joined together by cartilaginous joints that allow the ribs to move during breathing.
- **Synovial** joints are the most common type. They are flexible and move in a range of different ways. The hip joint (Figure 14.15) is a good example of a synovial joint.

> **Key term**
>
> **Cartilage:** another type of connective tissue that contains, among other components, collagen and the elastic protein elastin. Cartilage is more flexible than ligaments and muscles, but not as hard and rigid as bone.

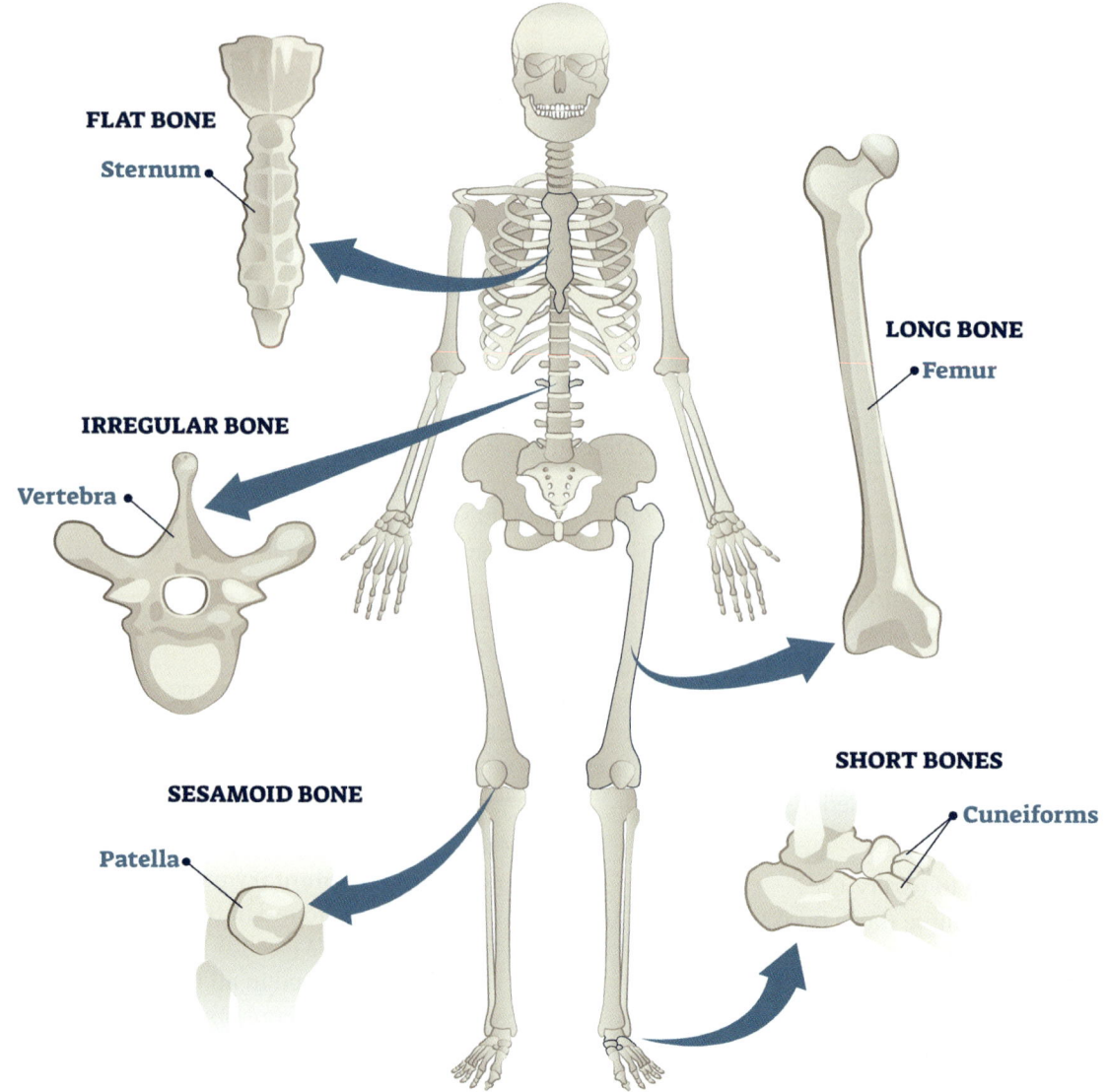

▲ Figure 14.14 The main types of bone in the human skeleton

B2: Further science concepts

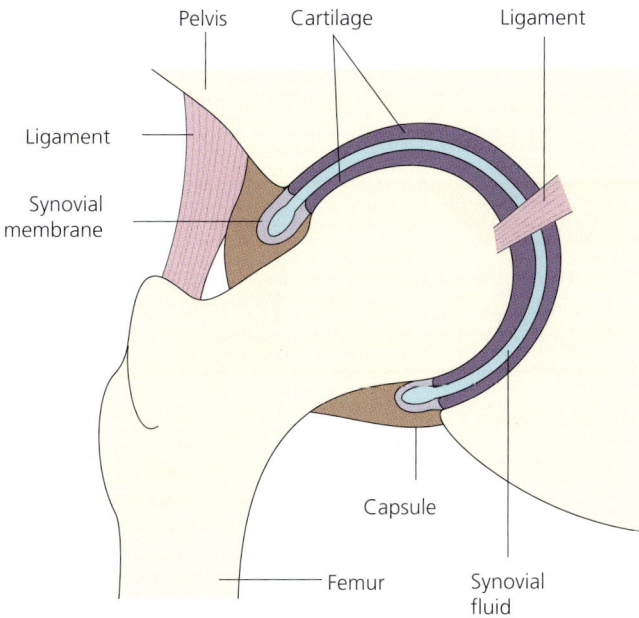

▲ Figure 14.15 The hip – a synovial joint

Synovial joints all have cartilage that provides cushioning between the bones that are joined. They also have a **synovial capsule** consisting of connective tissue containing **synovial fluid**. This helps to lubricate the joint, allowing smoother movement and reducing wear on the bones. **Ligaments** hold the bones together while allowing a degree of movement and flexibility.

Synovial joints can be classified according to their function. This functional classification of joints is based on the type and degree of movement they permit. Figure 14.16 shows the main types of joint in the human skeleton. You are not expected to know this amount of detail; this is provided only to show the context.

> **Key term**
>
> *Ligaments:* made of connective tissue containing the protein collagen. Their function is to join bones together and to strengthen joints.

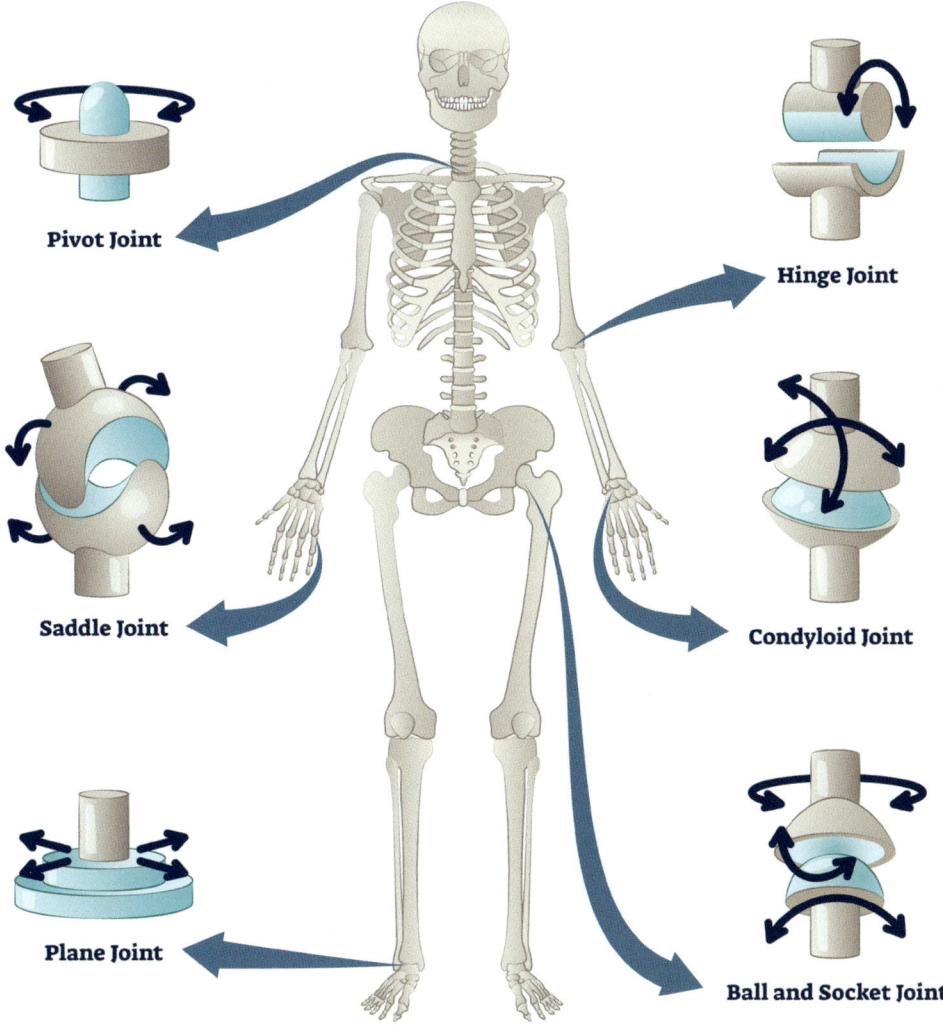

▲ Figure 14.16 The main types of synovial joint

297

The full skeletal structure is shown in Figure 14.17. You are not expected to know this amount of detail; this is provided only to show the context.

Besides bone and ligaments, the other main component of the musculoskeletal system are the muscles and associated **tendons**. These muscles are known as skeletal or striated muscles (Figure 14.18).

Muscle fibres are the individual muscle cells. They contain many **myofibrils**, which are responsible for muscle contraction. The muscle fibres are held together in bundles by a sheath of connective tissue and several of these bundles will make a single muscle. Tendons at each end of the muscle attach it to the bones.

Skeletal muscle viewed in the light microscope (Figure 14.19) has a characteristic striped appearance.

> **Key term**
>
> **Tendons:** similar in structure and composition to ligaments. Their function is to attach the muscles to the bones that make up the skeleton.

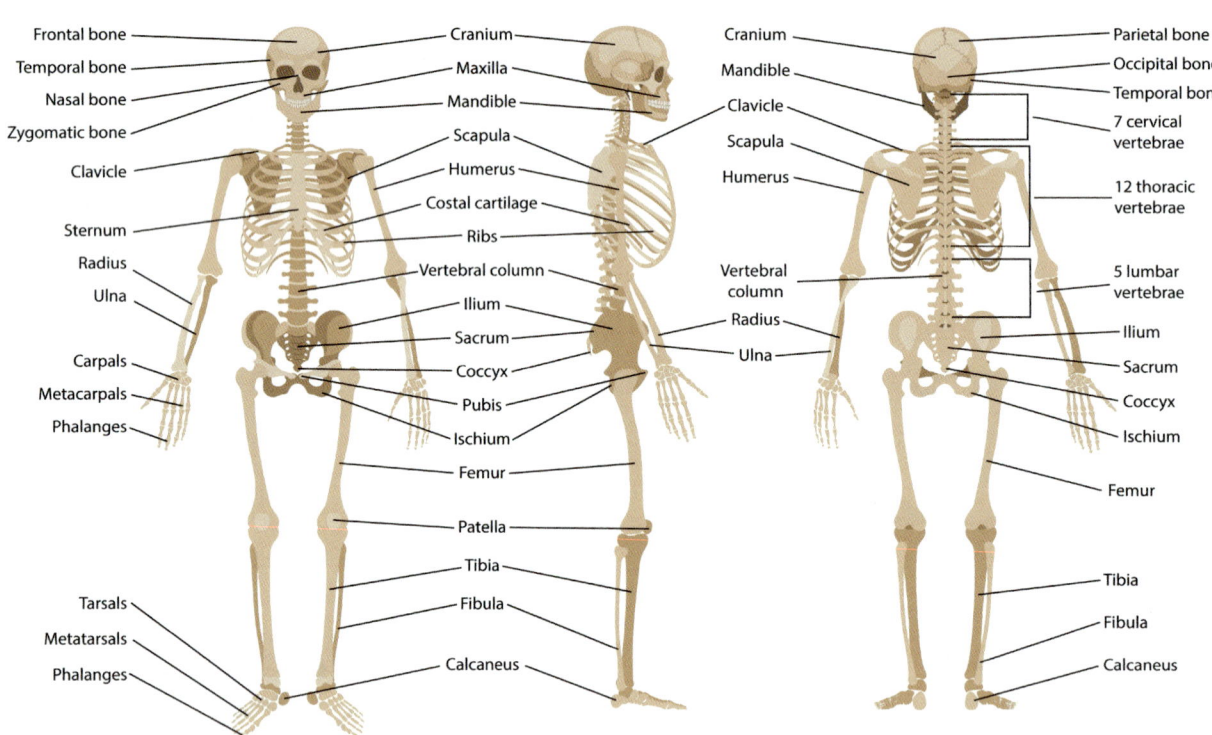

▲ Figure 14.17 The full skeletal structure

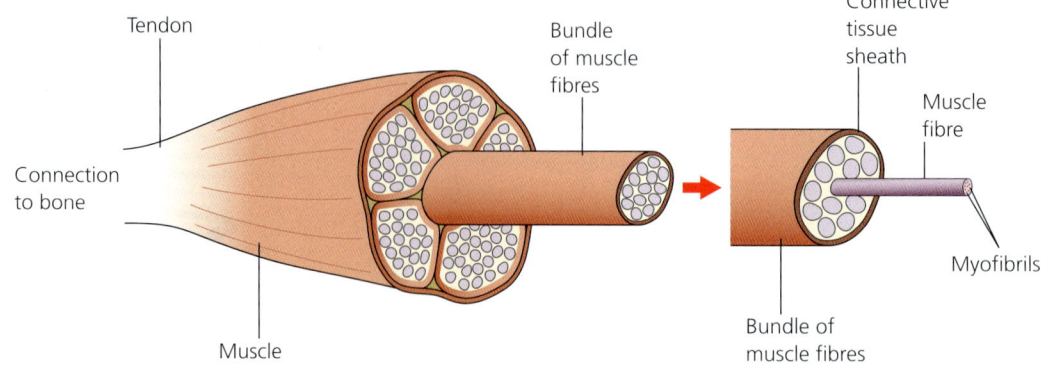

▲ Figure 14.18 The arrangement of muscle fibres in skeletal muscle

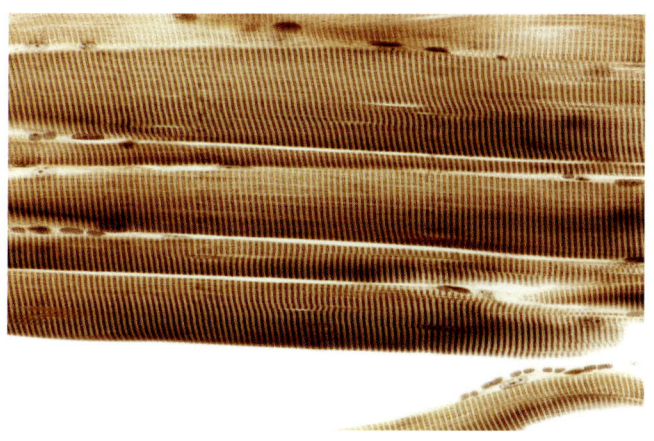

▲ Figure 14.19 Skeletal muscle fibres viewed through an optical microscope showing the striations

These striations give an insight into the way in which skeletal muscle contracts and forms the basis of the **sliding filament hypothesis**.

Functions of the musculoskeletal system

The skeletal system provides support for the body, protection of organs such as the brain, and also allows for attachment of the ligaments holding joints together and the muscles involved in movement.

> **Reflect**
>
> Think about how the following parts of the skeleton provide protection. Which organs do they protect?
> ▶ The skull.
> ▶ The backbone (vertebrae).
> ▶ The pelvis.
> ▶ The ribs.

There are also some less obvious functions of the skeletal system.

Blood production

The long bones (see Figure 14.14) contain a spongy tissue in the centre called the **bone marrow**. This contains many **stem cells** that can develop into all the different types of blood cells, including **erythrocytes** (red blood cells) and the various types of **lymphocytes** (white blood cells) that are involved in the immune response (covered in section B1.30).

Minerals

Bone is a complex structure of cells embedded in a hard material consisting of the protein **collagen** and the inorganic compound **calcium phosphate**. This makes bone a bit like the **composite materials** that we looked at in section B1.33.

The presence of large amounts of calcium phosphate allows bone to act as a reservoir of both of the minerals (calcium and phosphate ions) that are important for many processes in the body. Calcium is particularly important as it is involved in nerve conduction, muscle contraction and blood clotting. Phosphate is important as it is a major component of **DNA** and is also involved in energy metabolism. The main source of both calcium and phosphate is the diet. **Vitamin D** stimulates uptake of calcium from the gut and its incorporation into bone. However, the bones act as a **store** or **buffer** of both calcium and phosphate. The hormones **PTH** and **calcitonin** (section B2.1) regulate the levels of calcium and phosphate in the blood.

Movement (locomotion) and support

Figure 14.20 shows the two main muscles, **biceps** and **triceps**, involved in movement of the lower arm.

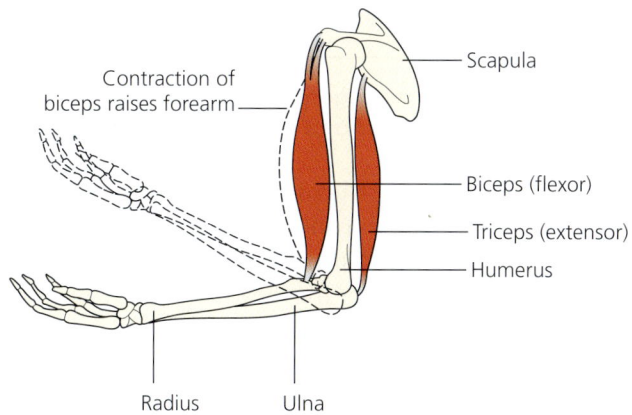

▲ Figure 14.20 Movement at the elbow showing the main bones and muscles involved

This shows an important principle of movement: muscles are generally arranged in **antagonistic** or **opposing pairs**. When the biceps contracts and the triceps relaxes, the forearm is raised. When the triceps contracts and the biceps relaxes, the forearm is lowered.

Sliding filament theory

Muscles contain two main proteins involved in muscle contraction, **actin** and **myosin**. These proteins make up the two types of **muscle filament** found in **myofibrils**:
▶ **thick** filaments contain myosin
▶ **thin** filaments contain actin, as well as two other proteins.

These filaments are arranged in the myofibrils in a repeating pattern known as **sarcomeres**. It is this repeating pattern that gives striated muscle its striped appearance.

When muscles contract, we can see that the sarcomeres **shorten**. You might expect, therefore, that the filaments shorten. However, this is not the case. We now know that the sarcomere shortens because the filaments slide over each other (Figure 14.21).

Relaxed

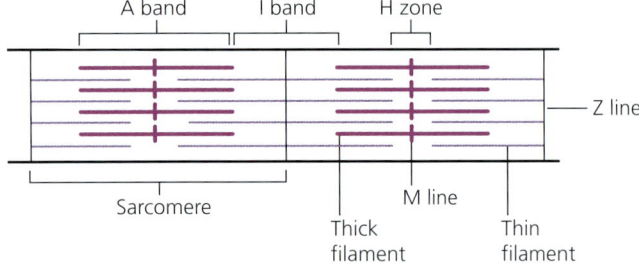

Contracted

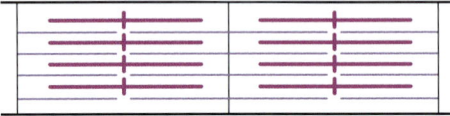

▲ Figure 14.21 The arrangement of thick and thin filaments in a relaxed and contracted myofibril

Figure 14.22 shows the structure of the thick and thin filaments. Thin filaments consist of long chains of actin molecules, while thick filaments are bundles of myosin molecules arranged so that the 'head' groups protrude all around the bundle. These head groups bind to actin molecules. When this happens, a change in the shape of the myosin head pulls the thin filament towards the centre of the sarcomere. The myosin head then detaches and energy transferred from the hydrolysis of adenosine triphosphate (ATP, see section B1.3) is used to change the myosin head back to its original shape ready to bind to another actin molecule. This process is repeated many times leading to shortening of the sarcomere. As a result of shortening of all the sarcomeres, the muscle contracts.

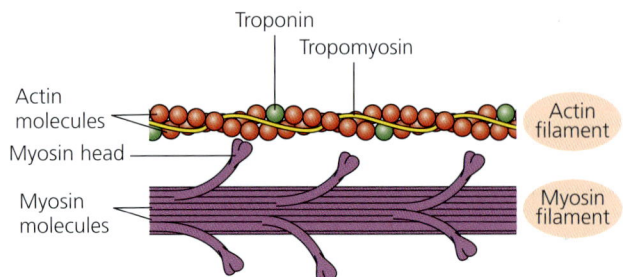

▲ Figure 14.22 The structure of thick and thin filaments

> **Test yourself**
>
> 1 Name and describe the three types of joint structure.
> 2 Give one example of each of the following types of joint:
>   a ball and socket joint
>   b hinge joint
>   c condyloid joint
>   d pivot joint.
> 3 Describe one similarity and one difference between ligaments and tendons.
> 4 Name the three types of muscle.
> 5 Name the main protein found in each of:
>   a thick filaments
>   b thin filaments.

B2.5 The digestive system

The components and organisation of the digestive system

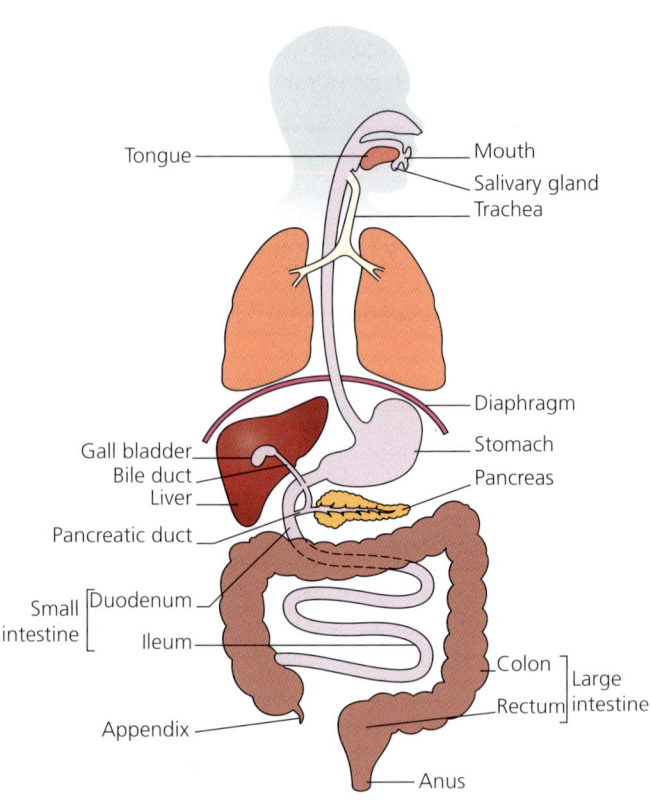

▲ Figure 14.23 The human digestive system

Figure 14.23 shows the human digestive system. You need to be familiar with the following parts:
- mouth
- oesophagus
- stomach
- pancreas
- liver
- small intestine, consisting of:
  - duodenum
  - ileum
- large intestine (colon).

The **gastrointestinal tract** (**GI tract**) consists of the oesophagus, stomach and small and large intestines. The wall of the GI tract has four layers (Figure 14.24). The figure shows the stomach wall, but other parts of the GI tract have a similar arrangement of layers.

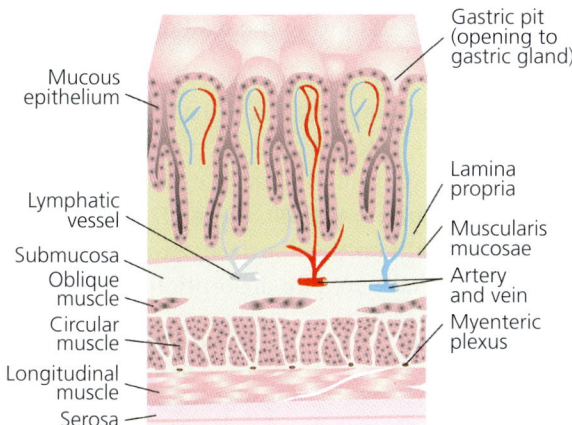

▲ Figure 14.24 The four layers of the wall of the GI tract: the mucosa, submucosa, muscularis and serosa

- The **mucosa** is the innermost layer, surrounding the **lumen** – the open space within the tube of the GI tract. The structure of the mucosa varies in the different parts of the GI tract, according to the function of each part.
- The **submucosa** consists of a dense layer of connective tissue with large blood vessels, **lymphatic vessels** and nerves.
- The **muscularis** or muscle layer has an inner oblique layer, a middle **circular** layer and outer **longitudinal** layer.
- The **serosa** forms the outer layer and consists of several layers of connective tissue.

There are also glands linked to the components of the GI tract that play an important part in digestion, including **salivary glands** in the mouth, the **gall bladder** and **bile duct**.

The functions of the digestive system

The digestive system breaks down food by **chemical** and **mechanical** digestion.

Mechanical digestion

This refers to the way in which food is broken up into smaller pieces, which increases the efficiency of chemical digestion.

The process starts with chewing the food (**mastication**). This begins the mechanical breakdown and mixes the food with **saliva**. The saliva helps lubricate the chewed food and contains the enzyme **salivary amylase**.

Mechanical digestion continues in the stomach where contraction of smooth muscle in the stomach wall causes a churning action, continually mixing the food with digestive enzymes and acid. This process can last for several hours.

Peristalsis describes the rhythmic movement of the wall of the gut that moves the food along the whole length of the GI tract. Circular muscle behind a mass of food contracts, pushing it forward. At the same time, longitudinal muscle around and ahead of the mass of food also contracts. This shortens the passage in front of the food. This process is controlled by the autonomic nervous system.

> **Key terms**
>
> **Smooth (involuntary) muscle:** Muscle that is not under conscious control. It is controlled by the **autonomic nervous system** and **hormones**.
>
> **Autonomic nervous system:** The part of the peripheral nervous system that controls many of the processes in the body over which we have no conscious control.

Chemical digestion

This involves digestive **enzymes** that catalyse (speed up) the **hydrolysis** reactions that break down the large molecules in food (proteins, lipids and polysaccharides such as starch) into smaller, simpler molecules. In sections B1.7 and B1.8, we saw how proteins and polysaccharides are formed by joining smaller molecules (amino acids and sugars) in **condensation** reactions. Hydrolysis is the reverse process.

Each type of food molecule is broken down by a specific type of enzyme, as shown in the following table. A major source of digestive enzymes is the pancreas. Pancreatic fluid is made by the pancreas and released into the duodenum via the pancreatic duct.

Enzyme	Location/source	Action
Salivary amylase	Saliva (in the mouth)	Begins the digestion of starch (a polysaccharide) into maltose (a disaccharide)
Pancreatic amylase	Pancreatic fluid	Completes digestion of starch into maltose
Disaccharidases: • maltase • sucrase • lactase	Duodenum	These convert disaccharides into their constituent monosaccharides **Maltase** completes the digestion of starch by converting maltose into two molecules of glucose **Sucrase** converts sucrose into glucose and fructose **Lactase** converts lactose into glucose and galactose
Proteases	Pepsin is located in the stomach Trypsin, chymotrypsin and carboxypeptidase are contained in pancreatic fluid	Proteases convert proteins into smaller fragments: peptides and eventually amino acids
Lipases	Pancreatic fluid	Break down lipids into fatty acids and glycerol

> **Reflect**
>
> **Enzymes – what's in a name?**
>
> If you look at the enzymes listed in the table above, you may notice a pattern. Most of them end in '-ase' and the first part of the name is linked to the function of the enzyme, for example we have maltase, sucrase and lactase. Amylase is so called because it digests a type of starch called amylose. Protease and lipase are general names that follow the same pattern. Pepsin, trypsin and chymotrypsin are exceptions to this rule – but you can usually tell what an enzyme does from its name.
>
> Find other enzyme names and see if you can match the name and the function.

There are two other important components of chemical digestion:
- **Hydrochloric acid**, secreted by glands in the stomach wall. This helps to sterilise the food and provides the acidic conditions required by stomach proteases such as pepsin.
- **Bile**, which is produced in the **liver**, is stored in the **gall bladder** and released into the duodenum via the **bile duct** and **pancreatic duct**. Bile acts as a surfactant (like a detergent) and helps to break up large fat globules into smaller droplets so that lipases can work more effectively.

Absorption processes

Digestion of the main food types can be summarised as:
- proteins → amino acids
- polysaccharides → monosaccharides
- lipids → fatty acids and glycerol

Absorption of the products of digestion occurs mainly in the **epithelial cells** lining the wall of the ileum.

Section B1.10 covered the principles of efficient exchange surfaces, in particular the need for a large surface area. This is achieved in the ileum by folding of the wall of the gut into finger-like projections called **villi** (singular = **villus**). The epithelial cells on villi have microvilli on their surface, which further increases the surface area for absorption (Figure 14.25).

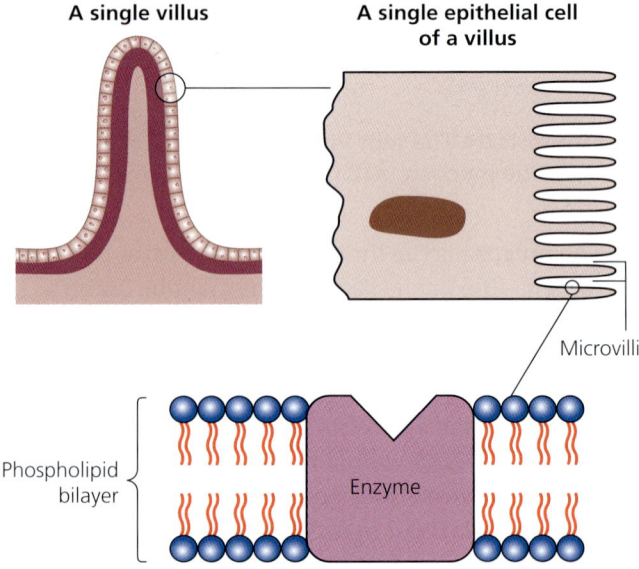

▲ Figure 14.25 The lining of the small intestine showing a villus, microvilli on the surface of an epithelial cell, and its cell surface membrane incorporating an enzyme, such as maltase

Section B1.11 covered the principles of transport across membranes.

Remember that polar molecules cannot cross the phospholipid bilayer, such as the one in the plasma membrane of the epithelial cells lining the ileum. Fatty acids are non-polar and can, therefore, pass into the epithelial cells by simple diffusion.

All the other products of digestion are polar molecules (monosaccharides, amino acids, etc.) and are absorbed into the epithelial cells by **active transport** and **facilitated diffusion**. The process of glucose absorption is covered in section B1.11; amino acids are absorbed by a similar mechanism.

The role of micro-organisms

A recent study estimated the total number of cells in the human body to be 3.0×10^{13}, while there are about 3.8×10^{13} bacterial cells. In terms of number of cells, we are all more bacteria than human!

Most of these bacteria reside in the **colon** and make up what is known as the **microbiome**. In **herbivores** such as cattle, horses and sheep, these gut bacteria play an important role in digestion of **cellulose** (the structural polysaccharide of plant cell walls) that cannot be digested by the animal's own enzymes. However, it is now understood that gut bacteria in humans also aid digestion, particularly for complex carbohydrates that are not broken down by enzymes such as amylase.

> **Test yourself**
>
> 1. Name the four parts of the gastrointestinal tract.
> 2. Name the four layers of the wall of the gut.
> 3. Name two sites of mechanical digestion.
> 4. State the location and function of each of the following digestive enzymes:
>   a salivary amylase b lactase c pepsin.
> 5. State the precise location of the absorption of the products of digestion.

B2.6 The cardiovascular system

Components and organisation of the cardiovascular system

The cardiovascular system consists of the heart and blood vessels.

Blood vessels

Figure 14.26 illustrates the structure of each of the three main types of blood vessel.

Arteries

The **arteries** carry blood away from the heart. The largest artery is the **aorta**, which leads directly from the left ventricle (see Figure 14.27) of the heart. The aorta divides into smaller arteries supplying all the organs of the body. The smallest arteries are called **arterioles**. Arteries have an outer layer of connective tissue that provides strength and support. However, they also have a thick layer of **muscle** and **elastic tissue**. The muscle allows **constriction** (narrowing) or **dilation** (widening) of the arteries to regulate blood flow to different parts of the body. The elastic tissue allows the artery to expand, helping it to withstand the pressure caused by the pumping of the heart.

Capillaries

The arterioles lead to the **capillaries**. These are the smallest vessels in the cardiovascular system and have a wall that is just a single cell thick.

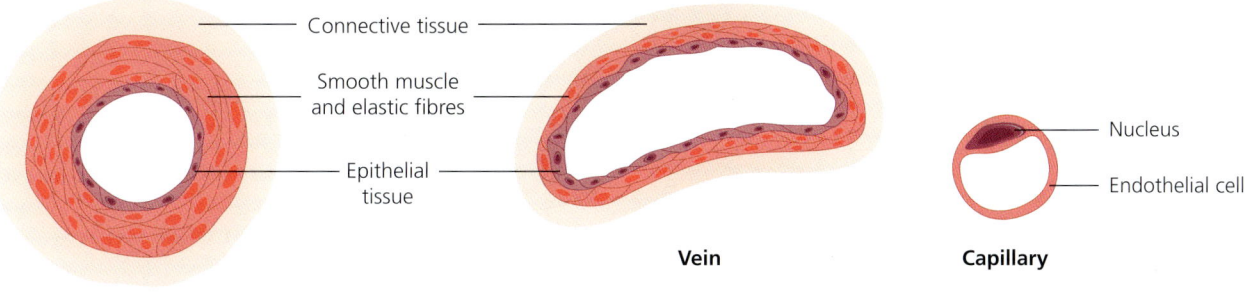

▲ Figure 14.26 Cross sections of an artery, a vein and a capillary; capillaries are often single cells wrapped into a tubular shape

Veins

The capillaries come together to form **venules**, which merge to form larger **veins**. The blood is at a much lower pressure in the veins because it has had to force its way through the narrow capillaries), so the **lumen** (the space in the middle) of a vein is much larger than that of an artery. Veins also have thinner walls as they do not need to absorb the pressure of the pumping of the heart.

The heart

The heart is a pump. The blood enters via the **atria** and passes into the **ventricles**. The ventricles have thick muscular walls that contract to pump the blood to the lungs (right ventricle) or around the body (left ventricle). To ensure that blood only flows in the right direction, the heart also contains **valves** that prevent back-flow. Figure 14.27 illustrates the structures of the heart that you need to be familiar with.

You should take note of some of the features of the heart.

- The right ventricle is on the left as you look at the diagram and the left ventricle is on the right. That is because we label them from the viewpoint of the animal (in this case, the human). This is just like when you face someone and their left arm is on the right as you look at them.
- The left ventricle has a thicker, stronger muscle wall. This is because it has to pump blood around the whole body. The right ventricle only has to pump blood a short distance to the lungs.
- The **atria** have relatively thin walls as they only need to pump blood into the adjacent ventricle.
- The **bicuspid** and **tricuspid** valves (also known as **atrioventricular** or **AV** valves) prevent blood flowing backwards from the ventricle into the atrium. When the pressure is higher in the atrium than in the ventricle, the valves are pushed open. When the pressure is higher in the ventricle than in the atrium, the valves are pushed closed. The tendons prevent the valves from being pushed too far so that they make a good seal.
- The **semi-lunar valves** have a different structure, but they perform a similar function to the bicuspid and tricuspid valves. Because the semi-lunar valves are located at the entrance to the pulmonary artery and the aorta, they prevent back-flow from these blood vessels into the ventricles.

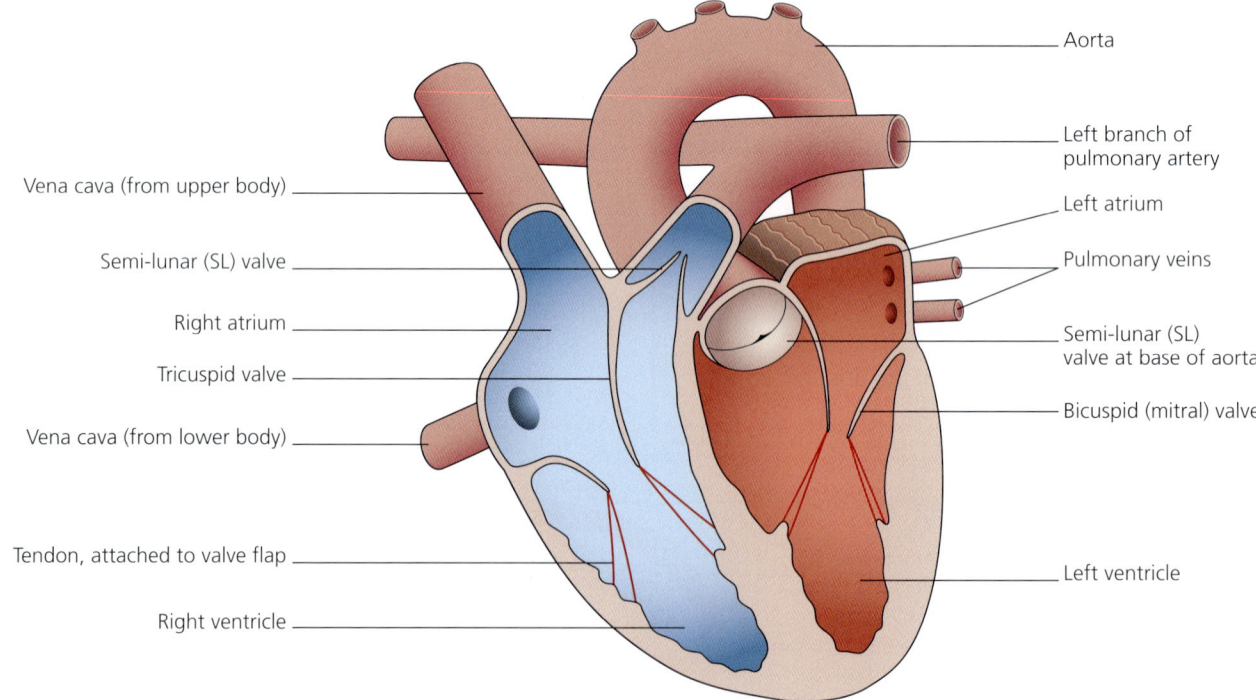

▲ Figure 14.27 Cross section through the human heart

Composition of the blood

The blood is made up of:
- plasma
- platelets
- red blood cells
- white blood cells.

Plasma is the straw-coloured fluid that is left if all the cells in blood are removed. It contains proteins, known as **plasma proteins**, and hormones, as well as all the small molecules (carbon dioxide, glucose, amino acids) and ions transported in the blood.

Platelets are small disc-shaped cell fragments without nuclei that are also called **thrombocytes**. They are present in large numbers in the blood and play an important role in blood **clotting**.

Red blood cells, or **erythrocytes**, are differentiated cells without a nucleus or the majority of their organelles. They are filled with **haemoglobin**, the protein that transports oxygen from the lungs to the tissues.

White blood cells, or **leucocytes**, are cells that are mostly involved in protection against infection including the immune response (see section B1.30).

The functions of the cardiovascular system

The cardiovascular system facilitates the circulation of blood to transport:
- nutrients (glucose, amino acids, lipids, vitamins, etc.), required for cell growth and repair
- oxygen, required for cellular respiration
- carbon dioxide, transported to the lungs to be eliminated from the body
- hormones (see section B2.1), transported to target cells
- blood cells
  - erythrocytes for the transport of oxygen
  - leucocytes as part of the immune system.

The human circulatory system is known as a **double circulatory system**. This is because the blood passes through the heart twice for every circuit of the whole body.

The first loop is from the heart to the lungs, then back to the heart. The second loop is from the heart, through all the other organs and back to the heart again (Figure 14.28). This means that, with very few exceptions, the heart will only have to pump through one set of capillaries at a time.

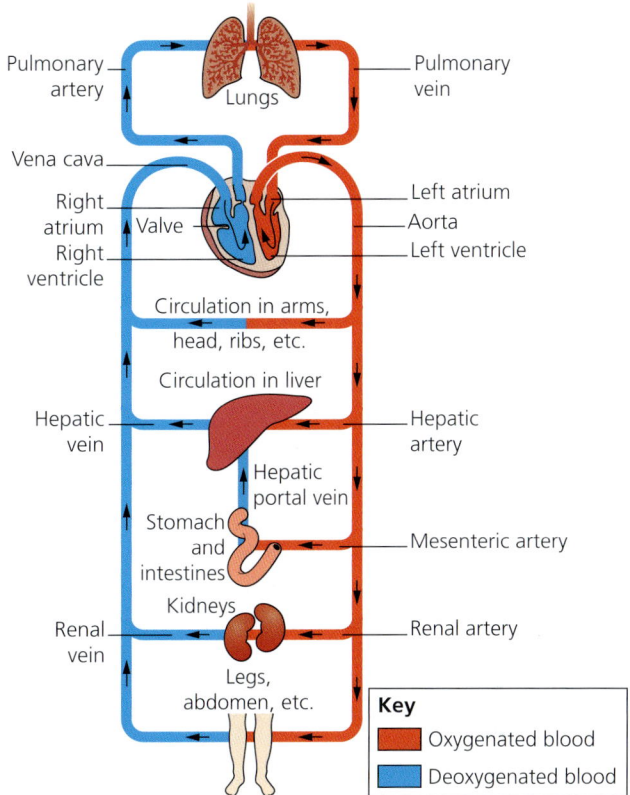

▲ Figure 14.28 The organisation of the human cardiovascular system

The main exception to this is the digestive system, where blood flows via the **mesenteric artery** to the capillaries surrounding the **gut**. It then flows via the **hepatic portal vein** to the **liver**, which is where most of the products of digestion are processed and **metabolised**. The **hepatic vein** then takes blood from the liver back to the heart.

The cardiac cycle

The heart pumps blood through a series of muscle contractions and relaxations called the **cardiac cycle**. One way to understand this is to trace the path taken by the blood through the heart:
- the blood enters the right atrium from the vena cava
- it then flows into the right ventricle
- from the right ventricle, it is pumped into the pulmonary artery to the lungs
- returning from the lungs via the pulmonary vein, the blood enters the left atrium
- it then flows into the left ventricle
- from the left ventricle, blood is pumped into the aorta and around the body.

You can trace this 'journey' taken by the blood using a very simple diagram like Figure 14.29.

Healthcare Science T Level: Core

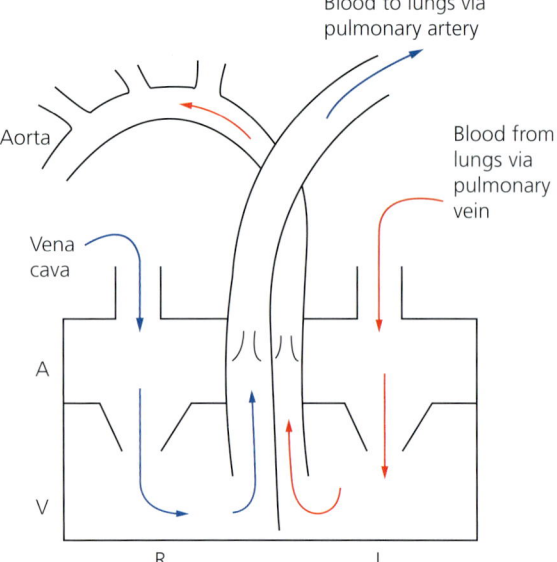

▲ Figure 14.29 Simplified diagram of the heart showing the main chambers, valves and blood vessels, illustrating the route taken by blood through the heart; A = atria, V = ventricles, R = right, L = left

We can also understand the working of the heart by thinking about the pressure changes that occur during the cardiac cycle. This is illustrated in Figure 14.30.

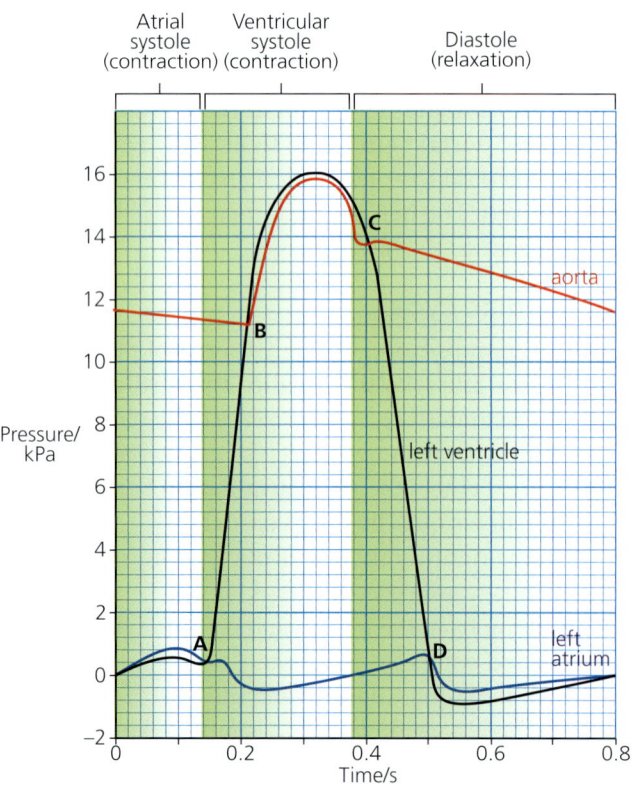

▲ Figure 14.30 A graph showing how pressure changes in the left atrium, left ventricle and aorta during one cardiac cycle

> **Key terms**
>
> **Systole** refers to the contraction of either atrium or ventricle: hence the terms **atrial systole** and **ventricular systole**, respectively.
>
> **Diastole** refers to the relaxation of either atrium or ventricle.

This might appear complicated at first. However, once you learn to read the graph it really does help understand what is happening. The graph shows how the pressure changes in the left atrium and left ventricle during one complete cardiac cycle.

It is probably easiest to follow what is happening if we start towards the end of cycle, at about 0.6 s on the graph.

▶ Blood is flowing back from the lungs into the left atrium. The pressure in the **atrium** is higher than in the **ventricle**, so the **bicuspid** valve is open and blood flows into the ventricle. We can think of this as the heart filling with blood.

▶ During **atrial systole**, the atrium contracts. This completes the emptying of blood from the atrium into the ventricle in preparation for the next stage.

▶ **Ventricular systole** is when the ventricle contracts. Its thick muscle wall means that the pressure in the ventricle rises rapidly. At point **A** on Figure 14.30 the pressure in the ventricle is higher than in the atrium and this pushes the **bicuspid valve** closed, preventing back-flow.

▶ As the pressure in the ventricle rises, it quickly exceeds the pressure in the **aorta**. This has happened at point **B** on Figure 14.30, and this pushes the semi-lunar valve open so that blood flows into the aorta.

▶ This causes the ventricle to empty.

▶ The cycle then moves to **diastole** (relaxation) and, at point **C** on Figure 14.30, the pressure in the ventricle falls below that in the aorta.

▶ This causes the semi-lunar valve to close, again preventing back-flow.

▶ Closure of the semi-lunar valve causes a drop in pressure in the aorta (the **dicrotic notch**) followed immediately by a slight increase in pressure (the **dicrotic wave**) that is caused by recoil of the elastic tissue in the wall of the aorta.

▶ The pressure in the ventricle continues to fall until, at point **D** on Figure 14.30, the pressure falls below that in the atrium. This causes the bicuspid valve to open, allowing blood to flow into the ventricle and the whole cycle can begin again.

Something else you will notice in Figure 14.30 is the spike in pressure in the aorta as the left ventricle contracts and forces blood into it and around the body. This spike can be felt as the **pulse** in many arteries, for example in the wrist or neck. As there is one spike in pressure for each heart contraction, the pulse can be used to measure heart rate.

You will also see how the pressure in the aorta reaches a maximum during ventricular systole and falls during diastole. This pressure can be measured and forms the basis of widely used blood pressure measurements (see section B2.11).

The regulation of heart rate

The heart contains a specialised type of muscle known as **cardiac muscle**. Other types of muscle (skeletal and smooth muscle) require nerve impulses to cause them to contract. In contrast, cardiac muscle is **myogenic** – it will contract in a regular pattern without any nerve input.

Contraction of heart muscle is initiated by a small patch of specialised cardiac muscle on the wall of the right atrium known as the **sinoatrial node** or **SAN** (Figure 14.31). This is also known as the pacemaker because it maintains the regular contraction of the heart.

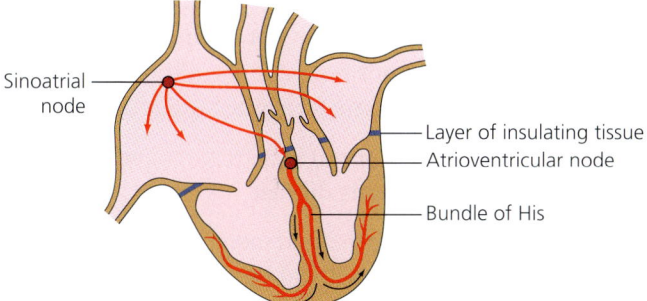

▲ Figure 14.31 Electrical activity in the heart that co-ordinates the heartbeat

The SAN generates electrical signals that spread out over the surface of the right and left atria, causing them to depolarise and leading to contraction (atrial systole). This electrical activity is unable to pass directly to the muscle of the ventricles as there is a layer of collagen that acts as an insulator between the atria and the ventricles.

However, these electrical signals reach another patch of specialised cardiac muscle known as the **atrioventricular node** or **AVN**. After a brief pause, the AVN generates more electrical signals that pass along another type of specialised muscle cells that act like nerve fibres. These are known as the **bundle of His** because they were discovered by the anatomist Wilhelm His. The electrical activity (depolarisation) generated passes down the muscle separating the two ventricles and then passes up the walls of the two ventricles. As it does, it initiates contraction of the ventricles.

There are two important consequences of this complex arrangement:
1. the pause caused by the AVN means that the atria can complete their emptying into the ventricles before the ventricles start to contract
2. contraction of the ventricles from the base of the heart upwards, towards the pulmonary artery and aorta, means that the ventricles are not trying to pump blood against a blind end.

Left to itself, the heart would maintain a regular heartbeat. However, we know that heart rate increases in times of stress or when we exercise. This is under nervous control, co-ordinated by the **cardioregulatory centre** in the medulla, as shown in Figure 14.32. Two types of receptor, **chemoreceptors** and **pressure receptors**, detect changes in the acidity of the blood and blood pressure. These are located in the aorta and in the **carotid arteries** that pass through the neck to the brain. The cardioregulatory centre responds to inputs from these receptors and sends nerve impulses to the SAN that either speed up or slow down the heart rate.

Use of electrocardiography (ECG) to monitor heart activity

The electrical activity of heart muscle that causes the heartbeat can be detected using electrocardiography (ECG). This uses electrodes placed on the skin to detect electrical signals and produce an electrocardiogram (also abbreviated to ECG). Figure 14.33 shows an ECG of a healthy heart.

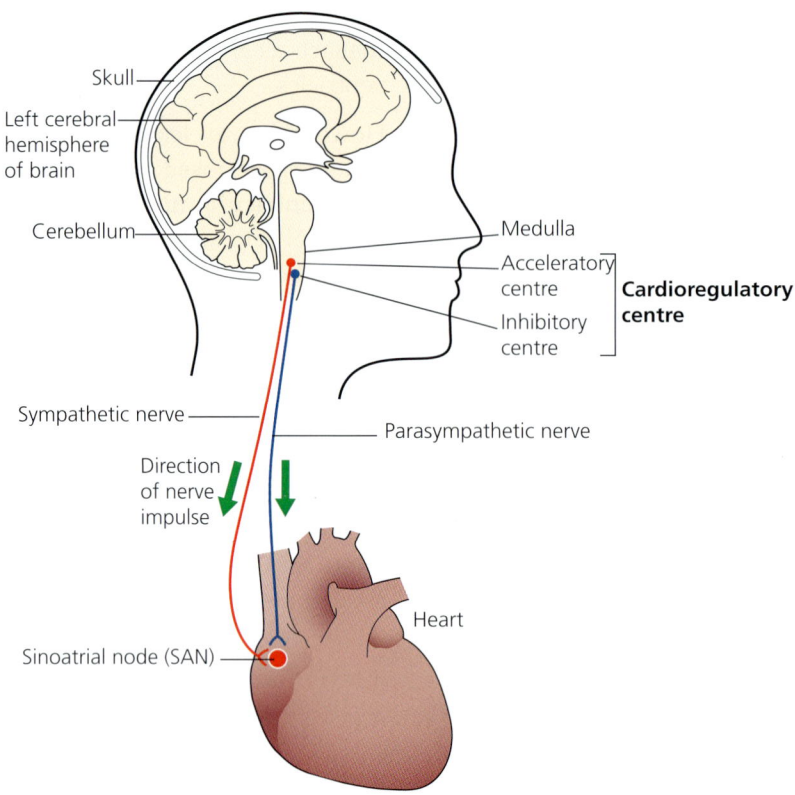

▲ Figure 14.32 Role of the medulla in the regulation of heartbeat

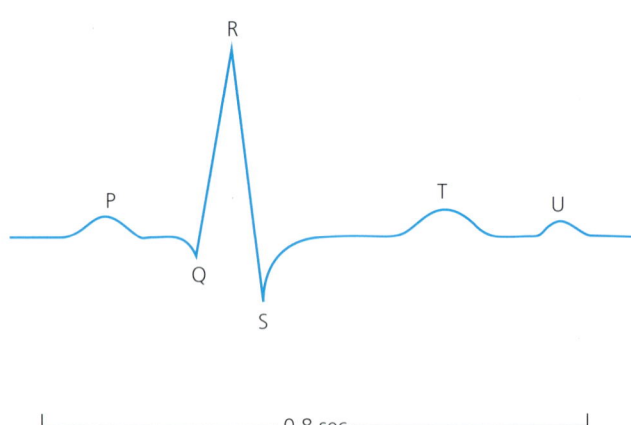

▲ Figure 14.33 ECG showing one beat of a healthy heart

The ECG shows several distinctive waves caused by the heart activity:
- The **P wave** is caused by depolarisation of the atria initiated by the electrical signals generated by the SAN (atrial systole).
- The **QRS complex** is caused by depolarisation of the ventricles initiated by the electrical signals generated by the AVN and transmitted along the bundle of His (ventricular systole).
- The **T wave** is caused by repolarisation of the ventricles (diastole).
- The cause of the **U wave** is not certain and it is not always present in normal patients, although it can be exaggerated in some forms of cardiac disease.

Figure 14.34 shows a normal ECG trace together with examples of types of heart disease.

Atrial fibrillation is a faster and more irregular heartbeat caused by disorganised electrical signals in the atria. It is the most common serious abnormal heart rhythm and affects more than 33 million people worldwide.

Ventricular fibrillation is caused by disorganised electrical signals in the ventricles, which causes them to twitch randomly rather than contracting in an organised way. If it is not treated it can rapidly lead to cardiac arrest (the heart stops beating) and death.

B2: Further science concepts

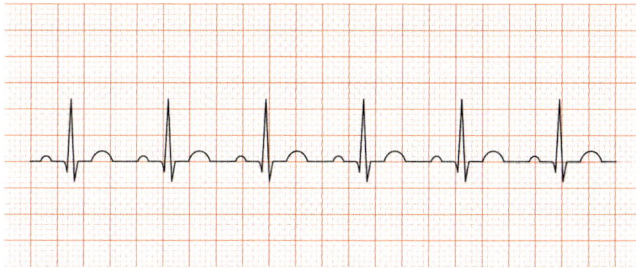

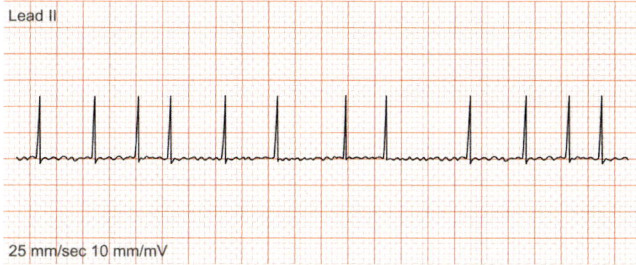

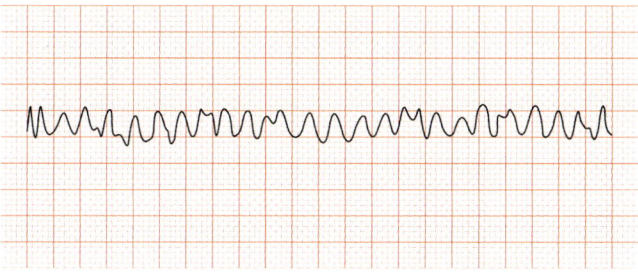

▲ Figure 14.34 ECGs of normal heart rhythm (top), atrial fibrillation (middle) and ventricular fibrillation (bottom)

Other abnormalities can also be diagnosed by ECG, including:
- **tachycardia**, where the heart beats too rapidly – a resting heart rate greater than 100 beats per minute (bpm): the peaks on the ECG are too close together
- **bradycardia**, where the heart beats too slowly – a resting heart rate less than 60 bpm: the peaks are too far apart
- **ectopic heartbeat** where the heart beats too early, followed by a pause: this is quite common and usually does not require any treatment.

Note that a resting heart rate of less than 60 bpm is not necessarily a sign of heart disease. Highly trained athletes can have resting heart rates of 50 bpm or less.

Blood groups

We saw in section B1.29 how all body cells have **antigens** on their plasma membranes that allow the immune system to distinguish between self and non-self.

Two types of these antigen are found in the plasma membranes of erythrocytes and form the basis of the two most important types of blood group: **ABO** and **Rhesus (Rh)**.

The **ABO system** is used to indicate the presence of one, both or neither of the A and B antigens on erythrocytes.
- group A blood only has the A antigen
- group B blood only has the B antigen
- group AB blood has both antigens
- group O blood has neither antigen.

This system is of great importance in **blood transfusion**. You would normally be given blood of the same **blood type** as your own, otherwise your immune system will see it as foreign. However, a person with type AB blood will have both antigens, so their immune system will not recognise A, B or O types of blood as foreign. Similarly, because type O blood does not contain either antigen, it can be given to recipients of any ABO blood type. Fortunately, type O blood is the most common type in western Europe.

The **Rh system** is based around another set of antigens on erythrocytes. There are 49 defined Rh antigens, of which the **RhD** is by far the most common. According to the NHS (**www.nhs.uk/conditions/blood-groups**), about 85 per cent of the UK population have the RhD antigen and are described as **Rh positive** while about 15 per cent lack the antigen and are described as **Rh negative**.

As group O and Rh positive are the most common, it is not surprising that O positive is the most common blood type. However, O negative is probably the most useful. Because these individuals do not carry ABO or Rh antigens, they are known as 'universal donors' as their blood can be given to almost all recipients. Although they only form about eight per cent of the UK population, about 13 per cent of blood donors in the UK have O negative blood, so the donation rates are higher than average in response to this demand for their blood type.

Healthcare Science T Level: Core

> **Test yourself**
>
> 1. Blood vessels have similarities and differences. Name one feature that is common to arteries, veins and capillaries.
> 2. Give one difference between the structure of arteries and veins.
> 3. Describe the path through the heart taken by blood from the vena cava via the lungs to the aorta. Include all the valves and the main blood vessels in your answer.
> 4. Explain why the human cardiovascular system is described as a double circulation system.
> 5. Describe:
>   a. the role of the sinoatrial node (SAN) in how the heart maintains a steady rate of contraction without nerve impulses
>   b. the role of the AVN and bundle of His.

B2.7 The reproductive system in males and females

At its simplest, **sexual reproduction** involves formation of male and female **gametes**. Male gametes are **sperm cells** (also known as **spermatozoa**). Female gametes are **egg cells** (also known as **ova**). In the process of **fertilisation**, the gametes fuse to form a **zygote** (fertilised egg cell). The zygote develops into an **embryo** and then a **fetus**. This is covered in more detail next.

First, we have to consider the components of the female and male reproductive systems (Figure 14.35).

> **Key terms**
>
> **Gametes:** haploid cells (half the number of chromosomes) that are produced by **meiosis**, a type of cell division that halves the number of chromosomes.
>
> **Fertilisation:** The fusion of haploid gametes (sperm and egg) to form the **diploid** zygote with the full number of chromosomes.

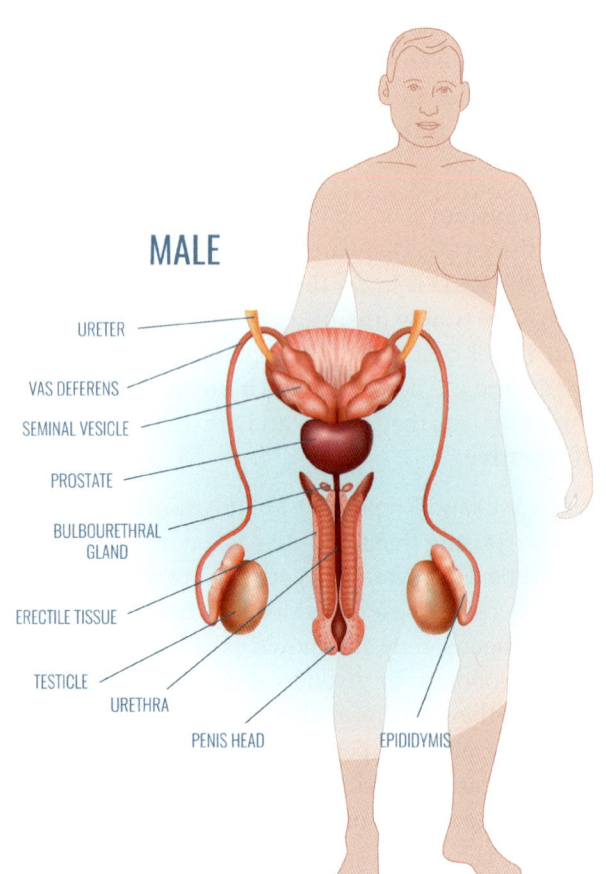
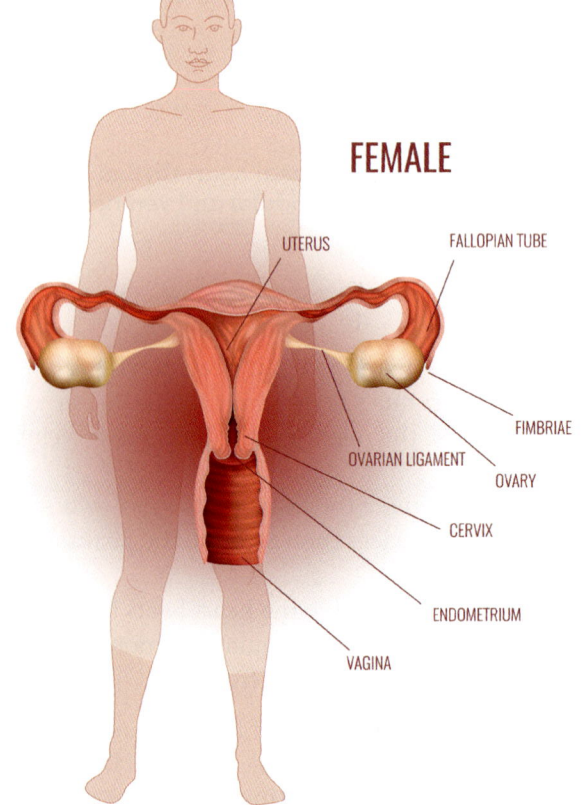

▲ Figure 14.35 The human reproductive system

The components and organisation of the female reproductive system

Ovaries

The ovaries produce the female **gametes** (egg cells). Usually, one egg is released in every menstrual cycle. For more detail on the hormones that control the menstrual cycle, see section B2.1.

Fallopian tubes

The fallopian tubes connect the ovaries with the **uterus**. An egg cell that is released from the ovary is drawn into the fallopian tube where it may meet a sperm cell and fertilisation may occur. The fertilised or unfertilised egg cell passes down the fallopian tube to the uterus. A fertilised egg will have become an embryo by this stage and will become implanted in the wall of the **uterus**. An unfertilised egg will pass out of the uterus with the **menstrual flow**.

Uterus and cervix

The **cervix** is a ring of muscle that acts as a barrier to the **uterus**. Cervical mucus helps to either block or promote the passage of sperm from the vagina to the uterus at different stages in the menstrual cycle.

If an egg is fertilised and becomes an embryo, it will implant in the wall of the uterus and will develop into a fetus. The cervix remains closed during pregnancy and a plug of cervical mucus helps keep pathogens from infecting the fetus. At the end of pregnancy, the hypothalamus (see section B2.1, page 284) releases the hormone **oxytocin**. This stimulates contraction of the muscular wall of the uterus which, along with the pressure of the baby's head on the cervix, causes the cervix to start to **dilate** (get wider). This leads to the release of more oxytocin, stimulating even more contraction of the uterus. This is an example of **positive feedback**, where movement away from a normal level (in this case, contraction of the uterus) leads to movement even further away from the normal level. This normally leads to rapid delivery of the baby.

Vagina

The **vagina** is the elastic, muscular part of the female reproductive system. It stretches from the **external genitalia** or **vulva** to the cervix. The vagina fulfils three functions:
- it receives sperm during sexual intercourse
- it forms the **birth canal** along which the baby moves during childbirth
- it allows the loss of menstrual blood when the lining of the uterus breaks down during each cycle.

> **Key term**
>
> *Genitalia:* the male and female sex organs.

The components and organisation of the male reproductive system

While the female reproductive system is mostly internal (inside the body), the male reproductive system is largely external (on the outside of the body).

External organs

Penis and urethra

The **penis** has a dual function. The **urethra** connects to the **bladder** and provides an exit from the body for **urine** (see section B2.8). The urethra is also connected, via the **vas deferens**, to the testes (see section B2.1), which is where sperm is produced. During sexual arousal, the erectile tissue of the penis fills with blood, which causes it to become erect. This allows it to be inserted into the vagina of the female during sexual intercourse. **Semen**, which contains sperm, is expelled through the end of the penis (a process called **ejaculation**) when the man reaches a **sexual climax** or **orgasm**. (When the penis is erect, the flow of urine into the urethra is blocked so that only semen is ejaculated.)

Scrotum and testes

The **testes** produce sperm and are contained within the **scrotum**. This is a relatively loose sac of skin that hangs below and behind the penis. By holding the testes outside of the core body, they are maintained at a slightly lower temperature than normal body temperature; this is essential for normal sperm development.

Internal organs

Vas deferens and seminal vesicles

The **vas deferens** is a long, muscular tube that carries sperm from the testis to the urethra. There is one on each side. Each vas deferens meets the **seminal vesicles** just before it enters the urethra at the base of the bladder. The seminal vesicles produce a fluid rich in the sugar fructose that provides sperm with a source of energy to help them move once they reach the vagina.

Prostate

The **prostate gland**, which surrounds the urethra just below the bladder, also contributes fluid that helps to nourish the sperm. The combination of sperm with the seminal fluid and fluid from the prostate forms **semen** (also known as **ejaculate**).

> **Practice point**
>
> The prostate gland is often misspellt as the 'prostrate gland'. **Prostrate** means 'lying face down' and has nothing to do with the male reproductive system.

The functions of the reproductive system

Sexual reproduction involves male and female gametes fusing in the process of fertilisation. In one sense, it provides a mechanism for the survival of the species by producing offspring through the combination of gametes (eggs and sperm). However, you will have learned from studying genetics in Chapter B1 (section B1.13, page 225) that sexual reproduction means that offspring inherit characteristics from both parents. This leads to greater variation, meaning that some organisms can become better adapted to their environments. This gives some a survival advantage and is the basis of **evolution**.

The **male** reproductive system has one function: to produce and deposit sperm as described before.

The **female** reproductive system has two functions:
- to produce egg cells; this occurs during the menstrual cycle and was discussed in section B2.1
- to protect and nourish an offspring until birth.

The second function is carried out by the **uterus** and **placenta**. As the embryo develops, part of the embryo grows into the wall of the uterus. This is the placenta, and it has a rich blood supply that is in very close contact with the mother's blood supply. This allows for exchange of gases (oxygen and carbon dioxide), supply of nutrients (glucose, amino acids, etc.) and removal of waste products via the mother. The fetus is also contained within membranes in the fluid-filled amniotic sac, which provides additional protection.

Stages of embryofetal development

This begins with the process of fertilisation and ends with the birth of the baby. Fertilisation of the egg cell occurs in the fallopian tubes and forms the **zygote** (fertilised egg), which travels down the fallopian tubes towards the uterus, dividing several times to form a ball of cells known as the **morula**. Cell division continues forming, after about four days, the **blastocyst**. At this point differentiation has occurred and the blastocyst consists of an outer layer of cells that will form the extra-embryonic structures (placenta and membranes) and an inner layer that will develop into the fetus. The blastocyst reaches the uterus after about five days and the outer layer of cells adhere to the cells lining the uterus. This initiates the process of implantation that is complete about eight to ten days after ovulation. Once implanted, the embryo grows rapidly and cell differentiation begins (see section B1.5).

Pregnancy begins when the zygote becomes implanted in the uterus. In humans it is divided into three **trimesters**, each approximately three months long. Gestational age is a measure of the age of a pregnancy taken from the beginning of the mother's last menstrual period; this will typically be about 14 days before the date of fertilisation. By the 10th week of gestation (8th week of development) the developing organism is known as a fetus. The growth rate is linear up to 37 weeks of gestation, after which it reaches a plateau. This is illustrated in Figure 14.36.

> **Test yourself**
>
> 1. Give a simple description of sexual reproduction.
> 2. Describe the function of the following parts of the female reproductive system:
>   a. fallopian tubes
>   b. cervix
>   c. vagina.
> 3. Describe how semen is formed.
> 4. Describe the two functions of the female reproductive system.

B2: Further science concepts

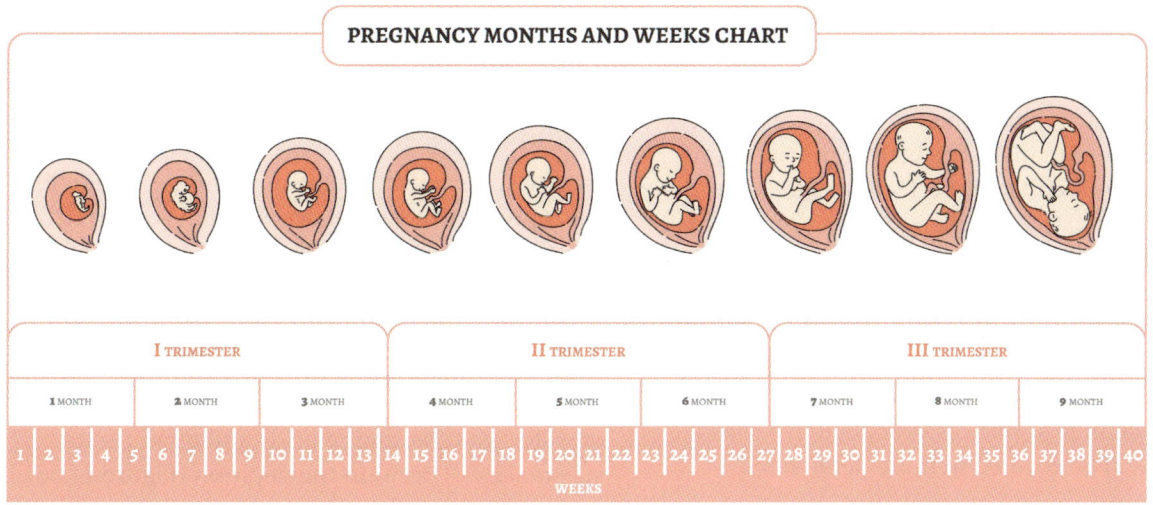

▲ Figure 14.36 The stages of human pregnancy

B2.8 The renal system

The renal system has two main functions:
▶ **excretion** or removal from the body of **nitrogenous waste** in the form of **urea**
▶ **osmoregulation** or regulation of the water balance of the body. This aspect was discussed in section B2.1.

Proteins and nucleic acids both contain nitrogen. We normally take in more nitrogen-containing compounds in our food that we need daily. Any excess is converted to **urea** by the **liver**. The urea is transported in the blood to the kidneys where it is removed during the process of formation of **urine**.

The renal system is sometimes called the **urinary system** and is closely connected with the reproductive system. For this reason, the two systems are sometimes referred to as the **genitourinary system**.

The components and organisation of the renal system

The **kidneys** form the main part of the renal system. If you look at Figure 14.37, you will see that the kidneys are supplied by the left and right **renal arteries**. Blood leaves the kidney via the **renal veins**. Urine, formed in the kidney, is transported via the **ureter** to the **bladder** where it is stored prior to **urination**.

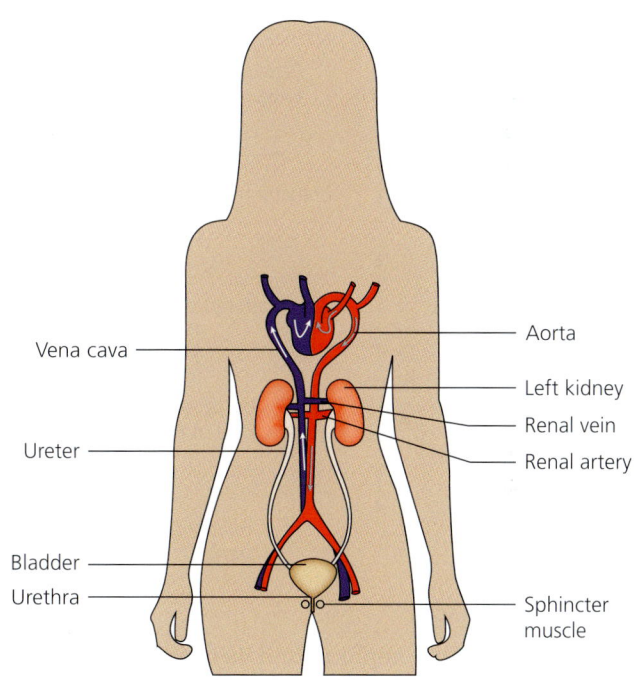

▲ Figure 14.37 The urinary system

Glomerulus

The **glomerulus** is a knot or tangle of capillaries in the space surrounded by Bowman's capsule (see Figure 14.38) and is the site of **ultrafiltration**; this is described in the next section.

Nephron

Each kidney contains about one million nephrons. The **nephron** is the main functional unit of the kidney. It is like a long, U-shaped tube surrounded by capillaries. The nephron is where the blood is filtered and where water and other useful substances are reabsorbed leading to the production of urine. Many nephrons connect with collecting ducts that take what has become urine towards the ureter and then the bladder. The length of the nephron means that there is a large surface area for exchange. The wall of the nephron is a single layer of **epithelial** cells that is in close contact with capillaries whose walls are a single layer of **endothelial** cells. This means that there is a short diffusion pathway. Finally, the unusual layout of the nephron, with **the loop of Henle** (Figure 14.38), helps to maintain a concentration gradient. We can see, therefore, that the nephron has all the characteristics of a good exchange surface as described in section B1.10. This will be covered in more detail next.

Ureter, bladder and urethra

The left and right ureters take urine from each kidney to the bladder where it is stored until the bladder is emptied via the urethra in the process of **urination**.

In males, the urethra is intimately connected with the reproductive system described in section B2.7. In females, the urethra is shorter and leads to an opening within the vulva next to the vaginal opening.

The functions of the renal system

Filtration of the blood to remove urea and reabsorption of water, glucose, amino acids and other useful substances all occur in the nephron (Figure 14.38).

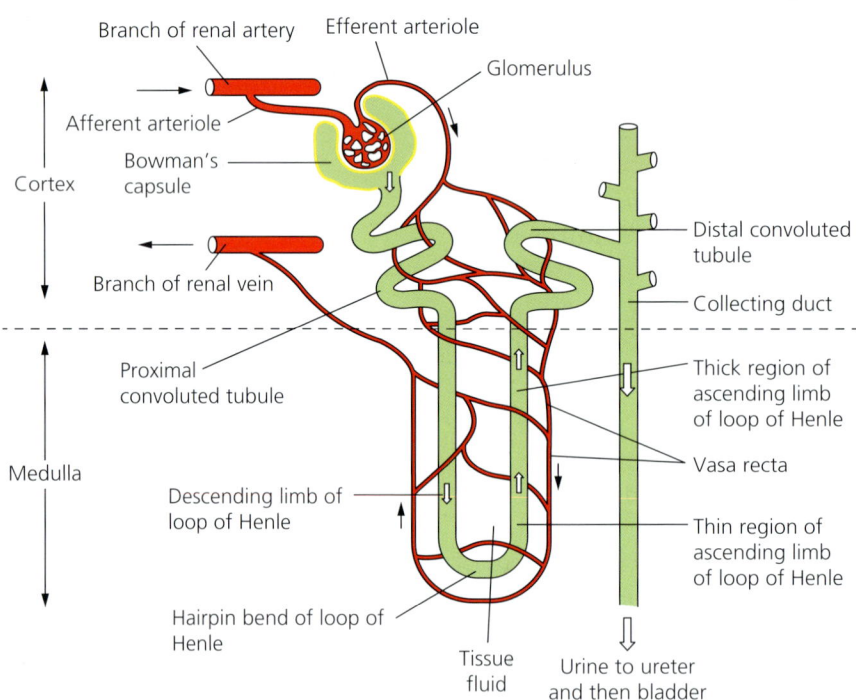

▲ Figure 14.38 One nephron and its associated blood vessels; the flow of blood is shown with black arrows and the flow of filtrate and urine with white arrows

Practice point

The term **medulla** means the inner part of an organ. In this chapter, you will encounter the medulla oblongata (in the brain), the adrenal medulla (in the adrenal gland) and the renal medulla, which is the one we are considering here. You might find the term medulla used on its own and will need to check the context to be sure which medulla is being referred to. Throughout section B2.8, the term medulla refers to the renal medulla.

Removal of waste products from the body

Urea is removed from the blood by the process of **ultrafiltration**. This occurs at the start of the nephron in **Bowman's capsule**. If you look at the blood vessels in Figure 14.38, you will notice how a branch of the renal artery leads to an **afferent arteriole**. This then divides into many capillaries in the space surrounded by Bowman's capsule. This knot or tangle of capillaries is known as the **glomerulus**. The capillaries of the glomerulus come together to form the **efferent arteriole**. The efferent arteriole leads to another network of capillaries that surround the rest of the nephron before joining a branch of the renal vein. The term afferent means 'leading in' and efferent means 'leading out'.

Because the diameter of the efferent arteriole is smaller than that of the afferent arteriole, a high pressure develops in the glomerulus. This pressure forces out fluids from the capillaries and into the lumen (space inside) of the nephron, forming the **filtrate** (i.e. the product of filtering). The filtrate contains water; small molecules such as glucose and amino acids; mineral ions such as sodium, potassium and chloride; and also urea. Only red blood cells and large proteins are unable to pass into the filtrate.

Process of urine production

The filtrate then moves along the length of the nephron. The changes to the composition of the filtrate in the nephron lead to it eventually becoming urine. The urine enters the collecting duct and from there is taken via the ureter to the bladder.

Reabsorption

Many of the substances dissolved in the blood are required by the body and so must be reabsorbed. These include glucose and amino acids. These are reabsorbed by a mechanism of co-transport, which is very similar to the mechanism illustrated in Figure 11.17 (page 223 in section B1.11). This occurs in the first part of the nephron called the **proximal convoluted tubule (PCT)**.

Mineral ions, such as sodium, potassium, calcium and chloride may also need to be reabsorbed. This depends on whether there is an excess of them present in the blood or not. This reabsorption takes place mostly towards the end of the nephron in the **distal convoluted tubule (DCT)** and is controlled by the mineralocorticoid hormones (mentioned in section B2.1) that regulate the concentrations of mineral ions in the body.

Water is also reabsorbed. However, how much water is reabsorbed depends on the water balance of the body and the part of the system known as **osmoregulation**.

Role in osmoregulation

Reabsorption of glucose and amino acids occurs in the PCT. As a result of the molecules entering the epithelial cells, the water potential of those cells falls. Therefore, water moves out of the filtrate down a water potential gradient by **osmosis** (see sections B1.11 and B2.1). Most of the reabsorption of water occurs in the **collecting duct** that passes through the **medulla**. If you look at Figure 14.38, you will see that the loop of Henle is shaped like a hairpin, i.e. folded back on itself. As the filtrate passes **up** the **ascending limb**, Na^+ and Cl^- ions are pumped out into the surrounding medulla, from where they diffuse into the **descending limb**. The effect of this is to cause the highest concentration of ions in the filtrate at the bottom of the loop of Henle. This means that, moving down the medulla, the concentration of ions in the medulla surrounding the collecting duct **increases**. This means that the water potential **decreases** in the same direction.

As a result, there is a constant water potential gradient from the collecting duct to the surrounding medulla. As water moves out of the collecting duct by osmosis, the water potential of the filtrate in the collecting duct falls. However, as it moves further down the collecting duct it meets the medulla where the water potential is even lower. Therefore, there is a constant water potential gradient that moves water out of the filtrate by osmosis.

At the end of this process the filtrate has become **urine**. The urine will be more or less concentrated, depending on how much water is reabsorbed. This is controlled by the hormone **ADH**; the mechanism of this has been described in section B2.1. ADH acts by stimulating an increase in aquaporins in the epithelial cells of the collecting duct, thereby increasing the permeability of the collecting duct leading to greater water reabsorption. This also explains how drinking alcohol can lead to dehydration as alcohol inhibits ADH and so inhibits reabsorption of water.

Role in homeostasis

Homeostasis is the regulation of the internal environment of the body. **Osmoregulation** is an important part of this. Regulating the water balance of the body also plays a part in maintaining blood pressure. A rise in blood pressure can be caused by a rise in blood volume. More water is removed by the kidney when release of ADH by the pituitary is inhibited, and this leads to reduction in blood pressure.

Another mechanism is the **renin–angiotensin** system. Renin is an enzyme produced in the kidney when there is a fall in blood pressure. The renin–angiotensinogen system operates to stimulate release of ADH from the pituitary and this leads to an increase in reabsorption of water, resulting in an increase in blood pressure.

Production of hormones

The kidney produces the hormone erythropoietin (EPO), which stimulates production of erythrocytes by the bone marrow.

Healthcare Science T Level: Core

The kidney also produces the enzyme **renin**. This catalyses the conversion of the peptide angiotensinogen, produced in the liver, into the hormone **angiotensin** (see previously).

> **Test yourself**
>
> 1. Describe the process of ultrafiltration.
> 2. Describe how the loop of Henle assists in the reabsorption of water from the collecting duct.
> 3. Describe the role of ADH in osmoregulation.
> 4. Describe the role of the renin–angiotensin system in homeostasis.

B2.9 The integumentary system

If you were asked to name the organs of the human body you would probably focus on the internal organs and overlook the skin. However, as well as being the heaviest organ, the skin has a number of important functions. It is a part of the **integumentary system**, which also includes hair and nails.

> **Key terms**
>
> **Integumentary system:** this includes the skin, exocrine glands, hair and nails; An **Integument** is a tough outer protective layer.

The components and organisation of the integumentary system

Skin

The strong surface layer of the skin is the **epidermis** (Figure 14.39) that consists of **squamous** (flattened) **epithelial** cells. These are continually worn away and so the epidermis is regenerated by division of **stem cells** in the lowest layer of the epidermis. There are no blood vessels in the epidermis, so it obtains nutrients from the underlying dermis. The protein **keratin** (the main fibrous protein of **hair** and **nails**) helps to waterproof the epidermis.

Lying below the epidermis is the **dermis**. This is a layer of connective tissue that helps to support the epidermis as well as making the skin elastic. There are many blood vessels and nerve endings in the dermis, as well as the **hair follicles** and **exocrine glands** (**sweat glands** and **sebaceous glands**). See section B2.1 for a description of exocrine glands.

Hair consists of the fibrous protein **keratin** and grows outwards from **hair follicles** that are lined with epithelial cells.

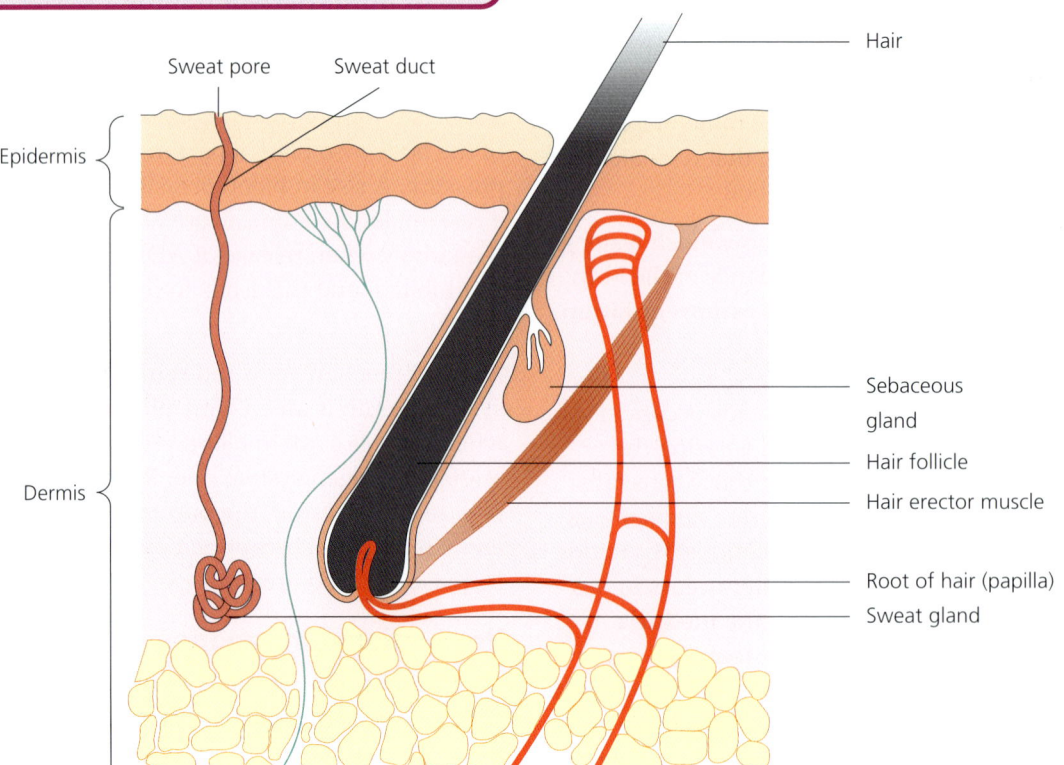

▲ Figure 14.39 Cross section of human skin

The functions of the integumentary system

Protection

An essential function of the skin is to act as a physical barrier to infection. This was mentioned in section B1.30 (page 236, Immunology). However, the skin is not just a physical barrier. Antimicrobial peptides are produced by skin cells and exocrine glands and help to protect against infection by bacteria and fungi. In addition, we have a population of benign bacteria that live on our skin and help to prevent infection by pathogens such as other bacteria or fungi.

Temperature regulation

The importance of the **hypothalamus** in homeostasis was mentioned in section B2.1 and homeostasis will be discussed in more detail in section B2.12. Regulation of body temperature is controlled and co-ordinated by the hypothalamus, but the skin is an important **receptor** and **effector**.

The main temperature receptors are in the hypothalamus itself and monitor core body temperature (the temperature of the internal organs, which is often higher than the temperature of the body surface). However, **peripheral temperature receptors** are located in the skin and monitor the external temperature. The hypothalamus uses inputs from both types of receptor.

There are three main mechanisms under the control of the hypothalamus by which the skin helps to maintain an almost constant body temperature.

Sweat glands release sweat when the body temperature rises. Thermal energy from the skin and blood in capillaries close to the surface of the skin is transferred to the water in sweat, causing it to evaporate. This transfer of thermal energy cools the skin.

Arterioles supplying the capillaries near the surface of the skin can constrict (**vasoconstriction**) or dilate (**vasodilation**) as shown in Figure 14.40.

When the core body temperature rises, nerve impulses from the hypothalamus cause the muscles in the walls of the arterioles in the dermis to relax. This causes **vasodilation** – the diameter of the arterioles increases. As a result, more blood can flow through the capillaries close to the surface of the skin and more thermal energy is transferred to the surroundings.

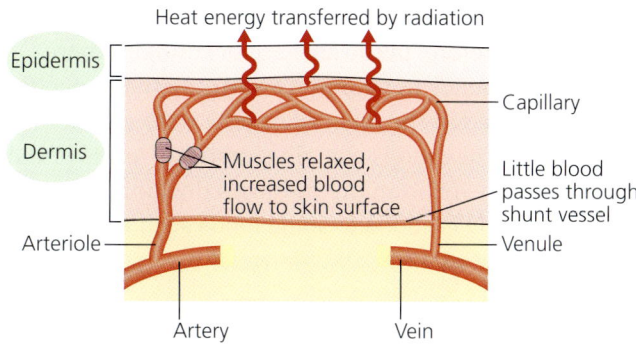
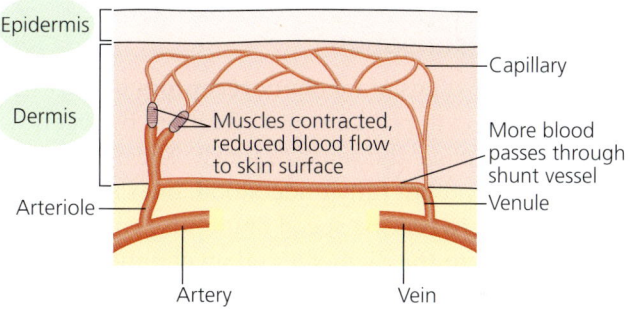

▲ Figure 14.40 Vasodilation (top) and vasoconstriction (bottom) in the skin

When the core body temperature falls, nerve impulses from the hypothalamus cause contraction of the muscles in the walls of the same arterioles. This causes **vasoconstriction** – the diameter of the arterioles decreases. As a result, less blood flows through the capillaries close to the surface of the skin; instead it is diverted through a **shunt vessel** to a venule. A shunt vessel is a small vessel connecting an arteriole to a venule, bypassing the capillaries. This means that less thermal energy is transferred by radiation.

The final mechanism involves **hairs** on the skin. A fall in core body temperature causes the hypothalamus to send nerve impulses to the **hair erector muscles**. This causes them to contract, which raises the hairs. As a result, a thicker layer of air is trapped next to the skin and forms an insulating layer, reducing heat loss. If the core body temperature rises, nerve impulses from the hypothalamus cause the erector muscles to **relax** and so the hair lies flat, reducing the thickness of the insulating layer. During human evolution, thick body hair has been replaced by clothes, so this mechanism is more important for other mammals than for us. We can still see the mechanism in action when we are cold and get 'goosebumps' – this is caused by contraction of the erector muscles.

Vitamin D synthesis

Strictly speaking, **vitamin D (cholecalciferol)** is not a vitamin. This is because it is made in the lower layers of the skin epidermis. This reaction is dependent on sunlight. Therefore, in the absence of sunlight, there can be a deficiency in vitamin D meaning that it needs to be consumed in the diet. Vitamin D is fat soluble and relatively few foods contain significant levels of the vitamin. However, in many countries (including the UK), vitamin D is added to some foods such as milk and breakfast cereals.

Vitamin D works together with PTH and calcitonin to regulate the calcium balance of the body (see section B2.1).

Cutaneous sensation

Four different types of **mechanoreceptors** in the dermis respond to pressure and vibration. Between them they produce the sense of touch. The details are complex and not fully understood, but there are differences between the speed of impulse conduction that is related to the diameter and myelination of the neurones. Some of these respond to skin movement whereas others respond to static indentation of the skin. They have a large diameter and high degree of myelination and so conduct nerve signals quickly. Neurones responsible for rapid pain sensation are the most sensitive. Finally, the most common type is the group known as C fibres. They are activated by mechanical and thermal stimuli as well as chemicals, such as capsaicin (the chemical in chilli peppers that produces a burning sensation).

Excretion

Sweat glands (Figure 14.39) are an example of exocrine glands because they secrete their products on to a surface rather than into the blood. Although the main function of sweat is to help reduce body temperature, sweat contains inorganic ions and urea, and so plays a part in excretion.

Sebaceous glands are another exocrine gland. They excrete an oily substance called sebum that helps to lubricate the skin and hair. Sebum also keeps the skin slightly acidic, which helps protect against microbes.

> **Test yourself**
>
> 1 Describe two functions in the skin of the protein keratin.
> 2 Describe two functions of sweat glands.
> 3 Explain why vitamin D is often added to foods in northern European countries.

B2.10 The basic function of the eye and visual system

The **ocular** (eye and visual) **system** includes the eye and optic nerve. In simple terms, the eye processes light into electrical signals which are then processed by the brain into images to allow us to see and interpret the outside world.

Figure 14.41 shows the structure of the eye.

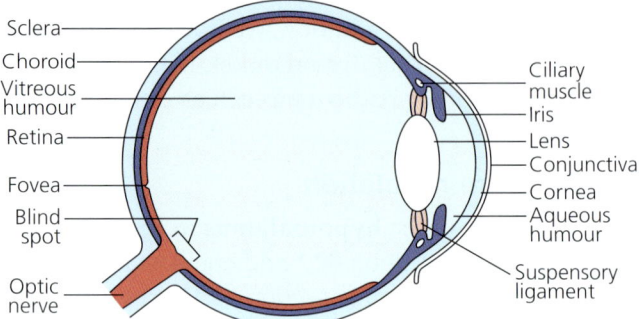

▲ Figure 14.41 The structure of the eye

Lids

The eyelids are thin folds of skin that cover and protect the eye. Eyelids have eyelashes along the edges that increase protection from dust and debris, as well as from sweat. The conjunctiva is a thin tissue of epithelial cells covering the cornea; the eyelids keep this moist by spreading tears and other secretions over the surface. The eyelids close during sleep to prevent the eyes from drying out, while the blink reflex helps protect the eye from impact by foreign bodies.

Cornea

The **cornea** is part of the tough outer layer of the eye. Unlike the whitish sclera, the cornea is transparent and is more curved, covering the front of the eye and allowing light to pass through, but protecting the inner part of the eye.

Iris

The **iris** is the coloured part of the eye with a central hole, known as the pupil, through which light passes into the main part of the eye. Radial and circular muscles in the iris control the **pupillary response**. In bright light the iris constricts, reducing the amount of light entering the eye. In dim light the pupil dilates, increasing the amount of light entering the eye.

Lens

The **lens** focuses light rays on to the retina so that an image can be formed. This involves refraction of light, but this function is aided by the curvature of the cornea and the refractive effect of the aqueous humour.

Retina

The **retina** is the innermost, light-sensitive layer of the eye. Photoreceptors (light-sensitive cells) are of two types: **rods** and **cones**. These are located at the back of the retina, so that light rays have to pass through layers of blood vessels and neurones before reaching the photoreceptor cells. A third type of light-sensing cell, the **photosensitive ganglion cell**, is important in reflexes such as constriction and dilation of the pupil in response to changes in light intensity.

Rod cells are sensitive to light intensity, but not to colour (wavelength) of light, so they provide a monochrome image to the brain. Cone cells are of three types, sensitive to either red, green or blue wavelengths of light. The brain combines the inputs from each of these to generate a colour image. Cone cells are less sensitive than rod cells, explaining why we perceive monochrome images in low light intensities. The centre of the retina is called the **fovea**. This area receives most of the light rays passing through the lens and has the highest concentration of cone cells. The fovea is responsible for the sharp central vision in humans.

In summary, the photosensitive cells (rods and cones), convert the light into the electrical signals which are then transmitted by the optic nerve to the visual cortex.

Optic nerve

The optic nerve carries the neurones from the retina and connects to the brain. In fact, the optic nerve and retina are technically part of the CNS rather than the PNS. Because of the inverted arrangement of the retina, the optic nerve must pass through the light-sensitive layer of the retina. This means there are no light receptors in this region, giving rise to the **blind spot** – we do not see any images that are focused on that part of the retina.

Visual cortex

The **visual cortex** is part of the cerebral cortex, which is the outer layer of the cerebrum (the largest part of the brain in humans). The visual cortex receives nerve impulses via the optic nerve and processes these to create the images that we see.

B2.11 The use of physiological measurement tools and techniques in monitoring the action of physiological systems

Cardiovascular system

Electrocardiogram (ECG)

The use of an ECG to measure the electrical activity of the heart was described in detail in section B2.6.

Arterial blood pressure can be monitored, for example in the course of an electrocardiogram (ECG). This makes it possible to observe the dicrotic notch and dicrotic wave (see section B2.6). As we age, these tend to come later after the peak arterial pressure. However, in some forms of cardiovascular disease, the dicrotic notch becomes less distinct. In severe cardiovascular disease this can be detected as a second or **dicrotic pulse**.

Sphygmomanometer

Blood pressure has traditionally been measured using a **sphygmomanometer** and **stethoscope** (Figure 14.42). The measuring device shows the pressure in the arm cuff. The cuff is inflated to well above the expected systolic pressure. A valve on the cuff is opened and the cuff pressure slowly decreases. When the cuff pressure equals the systolic pressure, blood begins to flow past the cuff causing sounds that can be heard with the stethoscope. These sounds continue until the cuff pressure falls below the diastolic pressure.

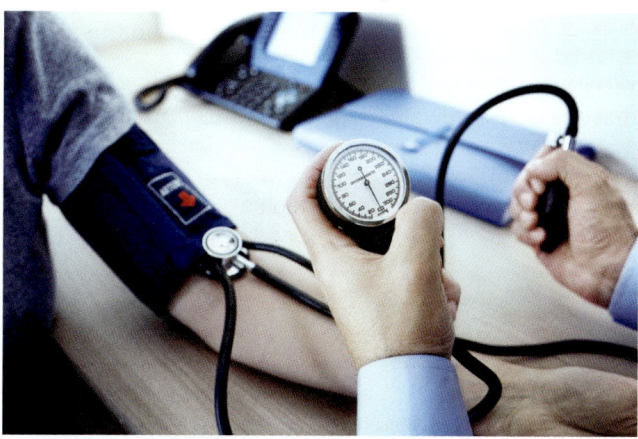

▲ Figure 14.42 Measuring blood pressure with a sphygmomanometer and stethoscope

An earlier type of sphygmomanometer used a column of mercury to measure the pressure – hence the units mmHg. Some practitioners still prefer these older types. Unlike the newer type, they do not need periodic recalibration to remain accurate.

More recently, electronic blood pressure monitors have become widespread. They require less skill to use, measure pulse rate at the same time and can be used in continual monitoring, e.g. in the intensive care unit (ICU). Some types are not very expensive and can be used to monitor your own blood pressure (Figure 14.43).

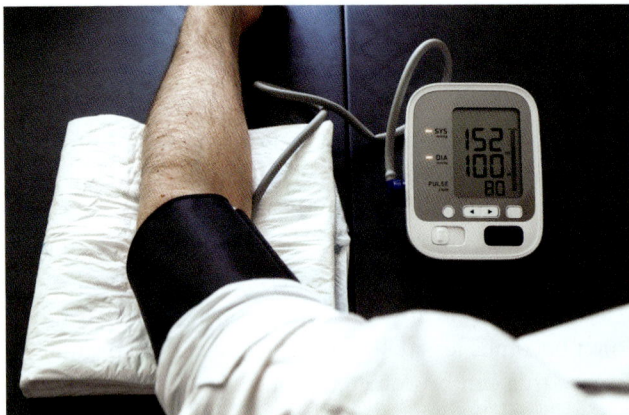

▲ Figure 14.43 A person using a blood pressure monitor to measure their own blood pressure

Stopwatch/clock

The simplest way to measure heart rate is to measure the **pulse** (see section B2.6). The **radial pulse** is measured using two fingers placed on the wrist and a watch to count beats per minute. The **apical pulse** is measured using a stethoscope placed on the chest directly above the top of the heart. It is generally simpler to measure the radial pulse, although it can be difficult to measure in newborn babies and children under five years. The apical pulse is therefore better used for individuals in this group.

Wristwatches are not usually allowed, for hygiene reasons, so a fob watch worn on the uniform is used instead (Figure 14.44).

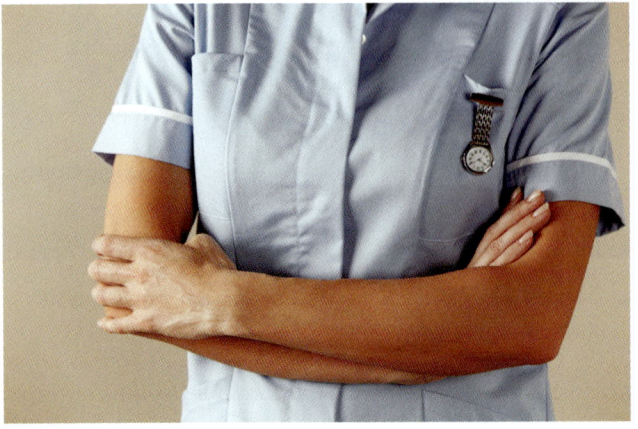

▲ Figure 14.44 A fob watch worn on the uniform

Respiratory system

Spirometry

A spirometer can be used to make a number of measurements related to breathing. Mechanical or electronic versions are available (Figure 14.45).

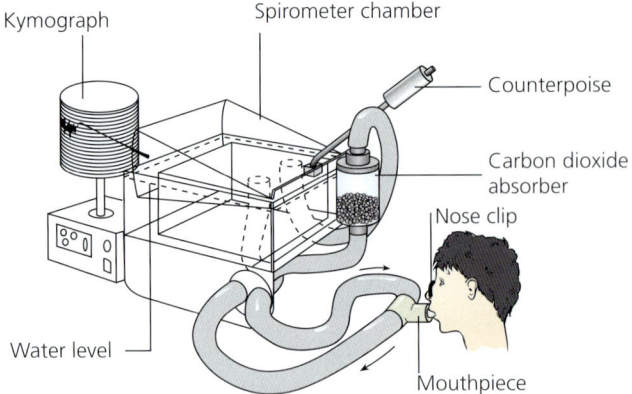

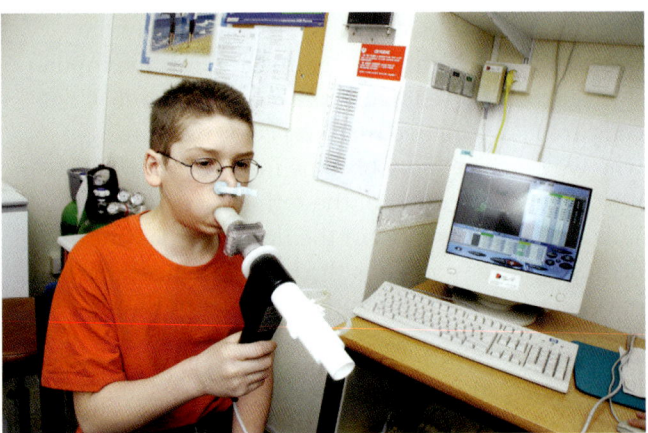

▲ Figure 14.45 A mechanical spirometer (top) and an electronic spirometer (bottom)

You are not expected to know the details of how a spirometer works, but some information has been included here in case you come across this equipment in your work. The spirometer produces a trace on a revolving drum (kymograph) or on a screen. The subject breathes in and out through the spirometer and carbon dioxide is removed from the re-breathed air by absorption with soda-lime. This is because high levels of carbon dioxide can cause respiratory distress.

You need to know about the use of a spirometer to measure the **vital capacity**, which is the maximum volume of air that can be breathed out after taking a maximum breath in. As well as this, the spirometer can measure the **breathing rate** and **tidal volume** (volume of air breathed in or out at rest). These are illustrated in Figure 14.46.

B2: Further science concepts

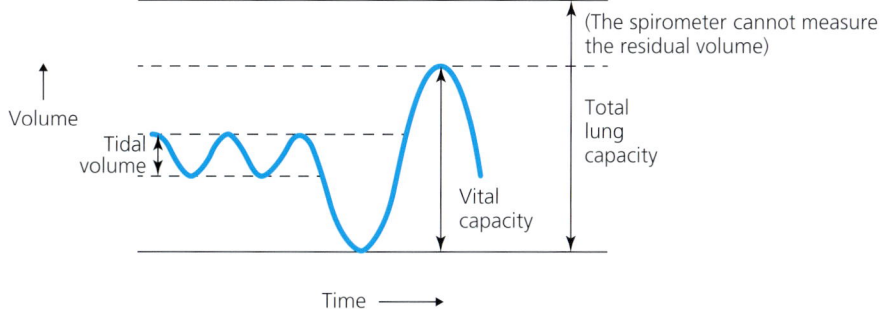

▲ Figure 14.46 A spirometer trace showing various measurements that can be made

In adults, the average total lung capacity (volume) is about 6 litres in males and 4.2 litres in females. The average vital capacity is 4.8 litres in males and 3.1 litres in females; the difference is the residual volume, which cannot be measured with a spirometer as it is impossible to completely empty the lungs.

Source: Tortora's Principles of Anatomy and Physiology, by Bryan H. Derrickson and Gerard J. Tortora, Wiley, 2017

Peak expiratory flow meter

Also known simply as a peak flow meter, this is used to measure a person's **peak expiratory flow** (**PEF**) or maximum speed of expiration (Figure 14.47). This gives an indication of the airflow through the bronchi. Any reduction in peak flow can indicate possible obstructions. For example, asthma leads to a reduction in PEF as a result of inflammation leading to constriction of the bronchioles.

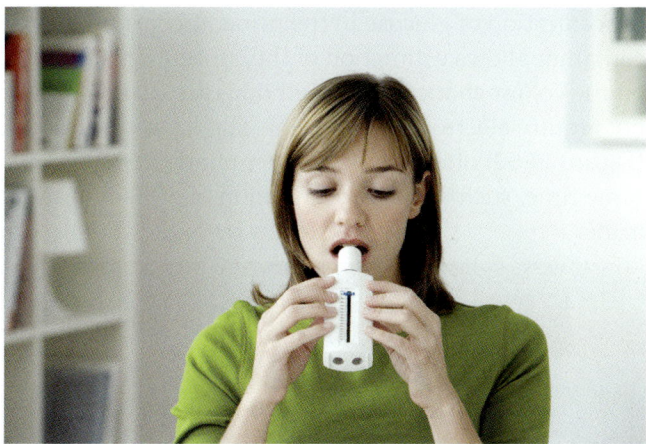

▲ Figure 14.47 A peak expiratory flow meter

Pulse oximetry

A **pulse oximeter** is used to measure the oxygen saturation of the blood. This is typically placed on a finger and shines light through the skin. The oximeter measures how much light is absorbed and then uses this to calculate both pulse and the oxygen saturation of the blood.

▶ During each contraction of the heart blood is forced through the capillaries. This increases their volume. The volume decreases between heartbeats. More light is absorbed when the volume increases and so the pulse can be detected and counted.

▶ Blood that is saturated with oxygen absorbs less red light and more infrared than blood that is less saturated. This difference in absorbance is measured by the pulse oximeter and converted to a figure for percentage saturation.

Pulse oximeters can be connected to computers or data loggers to provide continual monitoring.

Practice point

Pulse oximeters have been widely used during the COVID-19 pandemic and have been given to patients infected with SARS-CoV-2 who are not sufficiently ill to need hospital treatment to enable them to monitor their own condition from home. The normal range for oxygen saturation of the blood is 95–100 per cent. Patients are told to call 111 if the pulse oximeter reading falls to 94 or 93 per cent and to call 999 if it falls to 92 per cent or less.

There have been reports (for instance **www.bbc.co.uk/news/health-58032842**) that pulse oximeters can overestimate the oxygen saturation in patients with dark skin. This is most likely because pigment in dark skin absorbs more light than light skin. As a result, patients with dark skin, particularly those of black and South Asian ethnic backgrounds, are being advised to continue to use pulse oximeters, but to seek advice from a health professional on doing so. This group of patients has also been found to be at greater risk of contracting severe COVID-19.

Endocrine system

You will see from section B2.1 that the endocrine system is complex and involves many hormones. The part of this system that you are most likely to encounter in your professional practice is the regulation of blood glucose concentration by insulin and glucagon. This system does not function correctly in diabetes and can be monitored by measuring the concentration of glucose in the blood or urine.

> **Practice point**
>
> Strictly speaking, we should refer to blood glucose concentration rather than blood sugar level. There are many sugars, of which glucose is just one. Nevertheless, it has become established practice to refer to blood sugar levels when we mean blood glucose concentration, and that is the form we will use here.

Glucose meter

This is used to measure blood sugar levels in a blood sample taken from a finger prick. Most types use a test strip on to which the blood sample is placed (Figure 14.48). Chemicals in the strip react with the glucose and the meter then reads the glucose concentration.

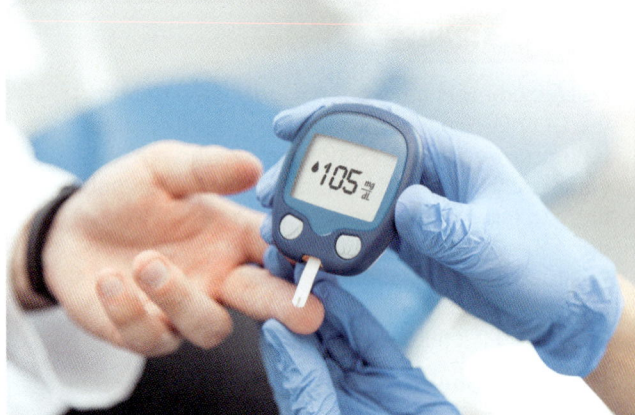

▲ Figure 14.48 A blood glucose meter

More recently, it has become possible to continually monitor a patient's blood sugar level using a disposable sensor that is placed under the skin and connected to a transmitter that communicates with a reader. The reader can be a dedicated device or a mobile phone app (Figure 14.49).

The advantage of continuous monitoring is that it allows the patient to control their blood glucose more accurately by adjusting their dose of insulin. It also removes the need for regular finger prick testing. However, the sensor must be replaced every few days.

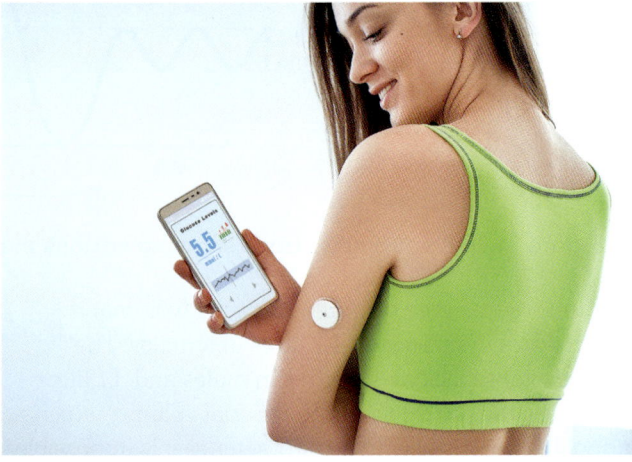

▲ Figure 14.49 A continuous blood glucose monitor

Insulin

The concentration of insulin in a blood sample can be measured in the laboratory. This can be used to confirm a diagnosis of Type 2 diabetes, where fasting insulin concentrations are raised above normal levels.

Dipstick (urine tests)

These are test strips like the ones used for measuring blood sugar levels. They change colour according to the concentration of glucose in the urine. A chart on the container allows estimation of the concentration based on the colour change. This method is rapid and does not require electronic equipment. The dipsticks used (Figure 14.50) often measure other parameters at the same time, such as the concentration of protein in the urine.

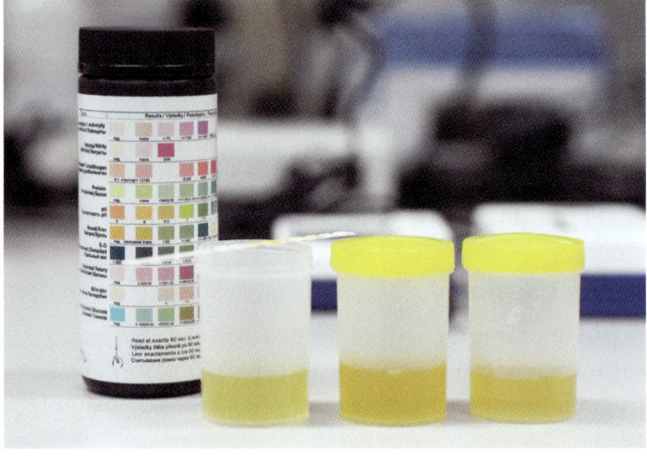

▲ Figure 14.50 Dipsticks used for urine testing

Similar test strips can be used to estimate blood glucose levels, although they are not as accurate as blood glucose meters.

Body temperature

Body temperature is measured using a clinical thermometer. Traditionally these were made of a long glass tube with a bulb of mercury at one end and marked in 0.1 °C divisions from 35 °C to 42 °C. The thermometer is placed under the tongue, in the armpit or in the rectum. After a few minutes, the temperature can be read. The disadvantage of this type of thermometer is that they require sterilisation between patients (or each patient should have their own) and they can be difficult to read. Moreover, glass is easily broken and mercury is toxic.

This type of clinical thermometer has now been replaced almost completely by electronic thermometers, particularly ones that measure the temperature of the **tympanic membrane** (ear drum) as shown in Figure 14.51.

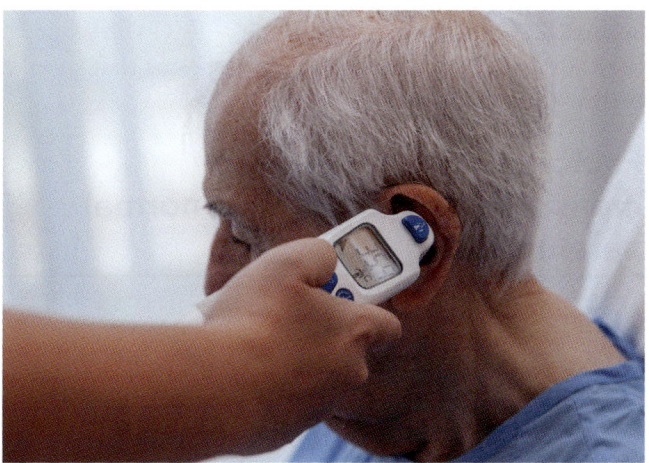

▲ Figure 14.51 A nurse using an electronic thermometer to measure a patient's body temperature

Electronic thermometers give a much quicker reading than traditional clinical thermometers. Another advantage is that they give a reading much closer to the core body temperature because the hypothalamus (which regulates body temperature) and the tympanic membrane share a blood supply. Other sites where temperature is measured can give a reading that might be less accurate.

Electronic thermometers also need to be sterilised between patients, although it is possible to avoid this by using disposable single-use sleeves on the probe.

Body temperature measurements can be used:
▶ as an indication of infection or fever
▶ to monitor blood flow, particularly to the extremities; this can be important in patients with diabetes or other conditions where circulation is impaired.

Pupil dilation and constriction

The pupillary response (see section B2.10) to bright light can be used as part of general clinical observations but particularly in the case of:
▶ eye injury
▶ brain injury
▶ use of recreational drugs
▶ treatment with various prescription or non-prescription medications.

Abnormal response can indicate underlying issues that should be referred to a senior medical practitioner, such as a neurologist or neurosurgeon.

> **Test yourself**
>
> 1. Describe two ways of measuring heart rate.
> 2. Give two disadvantages of a traditional glass clinical thermometer.
> 3. Give one advantage of an electronic thermometer.
> 4. What precaution should be taken when using a thermometer for more than one patient?

B2.12 The normal expected ranges for physiological measurements and how to identify when measurements fall outside the ranges, including factors that can contribute to measurement outside of usual parameters

So far in this chapter, we have covered the key areas of human physiology, particularly how blood pressure, heart rate, respiratory (breathing) rate and body temperature are regulated. Therefore, in any situation where we are monitoring the health or disease state of an individual, we need to be able to measure those and compare them to the **normal** or **average range**. We also need to understand the factors that can contribute to measurements falling outside the usual parameters.

Normal expected ranges for physiological measurements

Blood pressure

> **Key terms**
>
> **Blood pressure:** the pressure the blood exerts on the walls of the arteries when the heart beats; it is usually measured in mmHg (millimetres of mercury). Although the units of pressure are kPa, the unit mmHg relates to how blood pressure was (and often still is) measured – see section B2.11.
>
> **Systolic blood pressure:** the pressure when the heart contracts.
>
> **Diastolic blood pressure:** the pressure when the heart relaxes; it is always lower than the systolic pressure.

The World Health Organization (WHO) classifies **blood pressure** as shown in the following table.

	Systolic mmHg	Diastolic mmHg
Low blood pressure (hypotension)	< 90	< 60
Normal blood pressure	90–120	60–80
Pre-high blood pressure	120–139	80–89
High blood pressure (hypertension)	≥ 140	≥ 90

Blood pressure is always shown as **systolic** then **diastolic**, for example 120/80 mmHg. This is often referred to verbally as '120 over 80'.

Other parameters

The following table shows the average range of three other key physiological measurements in adults. These ranges can be significantly different in children.

Physiological measurements	Average range for an adult
Heart rate	60–100 beats per minute (bpm)
Peak expiratory flow	400–700 litres per minute
Blood sugar concentration	4.0–5.9 mmol/L (fasting, i.e. before a meal) to < 7.8 mmol/L (after a meal)

How to identify abnormal physiological measurements

If you have ever spent time in hospital, as a patient or otherwise, you will be aware of nurses taking regular **obs** or **observations**. These will usually cover blood pressure, pulse (heart rate) and temperature although other factors may be monitored in specific cases, such as **neurological observations** in patients who are unconscious or have a suspected neurological disorder. The frequency of these observations will depend on the status of the patient.

By regularly recording these physiological measurements it is possible to identify if any of them fall outside the normal range (are **abnormal**). More importantly, they can indicate a possible worsening in the patient's condition or an improvement.

The techniques used are covered in section B2.11, but they can include manual measurements, electronic monitoring equipment used by the health practitioner or continuous automated monitoring equipment, often linked to a computer, of the type seen in an **intensive care unit** (**ICU**).

The use of electrocardiography to monitor heart function and identify abnormalities was covered in section B2.6. Changes to the shape of ECG waves, or their absence, can indicate heart conditions that should be investigated further.

Factors that contribute to measurements outside of normal parameters

Age

Blood pressure in children is lower than in adults, increasing to the adult 'normal' of 120/80 mmHg by the age of 17–18 years. Blood pressure tends to increase with age as artery walls become less elastic.

In children, there are slight differences between boys and girls, with boys having a slightly higher normal blood pressure. However, the height of a child may determine blood pressure more than actual age.

The normal resting heart rate for children is higher than for the typical adult. The normal resting heart rate for babies up to three months is 107–81 bpm.

Resting heart rate remains fairly constant in adults with little change as we age. Other factors have more effect than age.

Smoking

Cigarette smoke contains over 4000 chemicals, many of which are **carcinogens** (cause cancer), so it is not surprising that smoking affects all of the physiological parameters we have covered.

- Damage to the respiratory tract, including inflammation, fibrosis and congestion of the bronchioles leads to a reduction in peak expiratory flow. Limitation of airways can be assessed using spirometry to measure forced vital capacity and FEV1 (the forced expiratory volume in one second).
- Nicotine in tobacco smoke increases blood pressure and heart rate.

Exercise

If you do regular weight training your muscles become bigger and stronger. The same is true of the heart muscle if you regularly undertake so-called *cardiovascular* or *cardio* exercise, such as running or cycling. The heart needs to pump harder to provide the body with oxygen and nutrients when doing strenuous exercise and responds by becoming larger. This means that it pumps more blood with each stroke – the **stroke volume** increases – so it does not need to beat as fast when at rest. Therefore, the resting heart rate of a well-trained athlete will be below 60 bpm, perhaps even as low as 40 bpm.

Sex

It is only in recent years that sex-based differences in normal physiology have been fully recognised. The differences between **body mass** and **body composition** in men and women are better known. The sex hormones also have an obvious effect on the different development of men and women. However, there are also less obvious differences.

Men have, on average, larger lungs than women, even when adjusted for height differences. This means that the maximum exercise capacity in women may be limited by lung capacity, especially as they age.

Men also tend to have larger left ventricles, which makes the stroke volume greater in men. There are even sex-related differences in the types of muscle proteins.

During pregnancy the **functional residual capacity** (**FRC**) of the lungs can fall. FRC is the amount of air left in the lungs after a normal passive exhalation. This is due to the increased pressure on the diaphragm by the uterus, and the reduction in FRC increases as pregnancy advances. However, there are other changes in the respiratory system during pregnancy, partly in response to increased levels of progesterone. These help to maintain the efficiency of the gas exchange system so that the fetus is provided with sufficient oxygen.

Pre-menopausal women tend to have a lower resting blood pressure and higher resting heart rate. However, blood pressure usually rises to equivalent levels to men after the **menopause**.

> ### Practice point
>
> In her book *Invisible Women*, Caroline Criado-Perez describes how safety equipment and items such as crash test dummies are often designed with reference only to the measurements of the average adult male body (i.e. excluding female averages). This means that women may be at greater risk of serious injury if involved in a car crash because cars are not designed with their bodies in mind. Likewise, differences in body type are not always recognised in the design of medical and scientific equipment. For instance, they are mostly designed by men and, in many cases, for men.
>
> Here are some examples of how this can cause problems:
> - Surgical instruments are mostly designed for larger male hands, making them less suitable for use by female surgeons.
> - PPE such as gowns are often provided in a single size (extra-large) on the assumption that these will fit everyone. Smaller team members, predominantly women, will be working in clothing that is several sizes too large and this can affect their work.
> - Cardiopulmonary resuscitation (CPR, see section A4.6) is taught and practised using mannequins (dummies) that are based on the male torso. Research has shown first aiders therefore feel less equipped to perform CPR on females.
>
> When using equipment or other items in the healthcare profession, it is important to consider when it may be necessary to make adjustments for people from certain groups, for instance whose body measurements do not fall within the average range.

Height

Both height and body mass can affect physiological measurements such as blood pressure, heart rate and respiratory parameters, such as peak expiratory flow, tidal volume and vital capacity.

Stress

Stress is associated with higher circulating concentrations of the hormone cortisol, which increases blood pressure and raises the blood glucose level. These responses can help survival of short periods of stress, such as an infection or a dangerous situation. However, they can have negative effects if stress becomes chronic (long term).

Type 1 and Type 2 diabetes

Type 1 diabetes is caused by lack of insulin produced by the pancreas. Therefore, blood insulin concentrations will be zero, or very low. Because insulin stimulates the uptake of glucose by the liver, muscles and adipose (fat) tissue, the blood glucose level after a meal will be very high – well above the normal range (**hyperglycaemia**). This leads to removal of glucose by the kidney and, as a result, the blood glucose level drops rapidly below the normal range (**hypoglycaemia**). Hypoglycaemia, or a 'hypo', can be very dangerous leading to unconsciousness, coma or even death if not treated quickly. Type 1 diabetics often carry sweets or biscuits to eat if they feel the early stages of hypo.

Type 2 diabetes is generally caused by resistance to insulin, so the concentration of insulin in the blood will be raised. Blood sugar levels are also elevated.

> **Research**
>
> Think about what we have covered so far on human physiology and physiological measurements.
>
> Can you see any common themes emerging?
>
> How do physiological measurements give a picture of a person's overall health and level of fitness?
>
> Choose an area of interest to you – such as sport science, ageing, mental health or wellbeing – and research how understanding of physiology and use of physiological measurement can enable us to do things like:
> ▶ assess patients and/or healthy individuals
> ▶ monitor patients, athletes and others
> ▶ diagnose disease and predict outcomes.
>
> You could use an internet search to help you, although you need to be careful. This is an area where not everyone is giving impartial or even informed advice or information. There are many who have a product to sell or an agenda to promote.
>
> One good place to start is the Public Health Action Support Team (PHAST) website at www.healthknowledge.org.uk. This is from the Department of Health and is aimed at supporting the continuing professional development of those working in the fields of health and social care.

Summary

You will see that the overall state of health of an individual will contribute to whether their physiological measurements lie within or outside normal parameters. Therefore, as a general rule, a person who takes regular exercise, eats a balanced diet and has no underlying health conditions is likely to have physiological measurements within the normal range, whereas lack of exercise, poor diet or poor health can all lead to measurements outside the normal range.

> **Test yourself**
>
> 1 For each of the following, explain whether the physiological measurements fall outside the normal range and would require further investigation.
>   a an elderly woman with blood pressure of 120/80 mmHg, resting heart rate of 90 bpm and resting respiration rate of 30 bpm
>   b a young child with a resting heart rate of 110 bpm
>   c a middle-aged man with a sedentary lifestyle (i.e. takes very little exercise) who has a resting heart rate of 105 bpm and a blood pressure of 140/95 mmHg
>   d a female athlete with a resting heart rate of 50 bpm and a blood pressure of 120/80 mmHg.
> 2 Suggest how you could use a blood test to assess whether a patient was suffering from chronic stress.
> 3 What physiological measurements would you expect to lie outside the normal range in
>   a Type 1 diabetes
>   b Type 2 diabetes?

B2.13 Homeostasis – the principles and how this contributes to preserving a healthy body

In previous sections, we have looked at several systems that play a part in regulating the function of the body. We will now see how the different physiological systems all interconnect to maintain the healthy body.

The principles of homeostasis

Homeostasis is the maintenance of an **almost constant internal environment** despite fluctuations in the external environment.

By internal environment we mean the body temperature, concentration of the blood (e.g. water, glucose), levels of oxygen and carbon dioxide, among other physiological parameters. Note that we use the term 'almost constant' rather than 'constant'. The point about homeostasis is that the levels of all of these fluctuate, but they are maintained within a narrow range. This is because of the way in which negative feedback works (Figure 14.52).

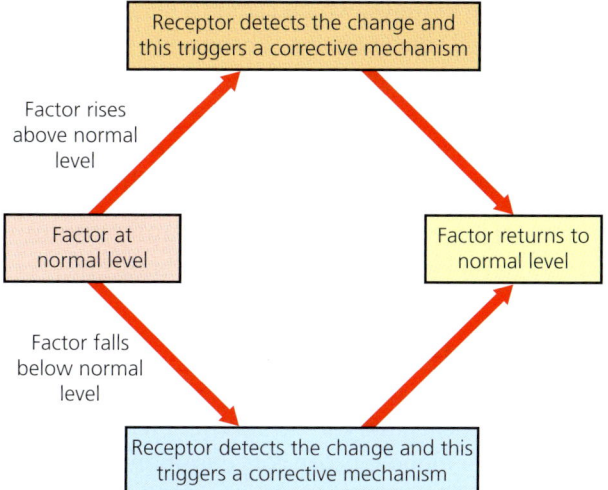

▲ Figure 14.52 Negative feedback

For negative feedback to operate, there has to be a movement (however small) away from the normal level. Negative feedback works in a way that returns the factor to the normal level.

Homeostasis covers several components, most of which have already been discussed in earlier sections.

- **Receptors**, such as those that detect the blood concentration of glucose, carbon dioxide or oxygen, or the core body temperature.
- **Effectors** – these are usually glands or muscles that make changes such as secretion of hormones or constriction of blood vessels that return the factor to its normal level.
- **Feedback systems** usually involve a control or co-ordination centre, such as the hypothalamus, that receives inputs from receptors and sends signals (hormones or nerve impulses) to effectors.

The role of the nervous system

We saw how the nervous system is involved in the regulation of body temperature (section B2.9) or heart rate (section B2.6). Nerve impulses travel quickly and so the nervous system is usually involved in the most rapid feedback mechanisms.

The role of the endocrine system

The endocrine system is involved in the regulation of blood glucose (section B2.1) and the water balance of the body (section B2.8) among others. Because hormones are released into the blood and transported to effectors (target organs), the response can be slower than mechanisms involving the nervous system. Therefore, the endocrine system is usually involved in more long-term homeostasis.

However, it is important to understand how the two systems work together in many homeostatic mechanisms, as you will have seen in the various examples in this chapter.

How homeostasis maintains stability and function

Homeostasis is the mechanism that maintains an almost constant internal environment ensuring the stability and function of the physiological systems and cells when there are changes to external conditions that would otherwise prevent normal physiological function.

How homeostasis contributes to preserving a healthy body

Bacteria that live in hot springs can survive perfectly well at temperatures close to the boiling point of water. Their enzymes seem remarkably heat stable when compared to our own, which start to **denature** at temperatures above about 40 °C. This is because human enzymes have evolved alongside the development of a body temperature around 37 °C. Any significant variation above or below that temperature will affect the rate of enzyme-controlled reactions: too low and reactions are too slow; too high and the enzymes lose activity as they start to denature. This explains the need for **thermoregulation**, as described in section B2.9.

The same is true about the water balance in the body. If you observe erythrocytes under a microscope and add pure water, you will see the cells swell and burst as water enters by osmosis. Similarly, if you add a drop of salt solution you will see the cells shrink and become crinkled as water leaves by osmosis. To function properly, our body cells need to be bathed in a fluid (called **tissue fluid**) that maintains a constant concentration of water. This explains the need for osmoregulation, as described in section B2.8.

Cells need a constant supply of glucose and oxygen for aerobic respiration – this is particularly true of brain cells.

The brain is the organ with the highest consumption of glucose and second highest consumption of oxygen. This explains the need for regulation of blood glucose concentration (section B2.1), breathing rate (section B2.2) and heart rate (section B2.6).

The regulation of the pH of the blood is also an important homeostatic mechanism, as enzymes need a constant pH to function effectively. Carbon dioxide is an acidic gas and so the concentration of carbon dioxide in the blood is regulated by means of gas exchange in the lungs (section B2.2) and regulation of heart rate (section B2.6).

> **Test yourself**
>
> 1. Explain why homeostasis is described as maintenance of an **almost constant** internal environment.
> 2. Name the two systems involved in homeostasis.
> 3. Explain the importance of maintaining the following within a narrow range:
>   a. body temperature
>   b. water balance
>   c. blood glucose concentration.

B2.14 How failure of homeostasis mechanisms can impact the body and the subsequent development of disorders

We have seen the importance of homeostasis and the correct operation of homeostasis mechanisms. Therefore, it is not surprising that failure of any of these mechanisms can lead to a number of disorders of different degrees of seriousness.

Failure of homeostasis mechanisms

Failure in a homeostasis mechanism can lead to cells being deprived of key nutrients or being exposed to toxic substances and thus beginning to work incorrectly or abnormally. This can happen in a variety of different ways.

Disorders

Type 1 and Type 2 diabetes

Although they have different causes, both types of diabetes involve a breakdown in the homeostasis mechanisms regulating blood glucose concentrations.

Type 1 diabetes

In Type 1 diabetes, the body attacks its own beta cells within the pancreas. As these are the cells that produce insulin, this means that the body cannot produce insulin in response to a rise in blood glucose concentration, e.g. after a meal. This means that the liver and muscles will not take up glucose from the blood and so the blood glucose concentration rises sharply. This leads to excess glucose being excreted by the kidneys, which causes a sudden fall in blood glucose concentration. These wide swings in blood glucose concentration can have short-term consequences (coma, even death) or long-term consequences, such as nerve damage (**neuropathy**) and damage to blood vessels in the eye (**retinopathy**).

Treatment of Type 1 diabetes requires regular insulin injections to replace the insulin that the body does not produce.

Type 2 diabetes

Obesity is one risk factor for developing Type 2 diabetes (genetic factors can be another), with its associated high blood glucose concentration over many years. This can lead to liver and muscle cells becoming unresponsive to insulin and also to a reduction in the production of insulin, meaning muscle and liver cells do not take up as much glucose. This means the normal homeostasis mechanism breaks down.

Treatment of Type 2 diabetes begins with diet – reduced intake of food rich in starch and sugars, and increased intake of high-fibre foods – and increased exercise. If this is not successful, anti-diabetic drugs can be prescribed. In some cases, it might be necessary to prescribe insulin injections for Type 2 diabetes.

Heat stroke or hyperthermia

Hyperthermia occurs when the core body temperature rises above the normal range. **Heat stroke** is a sudden increase in body temperature. The normal thermoregulatory mechanisms described in section B2.9 can be overcome by a combination of excessive production of heat (strenuous exercise), high environmental temperatures and reduced heat loss – for example, when high humidity reduces the effectiveness of sweating as cooling mechanism.

Hot, dry skin is typical in heat stroke as blood vessels dilate in an attempt to increase heat loss from the skin.

Severe cases lead to:
- confusion and aggressive behaviour
- increased respiration rate and heart rate (**tachycardia**) as blood pressure drops and the heart tries to maintain adequate circulation
- eventually organ failure, unconsciousness and death may result.

Treatment of hyperthermia involves cooling the body, for example in an ice bath.

Hypothermia occurs when the body temperature falls below the normal level – in humans this means a body temperature less than 35 °C. This is an example of **positive feedback** – where a movement away from the normal level leads to a change even further away from normal. In the case of body temperature, a fall in temperature reduces the rate of metabolic reactions meaning less heat is generated. This causes the body temperature to fall even further. Positive feedback is not a part of homeostasis mechanisms as these are designed to return a factor to the normal level.

First-aid treatment of hypothermia involves passive warming, i.e. removing cold or wet clothing and keeping the patient insulated. Alcohol should never be given as this makes hypothermia worse. Severe hypothermia requires hospital treatment, often involving the infusion of warm fluids to raise the body temperature gradually.

Renal failure

Renal failure is the result of chronic kidney disease, which is usually caused by other conditions that put a strain on the kidneys, such as:
- high blood pressure putting strain on the capillaries in the kidney
- diabetes, where high glucose concentrations damage the filtration mechanism
- high cholesterol, leading to a build up of fatty deposits in the renal arteries
- inflammation or infection of the kidney.

We have seen that the kidney plays a key role in two important homeostasis mechanisms, which explains the key symptoms of kidney failure:
- The body retains water, leading to swollen ankles and production of small volumes of urine as a result of a failure in osmoregulation.
- Accumulation of urea in the blood as a result of the failure of the kidney to excrete urea. As urea is toxic this can lead to widespread organ damage.

Renal failure cannot be cured, other than by **kidney transplant**, although **renal dialysis** can control the disease by replicating some of the function of the kidney.

Graves' disease

Graves' disease is an autoimmune disease where the body's immune system creates antibodies that mimic TSH and so cause the thyroid gland to become overactive and over-produce thyroid hormones such as **thyroxine**.

Treatment of Graves' disease involves reducing the production of thyroid hormones. This can be with drugs that interfere with the thyroid's ability to take in iodine, which is used in synthesis of thyroid hormones. Alternatively, radioactive iodine (^{131}I) can be administered. This is taken up by the thyroid and destroys the cells that produce thyroid hormones. The size of the thyroid is gradually reduced, after which the treatment can be stopped.

Infection and sepsis

Infection has been covered extensively in this book – see, for example, Chapters A9 (covering health and wellbeing) and A10 (covering infection control), while Chapter B1 covered the basic biology of infection (sections B1.24–B1.26) and the role of the immune system in fighting infection.

Sepsis occurs when the immune system over-reacts to an infection, usually in the blood rather than a localised infection. If sepsis is not treated it can develop very quickly to **septic shock** involving damage to tissues throughout the body causing multiple organ failure and, if not treated very quickly, death. Sepsis is more common than heart attack and causes more deaths than lung cancer and more than bowel, breast and prostate cancer combined.

Treatment of sepsis involves giving intravenous antibiotics (injected into the blood stream) as quickly as possible. Septic shock can be very difficult to treat as multiple organ failure occurs extremely rapidly.

> **Practice point**
>
> Sepsis illustrates the importance of regular monitoring and recording of clinical obs as these can be the first sign that a patient is deteriorating rapidly.

Dehydration

Dehydration occurs as a result of the normal homeostatic mechanisms not working properly or being overwhelmed. This can occur as a result of:
- excessive sweating, particularly after prolonged exercise

- vomiting and/or diarrhoea – this can be particularly dangerous in infants and children
- decreased water intake
- extreme heat
- burns
- **diuretics** – drugs that increase urine production. These are frequently prescribed to treat hypertension (see page 324), heart failure and liver failure. As these often occur in older people, who have a smaller volume of water in their bodies, dehydration must be monitored particularly closely in such patients.

Nervous disorders

These include tremors and convulsions.

A **tremor** is an involuntary, rhythmic muscle contraction causing shaking in one or more parts of the body. This can be caused by neurological problems in the part of the brain that controls movement. It may occur on its own, or be a symptom associated with other neurological disorders, such as:
- multiple sclerosis (MS)
- a stroke
- a traumatic brain injury
- neurodegenerative diseases, such as Parkinson's disease.

Other known causes include:
- some medications
- alcohol abuse or withdrawal
- liver or kidney failure
- anxiety or panic.

A **convulsion** is more severe, involving rapid and repeated contraction of body muscles resulting in uncontrolled shaking and loss of consciousness. They are caused by abnormal electrical activity in the brain. What triggers this is not always clear, although convulsions have been linked to:
- presence of some chemicals in the blood
- infections such as meningitis or encephalitis
- head trauma
- a stroke or lack of oxygen to the brain
- brain tumours.

> **Test yourself**
>
> 1 Describe the differences between Type 1 and Type 2 diabetes in terms of:
>   a causes
>   b treatments.
> 2 Describe the two types of homeostatic mechanism involved hyperthermia and hypothermia.
> 3 Name two conditions that can lead to renal failure.
> 4 Suggest why injection of radioactive iodine is a more effective treatment of Graves' disease that other forms of radiation therapy.

B2.15 Different classification systems and their purpose

There is a saying in the world of business 'what you can measure, you can manage', and the same is true in healthcare, which is why classification systems for different types of disease or health conditions are important. The **World Health Organization** (**WHO**) is an agency of the United Nations that promotes health and monitors disease in an attempt to achieve good health for all. WHO has established a Family of International Classifications (FIC) to provide a common language for health information worldwide.

Classification systems

There are several different classification systems in use, but we will concentrate on just three, as shown in the table below.

Type of classification	The conditions are classified under this classification type	Example
Topographic	Bodily region	Cardiovascular
Anatomic	Organ or tissue	Heart
Physiological	Function or effect	Angina

From the table, you will see that angina is a symptom of heart disease, which is a type of cardiovascular disease.

Purpose

Good classification systems have multiple benefits.
- They provide a common language for reporting and monitoring of health and disease.
- They allow the sharing and comparing of data, making like-for-like comparison possible.
- They allow the rate and frequency of disease to be assessed.
- They support the development of possible treatments.

B2: Further science concepts

For example, COVID-19 (SARS-CoV-2) is an illness caused by a respiratory virus that infects the lungs. This means it can be compared with other respiratory illnesses such as flu. However, as we learned more about COVID-19, it became clear that there were differences between how the flu virus was transmitted and how SARS-CoV-2 was transmitted. One observation was that COVID-19 caused severe inflammation and this led to doctors trying the steroid dexamethasone. This cheap drug had been used for many years to treat inflammation and it was found to be effective in treating COVID-19.

Other classification systems

There are other systems besides the three described above, for example:
- **Pathological** classification is made according to the nature of the disease. For example, cancer is associated with uncontrolled cell growth, while some inflammatory diseases are related to autoimmunity.
- **Epidemiological** classification refers to the rate of occurrence and distribution of disease in a population – see section B2.18.

B2.16 Examples of diseases and disorders and their relationship to the classification systems, including the possible causes and symptoms

We are going to look at three examples of disease and how each one fits into the classification system.

Topographical: diverticulitis

Diverticulitis is a type of **gastrointestinal disease** or disease of the gut. This is an example of classification according to the part of the body affected.

The symptoms of diverticulitis include abdominal pain. This comes on suddenly (we say it has **sudden onset**) but it can be prolonged.

Diverticula are small pouches that develop in the wall of the large intestine as you get older. Most people who develop diverticula do not have symptoms and may only become aware of them if they have a body scan for another reason.

When diverticula cause symptoms, it is described as **diverticular disease**.

If the diverticula become inflamed or infected and cause more severe symptoms, it is known as **diverticulitis**.

Early diagnosis of diverticulitis is important in order to start treatment promptly. However, the symptoms can be similar to other abdominal conditions. For this reason, blood **biomarkers** are now being used to aid diagnosis. A biomarker is a protein, gene or other molecule that is associated with a particular disease. C-reactive protein (CRP) is a blood biomarker that is associated with diverticulitis and higher concentrations of CRP indicate more severe disease.

Anatomical: hepatitis (liver disease)

The term **hepatitis** is used to describe **inflammation** of the liver and so is an example of anatomical classification – disease linked to a particular organ. There are different types of hepatitis, some of which are more serious than others. This shows how an anatomical classification can cover a range of diseases.

The symptoms of hepatitis include:
- fatigue
- dark urine
- pale stools
- loss of appetite and unexplained weight loss.

Viral hepatitis is caused by five different types of virus (hepatitis viruses A to E).

> ### Health and safety
>
> Healthcare workers can be at risk from viral hepatitis, particularly hepatitis B and C, as these are spread by blood-to-blood contact. This could occur as a result of poor healthcare practice, unsafe injections or needle-stick injuries (i.e. when they are accidentally injected by used needles).
>
> Vaccination against hepatitis B is recommended for people in high-risk groups such as healthcare workers.
>
> There is currently no vaccine available for hepatitis C and it often causes no noticeable symptoms, although it can be successfully treated with anti-viral medication. About 25 per cent of people infected with hepatitis C will fight off the infection and remain virus-free. In the remaining 75 per cent the virus will stay in the body for many years. This leads to chronic hepatitis C and can cause **cirrhosis** (scarring of the liver) and **liver failure**.
>
> Antibody tests can show if you have been exposed to hepatitis C virus, while PCR tests can show if the virus is still present.

Alcoholic hepatitis is caused by excess alcohol intake over a period of many years. The condition does not usually cause symptoms, although it can cause sudden **jaundice** and **liver failure**. Stopping drinking will usually allow the liver to recover, otherwise there is a risk of developing **cirrhosis**, **liver failure** or **liver cancer**.

Hepatitis can also be caused by paracetamol overdose.

> **Practice point**
>
> Paracetamol overdose may be an act of deliberate self-harm, but it can also be accidental; many cold and flu remedies contain paracetamol, so it is possible to ingest a significant dose without realising it.
>
> Liver damage can be reduced if the patient is given N-acetylcysteine or methionine within 24 hours - ideally within 8 hours. Unfortunately, symptoms of paracetamol overdose can take up to 24 hours to appear.

Physiological: chronic obstructive pulmonary disease (COPD)

Chronic obstructive pulmonary disease (**COPD**) is the name for a group of respiratory diseases caused by smoking, including:
- emphysema
- chronic bronchitis.

In individuals with **emphysema**, chemicals in cigarette smoke cause inflammation of the alveoli (see section B2.2) that leads to break down of **elastic tissue** and destruction of the **alveoli walls**. This reduces the surface area available for gas exchange in the lungs.

Chronic **bronchitis** is an infection of the bronchi that causes them to become irritated and inflamed, causing obstruction of airways, which also affects gas exchange.

COPD can also be caused by chronic, severe asthma. Asthma does not automatically lead to COPD, but a person with severe, poorly controlled asthma is more likely to have inflammation of the airways and scarring of lung tissues that can increase the risk of developing COPD.

The symptoms of COPD include:
- shortness of breath
- wheezing
- chest tightness
- chronic cough.

Unfortunately, there are several respiratory diseases that have superficially similar symptoms, so further investigation is usually necessary to provide a diagnosis.

> **Test yourself**
>
> 1 Describe the two main types of hepatitis.
> 2 Suggest how physiological classification of various respiratory diseases can help in identifying causes and possible treatments.
> 3 Suggest what classification could be given to the following diseases:
>   a Type 1 diabetes
>   b coronary artery disease
>   c irritable bowel syndrome.

B2.17 Injury and trauma

Injury is defined as **damage** to the body caused by external force. Injury and **trauma** differ only in degree; trauma is defined as an injury that has the potential to cause **disability** or **death**. The body responds initially in the same way, but trauma is more severe so the response becomes greater.

How the body reacts in a response to injury

Some aspects of the body's response to injury are similar to the response to infection, namely the **inflammatory response**, which was described in section B1.30.

Involuntary inflammatory response

The initial response to injury involves an inflammatory response, similar to the response to infection:
- increased blood flow
- increased metabolic rate
- redness at the site of injury as a result of increased blood flow and rupture of blood vessels around the site of injury
- pain, caused by pressure on pain receptors as a result of accumulation of fluid
- swelling (**oedema**) caused by increased accumulation of tissue fluid around the site of injury
- the white cell response; this involves movement of phagocytes to the site of injury as well as other lymphocytes involved in the immune response (see section B1.31).

Proliferation phase

This is the phase where tissue repair takes place. The goal of tissue repair is to remove damaged tissue and

any associated toxins or waste products. The steps involved include:
- The antibody response (see section B1.31).
- Pus formation and exudation. The action of phagocytes in engulfing pathogens and removing dead or damaged body cells eventually leads to an accumulation of dead phagocytes and other lymphocytes, which forms pus.
- The site of the injury is usually bridged by a **clot** (see section B2.6) that helps to reduce blood loss and prevent pathogens entering the wound. The clotting process also helps to bind the edges of the wound together and creates **scar tissue.**
- The next stage is growth of new tissue to replace damaged tissues. This involves a type of cell known as **fibroblasts**. These replace the collagen lost by the injury. **Angiogenesis** (growth of new blood vessels) means that the new tissue is supplied with blood vessels (**vascularisation**). The new tissue formed is known as **granulation** tissue; this results in the wound being remodelled as new connective tissue is formed. This increases the tensile strength of the new tissue. The **maturation stage** is the final stage of wound healing. There is a reduction in vascularisation and the scar begins to fade. The collagen laid down begins to form cross links, which increase the **tensile strength** of the wound. Tensile strength is a measure of the ability of the wound to resist pulling apart.

How the body reacts as a response to trauma

With trauma, the initial **inflammatory response** is the same as in injury. However, because of the greater severity of trauma, there will be several additional responses. These can include, depending on the nature of the trauma:
- loss of organ function (i.e. it stops working in some way or even totally)
- bone structure deformity, damage or loss of structure, e.g. a fracture
- haemorrhaging:
  - bleeding, when the skin is broken and blood vessels are ruptured
  - skin bruising (caused by bleeding under intact skin).

The greater severity of trauma means that the inflammatory response is greater. Once it has begun, inflammation can become a disease process. This can lead to multi-organ failure or even death.

Ischaemia

Ischaemia (sometimes spelled ischemia) is also known as going into shock. Shock is not the same as having a fright – it is the medical term that describes the reduction in blood pressure following an injury, excessive bleeding (**hypovolemic shock**), severe allergic reactions (**anaphylactic shock**) or infection of the blood (**septic shock** – see section B2.14).

As a result of the fall in blood pressure, there is a reduction in blood flow through organs or tissues – this is known as **hypoperfusion** or **ischaemia**. As a result, less oxygen and nutrients can be delivered to the tissues – this is known as **circulatory shock**.

Proliferation phase

Provided the trauma or subsequent shock does not prove fatal, the body then goes through a similar recovery process to that described previously under injury.

> **Test yourself**
>
> 1. What are the two stages of the body's response to soft tissue injury?
> 2. Describe the role of phagocytes in the process of wound healing.
> 3. Describe the role of the blood in the response to injury.
> 4. State two possible causes of shock.

B2.18 Epidemiology and how its objectives provide information to plan and evaluate strategies to prevent illness

Having lived through a pandemic, we are probably all better informed now about epidemiology – as long as we have obtained our news and information from reliable sources!

The meaning of epidemiology

Epidemiology is the study and analysis of the distribution and patterns of disease in **populations** and why they occur. It also covers the application of this study and analysis in order to control health problems.

John Snow is sometimes called the 'father of the field of epidemiology' for his work in mid-1800's London to discover the cause of cholera outbreaks and to prevent recurrence. This work was covered in the case study in section B1.27. The development of epidemiological methods continued in the late nineteenth and early twentieth centuries, mostly focusing on infectious disease.

Epidemiology developed rapidly in the second half of the twentieth century and has been extended to cover non-infectious diseases such as cardiovascular disease and lung cancer and its link with smoking.

Epidemiology also involves the study of factors that influence the distribution and patterns of disease, such as:
- diet
- environment
- ethnicity
- age
- sex
- co-medications (other medicines being taken)
- recreational drugs.

How objectives and strategies prevent disease

Epidemiology is not just an academic exercise; its purpose is to help understand the cause and spread of diseases so that strategies can be developed to **prevent** them.

In simple terms, epidemiology uses a systematic approach to:
1. **count** the number of cases of disease
2. calculate the **rate** of disease
3. **compare** rates, either over time or between different groups.

Identify the cause of disease

This may not be the starting point for an epidemiological study. We saw how John Snow used what we would now describe as epidemiology to identify the source (contaminated water), if not the actual cause (a bacterium), of cholera. More recently, epidemiology has led to acceptance of cigarette smoking as a cause of lung cancer.

Determine the extent of disease

By measuring **incidence** and **prevalence** of a disease we get important insights into the extent of the disease – it gives us data to work with.

Identify trends and patterns

Equipped with data about the incidence and frequency of a disease, we can then look for:
- **trends** – is the incidence of the disease increasing?
- **patterns** – does it affect mostly the elderly, or is it related to factors such as poverty or living conditions?

Study the progression of disease

Looking for trends and patterns in a disease gives an insight into how it spreads and what type of action might be needed. Epidemiology helps track the **mortality rate** of a disease. This gives an indication of how many times the progression of the disease is fatal and also the effect of any therapeutics.

Plan and evaluate preventative and therapeutic measures

Once we have an understanding of the cause of a disease, how it spreads and how quickly it spreads, we can start to plan ways of treating the disease (**therapeutic measures** such as drug treatment) or ways to prevent the disease (**preventative measures** such as vaccination.

Epidemiological methods also allow us to monitor the effectiveness of those measures so that we can **evaluate** and, if necessary, change or **improve** them.

> **Key terms**
>
> *Incidence:* the number of new cases within a specific time period. This means that it is a measure of the rate at which new cases occur. In the case of communicable or infectious disease you could think of it as being the risk of getting a particular disease.
>
> *Prevalence:* the proportion of a population affected by a medical condition at a specific time. It is usually expressed as a percentage, fraction or number of cases per size of population.
>
> *Morbidity:* refers to any physical or psychological state that is thought to be outside of the normal wellbeing. More simply, it describes illness or ill health. Morbidity is often used in describing **chronic** (long-lasting) or **age-related** illnesses. The **morbidity rate** depends on the incidence **and** prevalence of a disease.
>
> *Mortality:* death caused by a particular disease. Like prevalence, mortality is often expressed per number of population.
>
> *Mortality rate:* a measure of the frequency of death in a defined population within a specific time period.

Develop public health policy and preventative measures

Public health policy covers a wide range of measures, not just medical interventions like drug treatment or vaccination. Reduction in **morbidity** and **mortality** rates in the last hundred years have been due partly to

medical advances such as the development of antibiotics or widespread vaccination campaigns. However, other factors that must be included in public health policy have also played an important part. These include:
- improved nutrition
- improved sanitation (availability of clean, fresh water and removal of sewage)
- improved housing – particularly reduction in overcrowding, where infectious diseases are more likely to spread
- improved access to basic healthcare (rather than just advances in medical technology)
- greater education and health promotion.

How this has contributed to the prevention of specific diseases

Coronaviruses

Having lived through a pandemic, we should all by now be familiar with at least one of the coronaviruses – the SARS-CoV-2 virus, the cause of COVID-19. As well as COVID-19 there have been two other serious disease outbreaks in recent years caused by coronaviruses:
- severe acute respiratory syndrome (SARS), caused by the SARS-CoV-1 virus
- Middle-East respiratory syndrome (MERS), caused by the MERS-CoV virus.

Unfortunately, public education about COVID-19 also had to contend with sources of misinformation, particularly that spread on social media.

Coronaviruses are widespread, being one of the viruses that cause the common cold. However, COVID-19, SARS and MERS are examples of zoonotic diseases caused by a pathogen that has transferred from animals to humans.

The COVID-19 pandemic has provided epidemiologists with a great deal of data. Different countries have managed the outbreak in different ways, with different degrees of success. It is important that we should learn from this experience, as it is highly likely that there will be more pandemics in the future.

Although vaccines for COVID-19 were developed very quickly, new viral diseases often do not have effective preventions or treatments, at least in the early stages. For this reason, prevention is often the only effective course of action. This was the case in the early stages of COVID-19 and underlines the importance of education about preventative measures. The message to the public changed over time as more was learned about the virus and how it spread. At first, the focus was on hand washing and the risk of **fomite** transmission (i.e. from surfaces, see section A9.5) as this is a major route of transmission of other respiratory viruses, including the flu virus. With time, it became clear that droplets (aerosols) were the main method of transmission. This led to greater emphasis on mask-wearing and ventilation.

Human immunodeficiency virus (HIV)

> **Practice point**
>
> **Acquired immune deficiency syndrome (AIDS)** refers to a range of diseases as a result of infection with HIV. These include opportunistic infections, such as tuberculosis, as well as certain cancers, as a result of the damage to the immune system caused by the virus. Do not confuse AIDS (the disease) with HIV (the virus).

Unlike COVID-19, at the time of writing it has not been possible to develop a successful vaccine for HIV, even after 40 years of research. The first reports of increases in previously rare infections and the rare cancer Kaposi's sarcoma among gay men in New York and California were published in 1981. A year later, epidemiological evidence had shown that AIDS was caused by a sexually transmitted infection. After another year, HIV was isolated at the Pasteur Institute in Paris and shown to be the virus causing AIDS. In 1986, the US FDA approved the first anti-viral drug, zidovudine (AZT) for use in preventing HIV replication. By 1995, several other similar drugs became available, all targeting the same part of virus replication – this was known as **monotherapy**. However, not all drugs were equally effective in all patients and HIV quickly developed resistance to a single medication. The development of anti-viral drugs that target different parts of virus replication made possible the use of combination therapies, using different classes of drugs and thereby reducing development of resistance by HIV.

Although none of these treatments will cure HIV infection, in most cases the progression of the disease can be slowed down or even halted.

As HIV is transmitted via bodily fluids such as blood, saliva or semen it can be a sexually transmitted infection (STI). Use of condoms or other 'safe sex' practices can help reduce transmission in this way.

HIV can also be spread by needle-sharing between intravenous drug users. This has led to use of needle exchange programmes to reduce needle sharing, which helps to limit the spread of HIV. In the early days of HIV, contaminated blood products led to haemophiliacs and others being infected by HIV by this route. Rigorous screening and testing of blood products, as well as a move towards synthetic replacements for blood products, has significantly reduced the risk of HIV infection in this group.

As with COVID-19, education about prevention has been of great importance. See the case study in section B2.19 for an example.

> **Reflect**
>
> Some viruses mutate and evolve rapidly. The viruses that cause the common cold, including the coronaviruses, are an example. This, together with the large number of different cold viruses, is why it has not been possible to produce a vaccine against the common cold. It also explains why young children, with relatively little immunity, get frequent colds – particularly when they start school – as they tend to keep reinfecting each other. As we age, we tend to catch fewer colds as we build up a broader immunity.
>
> Viral mutation also explains the need for flu vaccines to be updated each year, as different strains become prevalent. It also explains the development of the different strains of the SARS-CoV-2 virus, such as the Alpha, Delta and Omicron variants.
>
> Think about the importance of epidemiology in studying, tracing and predicting new strains of virus. Do you think that epidemiology has a part to play in dealing with future epidemics and pandemics? How can this provide information to support development of new vaccines and/or treatments for viral diseases?

> **Test yourself**
>
> 1. What is meant by epidemiology?
> 2. Explain the difference between the following terms:
>   a. incidence and prevalence
>   b. morbidity and mortality.
> 3. In an epidemiological study, once you have collected data about the incidence and prevalence of a disease, what would be the next steps?
> 4. Why is public health policy so important?

B2.19 How health promotion helps control of disease and disorders

We have just seen how education and health promotion have played a part in the reduction in morbidity and mortality rates over the last hundred years. Living through a pandemic, we have all seen how health promotion has helped to control the spread of the disease – to a greater or lesser extent in different countries. But health promotion is not just about infectious diseases – it applies equally, if not more, to the so-called **lifestyle** diseases of developed countries, for example:

▶ obesity and related conditions, including Type 2 diabetes
▶ cardiovascular disease
▶ cirrhosis and other liver diseases
▶ some types of cancer.

> **Reflect**
>
> **Is obesity a disease?**
>
> We have just listed obesity as a type of lifestyle disease, but is it actually a disease? In part, it depends on what we mean by 'disease'. One definition is 'a condition of the body or one of its parts that impairs normal functioning and has distinguishing signs and symptoms.'
>
> On this basis, is obesity a disease? It is not a simple matter. Obesity is certainly a condition where the body develops excess fat. Measurements such as body mass, height and build can be used to define obesity. Obesity can be linked to increased risk of cardiovascular disease and Type 2 diabetes.
> ▶ Does this mean that obesity itself is a disease or simply a risk factor in developing other diseases?
> ▶ Does obesity always cause health problems?
> ▶ Does calling obesity a disease risk 'fat shaming' those who are obese?
> ▶ The World Health Organization (WHO) classifies obesity as a disease – do you agree?

Communication

Whether or not you think 'Hands – Face – Space' was the right approach to promoting ways to control the spread of COVID-19, you will almost certainly have heard it many times during the start of the pandemic.

B2: Further science concepts

> **Case study**
>
> In 1986, the BBC showed a series of public information films (adverts) on primetime TV to promote awareness of AIDS. They were highly controversial at the time, featuring powerful tombstone images and the slogan 'don't die of ignorance'. It was the first government-sponsored national AIDS awareness campaign and has been hailed as the most successful, with the approach being replicated worldwide.
>
> At the time, about 90 per cent of the British public recognised the advert and many changed their behaviour because of it.
> ▶ Do you think it is justified to use powerful, even frightening images in health promotion?
> ▶ What examples of health promotion campaigns (not just on TV) have you been aware of? Have they influenced you?

In the 1980s, radio, television, print media (newspapers and magazines) and posters were the main ways in which health promotion messages could be communicated. The advent of the internet and social media has changed this enormously. It has provided many more channels of communication. However, in some ways it has made communication more difficult, because the audience is more fragmented.

Policy and systems

Government and public policy can play an important role in health promotion, particularly by changing procedures, regulations or laws to enforce required behaviour, for example:
- restricted access to drugs of abuse
- restrictions on the sale of goods based on age, such as alcohol or cigarettes
- restricted movement of people, such as into and out of cities, regions or whole countries during the COVID-19 pandemic.

Systematic change to procedures, regulations or law to enforce required behaviour

The UK Government had various sources of scientific advice about dealing with the COVID-19 pandemic, to which it responded in different ways. Among the scientists advising the government were behavioural scientists, illustrating the importance of changing human behaviour when dealing with public health emergencies.

You will be able to think of many examples of this, particularly during the earlier stages of the pandemic:
- restricted access, ranging from limiting access to locations with outbreaks, to closing national borders
- closure of places such as bars, nightclubs, restaurants, schools, theatres and cinemas where transmission was likely
- restricted movement of people, such as:
  - stay indoors ('lockdown')
  - work from home
  - travel restrictions within and between countries
- test, track and trace: this has been at the centre of public health practice for over a century. Following testing to confirm the presence of a disease, local teams have been used to track and trace contacts of people with HIV and STIs (sexually transmitted infections).

Education programmes

As was mentioned in section B1.27, ignorance can be deadly. An important part of health promotion is improving knowledge and empowering individuals to adapt their own behaviour.

People are increasingly turning to the internet to help diagnose their symptoms. Use of internet search engines is not an adequate substitute for visiting your doctor. Nevertheless, it shows how people are using the internet for information about all aspects of their lives, including health and wellbeing.

Many universities and other organisations are offering online courses (**e-Learning**). Many of these are aimed at health professionals, but others are suitable for the general public or non-specialist.

The NHS has a great deal of information on its website covering a range of topics:
- **Health A-Z**; this has articles on a huge number of medical conditions, symptoms and medicines arranged alphabetically. This is where many internet searches will lead you.
- **Live Well**; this covers advice, tips and tools to help make informed choices about health and wellbeing.
- **Mental Health**; this has a great deal of information and support targeted at mental health issues.
- **Care and Support**; this is a guide to services for those who need help with day-to-day living because of illness or disability.

Various health apps are also available to support the work of healthcare professionals and help individuals to manage their health.

Other examples of health promotion include targeted awareness raising and campaigns, such as:
- Change4Life, a social marketing campaign by Public Health England, aimed at reducing childhood obesity by giving parents the support and tools they need to make healthier choices for their families.
- The annual flu vaccine is promoted through a range of media, including posters in GP surgeries, radio adverts, emails and letters to vulnerable groups, as well as social media campaigns (Facebook, Twitter and Instagram).

PHE was disbanded in March 2021 and ceased operations in October 2021; it was replaced by the UK Health Security Agency (UKHSA) and the Office for Health Improvement and Disparities (OHID) covering health protection and improvement, respectively.

See Chapter A9 for more on these and other health and wellbeing campaigns and initiatives.

> **Research**
>
> The flu vaccine campaign is a good example of health promotion for specific diseases or disorders.
>
> Search for health promotion campaigns England to see more about all of the Public Health England campaigns (for instance, Change4Life).
>
> How many of these campaigns are you aware of?
>
> Have any of them made you more aware of health and wellbeing issues? Have any of them made you change your behaviour? If not, what more needs to be done?

Active vaccination and/or therapy programmes and research

Vaccination has probably saved more lives than any other medical discovery. For some diseases there are no effective treatments, so prevention is essential, and vaccination, where available, is the most effective form of this. Vaccines have achieved some major improvements in human health and wellbeing:
- the eradication of smallpox
- the near eradication of polio
- significant reductions in childhood diseases throughout the world, including measles, pertussis (whooping cough), diphtheria, tetanus and hepatitis B.

The response to the COVID-19 pandemic has shown that, with sufficient investment and a supportive medicines approval process, safe and effective vaccines can now be developed very quickly. New technologies, such as mRNA vaccines, allow rapid adaptation of vaccines to meet the threat of evolving and mutating pathogens.

Research into new vaccines is also accelerating. Recently, vaccines have been made available against:
- malaria
- dengue fever
- Ebola.

Research is also underway to develop vaccines against some forms of cancer. For example, a vaccine against human papilloma virus (HPV), a cause of cervical cancer, is now offered routinely to 12-year-old girls in the UK. It is anticipated that this will fully or partially remove the need for screening women for cervical cancer in the future. HPV vaccine is also routinely offered to boys in the UK for the prevention of other HPV-related cancers.

One of the biggest epidemics that many economically developed countries face is that of diseases linked to obesity, such as cardiovascular disease and Type 2 diabetes. While research is being undertaken into therapies to reduce obesity, this is an area where health promotion campaigns are now focused.

> **Test yourself**
>
> 1 Describe the advantages of health promotion campaigns.
> 2 Describe two ways in which government policy can reduce disease.

B2.20 The concepts of genome and genomics and why these are different to the concept of genetics

A **genome** is the complete set of genetic information for an organism, hence the term 'human genome'. This includes all the coding (genes) and non-coding DNA stored within a cell.

Genomics is the study of the structure and function of an organism's genome (all of its DNA). This field of study includes the use of DNA sequencing methods and bioinformatics to sequence, assemble and analyse the structure and function of genomes.

Genetics refers to the study of individual genes and their role in inheritance. The laws of genetics were worked out long before scientists had any understanding of chromosomes or DNA and their role in inheritance.

B2.21 The characteristics of the different study areas within genomics

Structural genomics

Structural genomics is a branch of structural biology. It is the study and description of the 3D structure of biological macromolecules, particularly proteins. Structural genomics uses the techniques of **genomics** (see next section) and links it with the 3D structure of every protein encoded by a specific **genome**.

Functional genomics

This is the study of the functions and interactions of all the genes (and therefore the proteins) in a cell. Structural genomics collects and interprets the information needed to understand the structure and function of proteins in the cell. Meanwhile, functional genomics focuses on dynamic aspects such as understanding how transcription, translation, and the regulation of gene expression all interact in normal healthy cells, as well as in disease processes. Studying interactions of proteins with each other and with nucleic acids and small molecules also contributes to understanding in this area.

Evolutionary genomics

This is the study of the changes that may occur in a genome over an evolutionary timescale. It is possible to compare the genomes of related species alive today to work out evolutionary relationships on the basis of the number of differences in their DNA sequences. It is also possible now to obtain DNA samples from extinct species, such as Neanderthals and mammoths, and examine the DNA sequence.

The principles of evolutionary genomics can also be applied to micro-organisms, which have much shorter generation times and higher mutation rates. This approach has been used to study the evolution of human pathogens such as flu and coronaviruses.

Epigenetics

This is the study of chemical modifications to DNA that do not change the DNA sequence but can affect gene activity. The genetic information needed to make a protein is contained in the sequence of bases in DNA. The processes of converting this information into a protein are known as **transcription** and **translation**, and we describe this process as **gene expression**. The enzyme RNA polymerase converts the DNA sequence into a sequence of messenger RNA (mRNA). Chemical changes to the DNA, known as **epigenetic tags**, can regulate the process of gene expression.

The two most common epigenetic tags involve **acetylation** of histone proteins and **methylation** of DNA (see next). Histones are the proteins that the DNA molecule is wound around in all eukaryotic chromosomes. Acetylation means the addition of acetyl groups to the histone proteins, which makes the DNA wind less tightly round the histones (see Figure 14.53). This allows RNA polymerase to access the DNA in this region and thus stimulate transcription. Removal of acetyl groups makes the DNA wind more tightly and so suppresses transcription.

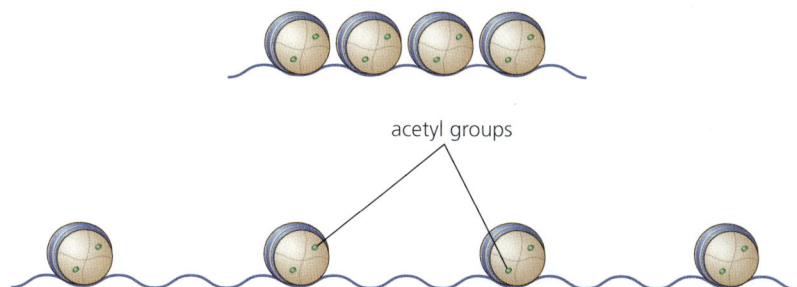

▲ Figure 14.53 Acetylation of histones makes the DNA wind less tightly round histones and so allows transcription to occur

Methylation of DNA suppresses transcription of the affected gene, usually by attracting the enzymes that remove the acetyl groups from histones.

Acetylation and methylation are two of the epigenetic tags that can be added to a genome. This can be the result of environmental factors, such as diet, stress, smoking or exercise, as well as in response to signals from other cells or within the cell. Methylation is an important mechanism in the 'switching on or off' of genes during embryonic development.

B2.22 How techniques in genomics are used to investigate, diagnose and treat disorders

Gene (DNA) sequencing

This is used to detect the order of bases (the **codons**) on the DNA within a genome, which corresponds to proteins that will be produced.

Sir Fred Sanger was responsible for developing a method to determine the sequence of amino acids in proteins and for developing the chain termination method for sequencing DNA. He later won a Nobel Prize for each.

Sanger's method of DNA sequencing was developed to increase the speed and throughput and, by 2001, a draft sequence of the human genome was published. This has now been replaced by new methods, known as **next-generation sequencing** (**NGS**) (Figure 14.54).

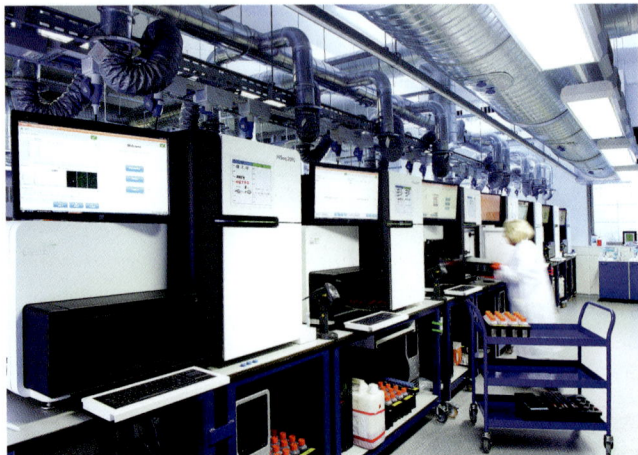

▲ Figure 14.54 High-throughput NGS machines at the Wellcome Sanger Institute near Cambridge

These methods allow the sequencing of thousands to millions of DNA molecules at the same time. As well as being a hundred to a thousand times faster than previous methods, NGS has made it possible to sequence an entire genome for less than $1000. Further developments will soon make it possible and cost-effective to have 'doctor's office' sequencing for use in personalised medicine (see next section).

During the COVID-19 pandemic, the Wellcome Sanger Institute was responsible for a large part of the sequencing of SARS-CoV-2 variants. Previously, genome sequencing of the Ebola virus contributed to greater understanding of its transmission during the 2015 epidemic in West Africa.

Because the DNA sequence determines the proteins that are produced, DNA sequencing will identify if a particular cell is unable to produce a specific protein for physiological function, such as an enzyme needed by the body in a metabolic reaction. This can be incredibly powerful as a research tool for studying the cause of a disease, as well as to develop new therapies. It can also be used in diagnosis (see next section).

Genome mapping

Genome mapping has been used for many years to identify and record the location of genes on a chromosome and distance between genes. While early techniques relied on genetic methods, it is now quicker and more cost-effective to use DNA sequencing to map a genome.

An important application is to identify specific chromosomal abnormalities, as well as to identify the physical location of genes on the chromosomes.

Genome editing

This is used to change the DNA within a cell, by adding or removing DNA sections or altering the DNA sequence. **Retroviruses** can be used to carry whole genes into a target cell and insert them into the cell's genome. This is the basis of gene therapy, which has the potential to treat disorders such as cystic fibrosis, which is caused by a mutation producing a defective protein. In this case, gene therapy allows the insertion of the normal gene so the cell is able to produce the functional protein. There are still many practical difficulties associated with this, however, and the method is still very much experimental.

More recently, the CRISPR–Cas9 system has allowed for more precise editing of the genome by replacing single bases or longer sequences at specific locations in the genome. This is also still experimental but has the potential to treat and even cure many inherited diseases caused by gene mutations.

It is also possible to use these techniques to modify non-coding sections of DNA that are involved in the regulation of gene expression. This offers the possibility of being able to switch on or off expression of one or more genes and, hence, the control the production of specific proteins.

B2.23 The applications of genomics within healthcare science

Pre-natal tests during pregnancy

Inherited (i.e. genetic) disorders can be screened for during pregnancy where there is a family history or other factors that increase the risk for some types of chromosomal abnormality, e.g. the age of the mother. Ultrasound scans are routine in pregnancy, and these can indicate the possibility of fetal abnormalities that require further investigation.

The next step is **non-invasive pre-natal testing (NIPT)**, which uses fragments of fetal DNA circulating in the maternal blood to exclude conditions caused by an atypical number of chromosomes. Trisomy, where there is an extra copy of a chromosome, is associated with inherited conditions such as Down's, Edwards' or Patau's syndromes.

If NIPT suggests a chromosomal or genomic variant or anomaly, invasive diagnostic testing such as chorionic villus sampling (CVS) or amniocentesis can be offered. If the woman chooses this option, the procedure provides a small sample of fetal cells for genomic analysis. However, there is a risk associated with either of these procedures, as they both increase the risk of spontaneous abortion (miscarriage) by about one per cent.

In some cases, analysis of fetal DNA in the maternal blood can detect the presence of single gene disorders, such as cystic fibrosis.

Some tests can be carried out before conception. Prospective parents can be tested to see if they are carriers of inherited disorders of which there is a family history. If this is carried out in conjunction with *in vitro* fertilisation (IVF), early embryos can be tested and only healthy embryos will be implanted.

Rapid fetal whole exome sequencing (RP-WES) sequences the whole of the fetal exome – these are the regions of the genome that code for proteins and make up about two per cent of the genome. Most mutations that cause inherited disorders are found within the exome.

Screening of individuals as a result of family history

Genomics can be used to screen individuals for inherited disorders that are the result of gene variants or mutations. This can be done before symptoms appear and can be used to decide on an appropriate course of treatment, where possible. While, in theory, it could be possible to screen everyone, in practice this is impossible. Besides the costs involved and the resources required (staff, equipment, etc.), screening such large numbers would produce too many false positives that could cause anxiety or lead to unnecessary treatment. For this reason, individuals are usually only screened when their family history indicates they might be at greater risk of inherited diseases and disorders.

Personalised/targeted cancer treatment

Genomics allows the use of targeted drug therapies based on the specific mutations in an individual's cancer. Tamoxifen is a drug that was commonly prescribed to women with breast cancers that carry the receptor for the hormone oestrogen (ER+). However, 65 per cent of women taking Tamoxifen developed resistance. There are several causes of resistance, but one group of women were found to have a mutation in the CYP2D6 gene that codes for the enzyme that metabolises Tamoxifen, so they were not able to convert it to the active form of the drug.

Other types of breast cancer are characterised by the presence of extra copies of the *HER2* gene and so produce higher than normal quantities of the growth-promoting protein HER2/neu, which stimulates tumour growth (this is known as an *HER2* positive tumour). The drug Herceptin® (trastuzumab) is a monoclonal antibody that targets the HER2 receptor. This blocks binding of the HER2/neu protein to the receptor and so growth of the *HER2* positive tumour is prevented. There is no benefit to patients who do not have the over-expression of HER2/neu in being treated with Herceptin. As Herceptin – like most monoclonal antibody drugs – is very expensive, it is not given to patients with *HER2* negative tumours.

Pharmacogenomics

Most people in a population will respond well to a drug, but others will respond less well or not at all, and some will experience side effects (adverse reactions). **Pharmacogenomics** helps us understand and hopefully address these issues.

The β2 adrenergic receptor is the drug target for bronchodilator drugs such as salbutamol, used in the treatment of asthma. Some individuals have reduced expression of these receptors and respond unpredictably to salbutamol. This is an example of a **polymorphism**, where different variants of drug targets exist in the population (i.e. there are different alleles).

However, variation in response to a drug is usually due to the interaction between many genes. For this reason, pharmacogenomics can be more useful, as it can use information from the whole genome rather than just individual genes to predict responsiveness. **Single nucleotide polymorphisms (SNPs)** underlie differences in susceptibility to disease.

A single SNP might be the cause of genetic disease. Sickle-cell disease is caused by a single base substitution in the β-globin gene. However, more complex diseases are often the result of interactions between several SNPs. To understand this, we need to prepare SNP maps that show the location of all the SNPs present in a single individual.

The prescription and dosage of medication can be based on this type of genetic profile to avoid adverse drug reactions or the use of prescription drugs that may not be effective.

> **Key terms**
>
> **Pharmacogenomics:** the study of how a person's genome affects their response to drugs.
>
> **Polymorphism:** the occurrence of two or more phenotypes as a result of there being two or more alleles, i.e. variants of a particular DNA sequence.
>
> **Single nucleotide polymorphism (SNP):** a change in a single base in a DNA sequence, e.g. C replaces G. This means that the two variants are **alleles**.

Assessing predisposition to illness or disease

Screening of the whole genome can identify the susceptibility of a person to certain disorders, such as heart disease, stroke or cancer. A pharmacogenomics study can be used to compare SNP maps and gene expression between normal and affected individuals. This is known as a genome-wide association study and can identify the genetic factors associated with the disease.

> **Research**
>
> **Genomics Education Programme**
>
> Health Education England has produced a Genomics Education Programme to deliver genomics education, training and experience for healthcare workers. It has a number of online learning resources, some of which are freely available while others require an OpenAthens, NHS or university login (your course tutor may be able to register your institution).
>
> Visit www.genomicseducation.hee.nhs.uk and look at a number of resources, such as the Bitesize genomics resources:
> - What is genomics?
> - What is epigenetics?
> - Where does our genome come from?
>
> You could also look at the 'Genomics in your profession' tab. Make a list of any resources that might be of use to you, either now or in the future.

> **Test yourself**
>
> 1. Why is NIPT described as 'non-invasive'?
> 2. Explain why there is a risk with invasive forms of pre-natal diagnosis.
> 3. Give two reasons why genome screening is usually only carried out on individuals with a family history of inherited disease.
> 4. Explain the benefits of using genomics in personalised cancer treatment.

B2.24 The importance of bioinformatics within the area of genomics

What is bioinformatics?

Bioinformatics brings together multiple disciplines to help us understand biological data. These disciplines include:
- biology (biochemistry, genetics, genomics, molecular biology)
- computer sciences
- mathematics/statistics.

Bioinformatics can be used to organise, analyse and understand, sometimes very large, biological data sets (big data) to make the data understandable and clinically actionable (see Figure 14.55).

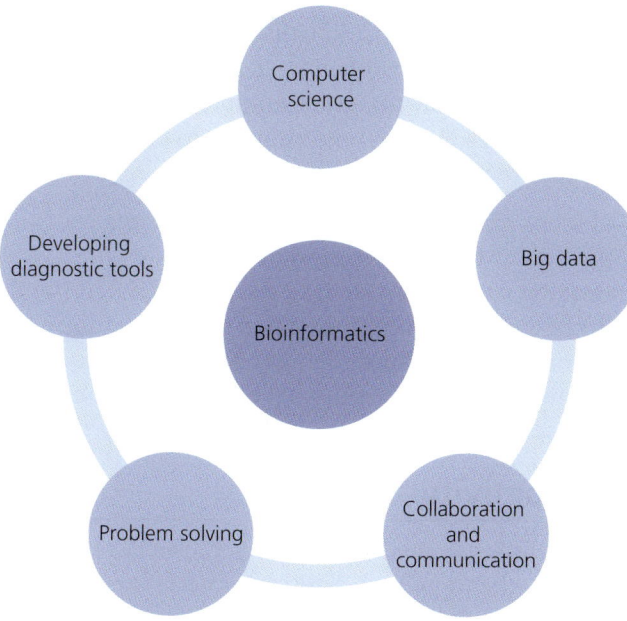

▲ Figure 14.55 Bioinformatics brings biology and IT together to make sense of big data

Developing software solutions for analysis of biological data

We saw, in the previous section, the importance of SNP and the ability to correlate various SNPs with an increased risk of disease, the basic disease mechanism (how it develops) and how disease can be treated, including on a personalised level.

To do this, it is necessary to work with 'big data' (extremely large data sets). By using larger data sets it is possible to obtain more accurate results.

Examples include:
- genome-wide association studies that can pinpoint the mutations responsible for complex diseases, such as:
  - infertility
  - breast cancer
  - Alzheimer's disease.
- the 100 000 Genomes Project, established to sequence 100 000 genomes from about 85 000 NHS patients affected by a rare disease or cancer. Combining genomic sequence data with medical records has enable investigation of the causes, diagnosis and treatment of disease.

Automation of analysis processes

Each sample from a participant in the 100 000 Genomes Project generates 100 Gb of data – that is, more than 20 HD movies. The sheer volume of data produced by genomic studies means that automation of analysis is essential. Automation allows faster analysis, with fewer manual tasks involved and can also be used for prediction modelling.

Case study

A pilot study for the 100 000 Genomes Project recruited 10 000 NHS patients across 57 hospitals. The whole genomes were sequenced, rather than just the better-studied **exome** (coding regions). This allowed investigation of regions of the DNA that regulate the expression of genes.

In total, 172 million genetic variants were identified, many of which had not been discovered before. As a result, it was possible to identify 95 genes that were associated with rare diseases, and at least 79 of these were shown to definitively cause the disease.

Why do you think this study focused on rare diseases? What would the next step be, having identified genes that causes these diseases?

Research

The Genomics Education Programme website (see section B2.23) has a Bitesize genomics section called 'what is bioinformatics?'

Genomics England (www.genomicsengland.co.uk) was set up by the Department of Health and Social Care to deliver the 100 000 Genomes Project. Their website contains a lot of information about genomics, DNA sequencing and the work done so far.

> **Reflect**
>
> **Is ignorance bliss?**
>
> One criticism that has been made of genetic screening in general and genomics studies in particular is that they can identify people who are likely or even certain to develop a life-limiting condition, but without offering the hope of a cure, or even treatment – at least for now.
>
> Some people have had other concerns:
> - What action would my employer take if this screening found something?
> - Would I be able to get life assurance?
> - Would my future employment prospects be affected?
>
> Do you think this is a reason why this type of research should not be carried out? Use the online resources listed in this section to research these aspects and form your own conclusions. Sometimes there are no right or wrong answers, only informed opinions.

B2.25 How physics principles are applied in the field of medical physics to support prevention, diagnosis and treatment of disease

Chapter B1 covered a number of aspects of physics that are of relevance in healthcare science, such as:
- electricity
- magnetism
- waves
- particles and radiation.

In this section, we will cover a few examples of how these are applied in the field of **medical physics**.

> **Key term**
>
> **Medical physics:** the application of physics concepts, theories and methods to medicine and healthcare.

Electric potentials

These are used to measure heart electrical activity in electrocardiographs (ECGs); the use of ECGs has been covered in sections B2.6, B2.11 and B2.12.

Transducers

A **transducer** converts one form of energy into another form. Transducers are used to produce and receive sound waves and to convert them into electrical signals to create a sonogram in an ultrasound scan. This was mentioned in sections B1.55 and B1.56.

Electromagnets and electromagnetic radiation

A magnetic field and radio waves are used to generate images in magnetic resonance imaging (MRI) scans.

Ionising (electromagnetic) radiation is the basis for X-ray imaging, with this radiation passing through the body but being absorbed by dense tissues such as bones to generate images. Computed tomography (CT scans) uses X-rays and computers to build up a 3D image of the body.

MRI scans and CT scans can both give 3D images of the body. MRI scans tend to be more useful in examining soft tissues, such as tendons, ligaments and internal organs. CT scans tend to be more useful in examining dense tissues such as bones (for fractures, for example) or tumours in diagnosing and monitoring cancers.

Radioactivity

Radiotherapy can be used to treat some cancers. Typically, a beam of high-energy X-rays is used to destroy cancer cells. This is known as external radiotherapy.

Brachytherapy involves placing small pieces of radioactive metal inside the body next to the cancer.

Radioisotopes can be attached to monoclonal antibodies that specifically target cancer cells. The radioisotope becomes concentrated near the cancer cells, allowing them to be destroyed while minimising damage to normal body cells.

There are more examples of the use of radioactive isotopes in healthcare and medicine in section B1.61.

B2: Further science concepts

Project practice

You are working as part of a multidisciplinary healthcare team and have been asked to prepare a report on the COVID-19 pandemic, focusing particularly on the lessons learned and how this could apply to potential future pandemics.

You need to carry out the following:

Background research

The NHS website aimed at patients (**www.nhs.uk**) may help; there is also additional information aimed at clinical staff about Coronavirus (**www.england.nhs.uk/coronavirus**).

- What is known about the mechanism of transmission of the SARS-CoV-2 virus?
- How has epidemiology contributed to this understanding?
- SARS-CoV-2 is not simply a respiratory virus. What is currently known about the effects of COVID-19 on the main physiological systems in the body?
  - respiratory system
  - endocrine system
  - nervous system
  - cardiovascular system.
- Some people infected with SARS-CoV-2 develop a post-viral syndrome known as 'long COVID'.
  - How does long COVID affect patients?
  - Is there a link between the severity of infection and the risk of long COVID?

Health promotion

What policies and systems were put in place to reduce the spread of the disease? How well did they work?

Consider the different ways in which bodies such as Public Health England promoted awareness and understanding, including areas such as:

- risk factors for severe disease (such as obesity, age, weakened immune system)
- precautions to take to reduce spread of the disease
- encouragement of vaccine take-up
- improving public awareness and countering misinformation.

Report

Prepare your report, either as a piece of extended writing or as a PowerPoint presentation. You should include the following points:

- how our understanding of COVID-19 developed
- the success, or otherwise, of health promotion campaigns
- what lessons can be learned and applied in future pandemics.

Group discussion

Have you given a balanced account? Are there any important areas that you have overlooked? Does the group feel that we will be better prepared for future pandemics?

Reflection

Write a reflective evaluation of your work.

Assessment practice

1. Patients with cardiovascular disease are sometimes prescribed exercise rather than medication. A middle-aged man recovering from a mild heart attack was recommended to monitor his heart rate while using a treadmill for walking at a moderate pace.
   a. Suggest advantages and disadvantages of using a wrist heart rate monitor (e.g. a Fitbit or other exercise watch) or a pulse oximeter for monitoring heart rate.
   b. Explain the physiological factors that the patient would experience if he exercised at too high an intensity.

2. In epidemiology, which of the following best describes the difference between morbidity and mortality?
   a. Morbidity is a measure of the frequency of illness and mortality is a measure of the number of people who die from the disease.
   b. Morbidity is a measure of the seriousness of illness and mortality is a measure of life expectancy.
   c. Morbidity describes the state of ill health and mortality means death caused by a disease.
   d. Morbidity measures the number of new cases of a disease and mortality measures the number of existing cases.

3 Of the three types of muscle (skeletal, smooth and cardiac), explain which has the highest and which has the lowest number of mitochondria.

4 Describe how the endocrine system contributes to chemical and mechanical digestion.

5 The table shows the concentrations of various substances in the blood plasma in glomerular capillaries, the glomerular filtrate and the urine.

Substance	Concentration in plasma of glomerular capillary (g/dm^3)	Concentration in glomerular filtrate (g/dm^3)	Concentration in urine (g/dm^3)
Proteins	80.0	0.005	variable
Glucose	1.0	1.0	0.0
Urea	0.3	0.3	8–10
Mineral ions	7.2	7.2	3–4

a Explain what the figures for concentration in plasma and filtrate of these substances show about the process of ultrafiltration.

b Explain the difference in the concentration of glucose in the filtrate and in the urine.

c Describe how the endocrine system influences the concentration of urea in the urine.

d Type 1 diabetes is often diagnosed by the presence of glucose in the urine. Suggest why glucose might be present in the urine of someone with Type 1 diabetes.

6 The walls of the vagina secrete peptides that can destroy micro-organisms such as bacteria, yeasts and viruses. These antimicrobial peptides (AMPs) are produced all the time, although secretion of AMPs increases in response to inflammation. Secretion of some AMPs by the walls of the uterus and vagina also increases in response to progesterone during pregnancy. Suggest explanations for these facts.

7 The 'fight or flight' response to danger is controlled by both the endocrine and nervous systems. Cells in the sinoatrial node (SAN) have receptors for adrenaline on their plasma membranes.

a Explain how release of adrenaline will help prepare the body for 'fight or flight'.

b Suggest how the endocrine and nervous systems work together in the 'fight or flight' response.

8 Describe the similarities in the body's responses to injury and infection.

9 During the COVID-19 pandemic, the UK Government was reluctant to make vaccination compulsory for care workers and healthcare staff. Suggest the reasons for this.

10 Explain why genomic screening for disease is usually only offered to individuals with a family history of the disease.

11 Explain what is meant by bioinformatics.

12 Give two reasons why bioinformatics involves automation of analytical methods.

13 The UK birth rate and death rate have changed significantly in the period since 1700.

a Between 1700 and 1800 there were fluctuations in death rate. Suggest two reasons why the death rate would fluctuate.

b The death rate declined steadily between 1800 and 1940. Explain reasons for this decline.

c There has been an increase in the death rate since 1980. Suggest one explanation for this.

Core skills

To pass the employer-set-project (ESP) and pass this qualification, you must show that you are able to apply core knowledge in context by demonstrating the following core skills.

CS1 Research skills

Research is an integral part of healthcare science; therefore, you must be able to carry it out effectively and gather sufficient evidence. Conducting research can lead to improvements in future practice and organisations within this sector.

CS1.1 Collect literature and introduce the scope of the review and the criteria for the selection of sources

Define the topic and scope of the research to be undertaken

Any researcher needs to plan, present and analyse their findings in a manner that is suitable for a research project. The process needs to include:
- choosing the subject area
- defining the topic or problem being investigated
- setting out the hypothesis, issue or research question
- writing the aims and objectives for the research
- selecting appropriate research methods
- identifying ethical considerations
- time management
- record keeping.

When choosing the subject area for a research project it is good practice to choose a subject that interests you. It is useful to make a list of possible topics. At this stage, broad subject areas are fine; they can be narrowed down at the decision stage. A spider diagram is a useful tool when trying to decide on the focus of the research. Remember to consider the amount of time available for the research to be carried out.

Identify relevant literature

- Identify what was included in the review.
- Identify what was not included in the review and why.

A sensible place to start with a research project is to gather background information. This is known as a **literature review** and was discussed in Chapter A8 (see CS1.2). A literature review enables the researcher to identify and define an area in their research topic. This will provide the reasons for the research paper and helps other healthcare professionals to understand why this new study was carried out. The researcher should summarise the previous studies so readers will understand the context of the investigation. For instance, there may be gaps in the previous findings that the researcher is attempting to address, or further data required to establish the limits of effectiveness of a certain treatment.

The researcher must identify data that will be useful to their project. A lot of information from secondary research and from colleagues may be interesting but it may not address the issue that they are examining in their project. They must ensure that they stick to the hypothesis that they have set. It will take careful reading and sifting through the information available to ensure it relates to their project.

Another key factor is to identify what has *not* been included within the research. A researcher identifying areas that have not been included should ask themselves why. If they recognise a gap within current information, they may set out to investigate the missing elements in the research.

Validate sources

Source and author bias

When carrying out any research, it is important that the researcher is objective. This means that they must examine any material that has been collected without any bias or prejudice. They must report only what they have found and must not add extra points that have not been demonstrated by their research. It is easy for personal opinions or views to affect research findings, therefore the researcher must try to ensure that any conclusions made are proved through the research for their research to be valuable. The author should not disregard other sources of information due to bias, for example information from a competing source.

The facts as they appear should be analysed and presented. Recognising that personal opinions and views can affect objectivity will help the research to be as objective as possible. **Subjectivity** is when personal opinion and views are allowed to influence the conclusions of the research.

Age and relevance of the source

Make sure the information used is current and up to date. It is no good using a book from 1952 if the topic is medical advances in the 2020s! Check the age of the research and statistics in any book.

Reliability of source

If the findings of research can be **replicated** (copied exactly) or repeated (by a different researcher at a different time) with the same or similar results, then the data is said to be **reliable.** Reliability depends on the researcher using appropriate research methods. It is therefore important to choose the best method for the study. Could other methods have been used? Would they give similar results? If the topic is the consumption of alcohol among teenagers, then it is likely that interviewing different age groups of people (for example, 14–19 year olds and 45–50 year olds) would give very different results. Researchers must target participants who are representative of the group they wish to target or serve. If not, the results will be unreliable.

Source citations

Source citations are essential to include within research. You must acknowledge the author, journal, article or website you sourced your information from. Citations throughout a report usually include the author's surname and the year the information was published.

Plagiarism means representing someone else's work as your own. Many educational establishments use anti-plagiarism software to check submitted work in case it has been copied (usually, but not always, from the internet). One way to avoid appearing to have plagiarised someone's work is to reference it properly, sometimes known as citing or giving a citation. Citing previous work is expected in science, particularly when you refer to a method or series of experiments done by someone else and you are basing your own work on it. Anyone reading your work can then go to the original publication if they want to get more information. You can validate sources by identifying citations in a piece of research and therefore finding the original research that the source has been based on.

A **bibliography** is a list of all of the sources you have used in researching your work. It should include:
- the authors' names
- the titles of the publications (i.e. the book, journal, newspaper, etc.)
- the names and locations of the publishers (usually just for books)
- the dates your copies were published.

For journal articles, the bibliography will include:
- the authors' names
- the title of the paper
- the title of the journal
- the year of publication, volume number and page numbers.

> ### Research
>
> There are many different styles for references or citations, so you must make sure you use the correct one. Your college, other educational establishment or employer may have a preferred style. If your work is published in an academic journal, you will find different styles are used.
>
> Find out whether your organisation uses a particular style for references. If it does not, then choose one of the common styles such as Harvard, Chicago or Vancouver as this will be easier to follow. Research your chosen style and how citations should be made in the body of your work (sometimes called **in-text citations**) as well as for reference lists or bibliographies. Try to keep to that style consistently in your work, including the ESP.

CS1.2 For each of the selected literature, identify and record through analysis

What was the research question of the literature?

When completing literature reviews, the literature needs to relate specifically to the topic area, and the easiest way to identify this is through the name of the secondary research article. Analyse the research question to ensure the information written within the report will relate.

What were the research methodologies?

Analyse literature review undertaken by the source, the sample and variables used, the results and the conclusions

Research involves exploring a topic to find out new information. In the healthcare sector, practitioners have a duty to ensure they keep up to date with the latest research; for example, doctors have a duty to follow medical research into prescription drugs and their side effects so they can use this information to make the best decision for the treatment of their patients.

Drawing conclusions means that the researcher reflects on everything that has been done during the project. They weigh up facts from primary and secondary research and they then come to a conclusion about how satisfactory the whole research project has been. Decisions are made about the hypothesis, aims and objectives, time planning, methodology, presentation, and analysis of results. Once conclusions are drawn, the natural next step is to make recommendations for future planning. You will need to analyse past and current literature based on the sample and variables used. You must analyse the sample size to identify whether it was representative and consider why it was or was not. It is also important to analyse whether the methods were correctly used.

In the conclusion to the research, all the findings of the report are pulled together, and conclusions are drawn. The researcher should not add any new information in this section. Conclusions should only be made based on the information that has been presented in the project. The hypothesis should be referred to and the researcher should state if the aims of the research have been met. As you analyse past research you will be able to draw conclusions in relation to the use of the research and whether the aim has been effectively met or not. During this, you will be able to identify future research that should be carried out.

Conflicting literature

There will be conflicting literature within any research as investigators may have opposing theories. Research will set out to investigate and identify different areas within a topic, therefore causing friction in relatable theories. As long as information is backed up with **reliable** sources and **repeatable** methods, there can be a range of possible conclusions evident.

Analysis of authors and their research

Literature must be cited as previously discussed, past research will also cite other authors and analyse their information and data. Trustworthy sources are important to establish effective data conclusions. Furthermore, reputable information should follow steps when information is reported. The layout within a report should involve clear analysis of the authors, methodologies, data collected, participants and conclusion. Within research it is essential to ensure we can successfully analyse information gathered.

> **CS1.3** Undertake a logically ordered discussion of themes, including how the literature relates to one another and to the specific research or innovation in an area of healthcare science practice

This includes:
- summarising key findings, using appropriate technical terms
- highlighting agreements and disagreements in findings
- organising material coherently
- identifying gaps or areas of study for the future
- identifying changes to make for future improvements
- using findings to contribute to research and innovation within a specific area of practice.

Scientists constantly research new and more effective treatments for diseases. For example, scientists developed several COVID-19 vaccines, which have been successful at helping to reduce the spread and effect of the virus on the population. Treatments evolve all the time with scientists trying to improve the outcomes for patients. Most patients with cancer, for example, now have a much better longer-term outlook thanks to advances in treatments.

This is one of the main objectives for carrying out any research. For example, if a healthcare professional has been looking at lowering the incidents of *Clostridium difficile* (*C. diff.*) on their ward and has found out that certain practices work in other hospitals, then it would be worth piloting the practice in their hospital.

Small changes introduced to improve practice could have a big impact on the working practices across the organisation. They could also improve the wellbeing of patients. For example, if the research helped to reduce the number of patients with C. diff. on the ward it would most certainly improve the health of the patients. The staff would benefit too as they would only have to nurse the patients for their original complaint.

Research papers have a specific layout when reporting their information and use the following subheadings:
- abstract
- introduction
- methodology
- presentation of data
- analysis of results
- conclusion
- evaluation of design and conduct of research
- recommendations for future research
- bibliography.

CS2 Communication skills

You need to be able to communicate effectively with patients, customers, carers and other healthcare science professionals using a range of techniques to overcome communication barriers.

CS2.1 Communicate clearly and effectively with a variety of stakeholders

It is important to communicate clearly and effectively with the following people:
- patients
- service users
- customers
- carers
- other health and social care professionals.

When communicating with other professionals, an interaction will probably be on a formal basis. Formal interactions can be one-to-one with other professionals or in a group. A group situation is more likely when several professionals are consulting together or when they are in a case conference. Interactions with patients can be formal or informal, but the message must be clear and unambiguous in both types of interaction.

CS2.2 Communicate effectively with a variety of stakeholders within the healthcare science setting

Communicate in a clear and unambiguous way, tailoring language and technical information to the audience

The effectiveness of your communication skills may depend on how far your approach meets the needs of the other person. For example, you will have to approach a 3-year-old child differently from the way you approach an older person. Language, posture, pace and tone all need to be adapted to the other person. You should not use technical language if you know the person would not understand you – instead you should present the information in simpler terms.

Select the most appropriate way of communicating, using images and other tools (for example, visualisations or infographics) to clarify complex information

When working in the healthcare science sector, there will be instances in which alternative methods of communicating, e.g. images, charts and diagrams, need to be used to clarify complex information to patients. Visual communication can benefit patients who have lower literacy skills and require information to be explained to them in more visual ways, making it easier for them to comprehend. The use of images and other visual tools helps to break down the otherwise complex information and present it in an alternative way. AAC communication boards can be used with adult patients who have suffered from a stroke and require additional help with communicating (see Chapter A5, page 104).

Ask appropriate questions to test understanding based on the task required

Open

Open-ended questions enable more in-depth conversation as healthcare science professionals and patients are not restricted to a yes or no answer and are able to discuss their concerns freely. They enable a much more thorough discussion to take place and give a clear, informative idea of a patient's current health.

An example of an open-ended question would be a professional asking a patient: 'How are you feeling today?'

Closed

Closed-ended questions limit a professional or patient's response to generally a yes or no answer. Closed-ended questions include direct questioning with the aim of receiving a quick response and to not facilitate long-winded dialogue.

An example of a closed-ended question would be a professional asking a patient, 'Have you had a drink in the last two hours?'

Leading

Leading questions are a type of closed question that suggests a particular answer because of the way they are phrased. They potentially encourage or lead a person to respond in a certain way.

An example of a leading question would be a professional asking a patient: 'So, you're not feeling well today?'

Probing

Probing questions allow a professional or patient to gather more information from an individual's previous answer. They are a type of follow-up question designed to seek clarification and further understanding.

An example of a probing question would be a professional asking a patient: 'And why do you think it is that you are not feeling well?'

> **Reflect**
>
> Think of a time either yourself or someone close to you was communicating with a healthcare science professional, or when you communicated with patients on placement. What type of questioning techniques were used? Do you feel they were appropriate for the conversation?

Actively and/or critically listen to the stakeholder's contributions

Actively and/or critically listening to the stakeholder's contribution is an important part of communicating effectively in healthcare science and achieving the best outcomes. If you do not give your full attention to the stakeholder, you could miss important information that could put a different slant on the conversation. Active and critical listening requires the listener to understand, interpret and evaluate what they hear through paraphrasing and summarising what the individual has said to them. Paraphrasing is useful here as it captures the main points that the individual has said. Further questioning may also be necessary to clarify or check points made. Active and critical listening also involves observing body language, gestures and facial expressions, as well as showing empathy by reflecting feelings.

Respond to the stakeholder's questions, using a tone and register that reflects the audience

Professionals should ensure that when responding to stakeholder's questions regarding generally sensitive health-related situations, they are doing so in an honest yet sensitive manner. It is important that stakeholders are responded to in an appropriate tone so that they can trust the advice and information they are being given, and so that professionals can build up a trusting relationship with stakeholders. The situations in which healthcare science professionals will be responding to stakeholders' questions may be tense and emotional, so it is essential that questions are responded to professionally and in a sensitive manner.

Speak clearly and confidently, using appropriate tone and register

Professionals communicating with stakeholders should ensure they are doing so in a clear and confident manner in order to gain the trust of the stakeholder and ensure they have full clarity of the information being communicated. A calm, slow voice can indicate an unhurried and friendly approach to the individuals. The tone of voice together with facial expression and body language can show interest and concern for the patient.

Display appropriate body language (for example, engaged, open)

Communication can be enhanced by positive and appropriate body language, which is also known as non-verbal communication. A professional can show through their body language if they are friendly and responsive to the needs of the patient. For example, if a patient asks the healthcare science worker a question and the worker looks at their watch and starts to move away, it demonstrates lack of engagement. To show engagement the healthcare science worker should make eye contact as a way of demonstrating interest in the conversation.

Communicate benefits to stakeholders, using calculations, diagrams and data to reinforce these assertions

When information needs to be presented to stakeholders, different diagrammatic presentations can be used to highlight commercial benefits, for example a good business relationship with suppliers. Even hospitals need to work with suppliers, such as companies that provide food for the hospital kitchen or remove their clinical waste products. The hospital management has to get the best deal and, after careful research into the possible benefits of the preferred company, the manager may have to present figures to the board of governors to demonstrate how the hospital budget is spent. Figures presented must be accurate and honest; they must not be changed to fit the hoped-for outcome.

CS2.3 Use a range of techniques to overcome communication barriers

Succinctness

If you are succinct, you clearly and concisely express what you want to say without unnecessary words. This means that the person listening to the conversation does not have to pick out the main points among a lot of unnecessary speech.

Avoid use of jargon/slang (for example, use non-clinical terminology)

As a healthcare professional you will use medical jargon that would make no sense to a non-medical individual. For example, a medical practitioner might say to a colleague that the operation was 'iatrogenic'. If that was repeated to a patient, it would probably be meaningless as most people would not know that it meant that the operation did not go as planned. You could lose patient confidence if you speak to them using medical terminology, especially if they misunderstand what you mean or what their condition or treatment involves.

Retain awareness of cultural differences

It is important to be able to communicate with individuals who have a different cultural background to your own. Individuals who are not fluent in English must have access to interpreters and advocates to act on their behalf when using health services. Interpreters will tell you what they are saying so that you can understand and respond, while advocates will help them gain access to services and act on their behalf to obtain their rights within a service. Family or friends can act as an advocate; if the person does not have family or friends to help them, however, the council (social services) must provide one free of charge. Many charities, such as POhWER, Age UK and VoiceAbility, can provide advocates free of charge.

Use of assistive technology and other communication aids where appropriate (for example, Braille)

If a patient requires alternative communication techniques, healthcare science professionals should be able to accommodate their needs. For example, individuals who are registered as blind may use Braille to read. Braille is a method of written communication that uses raised marks that can be felt with a person's fingers.

> **Research**
>
> Ask your mentor and/or manager on placement if they offer any courses on alternative methods of communication that you could complete, e.g. Braille.
>
> Courses such as the Braille courses offered through the Royal National Institute of Blind People may be available to you.
>
> www.rnib.org.uk/braille-and-moon-tactile-codes/learning-braille/braille-courses-adults

Collaborative working with other professionals (for example, carers)

Multi-agency working is an important aspect when overcoming communication barriers. Healthcare science professionals often work with other professionals to collaboratively assess and meet the needs of patients who have specialist communication needs. To remove potential communication barriers effectively, professionals working collaboratively must use formal and clear communication skills that enable others, such as carers, to have a full understanding of the necessary care needed and for patients to have full clarity of the treatment being implemented.

Identify when to refer to a colleague (for example, if sign language or translation services are required)

It is a good idea to refer to a colleague as soon as you recognise that you are out of your depth with a patient and need a signer or a translator to help you communicate. Rather than waste time and effort trying to communicate, it is better to admit you need assistance.

Use non-verbal communication such as gestures to imitate actions (for example, eating or drinking)

Gestures can be used to aid understanding but, when they are used in a haphazard way or there are too many of them, it can cause confusion. It is also important to be aware of what is acceptable for patients from different cultures. For example, in the UK the thumbs up is a sign that something is good but in other cultures this sign could be insulting or meaningless.

A frequent gesture for professionals to use with patients may be gesturing if a patient would like a drink or something to eat. While this is widely recognised and understood, some patients may not understand the gesture.

Use a quiet space free from distractions

For any conversation to be successful, the patient must be comfortable and able to concentrate on what is being said. If they are not comfortable, they may be uneasy and distracted. If the room is too noisy, the patient may not hear or may misinterpret what is being said, especially if they have problems with their hearing or ability to concentrate. If the door is left open there may be lots of people going past, particularly if they are in a busy hospital, so the patient may be distracted.

CS3 Team working skills

As part of your role in healthcare science, you will need to work collaboratively with a range of healthcare professionals both within and outside your specific team, as well as with other individuals such as carers.

CS3.1 Identify the functions of different teams/job roles as well as their own role within the wider team/working context

Stakeholder groups

Professionals working in healthcare science will work with a broad range of different professionals and patients daily. 'Stakeholder groups' refers to the broad range of individuals who are involved in or have an interest in decisions made in healthcare. Stakeholder groups include healthcare professionals and other multi-agency professionals working collaboratively with patients, their families and/or carers.

Identify structure of the team

Position within the team

When professionals are working among other professionals and in large teams within a healthcare science organisation, it is important that each individual's position within the teams is clearly understood so that they are aware of their own responsibilities and what is expected of them. By knowing an individual's position in a team, work can commence more effectively, which will result in better patient outcomes. Individuals are also able to recognise where they are excelling in their role and possible areas in which they could develop. They are not able to do this if they don't understand their position in the team.

Identify any direct reports

It is important that individuals know who to report to when they need help and/or advice. Reporting in healthcare science organisations enables practices to be carried out in a safe and effective manner. Direct reports might be from one healthcare professional team to another or within a team, such as a nurse providing the next nurse due on shift with information regarding a patient's current health status.

Identify relevant departmental organigrams

An organigram (sometimes called an organisational chart) is a diagram that highlights a department's or organisation's hierarchy and identifies its management structure and responsibilities. They can be as broad as an entire organisation or just one department. Organigrams in departments are important for the identification of management, which enables employees and even patients to recognise who to report to in the event of an incident. It clearly identifies an employee's authority and responsibilities within their job role so an individual knows who to go to.

> **Research**
>
> Look at the organigram for your work placement team. If one does not exist, gather information on your department's structure and create your own, ensuring you include in detail each department section's responsibilities and who is in charge at each section.

Define team responsibilities and accountabilities

Team responsibilities and accountabilities refer to the duties that a group of professionals are expected to be carrying out competently in their role. It is essential that professionals in teams are aware of the responsibilities attached to their roles; they can then strive to accomplish a common set of goals and objectives that they are accountable for.

Identify scope of practice of collaborators (for example, patients/carers)

Identify how scope of practice affects activities undertaken by different teams

Scope of practice is an essential factor to know about one's own job role as it identifies the procedures and tasks that professionals are permitted to carry out. This refers to their expertise, knowledge and professional experiences that enable them to carry out their role safely. When working in teams that include professionals with different areas of expertise and scopes of practice, it enables a wider range of activities to be carried out professionally and safely. It is very important that professionals stay within the limit that their scope of practice allows. A team of different collaborators with a range of scopes of practice enables a wide range of tasks to be carried out safely, lawfully and effectively.

Ask and respond to questions for clarification

Always ask questions if unsure about anything. It is good practice to ask another team member/manager for advice if you are in doubt as they will be able to address your query and clear up your uncertainties. Managers should encourage staff to seek clarification as it demonstrates that staff are committed to completing the job correctly and avoids confusion and time wasted doing the wrong thing. It also ensures that there is no duplication of effort across the team, with two members unknowingly carrying out the same task.

Recognise increased importance of communication when dealing with stakeholders outside of the sector and adapt communication accordingly (for example, reduce technical language/ jargon)

Positive and professional communication when working with any individual is imperative for ensuring effective practice; however, it is important to recognise that when communicating with stakeholders outside of the sector, communication and language may have to be adapted depending on their level of understanding. If an individual is not familiar with the jargon and technical language used by healthcare science professionals, there could be a lack of understanding of the message being discussed that could have serious implications for both patients and professionals.

> **Reflect**
>
> Can you remember a time when you were engaged in a conversation with a healthcare professional and you were unsure of the jargon/technical language used? How did it make you feel? How did you overcome this?

Identify own responsibilities

Tasks they are accountable for

Accountability means being answerable for something, primarily to your immediate boss, i.e. your line manager. To be accountable the individual needs to be clear about what they need to do, complete the tasks given to them within an agreed timeframe, then let the team or people involved know the task is finished. Failure to complete the work could lead to disciplinary action. Obviously, if there are extenuating circumstances, such as being absent through illness, then the deadline for the work would be extended. Similarly, if there is an unforeseen problem with the task, then a new timeline would be agreed, but this should be agreed as soon as possible rather than waiting until the deadline. Everyone is accountable within an organisation, from the top down to the bottom.

Position within wider healthcare organisation

It is important that an individual also recognises the role that they have within their wider healthcare organisation. When individuals understand their position within the wider healthcare organisation that they are employed by, they recognise the importance of their own specific job role and the tasks they carry out. They should feel empowered and motivated so that they carry out their tasks to the best of their ability to ensure they are meeting the aims of the organisation.

Deliverables they are accountable for

A **deliverable** is a product or service created at the completion of any project, but it can also refer to smaller components of a project. For example, five health care students have been asked to take part in a health promotion event at a primary school. They have decided to give a presentation on healthy eating for Year 3 pupils. In order to deliver this event, several components or tasks have to be completed before the presentation can take place. For example, one of the students needs to contact their local health promotion unit to obtain the latest available resources. Another needs to write a questionnaire for the Year 3 students to fill out prior to the visit so the group can see what they already know about healthy eating. Another person has to book the visit with the school. Then there is the actual presentation to design and write, and a slideshow presentation to produce. These are all deliverables and every one of them depends on all of the team members carrying out their agreed tasks so that the event can go ahead. In other words, they all know which deliverables they are accountable for.

Direct reports (if applicable)

Direct reports involve individual members of staff and a supervisor who is directly responsible for managing them. These individuals will have regular one-to-one meetings where the manager can build a supportive relationship with them. These help staff to feel part of the organisation and, therefore, a valuable member of the team. It also allows the manager to give constructive feedback to the worker on any of their projects. The worker can also discuss any issues they may have before they become a big problem. Praise can also be given for the successful completion of each project in these meetings rather than waiting months for an annual review.

CS3.2 Undertake collaborative working, demonstrating specific abilities

Establish a common purpose or goal

A goal or purpose brings a team together as they are all working towards a common aim. Setting goals allows everyone the opportunity to demonstrate and develop their skills. Good communication and collaboration are necessary to meet these goals. Once goals have been set, it is a good idea to draw up an action plan so that everyone knows what is required from them and the dates they should aim for. It will also allow the organisation time to gather together the resources required to meet the final objective or goal. It is often advisable to follow the SMART goal system:

- **S**pecific goals or purpose – objectives should be specific about what you want to achieve.
- **M**easurable – you should be able to measure whether objectives are being met or not.
- **A**chievable – it should be possible to achieve the objectives set.
- **R**ealistic – the goal should not be too ambitious given the resources available.
- **T**ime-bound – realistic time frame set with a clear end date.

Demonstrate respect towards others

Team members need to respect other members as well. All partners are unique and bring their own knowledge, skills, creativity and understanding for the advantage of the group. Additionally, if team members are not acknowledged for their contribution to the group, they are less likely to be fully committed to team objectives. Demonstrating respect requires every member of the team to take responsibility for their actions.

Delegate work when appropriate

Delegation is when a manager/supervisor gives an individual, who is lower on the management hierarchy, responsibility for a task. When a manager delegates they must be sure that the worker is capable of carrying out the task, i.e. they must be competent. This will partly depend on how long they have been doing the job. If the staff member is new to the role, the manager may not know them well enough to delegate important tasks to them or feel that they are too inexperienced. Smaller, less-involved tasks could be delegated to newer staff members to build up their confidence and demonstrate their competence. Delegating can motivate staff as they enjoy the opportunity to take control and make decisions. Managers must set clear outcomes when delegating tasks so that staff know exactly what is required and when it is required by.

Encourage contributions from other participants

If individuals are encouraged to contribute to projects they will work harder as they will feel that their contribution is valued. They will feel a sense of ownership of the project and want it to succeed. Everyone should be encouraged and have a chance to speak, and meetings should be structured to create equal opportunities for every staff member to have their ideas heard. It is a good management strategy to have a collaborative approach for projects rather than a hierarchical one. This is because it allows every member of the team to have a leadership role, even if it is for a very small part of the project.

Demonstrate clear communication skills, including making relevant and constructive contributions to move discussion forward

When working in a team, clear communication is vital. Good communication is needed both to give and obtain information and to share ideas. All members of the team need to be kept up to date with any developments on a project they may be working on. Failure to communicate can cause anger and a sense of mistrust. Poor communication can cause stress and anxiety as individuals may be unsure of what is happening.

To move things forward in discussions, it is a good idea to ask questions and give updates on progress after checking the latest status with other team members as they may have more up-to-date information. If you are the project leader for the part of the project being discussed then the importance of clear communication cannot be overemphasised. Everyone should be an active participant in the discussion, willing to share ideas and ready to help and support others in the team without monopolising the meeting.

Present information/ideas orally using non-digital and digital tools and other aids

Individuals working in healthcare science teams may be expected to present information and ideas to their team members. Depending on the size and complexity of this information, this could be done using non-digital tools, for example noting the main points on to a whiteboard and allowing for further questioning and clarification via a discussion. Alternatively, this could be done through the use of new analytical digital tools, for example the use of the cloud, analytics and data to present information digitally and visually to aid understanding.

Demonstrate adherence to relevant health and safety procedures

Managers must pay attention to health and safety as having and following effective health and safety policies and procedures is in everyone's interest. Employees also have a duty to follow any procedures laid down by the workplace. The procedures provide a framework for keeping everyone safe from potential hazards and risks. For example, each workplace will have a fire evacuation policy, which is explained to all staff and practised regularly, so everyone knows when and how to leave the building in the event of a fire. Other policies might be designed to ensure that all workers are carrying out their duties in a clean, well-ventilated, heated and well-lit environment.

The health and safety policy (shortened version) should be displayed on a notice board and published in any other relevant languages to make it accessible to all staff.

Follow standard operating procedures specific to the environment they are working in

Team members must follow standard operating procedures (SOPs; see sections A7.2 to A7.4) specific to the environment that they are working in, as there may be variation between different departments even for the same healthcare facility. If the healthcare worker has been moved to a different department, then it is up to them to find out about the policies and procedures of the new department and make sure they note any similarities and differences. They must then ensure that they follow them and, if they are unsure, they must ask another team member.

Make decisions

There should be a clear procedure within the team about decision-making with everyone involved. If the team has decided that a majority decision will stand then this should be followed wherever possible. If not, team members will feel left out of the process or that they do not have to follow the decision. This could also alienate team members if they do not feel confident that the correct decision has been made or that their input is not valued. However, it should be noted that the manager may override a team decision if they feel it is in the best interest of the organisation.

CS4 Problem-solving skills

In healthcare science, it is important to be able to identify problems and propose innovative systems to implement where appropriate. A range of methods can be used to identify problems and overcome them effectively.

CS4.1 Identify a problem and conduct a typical root cause analysis

Identifying problems can be done through patient or employee feedback. The following process describes how to carry out a root cause analysis.

Define

When defining a problem, consider whether it is associated with fact or opinion. Once this is determined, the underlying cause can then be investigated to make the necessary changes. The problem must be specified before considering how to overcome the problem. Research can then be carried out to investigate the issue and its cause, therefore enabling future improvements with the use of other methods.

Measure and analyse

To measure a problem, appropriate tools and technology will be required. For example, during drug trial methods, participants will be asked to complete questionnaires. The participants' answers will then be measured against other corresponding data to enable the research to determine the effectiveness of the drug or whether it needs improvements.

Feedback is an imperative part of any investigation as it enables the researcher to understand and identify the strengths or limitations of the methods being used. Through measurement and analysis, the individual can gather and interpret evidence to make recommendations for the future.

Improve and control

Controlled methods to help improve problems such as training plans, performance measurements and organisational policies and procedures can help to minimise future issues. Following regimented requirements enables minimised problems occurring or, when an issue does arise, it can be resolved through the use of methods in place.

CS4.2 Plan how to implement and embed the identified solution

Define the strategy for implementing the change

To identify changes there needs to be an understanding of what is required such as:
- What changes are needed?
- What steps are required?
- What are the success criteria to measure changes?

Organisations can begin to establish measures that need to be taken to implement new methods and define how to identify the success of the change. For example, if an organisation was to use a new technological method to enable patients to order repeat prescriptions online, then the old system of coming into the organisation would need to be tested through patient feedback such as surveys. The organisation could then trial the new technological system against the old method to identify if patients were more likely to use the new system compared to the old and distinguish how satisfied they are with the new service. Again this could be tested through the use of surveys.

Define and document an implementation programme for the change to be embedded

Firstly, you will need to define the measures and feedback tools that will be used to measure the impact of the changes:

- feedback surveys
- departmental outputs
- efficiency changes.

Then comes defining control measures that will be required to embed the changes. This includes:

- training plans and tools
- performance management criteria defining the success criteria by which the change will be assessed.

Departments within organisations may be asked to discuss and identify areas of change or areas of current complications to determine better working practices. To determine and overcome problems, it is important to ask those using the systems or services what is working well and what isn't. Furthermore, involving the participants who use the services or technologies is a key step to discover areas that require improvement and how to improve them. This will allow changes to be made to ensure systems are more efficient. Efficiency of new products can also be identified through the use of focus groups and feedback surveys to gain views on departmental outputs (i.e. what the results of the department's work are).

Changes that are to be made need to be effectively measured against a time scale. This will be dependent on the type of issue and whether it can be measured short term or long term. Training plans and tools such as involvement from other similar organisations that may use a particular system can be useful in gaining ideas and information of how changes can be implemented effectively. The use of information from other organisations can also help to target performance outcomes to ensure they are not based solely on opinion but on facts instead.

To define control measures to measure the effectiveness, criteria will need to be considered and tested against. Changes will then be analysed against previous working systems and measures, to identify differences and whether there is a considerable improvement in effectiveness. If the analysis points to ineffective measures, then other measures must be considered.

CS5 Reporting and presentation skills

In healthcare science you need to be aware of how to interpret and analyse data sufficiently. Once data has been interpreted, it should then be reported, and there are a range of formats suitable for presenting the data, depending on the audience.

CS5.1 Interpret and analyse information and data

Data analysis consists of processing the information and establishing relevant themes. When reporting or publishing, these need to be identified clearly so the audience can make sense of the information. The data collected needs to be described and analysed within an investigative report. When results are presented, they should be demonstrated through statistics, graphs or charts to enable them to be clearly understood by the reader or audience. When interpreting data, conclusions need to be made clear through use of necessary titles, subtitles, graphs or imagery.

Identify and collect suitable data

A variety of methods can be used to collect healthcare data including medical records, surveys and databases (see Chapter A8 for more information on this). This data must be relevant to the hypothesis that is being tested, and will often therefore be restricted to a certain group, for instance a specific age range, or people with a certain condition or taking the same medication. Remember to be sure that all relevant data protection legislation is complied with (see page 94), for instance around storing data, and that consent has been given where required.

Process, interpret and apply data accurately as well as search for and gather evidence efficiently

Data must be processed accordingly through the use of analytical skills and methods. Once data has been collected and passed through statistical testing it can then be interpreted through the use of graphs, bar charts, tables and other methods to enable the audience to establish the meaning of the findings.

Data interpretation methods can be used to analyse and review relevant information to draw conclusions. These conclusions may be as predicted from a hypothesis, however, sometimes conclusions may differ from the original hypothesis.

For information and data collected, demonstrate an understanding of the nature, type, quality and reliability

The nature of data collection means the underlying process of how information is gathered. It includes the type of methodologies used to collect information, such as the use of secondary data from literature reviews, observation, laboratory experiments and other investigative methods. Hypotheses will then be tested to interpret and evaluate data.

Quantitative and qualitative data can both be used during investigative research, either individually or together, depending on the type of data to be gathered. Quantitative data is numerical and should be represented using statistics or graphs, whereas qualitative data is non-numerical and more descriptive.

Types of quantitative data collected include nominal, ordinal or interval. These represent the level of measurement:
- Nominal data can be categorised, for instance characteristics such as gender or eye colour.
- Ordinal data can be ranked in an order or with the use of a scale, for example, 1–10.
- Interval data is interpreted through the use of international units of measurement, such as time with the use of a stopwatch or weight with the use of scales.

The quality of data is dependent on the measurement and whether it is fit for purpose. Has the data met the specific needs of the investigation? Data needs to be accurate for it to be used for the purpose, and also relevant to the research investigation. This must be made clear when data is presented and related back to the research question. Ensuring data is reliable is a key factor within investigative research; this is to ensure it is trustworthy.

Use appropriate technology to record and analyse data

Professionals already working in the healthcare sector may find that there is already a lot of data, statistics, patient information and so on stored on their healthcare technology system (this data is unavailable to the general public). They may already have permission to access it, as they use the technology system in their everyday work, and they should be able to download it and add their own data to it. This will make research easier if raw data is available, but they may have to process it. They should, however, let their manager know that they intend to use the information if it is available, and how they intend to use it, and make sure that they comply with any guidance on data protection.

Select and implement the correct data analysis techniques

The following should be identified:
- the approach
- similarities and differences within information
- relationships between information
- how to combine different types of information (for example, quantitative and qualitative).

When presenting research ideas, the approach taken during the investigation should be clearly identified, and the selection process of the research techniques should be discussed to explain why they are appropriate. Similarities and differences should be represented clearly with reference to the question being investigated. Clear themes should be highlighted when presenting research to ensure the audience is aware that it is significant.

Follow correct policies and procedures to ensure confidentiality is adhered to

As discussed through the healthcare science components, confidentiality must be continually upheld to ensure effective and high-quality practice is being carried out. When reporting and presenting patient- or participant-related information from research investigations, individuals do have the right for their confidentiality to be upheld. All organisations have policies that must be adhered to in response to confidentiality queries and implications. Every professional must be thoroughly aware of their responsibilities by reviewing their organisation's policies in relation to confidentiality and maintaining good practice. When presenting patient-related information, codes such as, Patient A…' etc. can be used in place of patient names.

> **Research**
>
> Research the policies and procedures relating to confidentiality at your work placement.
>
> Explain the expectations of the policies and how professionals must adhere to these rules.
>
> Evaluate the importance of upholding confidential information to protect patient rights.

Share information in line with organisation's policies and procedures

All participants of research investigations must be made aware that their information will be shared across a professional team or the expected audience. This information must only be shared when relevant, such as during a presentation of medical advances of a treatment trial. When sharing patient information to stakeholders, the presenter must use their professional judgement to determine the facts that are necessary. The patient whose information is being used must be made aware of what information is being shared and who will have access to it. This is strictly controlled by data protection legislation, so you must be clear on this.

> **Research**
>
> Using the NHS's website, create a poster stating dos and don'ts when sharing patient information.
>
> www.nhs.uk/NHSEngland/keogh-review/Documents/quick-guides/Quick-Guide-sharing-patient-information.pdf

CS5.2 Effectively present or report on conclusions following the analysis undertaken

Use technical language correctly, using graphics and other tools to aid understanding

Medical professionals as well as those working within other healthcare industries will use particular technical terms or acronyms that relate to their work. If there is any use of technical terms, jargon or acronyms when discussing or presenting information, these terms must be explained clearly and detailed to ensure understanding.

The use of imagery or statistics can also aid understanding, such as the use of graphs to present data findings.

Demonstrate understanding of audience requirements

The presenter must be aware of their audience's needs, meaning they should be aware of their level of understanding and a range of communication methods that may need to be used. Furthermore, being aware of the audience enables the presenter to identify key content that should be discussed, to ensure it meets the audience's expectations and areas of interest. Before presenting information to stakeholders, the presenter should plan the message they are trying to convey carefully to ensure it meets the targeted audience's understanding.

Ensure data is presented in an appropriate manner

The way that data is presented will vary according to the type of data collected – qualitative or quantitative. If quantitative data is being discussed, a wide range of bar charts, graphs or statistics can be used to present these ideas effectively. Qualitative information can be displayed with the use of categories or themes relevant to the information.

Before presenting information to stakeholders, the presenter should ensure information is laid out clearly and can be easily understood by the audience. If graphs or charts are used, they should be labelled correctly, along with any other types of imagery. Clear presentation of data is imperative.

Select appropriate font types, styles, sizes, colours and documentation layout

Documentation layout needs to be considered carefully. Is the font style clear for the reader? Can the text size can be seen easily? Should any points in the text be bold, italic or highlighted in any way to help the audience to identify key information? Colours can be used within reports and documents to help co-ordinate information into particular categories and to draw the reader's eye to important information. However, it is important to not use colour in a way that distracts from the rest of the information.

Use appropriate communication skills to present the data findings

Communication can be verbal or non-verbal. You will use both when giving a presentation, speaking about your findings but also using body language and indicating more information on projected slides or handouts. It is important to decide which information should be communicated each way.

Reflective practice describes a way of working that involves keeping notes or a journal of what you do, as well as your observations and ideas. These notes can be in any format (on paper or digitally) as long as you can understand what they mean at a later date. This then becomes a resource for you to go back to, to think about and ask questions about. They are usually informal and for the writer's use only.

Documents written for the workplace are usually formal and concise. These factual documents need to be clear, well structured and well written. They should identify a problem then offer findings and research, recommendations and conclusions. An individual may be asked to produce one themselves or it could be a team effort.

Highlight information

Important information should be highlighted, which can help to identify any gaps within the data or areas that may need further investigation. The explanation of these highlighted areas should enable the audience to understand your reasoning.

Agreements and disagreements within the information can also be highlighted as the audience needs to be aware of other information that is currently accessible. The reasons for these agreements or disagreements needs to be explained effectively.

Manage time effectively

Effective time management when reporting and presenting is a useful skill. The main part of any report or presentation should focus on key information.

Demonstrate knowledge via questioning and answers

Before delivering a presentation, the presenter should review similar materials or documentation that may help to inform them of how to respond appropriately to any questions asked.

At the end of a presentation it is important to give the audience the opportunity to ask any final questions. This ensures the presenter has carried out their role effectively, but also helps them to identify strengths or areas for improvement in future reports and presentations.

Presenters can use question and answer techniques to gain further understanding from the audience and to identify any areas that may not have been clear.

Demonstrate correct referencing

Correct referencing techniques must be followed when using information from other sources. Citations should be given throughout a report or presentation to enable the audience to identify where information has been taken from. Finally, the documentation must conclude with a bibliography giving a full list of sources and references formatted using Harvard or Vancouver referencing systems, for example (see page 349).

CS6 Reflective evaluation

You should be able to reflect on your own practice and make improvements to it; for example, having completed a task, you can review and suggest improvements, and consider the lessons learned for your own professional development.

CS6.1 Select the appropriate evaluation theory to use when reflecting on the task

Kolb

Kolb's experiential learning cycle is used by professionals in healthcare science when reflecting on their cognitive abilities and the way in which they process information to reflect and make sense of situations. Kolb's experiential learning cycle is primarily used when reflecting on laboratory-based activities and consists of four stages (Figure 15.1).

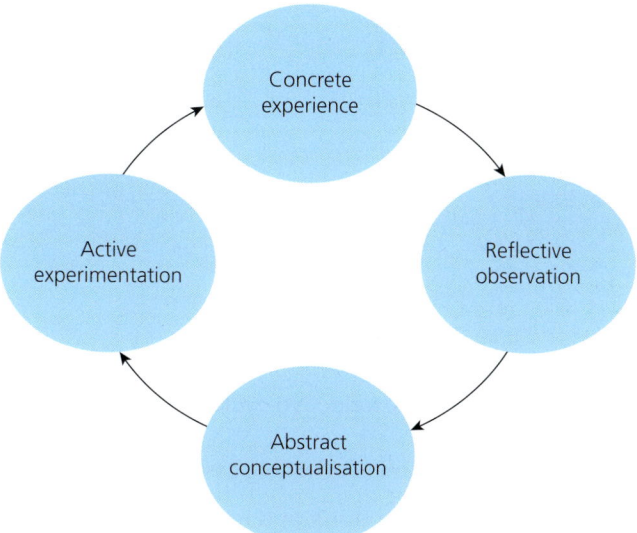

▲ Figure 15.1 The four stages of Kolb's experiential learning cycle

Stage 1 – Concrete experience: the stage in which the action is actually carried out.

Stage 2 – Reflective observation: reflecting on what happened during the concrete experience stage.

Stage 3 – Abstract conceptualisation: after reflecting on all of the information, the individual develops logical ideas to solve problems and make sense of the experience.

Stage 4 – Active experimentation: planning and then actively trying out the original action, however this time tackling aspects of the task differently, therefore demonstrating that they have learned from the experience.

Gibbs

Another model used by healthcare science professionals is Gibbs' (1988) reflective cycle, which is often used by professionals when reflecting on their practices with patients. This model is also straightforward to use and leads you through six different stages so that you can make sense of an experience and use it to improve your practice (Figure 15.2). It is a framework for examining experiences.

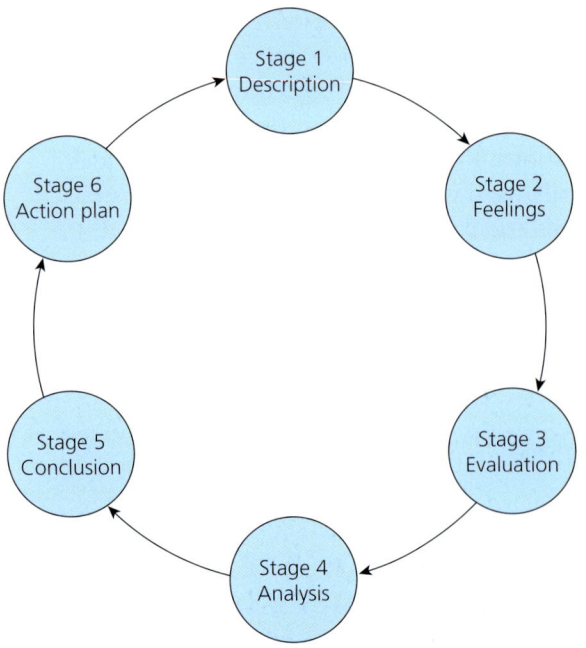

▲ Figure 15.2 Gibbs' reflective cycle

Stage 1 – a description of what happened.

Stage 2 – what did you think and feel? What was your reaction?

Stage 3 – what worked well and what did not?

Stage 4 – what happened and why?

Stage 5 – what else could be done? What have you learned?

Stage 6 – what would you do next time? What changes are you going to make?

CS6.2 Carry out appropriate evaluations of own practice within the task

Describe

Describe the situation or experience

Review the situation or experience by first of all considering in detail the actual events that happened in the order that they happened in. For example, what happened, where and when, was any other person involved, what was the outcome of the situation/experience?

Feelings

Describe thoughts and feelings during the task

After reviewing the details, an individual's thoughts and feelings during the situation/experience can be summarised, starting with what they were feeling throughout different stages of the situation. Did they feel differently than expected? How did they feel at the start of the situation in comparison to the end? What about the feelings of the other individuals involved? Do they feel the same regarding the situation as you do?

Evaluate

Summarise good and bad elements of the experience

An individual should evaluate the good elements of the situation or experience, e.g. what they felt worked well. They should also evaluate the bad elements of the situation or experience, for example anything that didn't work particularly well in hindsight.

Record individual actions taken within the task

It is important at this stage that the individual stays honest and unbiased so that they can reflect on events as objectively as possible. Individuals should be able to record their own individual contributions to events when evaluating so they can reflect on how they contributed to the overall result. Did their own actions work well? Were there any contributions that didn't work particularly well? When reflecting, do they feel positive regarding their own individual contribution or are there any thoughts looming over them as to what they felt they didn't do well?

Analyse

What might have helped and hindered the experience (for example, unclear instructions)

After evaluating what went well and what didn't, an individual is able to formulate changes that could occur to improve the bad elements of the situation or experience. An analysis of the good elements of the experience is just as important as analysing what could have hindered the experience, however. Academic literature and research could be used to support an individual in analysing why things did or didn't go well so that they can try to make sense of the situation.

Assess suitability of methods and techniques used

The techniques and methods used for the tasks throughout could also be assessed at this point. What impact did they have on the outcomes of the experience? Could another method or technique be used that could have led to a better outcome for all involved?

Conclude

What could be improved for future tasks?

A solid conclusion can be made at this stage regarding the whole experience, summarising what has been learned from the whole process. If they have reflected objectively, they should be able to say what actions they could change to further improve the elements that went well originally, as well as how they could improve the elements that they felt didn't go well to make them more successful.

Action plan

Summation of all previous elements of the cycle

Individuals should summarise all elements of the whole cycle of their reflection to come up with an action plan. An action plan needs to include anything that they need (or want) to improve for next time if they are to repeat this situation or in a similar situation in the future. Their action plan needs to include an identification and summary of what they are going to do differently and how they are going to do this.

Identification of improvements

As stated previously, action plans should be an identification of improvements that they want to be evident if they encounter a similar situation again. This should involve personal contributions and changes that they would adopt. An action plan should include an individual's recognition of what actions they would repeat in the future as well as actions for areas that they feel they would change and do differently, and how they can make sure they achieve this. If these changes require individuals to develop their own skills, how are they going to do that?

Evaluate fulfilment of objectives

This should consider whether the objectives that the individual set out to achieve have been fulfilled overall. Have some of the objectives been met while others would need to be altered through action plans to be achieved?

CS6.3 Use reflective evaluation to identify areas for improvement

Improvements that can be made to own performance within the task

Reflective evaluation is key for supporting professional development in the healthcare science sector. Individuals have a responsibility to review their own performance within tasks so that self-improvements can be acknowledged and developed. By using reflective evaluation, individuals can review their own performance and view it from the perspective of another individual, e.g. a patient receiving care from that individual or another professional observing, and acknowledge how their own performance could have been improved.

Improvements that can be made to team performance within the task

Reflective evaluation also includes the identification of areas in which team performance throughout a task could be improved. It is important that professionals can give and receive feedback on their performance as a team so that individuals can work together collaboratively to improve the team's performance as well as the outcomes of a task.

Alternative approaches that could have been taken

As an individual

Alternative methods and approaches could be learned to help develop skills that individuals already possess but need to improve on. It is important for individuals to attempt alternative methods so they are not making the same mistakes continuously and so that they can work towards improving their practice and contributions to a task.

As a team

When working in a team of professionals, potentially with different backgrounds and experiences, it can be difficult to collaboratively recognise that an alternative approach needs to be adopted or learned. Awareness of new approaches and developments in practice is essential. Teams of all experiences and specialisms need to review their own practice continuously and consider alternative approaches.

Appreciation of own knowledge limitations (for example, when to seek help)

Acknowledgement of an in individual's own scope and knowledge limitations within the healthcare science sector is very important for professional development and safe practice. Using reflective evaluation, individuals can identify areas in which their own knowledge base needs to be improved and where they need to upskill. It is important that individuals are able to seek help at this point from their line managers, so they are offered the opportunity to improve through training courses, shadowing and/or mentoring.

Assessment

Assessment overview

This qualification is assessed in the following ways:
- core component:
  - examination papers A and B
  - employer-set project (ESP)
- occupational specialism component:
  - synoptic assessment.

Core component

Paper A

This is a written examination; you will have 2 hours 30 minutes to answer all the questions.

The question types on Paper A are short-answer or extended writing.

The paper consists of four sections. Each section tests your knowledge of the content from two or three of the elements, each of which is covered by one chapter of this book. For instance, element A2 is covered in Chapter A2.

Paper A is worth 110 marks plus an additional 12 marks for quality of written communication (QWC), giving 122 marks in total.

Section A The roles and responsibilities within healthcare science

Element A1 – Working within the health and science sector

Element A2 – The healthcare science sector

Element A5 – Providing person-centred care when working in healthcare science

Section B Personal and patient safety

Element A3 – Health, safety and environmental regulations in the health and science sector

Element A4 – Health and safety regulations in healthcare science

Element A6 – Infection prevention and control in healthcare science settings

Section C Data handling and confidentiality

Element A7 – Managing information and data within the health and science sector

Element A8 – Managing information and data

Section D Regulatory and professional frameworks

Element A9 – Good scientific and clinical practice

Element A10 – Good scientific practice

Paper B

Again, this is a written examination in which you will have 2 hours 30 minutes to answer all of the questions.

The question types on Paper B are short-answer or extended writing.

This paper is composed of four sections:
- **Section A: Biology** – short-answer and extended writing
- **Section B: Physics** – short-answer and extended writing
- **Section C: Chemistry** – short-answer and extended writing
- **Section D: Science concepts** – short-answer and extended writing taken from any of the above content areas: biology, chemistry and physics

Paper B is worth 100 marks (including 10–16 marks for maths) plus 12 marks for QWC, giving 112 marks in total.

Healthcare Science T Level: Core

Question types

You can expect to find a range of different questions on the papers. These include:
- questions worth one mark requiring one-word answers or short sentences
- short-answer questions worth two to four marks
- medium-length answer questions worth five to six marks
- longer extended-response questions worth nine plus three QWC marks.

Paper B also includes some multiple-choice questions worth one mark each where you must select the correct answer from four options.

Questions worth one to two marks will usually require factual, knowledge based, one-word or short sentence answers that 'name', 'identify' or 'state' the required information.

Medium mark questions (four to six marks) generally require a short description or short explanation with reasons, for example.

Three QWC marks are awarded based on your ability to produce answers for extended writing questions where you:
- use a good standard of English
- express and organise ideas clearly and logically
- use a range of appropriate technical terms.

None of the individual parts of a question will be worth more than 12 marks: this is about your overall ability to write well.

Longer extended-response questions require answers that are well-structured into paragraphs with developed reasoning. The information will need to be accurate and use appropriate terminology. Accurate use of grammar, punctuation and spelling in these longer questions will support the overall quality of your response, as well as earning you QWC marks.

ESP tasks

In completing the ESP you will demonstrate six core skills, supported by underpinning knowledge and understanding from the core elements.

Core skills are covered in detail on pages 347–64.

Task 1: research/literature review – 5 hours

The first task of the ESP requires you to research and collate information and data from a range of literature sources that will be provided. This should be refined and focused on the details of the brief you are given. You will need access to the internet to use the literature sources/links provided.

After you finish Task 1, your tutor should take screenshots of your internet browsing history as evidence of your research, so remember to make sure you do not use private browsing or delete your history.

Task 1 must be completed within a single scheduled assessment period over a maximum of one day, and under supervised conditions.

Task 2: quality improvement report – 3 hours

For the second task you will need to produce a report that outlines how you would approach resolving the problems that are described in the brief. Some marks are allocated for good use of English, so pay attention to your spelling, grammar and punctuation, and how you demonstrate maths and digital skills. Again, you will need to show your browsing history so pay attention to all instructions you are given.

Task 3: peer discussion – maximum of 5 hours 25 minutes

This task is divided into two parts and will take place when all the students in your centre have completed Task 2.

Task 3(a)(i): preparing for peer discussion – 2 hours

Using a printout of evidence from each member of your group for Task 2, and a form to help you give feedback, you will be asked to prepare for a peer discussion group. The group will discuss how you can improve each other's proposals.

Task 3(a)(ii): exchanging feedback during peer discussion – between 1 hour and 5 minutes and 2 hours and 25 minutes (based on group size)

In groups of three to five students, you will now hold the discussion.

You will be able to refer to your own quality improvement report and your preparation form, and will have 20 minutes at the start to review these before the discussion starts. After that, taking it in turns, you will share feedback with each other and make notes by hand (unless you require reasonable adjustments) on the feedback you have received on your plan.

Task 3(b): quality improvement report v2 – 1 hour

After the peer discussion, using your feedback, you will reflect on what you have heard and write a summary of how you plan to amend your quality improvement report. You will be given a copy of your submitted report from Task 2 and you must reference the feedback you have received during the peer discussion, justifying your decisions and what you choose to do or not do as a result.

Task 4: present an overview of your quality improvement report – maximum of 2 hours 20 minutes, consisting of:

Task 4(a): preparing to present your quality improvement report – 2 hours

You will be supervised as you prepare for a discussion with your tutor, using a form provided. Part of this may include preparing how you will phrase or deliver your presentation. You cannot change what you have done in the first three tasks at this stage.

Task 4(b): presenting and discussing your quality improvement report – 20 mins

You will now present a summary of the key parts of your evidence from Task 2, as well as any appropriate comments from Task 3(b) and your justifications. Your tutor will be acting as if they are a supervisor in the area described in the brief and they will ask you questions to allow you to further justify your approach.

Task 5: reflective account – 2 hours

Having completed this project, you now need to write a reflection of how it went. Make sure you talk about all tasks and how well you think you have done at the outcomes you set out to achieve. This should include evidence from your completion of the tasks and an explanation of how these reflections will help you in your professional career. You should also consider the impact that your actions would have had in real-life practice, for instance on patients' care.

Occupational specialism components

These are synoptic task-based assignments linked to your chosen occupational specialism.

Examples of Occupational Specialism synoptic assessments:
- Practical activities such as assisting with physiological measurements and specimen collection.
- Lab based practical activities such as microscopy and specimen analysis.
- Written assessments based on work-based scenarios.

The occupational specialisms are:
- optical care services
- assisting with healthcare science.

You will choose one of these and the assignments will be focused on this occupation. 'Synoptic' means that it is an assessment of the overall specialism, rather than particular areas within it.

The assignments will comprise task-based assignments including observations.

Time allowed to complete the assignments:
- optical care services – 4 hours 40 minutes
  - assignment 1: 20 minutes
  - assignment 2: 30 minutes
  - assignment 3: 1 hour 50 minutes
  - assignment 4: 2 hours
- assisting with healthcare science – 6 hours 25 minutes
  - assignment 1: 1 hour
  - assignment 2: 55 minutes
  - assignment 3: 2 hours 30 minutes
  - assignment 4: 2 hours.

Healthcare Science T Level: Core

Command verbs

T Level Technical Qualifications delivered by NCFE use the following command words at the start of questions. These tell you what you must do to answer the question.

Command word	Use
Assess	Evaluate or estimate the quality of a given topic to make an informed judgement; may include advantages and disadvantages.
Analyse	Separate information into component parts; make logical, evidence-based connections between the components.
Calculate	Work out the value of something, showing relevant working.
Choose	Select from a range of alternatives (MCQ).
Complete	Finish a task by adding to given information.
Consider	Review and respond to given information.
Define	Give a definition or specify meaning of an idea or concept.
Describe	Give an account of or set out characteristics or features.
Discuss	Present key points about different ideas or strengths and weaknesses of an idea; there should be some element of balance, although not necessarily equal weighting.
Evaluate	Review information and bring it together to make judgements and conclusions from available evidence; students may also use their own understanding to consider evidence for and against.
Explain	Set out purposes or reasons or make something clear in relation to a particular situation; an explanation requires understanding to be demonstrated.
Explain how	Give a detailed account of a process or way of doing something.
Give examples	Answers should include relevant examples in the context of the question.
Identify	Name or otherwise characterise.
Justify	Support a case or idea with evidence; this might reasonably involve discussing and discounting alternative views or actions.
Label	Add names, indicating their correct position to an image or diagram.
List	Give a selection of answers, as many as the question indicates.
Name	Identify using a recognised technical term.
Outline	Set out the main characteristics or features.
Show	Provide structured evidence to reach a conclusion.
State	Express in clear, brief terms.
Summarise	Brief statement of the main points.
Suggest (what/why/how)	Present a possible cause or solution; apply knowledge to a new situation to provide a reasoned explanation.
Use or using (Figure 1, Table 2, the information above/in the scenario, your own knowledge and understanding)	Answer must be based on information given in the question; in some cases, students may be asked to use their own knowledge and understanding.
Work out	Perform one or a set of steps or calculations to arrive at an answer.

Source: www.qualhub.co.uk/media/22144/t-level-support-materials_command_verbs_v10.pdf

Preparing for the examinations

- ▶ Use the 'assessment practice' questions at the end of each chapter to help with your revision.
- ▶ Always ask your tutor if you don't understand something or are not sure – they are there to help you.
- ▶ It is never too early to start revising – begin your revision by going through your handouts and notes after each session – don't just file them away!
- ▶ Remember, the more times you go through a topic the more you will remember.

Assessment

- Make a revision plan – a timetable with dates – and tick off each topic you have revised.
- Use the practice 'test yourself' questions and 'research' and 'reflect' activities suggested in this book as another way to revise and to extend your knowledge.
- Learn the key terms for each topic so that you can use specialist terminology correctly in your answers.

Exam technique

There is more to producing a good answer to an exam question than simply knowing the facts. The quality of your response, such as how you organise your answer and whether it is fully relevant to the question, all help you gain extra marks.

Top tips

- Read each question through carefully at least twice before you start your answer.
- Underline or highlight the command verb so that you are clear about what you must do.
- Be guided by the number of marks and space provided for the length of your answer. The more marks available, the more space will be provided.
- Many questions will include the number of points they require, for instance: 'List **three** reasons …' Make sure you pay attention to this and provide enough information.
- If a question asks for 'ways', without saying how many ways, you must give a minimum of two as 'way**s**' is plural. The same applies to 'methods' 'reasons', etc.
- For higher-mark questions (for example, 6 or 12 marks) write your answer in paragraphs. Each paragraph should focus on a specific aspect of the answer. This ensures your answer is organised and logical.
- Make sure the information in your answer is accurate and relevant to the question – don't just write everything you know about a topic – answer the question!
- Do not leave any questions unanswered. Have a go even if you feel you don't know the answer – you probably know more than you think you do!

Sample practice questions and commentaries

Extended-response question

David discloses to healthcare worker Anna that he does not feel safe when he is at home. David reports his father has been hitting him. David also explained some comments his father repeatedly says to him, which insult and belittle him for being afraid or having an emotional reaction. David pleads with Anna not to tell anyone. Anna fears if she is to raise the concern that David will be subjected to further, more serious harm.

Explain Anna's duty of care within this scenario.

Consider Anna's responsibilities and the actions she should take, and how the right of confidentiality interacts with the right to be protected from harm in this situation.

Example medium-level response

Duty of care relates to ensuring service users are cared for effectively with the use of good professional practice. David is being abused at home and Anna must report this to her workplace's safeguarding officer. If Anna did not report this, David will receive further harm. This scenario conflicts with confidentiality because David has asked Anna not to discuss this further, but if Anna does not report this then David will be subjected to more harm. Anna is responsible for keeping David safe and preventing any risk of harm.

David is being physically and emotionally abused by his father. Although he is fearful of the repercussions of this being reported, it is Anna's duty of care to report this immediately. Although David has the right to discuss this matter confidentiality with Anna, because this puts him at risk of harm, Anna must inform David she will have to report this incident immediately. Anna has to comply with her duty to report this matter to the necessary people, such as her line manager or a safeguarding officer within her organisation. If Anna did not report this immediately, as David has begged her not to, Anna would be putting David at further risk of harm therefore not complying with her responsibilities to adhere to her duty of care. Furthermore, David's welfare would majorly be at risk and, therefore, this could result in severities such as death.

Commentary

This is a medium-level response. It is somewhat clear and developed, and the candidate demonstrates good knowledge and a good understanding of duty of care. The response directly considers the scenario, showing application of theoretical knowledge to a practical scenario throughout. The explanation uses some relevant terms, e.g. 'welfare', 'safeguarding' and 'comply with', demonstrating accurate use of appropriate terminology, and these are all relevant concepts that Anna should consider when adhering to her duty of care.

This explanation does not extend on the points provided. Each sentence provides a short description of reasoning but does not go into enough detail in providing specific examples or evidence of reasoning. However, the answer is clear and shows clear reference to the concept of confidentiality. The use of written communication is good with no errors of grammar, spelling or punctuation.

How it can become a higher-level response

To become a higher-level response, the answer needs to be further developed to ensure it explains the concept of duty of care thoroughly and considers the implications of confidentiality policies within organisations.

Further explanation and structure would be required for a higher-level response. For example, where the answer states 'Anna is responsible for keeping David safe and preventing any risk of harm', this answer could be further extended by specifically outlining Anna's responsibilities of duty of care, such as an explanation of minimising David's risk through instant reporting and investigative methods of the abuse.

The second paragraph is repetitive and could have focused on further specific requirements of Anna's job role in relation to duty of care. More accurate detail should be considered where it states 'Anna has to comply with her duty to report this matter to the necessary people, such as her line manager or a safeguarding officer within her organisation'; this is vague and further knowledge could be demonstrated, such as Anna's particular role of recording and reporting this conversation by following organisation policies and procedures effectively. The answer does not explain the role and, therefore, cannot achieve a higher-level mark.

Extended-response question

Analyse ways that national regulations and policies related to first aid influence the requirements of a local organisation's first aid policies.

Your response should include:
▶ reference to appropriate legislation
▶ having an appropriate number of first aiders
▶ needs assessment being carried out.

Example high-level response

The Health and Safety (First Aid) Regulations 1981 set out legal requirements for employers to provide adequate first aid provision for their employees. It requires that all workplaces adhere to first aid practices and have their own organisational policies in place to ensure that staff, clients and visitors are minimised from harm at all times, e.g. always having first aiders and well-stocked first aid boxes on site so that the appropriate first aid treatment can be administered in the event of an accident, as well as needs assessments being carried out. Organisations following the requirements set out by national regulations and creating their own first aid policies in line with those regulations are ensuring that employers are aware of their responsibilities, and minimising further harm to an individual in a circumstance in which first aid is needed.

National regulations and policies such as the Health and Safety (First Aid) Regulations 1981 ensure that local organisations have first aid policies in place that take the necessary steps in ensuring staff, clients and the public's safety through actions such as having the appropriate number of first aiders in ratio with the number of employees within the organisation. This will differ depending on the size of an organisation in terms of number of staff and will be unique to the risk associated with the organisation. However, by following national regulations, local organisations can implement their own first aid policy which meets regulations and is appropriate for their setting. For example, under the Health and Safety (First Aid) Regulations 1981, local organisations such as a dental laboratory would appoint the appropriate number of first aiders that was deemed relevant and safe for that organisation. If more than 25 employees worked in a dental laboratory, then at least one first aider must be appointed.

Needs assessments are taken out by local organisations when implementing their own first aid policy to stay in line with national regulations. This is because they are able to assess the nature of the work, any potential risks and hazards, and the history of accidents in that organisation. By completing needs assessments, local organisations are able to ensure that they are providing adequate facilities, informing staff about first aid arrangements, and have suitably stocked first aid kits. By national regulations setting out first aid requirements such as these, local organisations can protect the public by always having prompt and effective first aid policies in place.

Commentary

This response achieves full marks.

The full three marks for QWC were awarded as the answer is clearly expressed and well structured. The answer is presented using three paragraphs to organise the analysis. Paragraph one focused on the impact of national regulations on local policies, paragraph two focused on organisations having the appropriate number of first aiders in ratio with the number of employees within the organisation, and paragraph three covered needs assessments. This structure is to be recommended as it ensures all aspects of the question are covered. There were no issues of spelling, punctuation or grammar.

The response clearly and correctly references the Health and Safety (First Aid) Regulations 1981 as an appropriate national regulation, and how national regulations can impact on local organisations implementing their own policies. The candidate goes on to provide a detailed analysis of the importance of needs assessments and having the appropriate number of first aiders on site. The answer relates to the scenario as it links appointing the appropriate number of first aiders in a dental laboratory setting. A range of appropriate technical terminology is used confidently and effectively.

Short-answer question

State one purpose of the Health and Social Care Act 2012.

Response

- To improve the quality of care for patients.
- To create a more patient-centred care and facilitate choice of health service provision.

Commentary

This response is correct. The command verb is 'state' so no further information is required for this question.

Other valid responses are:
- To improve the quality of care for patients.
- To establish an independent NHS board to provide guidance and allocate resources.
- To increase the role of GPs in commissioning services on behalf of their patients.
- To cut NHS administration costs.
- To improve individuals' independence and wellbeing.
- It makes clear that local authorities must provide or arrange services that help prevent individuals developing needs for care and support, or delay people deteriorating such that they would need ongoing care and support.

Short-answer question

Outline **two** purposes of the Misuse of Drugs Act 1971.

Response

Award one mark for any valid requirement, to a maximum of two marks.
- to prevent the misuse of controlled drugs
- provide legislative framework for the regulation of dangerous drugs imposing a complete ban on the possession, supply, manufacture, import and export of controlled drugs except as allowed by regulations or by licence from the Secretary of State.

Accept any other suitable response.

Commentary

The command verb here is 'outline' so one mark is awarded for each valid and suitable response that clearly shows a purpose of the Misuse of Drugs Act 1971, up to a maximum of two.

Glossary

Abscess An infection in a tooth that causes the build-up of bacteria and pus.

Accident A separate, identifiable, unintended incident, which causes physical injury. This specifically includes acts of violence to people at work.

Accuracy Measurements that are close to the true value.

Acid A proton (H+ ion) donor. An acidic solution contains H+ ions.

Activity The rate at which a radioactive source decays. The unit of activity is the becquerel (Bq) where 1 Bq = 1 decay per second. Count-rate is the number of radioactive decays recorded each second. You can see that activity and count-rate can be used interchangeably.

Adsorbent Often used to describe the stationary phase in chromatography because substances become adsorbed to it during separation.

Adsorption When a substance (e.g. a gas, liquid or solute) binds to or attaches to another, usually solid.

Algorithm Instructions for solving a problem, especially by a computer.

Alkali A water-soluble base, such as sodium hydroxide. An alkaline solution contains hydroxide (OH−) ions.

Allele A variant of a gene.

Amino acid A molecule with both an amino group and a carboxyl group. Amino acids are the small molecules (monomers) from which all proteins are made. There are 20 naturally occurring amino acids found in proteins and all have the amino and carboxyl groups attached to the same carbon. This carbon also has a hydrogen and another substituent – the side chain, or R-group – which is different in each different amino acid. Amino acids are the monomers from which all proteins are made.

Ammeter Measures the flow of current; always connected in series. Voltmeters measure the potential difference in a circuit and are always connected in parallel.

Amplitude The maximum displacement of any point from the equilibrium position.

Analyte The solution of unknown concentration in a titration.

Anatomical waste Waste that involves human or animal tissue, for instance placenta. It also includes materials soaked in anatomical waste, such as swabs, blood bags, PPE, catheters, IV tubes and dressings.

ANOVA (analysis of variance) A checking system for groups.

Antibody A blood protein that is produced in response to a specific antigen. An antibody binds specifically to an antigen in a similar way to an enzyme binding specifically to its substrate.

Antigen A substance that is recognised by the immune system as self (the body's own cells) or nonself (foreign cells and pathogens) and stimulates an immune response. Antigens are found on pathogens but also on the surfaces of all body cells.

Artificial intelligence The simulation of human intelligence in machines. These machines are programmed to think like humans, e.g. learning and problem solving.

Asbestos Naturally occurring fibres that provide heat and chemical resistance to environments. Often used in older buildings, but we now know that it poses risks of serious illnesses if inhaled over a long period of time, e.g. years.

Ascities The abnormal build-up of excessive fluid in the abdomen causing swelling and bloatedness.

Aseptic Free from contamination caused by harmful bacteria, viruses or other micro-organisms; surgically sterile or sterilised.

Astigmatism A type of refractive error that can bring about blurry vision due to the lens of an eye being more of an oval shape, which means light is more focused on one part of the eye.

Atomic number Refers to the number of protons in the nucleus.

Automation A range of technologies that conduct healthcare services for patients with minimal human intervention.

Autonomic nervous system The part of the peripheral nervous system that controls many of the processes in the body over which we have no conscious control.

Base A proton (H+ ion) acceptor. Examples include hydroxides as well as ammonia and amines.

Blood pressure The pressure the blood exerts on the walls of the arteries when the heart beats; it is usually measured in mmHg (millimetres of mercury). Although the units of pressure are kPa, the unit mmHg relates to how blood pressure was (and often still is) measured.

British National Formulary (BNF) A pharmaceutical reference that informs and gives advice on prescribing medicines available on the NHS. It is jointly authored by the Royal Pharmaceutical Society and the British Medical Association (BMA).

Burette A long glass tube that has a tap at the bottom and is marked in 0.1 cm³ divisions. It is used to deliver an accurate volume of liquid (the titre) to reach the end point.

Calibration The process of comparing measurements, usually against a reference standard.

Cartilage Another type of connective tissue that contains, among other components, collagen and the elastic protein elastin. Cartilage is more flexible than ligaments and muscles, but not as hard and rigid as bone.

Categorical data is divided into groups or categories, such as male and female, ethnic group, city or country of residence.

Cell-signalling The process by which cells communicate with each other, usually by release of chemicals such as histamine, cytokines and interleukins.

Charge A fundamental property of many subatomic particles. Electrons, by convention, have a negative charge. The unit of charge is the coulomb (C) and the symbol is Q.

Chromatography The separation of the components of a mixture dissolved in a liquid or gas (the mobile phase) carrying it through a structure holding the stationary phase.

Cilia (singular cilium) Hair-like structures found on the plasma membranes of some types of cells, particularly in the lungs. These are known as ciliated epithelial cells.

Clinical bioinformatics The development of methods for acquiring, storing, organising and analysing biological data that affect patients' responses to drug treatments to aid in their prognosis.

Clinical commissioning groups (CCGs) NHS services that provide care that is specifically needed in local areas. When specific health needs have been identified, CCGs plan and commission the appropriate care that needs to be invested in and implemented to meet these.

Condensation reaction A reaction between two small molecules to produce a larger molecule and water; most large biological molecules are formed by condensation reactions.

Confidentiality To not disclose service user information to those who do not need to know. Information should only be shared with the relevant professionals on a need-to-know basis. Confidentiality upholds the rights of the service user to ensure their privacy is protected and respected.

Consent Permission or agreement, usually for someone to participate in something or to be subject to an activity, such as surgery.

Consumables Items that are used and then disposed of. They are mostly single-use but might be reused in some circumstances.

Containment barrier A physical barrier that prevents the spread of infections by enclosing and managing the infectious agents, therefore reducing or eliminating exposure.

Continuous data is numerical and can be measured. It is possible to have any intermediate value, for example, height, mass, length.

Controlled drugs Those licensed with a valid marketing authorisation for use within the UK and come within the Misuse of Drugs Act 1971.

Corrective action Putting right something that has gone wrong.

Corrosion The process where metals react with substances in the air to form oxides, carbonates, hydroxides or other compounds.

Cosmic radiation (also called cosmic rays) Originates from the Sun as well as from outside the solar system. It is a mixture of high energy protons (hydrogen nuclei), alpha particles (helium nuclei) and beta particles (electrons).

Coulomb (C) The unit of charge. Current is the rate of flow of charge past a given point in a circuit, i.e. how fast it flows past. The unit of current is the ampere (A), often shortened to 'amp', and the symbol is I.

Cytotoxic and cytostatic waste Hazardous or toxic medicines, often used in the treatment of cancers, that pose a serious risk to health.

Cytoplasm The fluid component of the cell, enclosed by the cell membrane and surrounding the organelles.

Delocalised electrons 'Free' electrons that are not associated with any single atom.

Dental X-rays (radiographs) Digital images of a patient's teeth created by exposure to X-ray radiation that can be used to evaluate their oral health.

Dependent variable (often denoted by y) A variable whose value depends on that of another variable. In an experiment, we usually count or measure the dependent variable.

Depolarisation (of a nerve or muscle cell) The reversal of the charge difference.

Detergent Purifying or cleansing agent that increases the ability of water to break down grease or dirt. Detergents act like soap but, unlike soap, they are derived from organic acids rather than fatty acids. Common examples are laundry detergent and washing-up liquid.

Diastole Refers to the relaxation of either atrium or ventricle.

Diastolic blood pressure The pressure when the heart relaxes; it is always lower than the systolic pressure.

Diffusion The movement of a substance from a high concentration to a low concentration. For instance, if you drop a crystal of copper sulfate into a beaker of water and watch the blue colour spread then you can see diffusion occur.

Disaster recovery plan A plan created by an organisation that documents detailed instructions for how to respond and recover effectively to an unexpected event.

Discrete data is numerical and can be **counted**. For example, number of patients (you cannot have half a patient). This is sometimes referred to as **integer** (only whole numbers).

Disinfectant A substance that destroys, inactivates or significantly reduces the concentration of pathogens such as bacteria, viruses or fungi.

Dispensing optician A specialist who fits and supplies patients with the most appropriate spectacles and/or contact lenses from the prescription provided by an ophthalmologist.

Ducts Tubes that lead from an exocrine gland to the place where the products are used or needed. Examples include tear ducts in the eye, or salivary and pancreatic ducts in the digestive system.

Ecological validity Whether the results can be generalised to real-life settings.

Electromagnet Produced when a current flows through a coil of wire.

Electromagnetic spectrum Describes all the different types of electromagnetic waves. The properties of the different types of waves vary considerably, so we usually consider the spectrum as seven groups, with slight overlaps.

Electromagnetic waves Include gamma rays, X-rays, visible light, microwaves and radio waves. Their energy is carried by oscillating electric and magnetic fields.

Electromotive force (emf) Like potential difference, except that it refers to power supplies such as cells (batteries), generators or mains power supplies. These transfer other forms of energy, such as light energy or kinetic energy, into electrical energy. The unit of emf is also the volt (V).

Eluate The mobile phase, containing dissolved substances, as it emerges from a column.

Eluent The solvent (mobile phase) used to wash substances out of a column.

Elution To wash out. In column chromatography this means 'washing out' a substance that has become adsorbed to the column (stationary phase).

Emollient A medical moisturiser used to treat eczema and soften rough, dry and irritated skin.

Employment tribunals Responsible for hearing claims from people who think an employer has treated them unlawfully, for example, through unfair dismissal or discrimination.

End point The point in a titration where the indicator changes colour.

Endocrine glands Glands that secrete (release) their products directly into the blood. Examples are the alpha (α) and beta (β) cells in the pancreas, which secrete the hormones glucagon and insulin, respectively.

Endocrine system A system of hormones that control many aspects of physiology (the normal functioning of the body).

Energy from waste The burning of non-hazardous waste as a source of renewable energy.

Epithelial cells Cells that line structures in the body, usually in thin, single layers.

Equivalence point The point of neutralisation where the number of moles of acid and base are equal. This should ideally be the same as the end point.

Ethics Principles that determine morality.

Exocrine glands Glands that release (secrete) their products into ducts or onto the body surface.

Factor analysis Simplifies data by reducing the number of variables, therefore focusing on the most significant variables.

Fertilisation The fusion of haploid gametes (sperm and egg) to form the diploid zygote with the full number of chromosomes.

Flagella (singular flagellum) Similar in structure to cilia but are much longer and are involved in propulsion of the cell.

Fluid mosaic model Describes the structure of the plasma membrane and how its components are arranged. The proteins, lipids and carbohydrates that are found in the plasma membrane vary in shape, size and location which creates the mosaic pattern. Due to the relatively weak forces between phospholipids, the membrane can be considered to be fluid as these components can move throughout the membrane.

Frequency (Hz) The number of complete waves that pass a given point in one second. One complete wave is a cycle, so a frequency of 1 Hz corresponds to one cycle per second. This is a very low frequency, so you will often see frequency measured in kHz (kilohertz, 10^3 Hz), MHz (megahertz, 10^6 Hz) or GHz (gigahertz, 10^9 Hz).

Gametes Haploid cells (half the number of chromosomes) that are produced by meiosis, a type of cell division that halves the number of chromosomes.

Gene A sequence of bases in DNA that codes for (contains the information to make) a polypeptide, or, in some cases, functional RNA (this is involved in regulating how genes are expressed).

General Dental Council (GDC) The UK-wide independent organisation that regulates and sets standards for qualified dental professionals to ensure that high-quality dental services are being provided.

General Optical Council The UK's regulator for optical care services which ensures the registration of qualified optometrists and dispensing opticians, and that the highest of standards are being practised to protect the eye care needs of the public.

General Pharmaceutical Council The UK's pharmacy services regulator that ensures high-quality services and safe measures are being offered by pharmacy professionals. Pharmacy professionals must meet requirements to remain on the council's register.

General Sales List (GSL) Medicines that can be sold in smaller quantities in most retail shops and are not restricted to pharmacies as they do not require consultations with a pharmacist and/or a medical professional for example, paracetamol.

Genetics The study of how single genes, or a small group of genes, function and how they affect the appearance and functioning of the organism.

Generator effect When a potential difference (voltage) is induced in a wire that experiences a change in magnetic field.

Genitalia The male and female sex organs.

Genome The entire genetic material of an organism. This includes DNA that does not code for proteins as well as the coding DNA (genes).

Genomics The study of how all the genes in an organism interact, as well as the role of non-coding sequences of DNA.

Gland A group of cells that make chemicals such as hormones or enzymes.

Grievance Any concern, problem or complaint you may have at work. If you take this up with your employer, it is called 'raising a grievance'.

Group Refers to the columns in the periodic table. Elements in each group have the same number of outer shell electrons. Period refers to the rows in the periodic table. Elements in each period have the same number of shells.

Haematology The analysis, diagnosis and monitoring of blood-based disorders.

Haemovigilance A set of surveillance procedures that cover the blood transfusion process. This includes the donation process, the processing of blood and its components, the provision of transfusions to patients and their follow-up checks.

Half-life The time taken for half the unstable nuclei in a sample to decay.

Hazard Something that has the potential to cause harm.

Health and Care Professions Council (HCPC) A UK organisation that aims to protect the public through the regulation of registered healthcare science professionals, ensuring they are meeting clinical standards.

Healthcare-associated infections (HCAIs) Infections that occur as a result of having surgical or medical treatment in a hospital.

High efficiency particulate air (HEPA) filter A mechanical air filter that removes/eliminates harmful bacteria and toxins from the air.

Hormone A chemical messenger released into the blood by an endocrine gland that acts on target tissues elsewhere in the body.

Human Medicines Act 2012 An act which was designed to modernise and amend medicines legislation in the UK.

Hypothesis A prediction of the outcome that will be tested as part of the experiment.

Incidence The number of new cases within a specific time period. This means that it is a measure of the rate at which new cases occur. In the case of communicable or infectious disease you could think of it as being the risk of getting a particular disease.

Independent variable (often denoted by *x*) A variable whose value does not depend on that of another variable. In an experiment, the independent variable is usually what we change.

Indicator A substance that changes from one colour to another or from coloured to colourless depending on whether it is in acidic or basic solution.

Induced magnet An object that can become a magnet when it is placed in a magnetic field.

Infection The process of bacteria, viruses or other micro-organisms (such as fungi or parasites) invading the body, making someone ill or diseased.

Inferential statistics Statistics used to predict whether the results of medical trials can be generalised to the wider population.

Inflammation A local response to injury and infection.

Inpatients Patients who stay in hospital overnight or for a duration while receiving medical treatment.

Integumentary system This includes the skin, exocrine glands, hair and nails. An **integument** is a tough outer protective layer.

Ionisation The formation of charged particles from neutral molecules or atoms by adding or removing electrons.

Ionising radiation Any form of radiation that interacts with matter, resulting in ionisation of that matter.

Ions Atoms that have lost electrons (positive ions) or gained electrons (negative ions).

Irradiation When objects are exposed to different types of radiation. It may be used to penetrate various materials and can be used to sterilise surgical instruments.

Isotopes Atoms of the same element (they have the same number of protons) but with different number of neutrons.

Joint The area where two or more bones connect.

Laws Legislation passed by parliament that state the rights and entitlements of individuals and provide legal rules that have to be followed. The law is upheld through the courts. If an individual or care setting breaks the law by, for example, inappropriately sharing or inaccurately recording information, they can, in certain circumstances, be fined, dismissed or given a prison sentence.

Levels A way of grading a qualification or set of skills and the corresponding occupations. The levels used today are based on the National Vocational Qualifications (NVQ) levels 1 to 5 developed in the 1980s. Over time, more emphasis has been given to the degree of difficulty or challenge of the qualification rather than the level of occupational competence in the workplace. There are now eight levels, and they cover academic qualifications such as GCSEs, A Levels and undergraduate and graduate degrees, as well as vocational qualifications such as T Levels and apprenticeships.

Life sciences The study of living organisms, for example microbes, human beings and fungi.

Ligaments Made of connective tissue containing the protein collagen. Their function is to join bones together and to strengthen joints.

Lines of magnetic flux Indicate the direction and strength of a magnetic field.

Lymphocytes Small white blood cells. B lymphocytes, or B cells, are responsible for antibody production. Different types of T lymphocytes, or T cells, play different roles in the immune response.

Magnet A material or object that produces a magnetic field.

Magnetic field A region where magnetic materials experience a force.

Magnetic materials Such as iron, steel, nickel and cobalt will experience an attractive force when placed in a magnetic field.

Magnetism The force experienced by some types of metals in the Earth's magnetic field or in a magnetic field of a magnet. It is also defined as the attractive or repulsive force produced by a moving electric charge.

Magnification How much bigger the image is than the actual object we are viewing. It should not be confused with resolution.

Materials Include items such as ingredients or components used in the manufacture of a product.

Maxillofacial prostheses (singular: **prosthesis**) Products that will reconstruct and restore the function and improve the overall quality of a patient's oral health.

Maxillofacial surgery Specialised surgery to treat conditions, defects and injuries of the mouth, teeth, jaws and face.

Mean The average number; all the numbers should be added together, then the value divided by the number of numbers.

Median The middle number within an ascending or descending list.

Medical negligence When a patient has been directly or indirectly injured or harmed during treatment or care, for example misdiagnosis or mistakes in surgery.

Medical physics The application of physics concepts, theories and methods to medicine and healthcare.

Medicines Act 1968 The first act of parliament that provided a system for licensing medical products in the UK.

Medicines and Healthcare products Regulatory Agency (MHRA) An executive agency of the Department of Health that is responsible for ensuring that medicines are safely manufactured and supplied.

Membrane All membranes consist of a phospholipid bilayer together with proteins and other components. They are selectively permeable (meaning they let some things through and not others) and can control movement of substances across the membrane as well as being the sites of many important processes in the cell.

Mode The number that occurs most often.

Mole An amount of substance. This helps us to work out the reacting proportions in any reaction. We can also use the mole to work out reacting masses or volumes. The abbreviation is mol.

Motor effect When a current-carrying wire is placed between magnetic poles. The magnetic field around the wire interacts with the magnetic field it is placed in. This causes the wire and magnet to exert a force on each other and can cause the wire to move.

Morbidity Refers to any physical or psychological state that is thought to be outside of the normal wellbeing. More simply, it describes illness or ill health. Morbidity is often used in describing chronic (long-lasting) or age-related illnesses. The morbidity rate depends on the incidence and prevalence of a disease.

Mortality Death caused by a particular disease. Like prevalence, mortality is often expressed per number of population.

Mortality rate A measure of the frequency of death in a defined population within a specific time period.

Multidisciplinary team A range of professionals from a variety of disciplines working together to support a patient's care.

Multidisciplinary A combination of a wide range of professionals from different specialisms.

Mutation A change in the sequence of bases in DNA. This can occur in a number of ways. When a mutation occurs within a coding region of DNA a new allele can be formed.

National Insurance Mandatory payments made by employers and employees in the UK that fund certain state benefits, e.g. healthcare, a state pension and payments for sick and unemployed people.

Negligence When professionals breach their duty of care, which can cause harm to the patient.

Nerve A bundle of neurones.

Neurone A nerve cell.

NHS trust An organisational unit that provides specialised care in a specific community. Within any community there may be several NHS trusts providing healthcare, such as mental health trusts, community trusts, acute trusts and ambulance trusts.

NICE (National Institute for Health and Care Excellence) An independent agency of the NHS that offers guidance and recommendations on the appropriate treatment plans for specific diseases.

Non-hazardous medicinal waste Waste that poses no physical, biological, chemical or radioactive risk, for example plastic packaging, clean glass and plastic, paper and cardboard.

Non-invasive A medical procedure/treatment that does not break the skin or enter the body.

Norovirus A very infectious virus common in the winter that causes diarrhoea and vomiting.

Occupational maps A visual outline of the pathway an individual will study for technical, higher technical and professional occupations, which also shows potential progression routes.

Offensive/hygiene waste Non-infectious, unpleasant waste that poses a low risk to health, such as dressings and PPE that are not contaminated with bodily fluids, as well as hygiene and sanitary waste, e.g. incontinence pads. It is waste that is not hazardous but would be unpleasant to come into contact with.

Ophthalmologist A professional who specialises in the diagnosis and treatment of eye abnormalities and will prescribe the treatment needed.

Optometrist A trained professional who undertakes eye examinations to detect vision problems and eye abnormalities and defects. Optometrists provide primary vision care.

Orbitals Where electrons are located. Each orbital can be empty or can contain one or two electrons.

Organelles Specialised structures within plant and animal cells that have specific functions. Some organelles are also found within bacterial cells.

Organism An individual plant, animal or single-celled lifeform.

Outpatients Patients who visit a hospital for an appointment but do not stay overnight.

Palliative care This type of care can provide support to patients with terminal illnesses to ensure continual monitoring and relief from their symptoms. Palliative care may take place either within the patient's home, a hospital or hospice.

Parallel Circuits where the components are each connected separately to the positive and negative terminals of the power supply.

Pathogen A micro-organism that causes illness or disease by damaging host tissues and/or by producing toxins.

Pathology The scientific study of the causes, effects and treatment of disease.

Peptide A compound containing two or more amino acids joined together by peptide bonds. A dipeptide contains two amino acids bonded together.

Permanent magnet Produces its own magnetic field.

Phagocytes Produced in the bone marrow and circulate in the blood. Some leave the blood and are present in the tissues.

Phagocytosis The process of a phagocyte engulfing a pathogen or other foreign material.

Pharmacist In accordance with the Pharmacy Act 1954, a person who is on the register of pharmaceutical chemists with the General Pharmaceutical Council may be called a pharmacist.

Pharmacogenomics The study of how a person's genome affects their response to drugs.

Pharmacy medicines Also known as 'over-the-counter' medicines; medicines that can only be purchased from a registered pharmacy, are kept behind the counter and require discussion with a medical professional such as a pharmacist or a trained member of staff acting under the supervision of a pharmacist.

Phoropter A specialised instrument that is used during an eye exam to test patients' individual lenses.

Phospholipid bilayer A double layer of phospholipids with the hydrophobic tails arranged towards the middle and the hydrophilic head groups on the outside. It forms the basis of all biological membranes.

Phospholipid A large molecule formed from a glycerol molecule covalently bound to two fatty acid molecules and a phosphate group. It has a hydrophilic (can interact with water) head group (because of the phosphate) and a hydrophobic (repels water) tail (because of the fatty acids).

Photosynthesis The process that plants use to make complex organic compounds such as sugars from carbon dioxide and water using light energy.

Physical science and bioengineering Measuring what is happening in the body and devising advanced ways to diagnose and treat disease.

Physiological science The use of advanced technologies to evaluate the functioning of different body systems and to diagnose abnormalities.

Plant Any equipment used in the workplace, e.g. laboratory equipment.

Plasma membrane Sometimes called the cell-surface membrane, it is the membrane that surrounds all types of cell; animal, plant and bacterial. Like all membranes, the plasma membrane consists of a phospholipid bilayer together with proteins and other components.

Polarisation (of a nerve or muscle cell) The different electrical charges on either side of the plasma membrane caused by the active transport of ions.

Polymorphism The occurrence of two or more phenotypes as a result of there being two or more alleles, i.e. variants of a particular DNA sequence.

Polymer A long molecule made from many small molecules called monomers.

Polypeptide A polymer of amino acids joined together by peptide bonds.

Power of attorney A legal document whereby an individual gives another person, usually a family member or friend, the official authority to make decisions in relation to health and welfare on their behalf, such as types of medical and non-medical care. This legal document only comes into effect once an individual with dementia has lost their capacity to make their own decisions.

Precise Measurements that are close to each other, but they may be inaccurate.

Prescriber A registered healthcare professional with the legal authorisation to prescribe a medical product.

Prescription A written order that is presented to a registered professional who has legal authorisation to dispense a medicinal product.

Prevalence The proportion of a population affected by a medical condition at a specific time. It is usually expressed as a percentage, fraction or number of cases per size of population.

Preventative action Taking action to ensure that nothing goes wrong.

Professional Standards Authority (PSA) A body that sets and promotes standards of regulation for both voluntary and statutory registration for healthcare science professionals. The PSA ensure high standards are being practised to promote the health, safety and wellbeing of the public.

Prospective These studies take a group of people and observe them over a period of time. This could involve looking for correlations between factors such as diet or exercise and development of cardiovascular disease. The advantage is that the data collection methods can be tailored to the question being asked. The disadvantage is that these can take many years to complete.

Protein A polypeptide with a recognisable three-dimensional structure. It may contain more than one polypeptide chain.

Qualitative data Descriptive data, for example a patient's medical history.

Quality management systems (QMS) The implementation of systems, policies and procedures that are designed to ensure high-quality healthcare while minimising the risk of harm to both staff and patients.

Quantitative data Numerical data, for example a person's age, height or weight.

Radioactive decay The random process that occurs when an unstable nucleus loses energy by giving out alpha or beta particles or gamma radiation.

Radiocarbon dating The process that uses a radioactive isotope of carbon, carbon-14, to determine the age of an object containing organic material.

Radioisotopes Unstable isotopes that undergo radioactive decay emitting radioactivity as they do so.

Radiopharmaceuticals Therapeutic drugs (medicines) that incorporate radioisotopes. Some radiopharmaceuticals are used to treat disease whereas diagnostic radiopharmaceuticals are used to help in diagnosis of disease.

Recoil The process by which elastic tissues or fibres return to their original length after having been stretched or expanded. This is what happens to an elastic band when you stretch it and then let go. Be careful not to use the term 'contraction' to describe this process. Contraction is what muscles do, whereas elastic tissues recoil.

Reference standard Something of known size, mass, concentration, etc. that we can use to calibrate equipment or methods.

Refractive errors Also known as refraction errors. Vision problems that make it difficult for an individual's vision to focus.

Regression analysis Determines the relationship between the dependent variable and other variables to distinguish a strength within the data.

Repolarisation (of a nerve or muscle cell) The restoration of the original charge difference.

Reportable injuries The following injuries are reportable under RIDDOR when they result from a work-related accident:

▶ the death of any person

▶ specified injuries to workers (see the HSE website for more information)

▶ injuries to workers which result in them being unable to work for more than seven days

▶ injuries to non-workers which result in them being taken directly to hospital for treatment, or specified injuries to non-workers which occur on the premises.

Resolution The ability of a microscope to distinguish between two adjacent points. The resolution of a microscope is the smallest distance between two points that can be seen as separate. A high-resolution microscope can show a clearer image.

Retrospective These studies look backwards at data from a group of people over many years. This often involves examining published data classifying people according to risk factors or medical outcomes. Although these can give results more quickly than prospective studies, the disadvantage of retrospective studies is that there is little control over data collection. This type of study typically looks at published data from many different sources that might involve different methods of data collection or analysis.

Risk How likely a hazard is to cause that harm.

Semi-conservative replication When DNA replicates two new double helix molecules are formed, but each one consists of one of the original strands and one newly synthesised strand.

Series Circuits where the components are connected in line, end to end between the positive and negative terminals of the power supply.

Serious adverse event (SAE) Any occurrence associated with the transfusion process that might lead to death or life-threatening, disabling or incapacitating conditions for patients, for example a patient contracting HIV, and so result in or prolong hospitalisation or morbidity.

Serious adverse reaction (SAR) A response or reaction, for example anaphylaxis, to the transfusion at any stage for the donor or the recipient that could be life-threatening or worsen their health condition.

Sexually transmitted infection (STI) Caused by a pathogen that is passed from person to person during sexual contact.

Simulated experience A useful way to train healthcare professionals, for example through the use of virtual reality or mannequins for first aid purposes. These provide almost lifelike experiences to prepare students for the healthcare industry workplace.

Single nucleotide polymorphism (SNP) A change in a single base in a DNA sequence, e.g. C replaces G. This means that the two variants are alleles.

Skeletal muscle The main type of muscle involved in movement, because it is attached to the skeleton.

Smooth (involuntary) muscle Muscle that is not under conscious control. It is controlled by the autonomic nervous system and hormones.

Sputum Mucus or coughed-up material (phlegm) from the lower airways (trachea and bronchi).

Standard operating procedure (SOP) Written instructions compiled by an organisation that describe how to carry out routine operations efficiently and safely. Healthcare science settings must have SOPs for how to perform jobs that involve potential risks so that they can be carried out safely and in compliance with procedure regulations.

Standard solution The solution of known concentration in a titration.

Stem cells Undifferentiated (non-specialised) cells that can give rise to one or more types of differentiated (specialised) cell.

Superbugs Strains of bacteria, viruses, parasites and fungi that are resistant to several types of antibiotics and other medicines commonly used to treat them.

Systole Refers to the contraction of either atrium or ventricle: hence the terms atrial systole and ventricular systole, respectively.

Systolic blood pressure The pressure when the heart contracts.

Tendons Similar in structure and composition to ligaments. Their function is to attach the muscles to the bones that make up the skeleton.

Titre The volume of standard solution needed to neutralise the analyte (i.e. to reach the end point of the titration).

The UK Health Security Agency (UKHSA) An organisation of the Department of Health and Social Care that is responsible for protecting the nation from the impact of infectious diseases, chemical, biological, radiological and nuclear incidents and other health threats. UKHSA replaced Public Health England (PHE) in April 2021.

Variable A characteristic that can be measured; examples include age, gender and ethnicity.

Vector-borne diseases Infections that are transmitted by an infectious agent, e.g. mosquitoes, blackflies and ticks.

Wavelength The distance between the same point in successive cycles. For example, the distance from the peak of one wave to the peak of the next wave. The standard unit of wavelength is the metre, m. However, electromagnetic waves can have wavelengths from 10^4 m to 10^{-15} m, so you will often see wavelengths expressed in units such as nanometres, nm. (1 nm = 1×10^{-9} m).

Work-related An accident in the workplace does not always mean that the accident is work-related – the work activity itself must contribute to the accident. An accident is 'work-related' if any of the following played a significant role: the way the work was carried out; any machinery, plant, substances or equipment used for the work; the condition of the site or premises where the accident happened.

Index

A

A&E (accident and emergency) departments 115–17
absences 5
abuse
 signs and symptoms of 99–101
 see also safeguarding
Academy for Healthcare Science 43
Academy for Healthcare Science (AHCS) 75–6, 92
accidents 53
accreditation 43
accuracy 188
acids 249–50
active participation 109
ADHD (attention deficit hyperactivity disorder) 102
adrenaline 285, 287
adrenals 284, 285
adsorption 252
advanced care planning 81
Advisory, Conciliation and Arbitration Service (Acas) 6
advocacy 86, 97
age 324
air flow cabinets 124
alcohol 111
algorithms 153, 169
alternating current (AC) 260, 261–2
Alton Towers 7
Alzheimer's disease 105
ambulance trusts 15
amino acids 217–18
amplitude 267
analysis of variance (ANOVA) 167
anatomical diseases 330, 331–2
anatomical waste 136
anonymity 90
antibiotic resistance 131, 133–4
antibiotic stewardship 131, 133
antibodies 236–40
anti-discrimination policy 94
 see also discrimination
anti-diuretic hormone (ADH) 286–7
antigens 236–40
appraisals 44
apprenticeships 11–12
apps 48
aprons 120
arteries 303
arthritis 103
artificial intelligence (AI) 47, 153–4
asbestos 137
aseptic technique 186
asthma 115, 321
astigmatism 23
atomic number 247
atomic structure 244
audit processes 7, 184, 204
augmentative and alternative communication (AAC) 104
augmented reality (AR) 48
autism spectrum conditions (ASCs) 102, 165
autoclaving 128, 129, 208
autoimmune diseases 329
automation 47, 48
autonomy 8, 43, 79

B

bacteria 228, 234
bar charts 147, 179–80
B cells 238–40
belittling 100
beneficence 7–8, 43, 89
bibliography 348
big data 152–3, 343
bioengineering 36
biohazards 207–8
 see also hazardous substances
bioinformaticians 169
bioinformatics 153, 343
biomedical scientist 36
bladder 314
blood, composition 305
blood glucose 284–6, 326
 measuring 322–3
 normal range 324
blood groups 309
blood pressure 306–7
 measuring 319–20
 normal range 324
blood transfusion 69–71, 309
blood vessels 303–4
body language 87, 351–2
body temperature, measuring 323
bone marrow 215
bradycardia 309
Braille 104, 352
breast ironing 99
breathing 220, 289, 320–1
 see also respiratory system
bribery 176
Bribery Act 2010 176
British National Formulary (BNF) 25
British Sign Language (BSL) 87, 104
British Standard 6
budgeting 114
bullying 100
bursaries 12

C

calibration 188
candour 95
capacity 8, 82
 legal 106–7
 mental 91, 102–3, 165–6
 physical 103
 see also consent
capillaries 303
carbohydrates 218
carbon fibre 246
cardiac arrest 67–9
cardiac cycle 305–6
cardiopulmonary resuscitation (CPR) 67–9
cardiovascular system 303–9, 319–20
Care Certificate 85
career pathways 10, 40
career progression 10
care plan 83
Care Quality Commission (CQC) 79, 84, 92, 113–14, 163
catalysts 251
cell differentiation 215–16
cell theory 211–16
 in plants 214–15
Centers for Disease Control 138
centrioles 214
ceramics 246
cerebral palsy 103
certification 43
cervix 310
chaperones 86

charities 15, 16–17
charts 146–8
chemical analysis 252–6
chloroplasts 214
choice 82–3, 95
Cholera 235
chromatography 252–5
chronic obstructive pulmonary disease (COPD) 332
classification systems 330–1
cleaning 122, 127–8
clinical bioinformatics 36
clinical commissioning groups (CCGs) 15, 64
clinical observations 150
clinical scientist 35–6, 42
clinical trials 169
closed questions 141, 171, 351
Clostridium difficile 125
cloud computing 154
codes of conduct 9
cohort study 142, 151
collective agreements 4
collision theory 251
column chromatography 253
commitment 96
communication 86–8, 96, 103–4, 107, 109, 179–81, 350–3
　barriers 352
　body language 87, 351–2
　questioning techniques 141, 171, 350–1
　written records 163
community trusts 15
compassion 73, 86, 96
compensation 83
competence 96
compliance 79, 184
composite materials 245–6
computer-aided design (CAD) 47
computer-aided manufacturing (CAM) 48
concrete 246
condensation reaction 217–18
conductivity 244
confidentiality 9, 85–6, 90, 117, 156–7, 162–4
　breach of 174
　limits of 164–6
conflicts of interest 90
consent 8, 82–3, 89, 100, 104, 165
consultations, digital 47
consumables 190
containment barriers 124
contaminated materials 207

continuing professional development (CPD) 5, 12, 43, 79
continuous improvement 7
controlled drugs 20, 65, 192
Control of Substances Hazardous to Health (COSHH) Regulations 1994 (2002) 52–3, 127, 136–8
convulsions 330
coronaviruses 335
　see also COVID-19 pandemic
corrective and preventative action (CAPA) process 205
corrosion 245
corruption 176
cosmic radiation 276
courage 96
covert administration of medication 166
COVID-19 pandemic
　classification 331
　impacts of 44, 335
　policies 337
　protection 120
　track and trace 153, 337
　transmission 234
　vaccination trials 91
　vaccines 192, 338
　see also personal protective equipment (PPE)
criminal convictions 3
cross-contamination 192
CT (computerised tomography) scans 18, 162, 270, 275, 344
culture 95, 352
cyber attacks 159
cytoplasm 211
cytostatic waste 135

D

data
　analysis 148–9, 167–9, 176–8, 359
　big data 152–3, 343
　breach 164, 175
　collection 141–5, 171, 358–9
　descriptive statistics 176–7
　inferential statistics 167, 177–8
　interpretation 171–2
　presenting 146–8, 179–81, 360–1
　security 156–7, 159
　statistical databases 167–8
　storage 149–50, 164
　types 145
databases 167–8, 172
data protection 85–6, 94, 154–6, 163–4

Data Protection Act 2018 94, 155–6, 163–4
Data Protection Officer (DPO) 164, 174
data scientists 169
data visualisation tools 154
Datix form 137–8, 172
decision-making 357
decontamination 128, 207–8
DeepMind 153
defibrillation 67–9
dehydration 329–30
delegation 356
delocalised electrons 243–4
dementia 105–7, 165
density 244
dental laboratory assistant 38
dental moulds 162–3
dental nurse 38
dental services 15, 24–5, 32–3, 38
dental technician 38
　registration 42
dental X-rays (radiographs) 24
dentist 38
dependent variables 146
depression 100
Deprivation of Liberty Safeguards (DoLS) 165
descriptive statistics 176–7
detergents 122
developmental co-ordination disorder (DCD) 102
diabetes 326, 328
diet 111
diffusion 219–20, 222–3
digestive system 286, 300–3
digital information management systems 154
digital technologies 47–8
dignity 74, 85–6, 95
dipeptides 217–18
direct current (DC) 260, 261–2
disaccharides 218
disaster recovery plan 45–6
disciplinary procedure 5, 83
Disclosure and Barring Service (DBS) 3, 34
discrimination 2–3, 75, 88, 94, 175
disinfecting 122, 128
dismissal 83
dispensing optician 22, 37
　registration 41–2
diversity 2
diverticulitis 331
DNA (deoxyribonucleic acid) 211–12, 224–7, 339–41

Index

Down's syndrome 103
dress code 125
drug classifications 65
drug trials 105–6
  see also clinical trials
ductility 244
duty of candour 95
duty of care 91–3, 117, 165
dyslexia 102
dyspraxia 102

E

ectopic heartbeat 309
effective practice 76
electrical waste 134
electricity
  circuits 261
  current 260, 261–2
electrocardiography (ECG) 307–9, 319
electromagnetic spectrum 269
electromagnetism 262–5, 344
electronic health records (EHRs) 48, 154
electron microscopes 230–2
electrons 247–8
  delocalised 243–4
emergency care 115–17
emollient moisturiser 131
emotional abuse 100, 175
emotional intelligence 108
empathy 107
employment
  appraisals 44
  contracts 3–4
  disciplinary procedure 5, 83
  dismissal 83
  grievance procedure 5–6
  inductions 184–5
  job description 34, 35
  legislation 93
  person specification 34
  policies and procedures 5–6, 88–9
  probation period 4
  regulations 63
  tribunal 6
  see also occupations
Employment Relations Act 2004 93
Employment Rights Act 1996 93–4
empowerment 73, 101, 108–10
endocrine system 283–7, 322–3, 327
Environmental Protection Act (EPA) 1990 54
epidemics 44
epidemiology 333–6
epigenetics 339
equality 2, 9, 75, 88, 94

Equality Act 2010 2, 75, 88, 94
equipment
  calibration 188–90
  maintenance 187
equivalence point 256
ethical practice 7–9, 76, 82, 89–91
eukaryotic cells 211–16, 221
evidence-based practice 204
exchange mechanisms 219–22
excitation 274
exercise 325
exocrine glands 316–18, 317–18
experiments 150–2
  see also research
expiry dates 192
eye anatomy 23, 318
  see also ocular system
eye care services *see* optical care services

F

face masks 120, 121–2
factor analysis 167
fairness 9
fallopian tubes 310
fatty acids 219
feedback 113
female genital mutilation (FGM) 99
fertilisation 309, 312
fibreglass 246
financial abuse 101, 175
fire safety 55
first aid 63, 66–9
Fleming's left-hand rule 266
fluid mosaic model 221
focus groups 141
fomites 186
food processing 271
Freedom of Information Act 2000 163, 166
frequency 267–8
frequency diagrams 148
fungi 228–9, 234

G

gametes 309
gamma rays 270, 271
gas chromatography 254
gaseous exchange 289
gaslighting 100
General Data Protection Regulations (GDPR) 94, 155–6
General Dental Council (GDC) 24, 42, 92

General Medical Council (GMC) 92
General Optical Council (GOC) 22, 41–2, 93
General Pharmaceutical Council (GPhC) 20, 42, 92
general practitioners (GPs) 15, 30, 64, 66, 114–15, 116
General Sales List (GSL) medicines 21
genes 224
genetics 224, 227–8
genitalia 310
genomics 169, 227–8, 338–42
GHS (Globally Harmonized System) hazard pictograms 52
Gibb's reflective cycle 362
Giemsa staining 233
global development delay syndrome 103
gloves 120
glucose meter 322
Golgi apparatus 213–14
Golgi vesicles 213–14
good laboratory practice (GLP) 199–201
good manufacturing practice (GMP) 201–3
good scientific practice (GSP) 197–8
Gram staining 232
graphs 146–8, 179
Graves' disease 329
grievance procedure 5–6

H

haematology 36
haematoxylin and eosin (H&E) staining 233
haemovigilance 69
hair 316
hand washing 122–3, 131, 132
hazardous substances 52, 136–8, 207–8
hazards 55
  see also risk assessment
Health and Care Professions Council (HCPC) 19, 91–2
  registration 42
health and safety 6–7
  accidents 53
  first aid 63, 66–9
  legislation 51–5
  promoting 56–7
  regulations 63–6
  risk assessment 55–6
  spillages 136–8
  training 58–9
  see also infection; waste management

Health and Safety (Display Screen Equipment) Regulations 1992 55
Health and Safety (First Aid) Regulations 1981 63, 66
Health and Safety at Work etc. Act 1974 51, 75, 138
Health and Safety Executive (HSE) 51
Health and Social Care Act 2008 74, 127
Health and Social Care Act 2012 63–4, 97–8
healthcare-associated infections (HCAIs) 125, 127
healthcare science assistant 34–5
healthcare science associate 35
healthcare science practitioner 36
health informatics 153
health promotion 110–12, 336–8
health records 48, 154
health tracking 108
hearing loops 87
heart 304
heart rate 307–9
   measuring 320
   normal range 324
heat stroke 328–9
hepatitis 331–2
high efficiency particulate air (HEPA) filter 124
higher technical occupations 11
high performance liquid chromatography (HPLC) 254
histograms 148
hitting 100
holistic approaches 80
homeostasis 283, 315, 326–8
hormones 283–5, 315–16
hospitals
   clinics 28
   laboratories 29, 31, 124, 199
   wards 28–9
hospital trusts 15
human immunodeficiency virus (HIV) 335
Human Medicines (Amendment) Regulations 2019 64–5
Human Medicines Act 2012 20
hyperthermia 328–9
hypothalamus 284, 317
hypothermia 44
hypothesis 169

I

imaging techniques 18, 48
immunity 236–40
immunology 233

inclusion 2
independence 108–10
independent variables 146
indirect discrimination 3, 88
induction heating 266–7, 271
inductions 184–5
infection
   antibiotic resistance 131, 133–4
   causative agents 234
   defense mechanisms 236
   definition 120
   prevention and control 120–31
   sepsis 329
   spread of 185, 235
   transmission 234
   waste management 134–6
inferential statistics 167, 177–8
inflammation 237, 332
influenza 44
information, managing 172–3
Information Commissioner's Office (ICO) 155
information security management systems (ISMS) 164
informed consent 8, 82, 89
infrared 271
infrastructure 45
injuries 53, 332–3
inpatients 27
Institute for Apprenticeships and Technical Education (IfATE) 10, 39–40
insurance 173
integrity 94
integumentary system 316–18
international system of units (SI) 276–8
internships 12
inter-professional learning 97
interviews 142, 170
involuntary inflammatory response 332–3
   see also inflammation
ionisation 249, 273
ions 243–4
irradiation 128
ischaemia 333
ISO (International Organization for Standardization) 6
isotopes 275
IVF (in vitro fertilisation) 16

J

jargon 87, 352
job description 34, 35
job roles see occupations
justice 9, 43

K

key performance indicators (KPIs) 44
kidneys 286, 313–16, 329
kinetic energy 251
Kolb's experiential learning cycle 361–2

L

labelling 89
laboratories 29, 31, 124, 199
laboratory information management systems (LIMSs) 199
leading questions 351
leaflets 180
learning disabilities 103–4, 107
legislation
   compliance 166
   enforcing 206
   equality and inclusion 2, 88
   health and safety 51–5
   laws, definition 2
Liberty Protection Safeguards (LPS) 165
life sciences 36
lifting see manual handling
line graph 147
lipids 219
literature review 151, 347–50
liver disease 331–2
logarithmic scale 249
longitudinal research 90, 152, 170
lymphocytes 237
   see also B cells; T cells
lysosomes 214
lysozyme 236

M

machine learning 153–4
magnetism 262–6
magnification 230, 232
Making Every Contact Count (MECC) initiative 110–12
malaria 234
malleability 244
maltreatment 83
Management of Health and Safety at Work Regulations 1999 51–2, 58
manual handling 55, 57–8
Manual Handling Operations Regulations 1992 55
marginalisation 89
mass spectrometry (MS) 254–5
maternity leave 3
maxillofacial prostheses 38

Index

maxillofacial surgery 32–3
mean 167, 177
median 168
medical device manufacturing 29
medicines 20–1, 64
   abuse/overuse of 174
   covert administration of 166
   drug trials 105–6
   storage and stock management 191–4
   see also pharmacy services; prescriptions
Medicines Act 1968 20
Medicines and Healthcare products Regulatory Agency (MHRA) 20, 64–5, 90
Medicines for Human Use (Clinical Trials) Amendment Regulations (MHCTR) 90
memory, and dementia 105
Mendel's laws 224
menopause 325
Mental Capacity (Amendment) Act 2019 165
Mental Capacity Act 2005 91, 102, 166
mental health 102, 111
mental health trusts 15
metabolic rate 220, 284
metabolism 284
metallic bonding 244
metals
   chemical properties 244–5, 247–8
   physical properties 244
   transition metals 245, 251
methicillin-resistant *Staphylococcus aureus* (MRSA) 125, 133
microbiology 228
microscopes 230–2
microwaves 270, 271
Millennium Cohort Study (MCS) 143
mission statement 203
Misuse of Drugs Act 1971 65, 191
mitochondria 212–13
mitosis 211
mode 168
monosaccharides 218
moral values 91
motor effect 265–6
motor skills 103
MRI (magnetic resonance imaging) scans 18, 344
multi-agency working 96–7, 352–3
multidisciplinary teams 30, 74, 80, 97
multiple-use products 127
musculoskeletal injuries 103
musculoskeletal system 295–300

N

National Health Service (NHS) 15
   constitution 84
   Long Term Plan 203
   NHS 111 116
   NHS trusts 15
   urgent and emergency care 115–17
national insurance 15
National Living Wage 4
National Minimum Wage 4
National School of Healthcare Science (NSHCS) 20, 43
National Vocational Qualifications (NVQs) 10
needs assessment 63
negative correlation 147
neglect 101, 175
negligence 75, 83, 173
nervous disorders 330
nervous system 292–5, 327
neurodiversity 102, 104
neutralisation 249, 256
neutrons 247–8
NICE (National Institute for Health and Care Excellence) 15, 142
nonmaleficence 8, 43
norovirus 125
nucleus 212

O

observation 142, 143, 152
observations (obs) 324
occupational maps 10, 40
occupations 10–11, 34–9
ocular system 318–19
open questions 141, 171, 350–1
ophthalmic nurse 37
ophthalmologist 22
optical assistant 37
optical care services 22–4, 31–2, 37, 41–2
optical coherence tomography (OCT) 23
Opticians Act 1989 22
optometrist 22, 31, 37
orbitals 247
organelles 211–12
organisational abuse 101
organisms 211
orthodontists 32
   see also dental services
orthotic services 25–6, 33, 38–9
orthotists 39
osmoregulation 315

osmosis 223
outpatients 27
ovaries 284, 285, 310
over-the-counter medicines 21

P

palliative care 74, 81
pancreas 284, 285–6
pandemics 44
parasites 229, 234
parathyroid 284
partnership working 96–7, 110
pathogens 238–40
pathology 17, 19, 29
patients
   choice and preferences 95
   feedback from 113
   health records 48, 154
   history 151
   home environment 29
   improving lives of 74, 108–10
   needs of 73, 79–80, 91
   rights of 84
   see also person-centred care
peak expiratory flow (PEF)
   measuring 321
   normal range 324
peer review 151
penicillin 228–9
penis 310
peptide bonds 217–18
performance monitoring 113–14
performance reviews 4–5
periodic table 247–8
personal hygiene 123, 125
Personal Protective Equipment (Enforcement) Regulations 1992 (2018) 53
personal protective equipment (PPE) 31, 53, 120–2, 137
   laboratory-specific 124
person-centred care 80, 96–7
person-centred planning 80
person specification 34
PET (positron emission tomography) 18
pH 249–50
phagocytosis 237
pharmaceutical industry 31
pharmacist 36–7
   registration 42
pharmacogenomics 342
Pharmacy Act 1954 20
pharmacy services 20–2, 30–1, 36–7
pharmacy services assistant 36

pharmacy technician 36
phoropter 23
phospholipids 219
photosynthesis 214, 276
physical abuse 100, 175
physiological diseases 330, 332
physiological science 36
pie charts 148
PIES needs 73, 79, 91
pituitary 284, 285, 286
plagiarism 348
plasma membrane 212
point of care testing (POCT) 47, 108
policies and procedures 2–6
polymerase chain reaction (PCR) 186
polymers 246
polysaccharides 218
positive correlation 147
posters 180
power of attorney 106–7
powers of 10 278
practical investigations 144
   see also experiments
precision 188
prefixes 277
pregnancy 312–13, 325
prescriptions 15, 20–1, 25
presenting data 146–8, 179–81, 360–1
Prevent strategy 2011 99, 101
primary care organisations 15, 26–7
primary prevention 112
prions 234
prison services 30
privacy 85–6, 90
private sector services 16
probation period 4
probing questions 351
probity 197
problem-solving 357–8
professional bodies 9, 11, 12, 83, 91–3, 184
professional codes of conduct 9
professional occupations 11
professional registration 41–3, 83–4
Professional Standards Authority (PSA) 43
prokaryotic cells 211, 216
prostate 312
prosthetic services 25–6, 33, 38–9
prosthetists 39
protected characteristics 2–3, 88
proteins 217–18, 221–2
protoctists 234
protons 247–8
psychological abuse 100, 175
puberty 286

Public Health England (PHE) 15
Public Interest Disclosure Act 1998 94
public sector services 15
pulse oximeter 321

Q

qualifications 10–11
qualified person (QP) 184
qualitative data 145, 149, 171, 359
qualitative research 142
quality assurance (QA) 7, 75–8, 197, 203, 208
quality control (QC) 7, 78–9, 208
quality management 78
quality management systems (QMS) 19
quality standards 6–7, 197–205
quantitative data 145, 167–8, 171, 359
questioning techniques 141, 171, 350–1

R

radiation 271–2
   applications of radioactivity 274–6, 344
   excitation 274
   ionisation 249, 273
   radioactive decay 272–3, 276
   radiocarbon dating 276
radiation sterilisation 130
radicalisation 99, 101–2
radioactive decay 272–3
radiocarbon dating 276
radiopharmaceuticals 275
radio waves 270
rape 100
reference standard 188
referrals 97, 114–17
reflective practice 361–4
refraction errors 23
registration 41–3, 83–4
Regulatory Reform (Fire Safety) Order (RRO) 2005 55
religion 86, 95
   and discrimination 3, 89
renal failure 329
renal system 286, 313–16
reportable injuries 53
Reporting of Injuries, Diseases and Dangerous Occurrences Regulations (RIDDOR) 2013 53
reproductive system 309–13
reputation 83
research

clinical trials 169
ethical practice 89
peer review 151
qualitative 142
skills 347–50
sources of information 142–4, 151
see also data
respect 9, 74, 86, 95
respiratory system 288–91, 320–1
Resuscitation Council UK 67
resuscitation guidelines 67–9
retinal images 162
ribosomes 213
risk assessment 55–6
risk factors 111
RNA (ribonucleic acid) 225–6, 339
role modelling 109

S

safeguarding
   concerns 175
   definition 3
   duty of care 91
   policies 3, 165
   principles 97–9
   see also abuse
safe haven 175
scanning electron microscope (SEM) 231
scatter graphs 147
scholarships 12
scope of practice 41–2
scrotum 310
sebaceous glands 318
secondary care 27
self-care strategies 108–9
self-esteem 100, 110
self-harm 174
self-neglect 101
seminal vesicles 310
sensory impairment 87
sepsis 329
serious adverse event (SAE) 70
serious adverse reaction (SAR) 70
Serious Crime Act 2015 99
Serious Hazards of Transfusion (SHOT) haemovigilance scheme 69–70
sex-based differences 325
sexual abuse 100, 175
sexually transmitted infection (STI) 234
sharps waste 54, 134, 208
shock 333
sickness absence 5

significant figures 278–9
sign language 87, 104
simulated experience 79
single photon emission computerised tomography (SPECT) 275
single-use products 126–7
six Cs 73, 96
Six Sigma 205
skeleton (human) 296, 298
    see also musculoskeletal system
skin 316–18
SMART goals 44
smartphones 47, 108, 153
smart watches 108, 152
smoking 111, 112, 324–5
social enterprises 15
social media 157–8, 180
social prescribing 111–12
social values 91
specimen
    analysis 18–19
    collection 17
sphygmomanometer 319
spillages 136–8
spinal cord injury 103
spirometry 320
spreadsheets 169
staff resources 45
staining techniques 232–3
standard deviation 177
standard form 243, 278
standard operating procedures (SOPs) 19, 57, 138, 183–7, 203
statistical analysis 167
Statistical Analysis Systems (SAS) 168
Statistical Package for Social Sciences (SPSS) 167–8
Statistics and Data (STATA) 168
statutory registration 42–3
statutory training 58–9
stem cells 215
sterilisation 128–30
stethoscope 319

St John Ambulance 16
stock management 190–4
stress 325–6
subatomic particles 248
superbugs 133
surveys 113, 141, 170–1
sweat glands 317–18
synovial joint 297
Système international (SI) 276–8
systems biology 153

T

tables 146, 179
tachycardia 309, 329
T cells 237–40
team working 353–7
technical occupations 10–11
temperature regulation 317
tertiary care 27
testes 284, 285, 310
thermometers 323
thin layer chromatography (TLC) 252–3
thyroid 284, 285
titration 256
topographical diseases 330, 331
toxoplasmosis 234
transition metals 245, 251
transmission electron microscope (TEM) 231
transparency 95
transport mechanisms 221–4
trauma 332–3
triglycerides 219
trust 82, 86, 90–1, 94
truthfulness 9

U

UK Health Security Agency (UKHSA) 15
ultrasound 18, 270

underlying health conditions 114–15
uniforms 125
units 276–8
urethra 310
urgent and emergency care 115–17
urinary system *see* renal system
uterus 310, 312

V

vaccines 335–6, 338
vagina 310
values 73, 91
variables 167, 170
vas deferens 310
veins 303
verbal abuse 100, 175
viruses 229, 234, 335
vitamin D (cholecalciferol) 317–18
voice output communications (VOCAs) 104
volume 277–8
voluntary registration 42–3
voluntary sector services 16–17

W

waste management 54, 134–6
wavelength 268
waves 267–71
weather, extreme 44
web pages 180
working environments 28–33, 58
work-related accidents 53
written records 163

X

X-rays 18, 162, 270
    dental 24

Z

zygotes 215, 312